HEALTH
BEHAVIOR
AND
HEALTH
EDUCATION

HEALTH BEHAVIOR AND HEALTH EDUCATION

Theory, Research, and Practice

4TH EDITION

KAREN GLANZ
BARBARA K. RIMER
K. VISWANATH
Editors

Foreword by C. Tracy Orleans

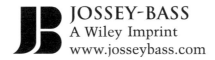

JOSSEY-BASS
A Wiley Imprint
www.josseybass.com

Published by Jossey-Bass
A Wiley Imprint
989 Market Street, San Francisco, CA 94103-1741—www.josseybass.com

Jossey-Bass books and products are available through most bookstores. To contact Jossey-Bass directly call our Customer Care Department within the U.S. at 800-956-7739, outside the U.S. at 317-572-3986, or fax 317-572-4002. Jossey-Bass also publishes its books in a variety of electronic formats. Some content that appears in print may not be available in electronic books.

Library of Congress Cataloging-in-Publication Data

Health behavior and health education : theory, research, and practice / Karen Glanz, Barbara K. Rimer, and K. Viswanath, editors. — 4th ed.
     p. ; cm.
 Includes bibliographical references and index.
 ISBN 978-0-7879-9614-7 (cloth)
1. Health behavior. 2. Health education. 3. Health promotion. I. Glanz, Karen. II. Rimer, Barbara K. III. Viswanath, K. (Kasisomayajula)
 [DNLM: 1. Health Behavior. 2. Health Education. W 85 H43415 2008]
 RA776.9.H434 2008
 613—dc22

2008021038

Printed in the United States of America

FOURTH EDITION
HB Printing 10 9 8 7 6 5 4 3

CONTENTS

FOREWORD

C. Tracy Orleans, Ph.D.

Health behavior change is our greatest hope for reducing the burden of preventable disease and death around the world. Tobacco use, sedentary lifestyle, unhealthy diet, and alcohol use together account for almost one million deaths each year in the United States alone. Smoking prevalence in the United States has dropped by half since the first *Surgeon General's Report on Smoking and Health* was published in 1964, but tobacco use still causes over 400,000 premature deaths each year. The World Health Organization has warned that the worldwide spread of the tobacco epidemic could claim one billion lives by the end of this century. The rising prevalence of childhood obesity could place the United States at risk of raising the first generation of children to live sicker and die younger than their parents, and the spreading epidemic of obesity among children and adults threatens staggering global health and economic tolls.

The four leading behavioral risks factors and a great many others (for example, nonadherence to prescribed medical screening and prevention and disease management practices, risky sexual practices, drug use, family and gun violence, worksite and motor vehicle injuries) take disproportionate tolls in low-income and disadvantaged racial and ethnic populations, as well as in low-resource communities across the world. Addressing these behavioral risks and disparities, and the behaviors related to global health threats, such as flu pandemics, water shortages, increasingly harmful sun exposure, and the need to protect the health of the planet itself, will be critical to world health in the twenty-first century.

In the past two decades since the publication of the first edition of *Health Education and Health Behavior: Theory, Research, and Practice* in 1990, there has been extraordinary growth in our knowledge about interventions needed to change health behaviors at both individual and population levels. This progress can be measured in the proliferation of science-based recommendations issued by authoritative evidence review panels, including the U.S. Clinical Preventive Services Task Force, the Centers for Disease Prevention and Control Task Force on Community Preventive Services, and the international Cochrane Collaboration. Today, there are evidence-based *clinical practice* guidelines for most major behavioral health risks, including tobacco use, unhealthy diet, sedentary lifestyle, risky drinking, and diabetes management. And there are parallel research-based guidelines for the health care system changes and policies needed to assure their delivery and use. New *community practice* guidelines offer additional evidence-based recommendations for a wide array of population-level school-, worksite-, and community-based programs and public policies to improve vaccination rates and physical activity levels for children and adults, improve diabetes self-management, reduce harmful sun exposure, reduce secondhand smoke exposure, prevent youth tobacco use and help adult smokers quit, reduce workplace and motor vehicle injuries, and curb drunk driving and family and gun violence.

Another success of the past two decades of theory-based research can be seen in the evolution of theories and models themselves—a move away from a major focus only on individual behavior change and toward broader multi-level behavior and social change models. By the late 1980s, the limited reach and staying power of even our most effective individual health behavior interventions, based on theories emphasizing intrapersonal and interpersonal determinants of health behaviors, made it clear that an exclusive reliance on individually oriented interventions would be inadequate to achieve our pressing population health and health care goals. These failures led to a fundamental "paradigm shift" in our understanding of what the targets of effective interventions needed to be, not just individuals but the broader contexts in which they live and work. This shift fueled the rise of ecological models of health promotion that have guided the development of powerful interventions in public health and health care arenas.

Related shifts in the models and strategies of public health and clinical health promotion opened the way for even broader population models that link health plans and community public health organizations, communities, clinicians, and public health practitioners. Examples are the Chronic Care Model promulgated by the Institute of Medicine and the similar framework promoted by the World Health Organization. And these frameworks energized efforts to refine and apply models and theories to translate effective clinical and public health interventions into practice and policy, including the diffusion of innovations model, community and organizational change theories, and social marketing and communications theories.

Tremendous parallel gains in what we have learned about the paradigms, processes, methods, and limitations of public health promotion and health care quality improvement over the past two decades illustrate the fundamental premise of this and previous editions of *Health Behavior and Health Education*—that a dynamic exchange between theory, research, and practice is critical to effective health education and promotion. Just as previous editions of *Health Behavior and Health Education* have provided essential stewardship for many of the advances described here, this fourth edition will help us navigate the new frontiers and challenges that lie ahead.

As this volume makes clear, using theory to craft and evaluate health behavior change interventions results in more powerful interventions and more robust theories. Like the previous editions, it presents in one place authoritative and highly readable summaries and critiques of the major theories and models of health education at multiple levels (individual, interpersonal, organizational, community, public policy) and in a wide variety of settings and populations. Thorough analyses of their strengths and weaknesses and helpful summaries of how their major constructs have been measured and operationalized—illustrated with clear practical applications and case studies—are features of the book designed to be helpful for researchers, practitioners, and program planners at all levels of experience, from those new to the field to its most seasoned leaders. The rigor and accessibility of these reviews reflect the extraordinary knowledge and vision of the editors and authors, who include many of the most respected and accomplished leaders in the field of health education and health behavior; together, they bring exceptional skill and experience in planning, implementing, and evaluating theory-based interventions for a diverse range of problems, settings, and populations.

In addition to describing important developments in theory and practice since the previous edition, this volume gives special attention to cultural and health disparities, global applications, and advances in health communications and e-health. It also prepares us for the urgent need to identify, extract, and replicate the critical "active" ingredients of effective interventions through theory-driven reviews and syntheses of past trials and studies, as well as formative early assessments of promising innovations and rigorous theory-based studies of "natural experiments." Theory is the essential "divining rod" in new efforts to learn rapidly about "what works" by evaluating grassroots efforts in schools and communities across the country and the world to implement programs, policies, and environmental changes to curb the rise in childhood obesity. For example, logic models that reflect lay conceptions of how programs can work are helping the Robert Wood Johnson Foundation to identify early on the more and less promising strategies being tried for obesity prevention. The strategies that align best with theory are often the most promising. This type of practical application of theory makes clear that, in the broadest sense, health education and health behavior encompass the processes of policy development, which are so critical to understanding and overcoming policy resistance to dissemination of the growing number of evidence-based interventions.

In short, readers will find that the fourth edition of *Health Education and Health Behavior* retains and builds on all of the features that have established it as the preeminent text and indispensable reference for our field—the first book we reach for to help us think about the foundations on which to design an intervention or research plan, inform a systematic evidence review, write or review an article or grant application, plan a course or presentation, and consult with other practitioners or researchers both within and outside our own disciplines.

As the editors state in Chapter Two, "the gift of theory" is that it provides the essential conceptual underpinnings for well-crafted research, effective practice, and healthy public policy. The gift of this volume is that it provides essential guidance for our efforts to realize the full potential of theory, as we build on our remarkable past progress in navigating the new frontiers and challenges that lie ahead.

February 2008   C. Tracy Orleans
                                                                Distinguished Fellow and Senior Scientist
                                                                Robert Wood Johnson Foundation
                                                                Princeton, New Jersey

In memory of my brother, David Glanz,
who contributed so much and so well to
his family, in his scholarship and
to the lives of older adults.
—K. G.

To my husband, Bernard Glassman, my parents,
Joan and Irving, and my sisters, Liz and Sara,
with gratitude for their unflagging support.
—B.K.R.

To my parents, whose life of hard work
and sacrifice allowed their children to
succeed in their endeavors.
—K. V.

TABLES AND FIGURES

TABLES

FIGURES

PREFACE

The Editors

Programs to influence health behavior, including health promotion and education programs and interventions, are most likely to benefit participants and communities when the program or intervention is guided by a theory of health behavior. Theories of health behavior identify the targets for change and the methods for accomplishing these changes. Theories also inform the evaluation of change efforts by helping to identify the outcomes to be measured, as well as the timing and methods of study to be used. Such theory-driven health promotion and education efforts stand in contrast to programs based primarily on precedent, tradition, intuition, or general principles.

Theory-driven health behavior change interventions and programs require an understanding of the components of health behavior theory, as well as the operational or practical forms of the theory. The first edition of *Health Behavior and Health Education: Theory, Research, and Practice,* published in 1990, was the first text to provide an in-depth analysis of a variety of theories of health behavior relevant to health education in a single volume. It brought together dominant health behavior theories, research based on those theories, and examples of health education practice derived from theory that had been tested through evaluation and research. The second (1996) and third (2002) editions of *Health Behavior and Health Education* updated and improved on the earlier volume. People around the world are using this book, and it has been translated into multiple languages, including recent Japanese and Korean editions.

It has been over five years since the release of the third edition; the fourth edition of *Health Behavior and Health Education* once again updates and improves on the preceding edition. Its main purpose is the same: to advance the science and practice of health behavior and health education through the informed application of theories of health behavior. Likewise, this book serves as the definitive text for students, practitioners, and scientists in these areas and education in three ways: by (1) analyzing the key components of theories of health behavior that are relevant to health education, (2) evaluating current applications of these theories in selected health promotion programs and interventions, and (3) identifying important future directions for research and practice in health promotion and health education.

The fourth edition responds to new developments in health behavior theory and the application of theory in new settings, to new populations, and in new ways. This edition includes (1) an enhanced focus on the application of theories in diverse populations and settings, (2) an expanded section on using theory, including its translation for program planning, and (3) chapters on additional theories of health behavior.

More global applications from both developing and developed countries are included. As new communication and information technologies have opened up an unprecedented range of strategies for health behavior change, this edition integrates coverage of e-health into health communications examples throughout the book. Issues of culture and health disparities are also integrated into many chapters, rather than covered as a separate chapter. These issues are of broad and growing importance across many theories and models.

AUDIENCE

Health Behavior and Health Education speaks to graduate students, practitioners, and scientists who spend part or all of their time in the broad arenas of health behavior change, health promotion, and health education; the text will help them both understand the theories and apply them in practical settings. Practitioners, as well as students, will find this text a major reference for the development and evaluation of theory-driven health promotion and education programs and interventions. Researchers should emerge with a recognition of areas in which empirical support is deficient and theory testing is required, thus helping to set the research agenda for health behavior and health education.

This book is intended to assist all professionals who value the need to influence health behavior positively. Their fields include health promotion and education, medicine, nursing, health psychology, behavioral medicine, health communications, nutrition and dietetics, dentistry, pharmacy, social work, exercise science, clinical psychology, and occupational and physical therapy.

OVERVIEW OF THE BOOK

The authors of this text bring to their chapters an understanding of both theory and its application in a variety of settings that characterize the diverse practice of public health education—for example, worksites, hospitals, ambulatory care settings, schools, and communities. The chapters, written expressly for the fourth edition of this book, address theories and models of health behavior at the level of the individual, dyad, group, organization, and community.

This book is organized into five parts. Part One defines key terms and concepts. The next three parts reflect important units of health behavior and education practice: the individual, the interpersonal or group level, and the community or aggregate level. Each of these parts has several chapters, and ends with a perspectives chapter that synthesizes the preceding chapters.

Part Two focuses on theories of individual health behavior, and its chapters focus on variables *within individuals* that influence their health behavior and response to health promotion and education interventions. Four bodies of theory are reviewed in separate chapters: the Health Belief Model, the Transtheoretical Model, the Theory of Reasoned Action/Theory of Planned Behavior/Integrated Behavioral Model, and the Precaution Adoption Process Model.

Part Three examines interpersonal theories, which emphasize elements in the *interpersonal* environment that affect individuals' health behavior. Three chapters focus on Social Cognitive Theory: social support and social networks, clinical-patient and interpersonal communication, and stress and coping.

Part Four covers models for the *community or aggregate level* of change and includes chapters on community organization, diffusion of innovations, organizational change, and media communications.

Part Five explores "Using Theory," which presents the key components and applications of overarching planning and process models, and a discussion of the application of theory in culturally unique and other unique populations. It includes chapters on the PRECEDE-PROCEED Model of health promotion planning, social marketing, ecological models, and evaluation of theory-based interventions.

The major emphasis of *Health Behavior and Health Education* is on the analysis and application of health behavior theories to health promotion and education practice. Each core chapter in Parts Two, Three, and Four begins with a discussion of the background of the theory or model and a presentation of the theory, reviews empirical support for it, and concludes with one or two applications. Synthesis chapters review related theories and summarize their potential application to the development of health education interventions. Strengths, weaknesses, areas for future development and research, and promising strategies are highlighted.

Chapter authors are established researchers and practitioners who draw on their experience in state-of-the-art research to critically analyze and apply the theories to health education. This text makes otherwise lofty theories accessible and practical, and advances health education in the process.

No single book can be truly comprehensive and still be concise and readable. Decisions about which theories to include were made with both an appreciation of the evolution of the study of health behavior and a vision of its future (see Chapter Two). We purposely chose to emphasize theories and conceptual frameworks that encompass a range from the individual to the societal level. We acknowledge that there is substantial variability in the extent to which various theories and models have been codified, tested, and supported by empirical evidence. Of necessity, some promising emerging theories were not included.

The first three editions of *Health Behavior and Health Education* grew out of the editors' own experiences, frustrations, and needs, as well as their desire to synthesize the diverse literatures and to draw clearly the linkages between theory, research, and practice in health behavior and education. We have sought to show how theory, research, and practice interrelate and to make each accessible and practical. In this edition we have attempted to respond to changes in the science and practice of public health and health promotion, and to update the coverage of these areas in a rapidly evolving field. Substantial efforts have been taken to present findings from health behavior change interventions, based on the theories that are described, and to illustrate the adaptations needed to successfully reach diverse and unique populations. *Health Behavior and Health Education* has now been established as a widely used text and reference book. We hope the fourth edition will continue to be relevant and useful, and to stimulate readers' interest in theory-based health behavior and health education. We aspire to provide readers with the information and skills to ask critical questions, think conceptually, and stretch their thinking beyond using formulaic strategies to improve health.

ACKNOWLEDGMENTS

We owe deep gratitude to all the authors whose work is represented in this book. They worked diligently with us to produce an integrated volume, and we greatly appreciate their willingness to tailor their contributions to realize the vision of the book. Their collective depth of knowledge and experience across the broad range of theories and topics far exceeds the expertise that the editors can claim.

We pay special tribute to Dr. Everett Rogers, a luminary in our broad field, whose work in the area of diffusion of innovations has taught and inspired us, and whose body of work cuts across several chapters in this book. Along with many colleagues, we were saddened by Ev's death in the fall of 2005 and know his work will continue to be influential in using theory to improve research and practice.

We also wish to acknowledge authors who contributed to the first three editions of this text. Although some of them did not write chapters for this edition, their intellectual contributions form an important foundation for the present volume. We especially appreciate the contributions of Frances Marcus Lewis, an editor for the first three editions. And we welcome K. "Vish" Viswanath, an internationally recognized health communication scholar, to the editorial team.

The staff at Jossey-Bass Publishers provided valuable support to us for development, production, and marketing from the time that the first edition was released through completion of this edition. Our editors at Jossey-Bass—Andy Pasternack and Seth Schwartz—provided encouragement and assistance throughout. Kate Harris provided exceptional technical editing support for this edition.

The editors are indebted to their colleagues and students who, over the years, have taught them the importance of both health behavior theories and their cogent and precise representation. They have challenged us to stretch, adapt, and continue to learn through our years of work at the University of Michigan, University of North Carolina at Chapel Hill, Emory University, Harvard University, the University of Minnesota, Ohio State University, The Johns Hopkins University, Temple University, Fox Chase Cancer Center, Duke University, the University of Hawai'i, and the National Cancer Institute (NCI). The updated review of theory use for this edition was completed by doctoral students at Emory University—Julia Painter, Michelle Hynes, Christina Borba, and Darren Mays.

We particularly want to acknowledge Kelly Blake and Jenny Lewis for their editorial and substantive contributions. Completion of this manuscript would not have been possible without the dedicated assistance of Kristen Burgess, Johanna Hinman, Jenifer Brents, Kat Peters, Terri Whitehead, Mae Beale, Suzanne Bodeen, Dave Potenziani, Elizabeth Eichel, Lisa Lowery, Shoba Ramanadhan, and Josephine Crisistomo.

Karen Glanz would like to acknowledge partial funding support from the Georgia Cancer Coalition for technical editing and production of this volume.

We also wish to express our thanks to our colleagues, staffs, friends, and families, whose patience, good humor, and encouragement sustained us through our work on this book.

Karen Glanz
Atlanta, Georgia

Barbara K. Rimer
Chapel Hill, North Carolina

K. Viswanath
Boston, Massachusetts

THE EDITORS

Karen Glanz is a professor and a Georgia Cancer Coalition Distinguished Research Scholar in the Rollins School of Public Health at Emory University, where she holds appointments in the Departments of Behavioral Sciences and Health Education and Epidemiology. She is also the founding director of the Emory Prevention Research Center. Prior to coming to Emory, Karen Glanz was professor and director of the Social and Behavioral Sciences Program at the Cancer Research Center of Hawai'i at the University of Hawai'i from 1993 to 2004. From 1979 to 1993, she was a professor in the Department of Health Education at Temple University in Philadelphia. She received her M.P.H. (1977) and Ph.D. (1979) degrees in health behavior and health education from the University of Michigan.

Glanz's research and academic interests have been in the area of health behavior change program development and evaluation, community nutrition environments, cancer prevention and control, ethnic differences in health behavior, and risk communication. She is currently principal investigator on five federally funded research grants that test health behavior change interventions for skin cancer prevention, colorectal cancer risk counseling, and chronic disease prevention; and on several grants that focus on translation and dissemination of effective interventions and measurement tools. Glanz's scholarly contributions consist of more than 270 journal articles and book chapters, and she serves on the editorial boards of several journals. She was recognized in 2006 as a Highly Cited Author by ISIHighlyCited.com, in the top 0.5 percent of authors in her field over a twenty-year period.

Glanz has been recognized with several national awards and was the 2007 recipient of the Elizabeth Fries Health Education Award from the James and Sarah Fries Foundation. She was honored by the Public Health Education and Health Promotion Section of the American Public Health Association (APHA) with the Early Career Award (1984), the Mayhew Derryberry Award for outstanding contributions to theory and research in health education (1992; with Barbara Rimer and Frances Lewis), and the Mohan Singh Award for contributions to humor in health education (1996). Her recent health education programs in skin cancer and underage drinking prevention have received national awards for innovation and program excellence. Glanz serves on numerous advisory boards and committees for scientific and health organizations in the United States and abroad, including the Task Force on Community Preventive Services at the Centers for Disease Control and Prevention.

■ ■ ■

Barbara K. Rimer is dean and Alumni Distinguished Professor of Health Behavior and Health Education in the School of Public Health at the University of North Carolina at Chapel Hill. Rimer received an M.P.H. (1973) from the University of Michigan, with joint majors in health education and medical care organization, and a Dr.P.H. (1981) in health education from The Johns Hopkins School of Hygiene and Public Health. Previously, she served as deputy director for Population Sciences at UNC Lineberger Comprehensive Cancer Center at UNC-Chapel Hill (2003–2005), as director of the Division of Cancer Control and Population Sciences at the National Cancer Institute (part of the National Institutes of Health), from 1997–2002, as Professor of Community and Family Medicine at Duke University (1991–1997), and as director of behavioral research and a full member at the Fox Chase Cancer Center in Philadelphia (1987–1991).

Rimer has conducted research in a number of areas, including informed decision making, long-term maintenance of behavior changes (such as diet, cancer screening, and tobacco use), interventions to increase adherence to cancer prevention and early detection, dissemination of evidence-based interventions, and use of new technologies for information, support, and behavior change.

Rimer is the author of over 280 publications and serves on several journal editorial boards. She is the recipient of numerous awards and honors, including the Healthtrac Foundation Award for Health Education (2004), the Secretary's Award for Distinguished Service from the U.S. Department of Health and Human Services (2000), the Director's Award from the National Institutes of Health (2000), and the American Cancer Society Distinguished Service Award (2000). Rimer was the first woman and behavioral scientist to lead the National Cancer Institute's National Cancer Advisory Board—a presidential appointment. She currently is vice chair for the Task Force on Community Preventive Services at the Centers for Disease Control and Prevention.

■ ■ ■

K. "Vish" Viswanath is an associate professor in the Department of Society, Human Development and Health at the Harvard School of Public Health (HSPH) and associate professor of population sciences at Harvard's Dana-Farber Cancer Institute (DFCI). He is also the director of the Dana-Farber Harvard Cancer Center's Health Communication Core and chair of the steering committee of the Health Communication Concentration of HSPH. Before coming to Harvard, Viswanath was the acting associate director of the Behavioral Research Program, Division of Cancer Control and Population Sciences, at the National Cancer Institute. He was also a senior scientist in the Health Communication and Informatics Research Branch. He came to the National Cancer Institute from Ohio State University where he was a tenured faculty member in the School of Journalism and Communication. He also held an adjunct appointment in the School of Public Health and was a Center Scholar with Ohio State's Center for Health Outcomes, Policy, and Evaluation Studies. Viswanath received his doctoral degree in mass communication from the University of Minnesota (1990).

Viswanath's research interest is studying how macro-social factors influence health communication, particularly strategic communication campaigns. His scholarly work focuses on health communication and social change in both national and international contexts, with a particular focus on communication inequities and health disparities and sociology of health journalism. He has been involved with planned social change projects in India and the United States. His current research examines the use of new communication technologies for health among urban poor, medical and health reporters and the conditions of their work, and social capital and health communications. Viswanath has published more than sixty-three journal articles and book chapters and coedited three books and monographs, including *Mass Media, Social Control and Social Change* with David Demers (Iowa State University Press, 1999) and *The Role of the Media in Promoting and Discouraging Tobacco Use,* a monograph to be published by the National Cancer Institute. He was also the editor of the Social Behavioral Research section of the *International Encyclopedia of Communication,* a ten-volume series to be published by the Blackwell Press.

An internationally recognized health communications expert, Viswanath holds leadership roles in professional organizations. He was chair of the Mass Communication Division of the International Communication Association, head of the Theory and Methodology Division of the Association for Education in Journalism and Mass Communication, and secretary and president of the Midwest Association for Public Opinion Research (MAPOR). He was recently elected a Fellow of MAPOR.

THE CONTRIBUTORS

Susan J. Blalock is associate professor of Pharmaceutical Outcomes and Policy in the School of Pharmacy at the University of North Carolina in Chapel Hill.

Lee R. Bone is associate professor at The Johns Hopkins University Bloomberg School of Public Health.

Noel T. Brewer is assistant professor in the Department of Health Behavior and Health Education at the University of North Carolina School of Public Health in Chapel Hill.

Frances Dunn Butterfoss is professor and director of the Division of Behavioral Research and Community Health in the Department of Pediatrics at Eastern Virginia Medical School, Norfolk, Virginia.

Victoria L. Champion is the Mary Margaret Walther Distinguished Professor and associate dean for research at the Indiana University School of Nursing.

Ronald M. Epstein is professor of Family Medicine, Psychiatry and Oncology and director of the Rochester Center to Improve Communication in Health Care at the University of Rochester School of Medicine and Dentistry.

Kerry E. Evers is director of health behavior change projects Pro-Change Behavior Systems, Inc., in Rhode Island.

John R. Finnegan Jr. is professor and dean of the School of Public Health at the University of Minnesota.

Edwin B. Fisher is professor and chair of the Department of Health Behavior and Health Education at the School of Public Health, University of North Carolina at Chapel Hill.

Vincent T. Francisco is associate professor in the Department of Public Health Education at the University of North Carolina in Greensboro.

Tiffany L. Gary is assistant professor of epidemiology at The Johns Hopkins Bloomberg School of Public Health in Baltimore.

Andrea Carson Gielen is professor and director of the Center for Injury Research and Policy at The Johns Hopkins Bloomberg School of Public Health in Baltimore.

Russell E. Glasgow is senior scientist at the Center for Health Dissemination & Implementation at the Institute for Health Research, Kaiser Permanente, Colorado.

Catherine A. Heaney is with the Stanford Prevention Research Center at Stanford University.

Barbara A. Israel is professor in the Department of Health Behavior and Health Education in the School of Public Health at the University of Michigan.

Danuta Kasprzyk is research leader at the Centers for Public Health Research and Evaluation, Battelle Memorial Institute, in Seattle.

Michelle C. Kegler is associate professor in the Department of Behavioral Sciences and Health Education in the Rollins School of Public Health at Emory University in Atlanta.

Laura A. Linnan is associate professor in the Department of Health Behavior and Health Education at the University of North Carolina, Chapel Hill, School of Public Health.

Alfred L. McAlister is professor of behavioral sciences at the University of Texas School of Public Health regional campus in Austin.

Eileen M. McDonald is associate scientist and MHS program codirector at The Johns Hopkins Bloomberg School of Public Health in Baltimore.

Meredith Minkler is professor of Health and Social Behavior in the School of Public Health at the University of California, Berkeley.

Daniel E. Montaño is research leader at the Centers for Public Health Research and Evaluation, Battelle Memorial Institute, in Seattle.

Brian Oldenburg is professor and chair of International Public Health at Monash University in Melbourne, Australia.

Neville Owen is professor and director of the Cancer Prevention Research Centre at the University of Queensland in Brisbane, Australia.

Guy S. Parcel is the John P. McGovern Professor in Health Promotion in the School of Public Health at the University of Texas Health Science Center, Houston.

Cheryl L. Perry is professor and regional dean at the University of Texas School of Public Health regional campus in Austin.

James O. Prochaska is professor and director of the Cancer Prevention Research Center at the University of Rhode Island.

Colleen A. Redding is a research professor in the Cancer Prevention Research Center at the University of Rhode Island.

Jose G. Rimón is at the Center for Communication Programs at The Johns Hopkins Bloomberg School of Public Health in Baltimore.

Gary B. Saffitz is deputy director of the Center for Communication Programs and senior associate faculty at The Johns Hopkins University Bloomberg School of Public Health.

James F. Sallis is professor of psychology at San Diego State University and director of the Active Living Research program in San Diego.

Peter M. Sandman is a risk communication consultant in Princeton, New Jersey.

Marc D. Schwartz is associate professor of oncology at the Lombardi Cancer Center at Georgetown University in Washington, D.C.

Celette Sugg Skinner is professor and chief of the Division of Behavioral and Communication Sciences at UT Southwestern Medical Center in Dallas.

J. Douglas Storey is associate director of the Center for Communication Programs at the Johns Hopkins Bloomberg School of Public Health in Baltimore.

Richard L. Street Jr. is professor and head of the Department of Communication at Texas A&M University and Baylor College of Medicine.

Nina Wallerstein is professor in the Masters in Public Health Program at the University of New Mexico in Albuquerque.

Neil D. Weinstein is research professor in the Department of Family and Community Medicine at the University of Arizona College of Medicine in Tucson.

Nance Wilson is a principal investigator with the Public Health Institute in Oakland, California.

HEALTH
BEHAVIOR
AND
HEALTH
EDUCATION

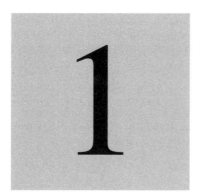

HEALTH EDUCATION
AND
HEALTH BEHAVIOR

The Foundations

CHAPTER

1

THE SCOPE OF HEALTH BEHAVIOR AND HEALTH EDUCATION

The Editors

KEY POINTS

This chapter will

- Discuss the importance of developing successful strategies to improve health behavior.
- Summarize the leading causes of death and disease burden in the United States and globally.
- Describe the scope and evolution of health education.
- Provide key definitions of *health education, health behavior,* and *health promotion.*
- Discuss the diverse settings and audiences for health education.
- Highlight progress and challenges in health behavior and health education research.

Perhaps never before have there been so many demands on those in health education and health behavior to facilitate behavior changes, or so many potential strategies from which to choose. Where professionals once might have seen their roles as working at a particular level of intervention (such as changing organizational or individual health behaviors) or employing a specific type of behavior change strategy (such as group interventions or individual counseling), we now realize that multiple interventions at multiple levels are often needed to initiate and sustain behavior change effectively. And where health education and behavior change professionals once might have relied on intuition, experience, and their knowledge of the literature, increasingly we expect professionals to act on the basis of evidence. In the time since the first edition of this book in 1990, the evidence base for health behavior change has grown dramatically.

A number of systematic reviews have shown that using theory in crafting interventions can lead to more powerful effects than interventions developed without theory (for example, see Ammerman, Lindquist, Lohr, and Hersey, 2002; Legler and others, 2002). It is an exciting time to contemplate behavior change. There are more tools and strategies and a better understanding of the role theory can play in producing effective, sustained behavior change. And the stage has changed from one that is primarily local and country-specific to one that is both global and local, in which we increasingly see the world as interconnected.

These exciting opportunities could not be taking place at a more propitious time. The positive changes of medical innovations, strong evidence base, and exciting and novel tools for health promotion are buffeted by countercurrents of increasing globalization, urbanization, industrialization, and inequalities that deter us from fulfilling the promise of advances in medicine and health promotion. Major challenges include heavy promotion of unhealthy lifestyles, such as tobacco use and fast-food consumption across the globe, increasing pollution, and health problems associated with poverty, such as overcrowding, lack of safe drinking water, unsafe neighborhoods, and limited access to health care services.

It is of little surprise that the number of topics on which health professionals and health education specialists focus has grown and evolved as health problems have changed around the world. Some professionals may counsel people at risk for AIDS about safe sex; help children avoid tobacco, alcohol, and drugs; assist adults to stop smoking; help patients to manage and cope with their illnesses; and organize communities or advocate policy changes aimed at fostering health improvement. Other health professionals may focus on environmental concerns. We expect that, over the next decade, more behavior change interventions will be directed at changing individual and community behaviors related to water consumption and to behaviors that may affect global climate change.

Health education professionals work all over the world in a variety of settings, including schools, worksites, nongovernmental organizations (including voluntary health organizations), medical settings, and communities. Since the first edition of this book, there has been increased recognition that what happens in other parts of the world affects us all, wherever we may be. To the extent that public health is global health and global health is local, we are committed in this volume to exploring the use of health behavior theories around the world and to discussing the potential relevance of what is learned in one setting to others. Although many of the examples are from research conducted in the United States, our perspective is decidedly *not* U.S.-centric.

Since the last edition of this book six years ago, there have been other changes as well. Part of what has made the world feel smaller and people more interconnected is the growth of new communication and information technologies, which have opened up an unprecedented range of strategies for health behavior change programs. Through the Internet, health behavior change interventions may reach people all over the world, regardless of their location. This means that health behavior change interventions can achieve scale never before imagined, potentially reaching millions of people rather than hundreds or thousands.

There is increased recognition that the fruits of research take too long to reach people who could benefit from them (Glasgow and Emmons, 2007; Viswanath, 2006). This has led to an increased emphasis on the dissemination of evidence-based interventions. Part of the rationale for this book is to speed the dissemination of knowledge about how to use theory, so that theory can inform those who develop and use health behavior interventions around the world.

Health experts are challenged to disseminate the best of what is known in new situations. They may also forge and test fundamental theories that drive research and practice in public health, health education, and health care. A premise of *Health Behavior and Health Education* is that a dynamic exchange among theory, research, and practice is most likely to produce effective health education. The editors believe fundamentally that theory and practice should coexist in a healthy dialectic; they are not dichotomies. The best theory is likely to be grounded in real lessons from practice. The best practice should be grounded in theory.

Kanfer and Schefft (1988) observed that "as science and technology advance, the greatest mystery of the universe and the least conquered force of nature remains the human being and his actions and human experiences." The body of research in health behavior and health education has grown rapidly over the past two decades, and health education and health promotion are recognized increasingly as ways to meet public health objectives and improve the success of public health and medical interventions around the world. Although this increasing amount of literature improves the science base of health behavior and health education, it also challenges those in the field to master and be facile with an almost overwhelming body of knowledge.

The science and art of health behavior and health education are eclectic and rapidly evolving; they reflect an amalgamation of approaches, methods, and strategies from social and health sciences, drawing on the theoretical perspectives, research, and practice tools of such diverse disciplines as psychology, sociology, anthropology, communications, nursing, economics, and marketing. Health education is also dependent on epidemiology, statistics, and medicine. There is increasing emphasis on identifying evidence-based interventions and disseminating them widely (Rimer, Glanz, and Rasband, 2001). This often requires individual health education and health behavior professionals to synthesize large and diverse literatures. Evidence-based groups like the Cochrane Collaboration (http://www.cochrane.org) and the CDC's (Centers for Disease Control and Prevention) Guide to Community Preventive Services (http://www.thecommunityguide.org) offer regular syntheses of behavioral interventions, some of which include theoretical constructs as variables in analyses of effectiveness.

Many kinds of professionals contribute to and conduct health education and health behavior (HEHB) programs and research. Health education practice is strengthened by the close collaboration among professionals of different disciplines, each concerned with the behavioral and social intervention process and each contributing a unique perspective. Although health behavior professionals have usually worked this way, there is increasing emphasis on an interdisciplinary or even a transdisciplinary focus (Turkkan, Kaufman, and Rimer, 2000). Psychology brings to health education a rich legacy of over one hundred years of research and practice on individual differences, motivation, learning, persuasion, and attitude and behavior change (Matarazzo and others, 1984), as well as the perspectives of organizational and community psychology. Physicians are important collaborators and are in key roles to effect change in health behavior (Grol and others, 2007). Likewise, nurses and social workers bring to health education their particular expertise in working with individual patients and patients' families to facilitate learning, adjustment, and behavior change, and to improve quality of life. Other health, education, and human service professionals contribute their special expertise as well. Increasingly, there are partnerships with genetic counselors and other specialists in this rapidly developing field.

THE CHANGING CONTEXT OF HEALTH AND BEHAVIOR

The most frequent causes of death in the United States and globally are chronic diseases, including heart disease, cancer, lung diseases, and diabetes (Yach, Hawkes, Gould, and Hofman, 2004). Behavioral factors, particularly tobacco use, diet and activity patterns, alcohol consumption, sexual behavior, and avoidable injuries are among the most prominent contributors to mortality (Schroeder, 2007; Mokdad, Marks, Stroup, and Gerberding, 2004, 2005). Projections of the global burden of disease for the next two decades include increases in noncommunicable diseases, high rates of tobacco-related deaths, and a dramatic rise in deaths from HIV/AIDS (Mathers and Loncar, 2006; Abegunde and others, 2007). Worldwide, the major causes of death by 2030 are expected to be HIV/AIDS, depressive disorders, and heart disease (Mathers and Loncar, 2006).

At the same time, in many parts of the world, infectious diseases continue to pose grim threats, especially for the very young, the old, and those with compromised immune systems. Malaria, diarrheal diseases, and other infectious diseases, in addition to AIDS, are major health threats to the poorest people around the world (The PLoS Medicine Editors, 2007). And, like chronic diseases, their trajectory may be influenced by the application of effective health behavior interventions. Substantial suffering, premature mortality, and medical costs can be avoided by positive changes in behavior at multiple levels. Most recently, there has been a renewed focus on public health infrastructure to plan for emergencies, including both human-made and natural disasters.

During the past twenty years, there has been a dramatic increase in public, private, and professional interest in preventing disability and death through changes in lifestyle and participation in screening programs. Much of this interest in disease prevention and early detection has been stimulated by the epidemiological transition from infectious to chronic diseases as leading causes of death, the aging of the population, rapidly escalating health care costs, and data linking individual behaviors to increased risk of morbidity and mortality. The evidence that early detection can save lives from highly prevalent conditions such as breast and colorectal cancer has also been influential. The AIDS epidemic has also contributed. Moreover, around the world communicable diseases and malnutrition exist alongside increasing problems, like obesity among the middle class (Abegunde and others, 2007).

Landmark reports in Canada and the United States during the 1970s and 1980s heralded the commitment of governments to health education and promotion (Lalonde, 1974; U.S. Department of Health, Education, and Welfare, 1979; Epp, 1986). In the United States, federal initiatives for public health education and monitoring populationwide behavior patterns were spurred by the development of the *Health Objectives for the Nation* (U.S. Department of Health and Human Services, 1980) and its successors, *Healthy People 2000: National Health Promotion and Disease Prevention Objectives* and *Healthy People 2010* (U.S. Department of Health and Human Services, 1991, 2000). Similarly, international agencies are drawing attention to the global burden of diseases and health inequalities (World Health Organization, 2007). Increased interest in behavioral and social determinants of health behavior change spawned numerous training programs and public and commercial service programs.

Data systems and surveillance initiatives now make it feasible to track trends in risk factors, health behaviors, and healthy environments and policies in the United States and developed countries and, in some cases, to tie these changes to disease incidence and mortality (http://www.who.int/research/en). Indeed, positive change has occurred in several areas. A major accomplishment in the United States has been surpassing the targets for reducing deaths from coronary heart disease and cancer (National Center for Health Statistics, 2001). Blood pressure control has improved, and mean population blood cholesterol levels have declined. Alcohol-related motor vehicle deaths and deaths due to automobile crashes and drowning have continued to decrease. Following major litigation against the tobacco industry and a multistate settlement, there are increased restrictions on tobacco advertising and enforcement of laws against selling tobacco to minors (Glanz and others, 2007). In the United States, fewer adults are using tobacco products—the reduction in adult smoking from 42.4 percent to 20.8 percent between 1965 and 2006 (Centers for Disease Control and Prevention, 2007b) is hailed as one of the top public health achievements of the past century. More adults are meeting dietary guidelines for higher consumption of fruits, vegetables, and grain products, as well as decreased dietary fat as a percentage of calories (National Center for Health Statistics, 2001). Rates of HIV/AIDS in the United States have leveled off, and transfusion-related HIV infections have decreased markedly. The proportion of women age fifty and older who have had breast examinations and mammograms exceeded the goal of 60 percent in forty-seven states in the past decade. Yet the recent leveling off of mammography use in the United States indicates just how fragile behavior change can be and points to the need for attention to maintenance of behavior changes (Centers for Disease Control and Prevention, 2007a; Breen and others, 2007). The collective efforts of those in health education and public health have indeed made a difference.

Although this progress is encouraging, much work remains to be done in these areas. More adults and children are overweight. Diabetes is increasing in near-epidemic proportions. More adolescents are sexually active. After major increases in seatbelt use in the early 1990s, rates have declined and remain at 67 percent—well below the target rate of 85 percent (National Center for Health Statistics, 2001). One-fifth of children under three years old have not received a basic series of vaccinations for polio, measles, diphtheria, and other diseases. Sixteen percent of adults under sixty-five years of age have no health insurance coverage. Ethnic minorities and those in poverty still experience a disproportionate burden of preventable disease and disability, and the gap persists between disadvantaged and affluent groups in use of preventive services (National Commission on Prevention Priorities, 2007).

The disease burden is not limited to the United States. Data from Popkin (2007) and others suggest that, like the tobacco epidemic, the obesity epidemic has taken on global proportions. One study of the burden of chronic diseases in twenty-three low- and middle-income countries posits that chronic disease is responsible for 50 percent of the disease burden in 2005 and estimates an economic loss of almost $84 billion (U.S. dollars) between 2006 and 2015 if nothing is done to address the burden (Mathers and Loncar, 2006).

Changes in the health care system provide new supports and opportunities for health education. Respect for patients' rights and more participatory patient-centered communication can lead to improved health outcomes (Arora, 2003; Epstein and Street, 2007), and shared decision making is now recognized as fundamental to the practice of medicine (Levinsky, 1996). Moreover, there is increased attention to issues of shared decision making (Edwards and Elwyn, 1999). Increasingly, patients are driving their own searches for health information by using the Internet (see, for example, Rimer and others, 2005; Hesse and others, 2005), though disparities remain in information seeking between those of higher and lower socioeconomic status (Ramanadhan and Viswanath, 2006). Clinical prevention and behavioral interventions are often considered cost-effective but are neither universally available nor equally accessible across race and socioeconomic groups (Schroeder, 2007; Gostin and Powers, 2006).

The rapid emergence of new communication technologies and new uses of older technologies, such as the telephone, also provide new opportunities and dilemmas. A variety of electronic media for interactive health communication (for example, the Internet, CD-ROMs, and personal digital assistants [PDAs]) can serve as sources of individualized health information, reminders, and social support for health behavior change (Viswanath, 2005; Ahern, Phalen, Le, and Goldman, 2007). These new technologies also may connect individuals with similar health concerns around the world (Bukachi and Pakenham-Walsh, 2007). This may be especially important for people with rare or stigmatized health conditions. However, the new products of the communications revolution have not equally reached affluent and more disadvantaged populations (Viswanath, 2005, 2006).

E-health strategies are becoming an important part of the armamentarium of strategies for those in health education and health behavior. Internet and computer-based applications, along with wireless technologies, can support many of the *Health Behavior and Health Education* strategies based on the theories presented in this book. Use of new technologies should be based on theories of health behavior and be evaluated (Ahern, Phalen, Le, and Goldman, 2007). Otherwise, we risk being technology-driven instead of outcome-driven.

At the same time, new technologies have the potential to cause harm through misleading or deceptive information, promotion of inappropriate self-care, and interference in the patient-provider relationship (Science Panel on Interactive Communication and Health, 1999), although the empirical evidence on harms remains to be documented. Interactive health communications provide new options for behavioral medicine and preventive medicine (Noell and Glasgow, 1999; Fotheringham, Owies, Leslie, and Owen, 2000) and are altering the context of health behavior and health education as they unfold and as their effects are studied (Hesse and others, 2005).

HEALTH EDUCATION AND HEALTH BEHAVIOR

The Scope and Evolution of Health Education

In the fields of health education and health behavior, the emphasis during the 1970s and 1980s on individuals' behaviors as determinants of health status eclipsed attention to the broader social determinants of health. Advocates of system-level changes to improve health called for renewal of a broad vision of health education and promotion (Minkler, 1989; see Chapter Twenty). These calls for moving health education toward social action heralded a renewed enthusiasm for holistic approaches rather than an entirely new worldview. They are well within the tradition of health education and are consistent with its longstanding concern with the impact of social, economic, and political forces on health. Focusing merely on downstream (individual) causes of poor health rather than the upstream causes risks missing important opportunities to improve health (McKinlay and Marceau, 2000).

Over the past forty years, leaders in health education have repeatedly stressed the importance of political, economic, and social factors as determinants of health. Mayhew Derryberry (1960) noted that "health education . . . requires careful and thorough consideration of the present knowledge, attitudes, goals, perceptions, social status, power structure, cultural traditions, and other aspects of whatever public is to be addressed." In 1966, Dorothy Nyswander spoke of the importance of attending to social justice and individuals' sense of control and self-determination. These ideas were reiterated later, when William Griffiths (1972) stressed that "health education is concerned not only with individuals and their families, but *also with the institutions and social conditions* that impede or facilitate individuals toward achieving optimum health" (emphasis added). Green and Kreuter's PRECEDE/PROCEED Model (2005; see Chapter Eighteen), which was first widely introduced over twenty-five years ago, addresses the multiple forces that affect health. Individual health does not exist in a social vacuum.

The view of health education as an instrument of social change has been renewed and invigorated during the past decade. Policy, advocacy, and organizational change have been adopted as central activities of public health and health education. Most recently, experts have explicitly recommended that interventions on social and behavioral factors related to health should link multiple levels of influence, including the individual, interpersonal, institutional, community, and policy levels (Smedley and Syme, 2000). This volume purposefully includes chapters on community and societal influences on health behavior and strategies to effect community and social policy changes in addition to the individual-level theories. In this context, definitions of *health education* and *health promotion* can be recognized and discussed as overlapping and intertwined.

Definitions of Health Education

According to Griffiths (1972), "health education attempts to close the gap between what is known about optimum health practice and that which is actually practiced." Simonds (1976) defined *health education* as aimed at "bringing about behavioral changes in individuals, groups, and larger populations from behaviors that are presumed to be detrimental to health, to behaviors that are conducive to present and future health."

Subsequent definitions emphasized voluntary, informed behavior changes. In 1980, Green defined *health education* as "any combination of learning experiences designed to facilitate voluntary adaptations of behavior conducive to health" (Green, Kreuter, Deeds, and Partridge, 1980). The Role Delineation Project defined it as "the process of assisting individuals, acting separately or collectively, to make informed decisions about matters affecting their personal health and that of others" (National Task Force on the Preparation and Practice of Health Educators, 1985).

Health education evolved from three settings: communities, schools, and patient care settings. Kurt Lewin's pioneering work in group process and his developmental field theory during the 1930s and 1940s provide the intellectual roots for much of health education practice today. One of the earliest models developed to explain health behavior, the Health Belief Model (HBM), was developed during the 1950s to explain behavior related to tuberculosis screening (Hochbaum, 1958).

As we already have noted, health education includes not only instructional activities and other strategies to change individual health behavior but also organizational efforts, policy directives, economic supports, environmental activities, mass media, and community-level programs. Two key ideas from an ecological perspective help direct the identification of personal and environmental leverage points for health promotion and education interventions (Glanz and Rimer, 1995). First, behavior is viewed as being affected by, and affecting, *multiple levels of influence.* Five levels of influence for health-related behaviors and conditions have been identified: (1) intrapersonal, or individual factors; (2) interpersonal factors; (3) institutional, or organizational factors; (4) community factors; and (5) public-policy factors (McLeroy, Bibeau, Steckler, and Glanz, 1988). The second key idea relates to the possibility of *reciprocal causation* between individuals and their environments; that is, behavior both influences *and* is influenced by the social environment (Glanz and Rimer, 1995; Stokols, Grzywacz, McMahan, and Phillips, 2003).

Health education covers the continuum from disease prevention and promotion of optimal health to the detection of illness to treatment, rehabilitation, and long-term care. It includes infectious and chronic diseases, as well as attention to environmental issues. Health education is delivered in almost every conceivable setting—universities, schools, hospitals, pharmacies, grocery stores and shopping centers, recreation settings, community organizations, voluntary health agencies, worksites, churches, prisons, health maintenance organizations, migrant labor camps; it is delivered through mass media, over the Internet, in people's homes, and in health departments at all levels of government. These settings are discussed later in this chapter.

Health promotion is a term of more recent origin than *health education.* As defined by Green, it is "any combination of health education and related organizational, economic, and environmental supports for behavior of individuals, groups, or communities conducive to health" (Green and Kreuter, 1991). A slightly different definition is suggested by O'Donnell (1989): "Health promotion is the science and art of helping people change their lifestyle toward a state of optimum health. . . . Lifestyle changes can be facilitated by a combination of efforts to enhance awareness, change behavior, and create environments that support good health practices." Definitions arising in Europe and Canada have yet another emphasis (Kolbe, 1988; Hawe, Degeling, and Hall, 1990). The *Ottawa Charter for Health Promotion* defines *health promotion* as "the process of enabling people to increase control over, and to improve, their health . . . a commitment to dealing with the challenges of reducing inequities, extending the scope of prevention, and helping people to cope with their circumstances . . . create environments conducive to health, in which people are better able to take care of themselves" (Epp, 1986).

Although greater precision of terminology might be achieved by drawing a clear distinction between health education and health promotion, to do so would be to ignore longstanding tenets of health education and its broad social mission. Clearly, health educators have long used more than "educational" strategies. In fact, the terms *health promotion* and *health education* are often used interchangeably in the United States. In some countries, such as Australia, health education is considered a much narrower endeavor than health promotion. Nevertheless, although the term *health promotion* emphasizes efforts to influence the broader social context of *health behavior,* the two terms remain closely linked and overlapping, share historical and philosophical foundations, and are often used in combination. In most cases, we consider the two terms too closely related to distinguish between them. In this book, the term *health education* is used most often. It is to be understood in the historical sense—as a broad and varied set of strategies to influence both individuals and their social environments, in order to improve health behavior and enhance health and quality of life.

Definitions of Health Behavior

The central concern of health education is health behavior, writ large. It is included or suggested in every definition of *health education* and is the crucial dependent variable in most research on the impact of health education intervention strategies. Positive, informed changes in health behavior are typically the ultimate aims of health education programs. If behaviors change but health is not subsequently improved, the result is a paradox that must be resolved by examining other issues, such as the link between behavior and health status or the ways in which behavior and health (or both) are measured. Informed decision making is a desirable endpoint for problems involving medical uncertainty, and studies suggest that shared decision making may lead to improved patient satisfaction and health outcomes (Rimer and others, 2004). Likewise, environmental or structural interventions to change presumed social environmental determinants of health behavior are intended to improve health by changing behavior (Smedley and Syme, 2000; Story, Kaphingst, Robinson-O'Brien, and Glanz, 2008). Thus, efforts to improve environments and policies should ultimately be evaluated for their effects on health behavior. If policy changes but does not lead to measurable changes in behavior, it may be either too weak or too short-lived, or it could be only a limited determinant of behavior.

In the broadest sense, *health behavior* refers to the actions of individuals, groups, and organizations, as well as their determinants, correlates, and consequences, including social change, policy development and implementation, improved coping skills, and enhanced quality of life (Parkerson and others, 1993). This is similar to the working definition of *health behavior* that Gochman proposed (though his definition emphasized individuals): it includes not only observable, overt actions but also the mental events and feeling states that can be reported and measured. He defined *health behavior* as "those personal attributes such as beliefs, expectations, motives, values, perceptions, and other cognitive elements; personality characteristics, including affective and emotional states and traits; and overt behavior patterns, actions, and habits that relate to health maintenance, to health restoration, and to health improvement" (Gochman, 1982, 1997).

Gochman's definition is consistent with and embraces the definitions of specific categories of overt health behavior proposed by Kasl and Cobb in their seminal articles (1966a, 1966b). Kasl and Cobb define three categories of health behavior:

1. *Preventive health behavior:* any activity undertaken by an individual who believes himself (or herself) to be healthy, for the purpose of preventing or detecting illness in an asymptomatic state.

2. *Illness behavior:* any activity undertaken by an individual who perceives himself to be ill, to define the state of health, and to discover a suitable remedy (Kasl and Cobb, 1966a).

3. *Sick-role behavior:* any activity undertaken by an individual who considers himself to be ill, for the purpose of getting well. It includes receiving treatment from medical providers, generally involves a whole range of dependent behaviors, and leads to some degree of exemption from one's usual responsibilities (Kasl and Cobb, 1966b).

SETTINGS AND AUDIENCES FOR HEALTH EDUCATION

During the past century and more specifically during the past few decades, the scope and methods of health education have broadened and diversified dramatically. This section briefly reviews the range of settings and audiences of health education today. We note that the ideas of "settings" and "audiences" have expanded and become more diversified over the past decade.

Where Health Education Is Provided

Today, health education can be found nearly everywhere. The settings for health education are important because they provide channels for delivering programs, provide access to specific populations and gatekeepers, usually have existing communication systems for diffusion of programs, and facilitate development of policies and organizational change to support positive health practices (Mullen and others, 1995). Seven major settings are particularly relevant to contemporary health education: schools, communities, worksites, health care settings, homes, the consumer marketplace, and the communications environment.

Schools. Health education in schools includes classroom teaching, teacher training, and changes in school environments that support healthy behaviors (Luepker and others, 1996; Franks and others, 2007). To support long-term health enhancement initiatives, theories of organizational change can be used to encourage adoption of comprehensive smoking control programs in schools. Diffusion of Innovations theory and the Theory of Reasoned Action have been used to analyze factors associated with adoption of AIDS prevention curricula in Dutch schools (Paulussen, Kok, Schaalma, and Parcel, 1995).

Communities. Community-based health education draws on social relationships and organizations to reach large populations with media and interpersonal strategies. Models of community organization enable program planners both to gain support for and to design suitable health messages and delivery mechanisms (see Chapter Thirteen). Community interventions in churches, clubs, recreation centers, and neighborhoods have been used to encourage healthful nutrition, reduce risk of cardiovascular disease, and use peer influences to promote breast cancer detection among minority women.

Worksites. Since its emergence in the mid-1970s, worksite health promotion has grown and spawned new tools for health educators. Because people spend so much time at work, the workplace is both a source of stress and a source of social support (Israel and Schurman, 1990). Effective worksite programs can harness social support as a buffer to stress, with the goal of improving worker health and health practices. Today, many businesses, particularly large corporations, provide health promotion programs for their employees (National Center for Health Statistics, 2001). Both high-risk and populationwide strategies have been used in programs to reduce the risk of cancer (Tilley and others, 1999a, 1999b; Sorenson and others, 1996) and cardiovascular disease (Glasgow and others, 1995). Integrating health promotion with worker safety and occupational health may increase effectiveness (Sorensen and Barbeau, 2006).

Health Care Settings. Health education for high-risk individuals, patients, their families, and the surrounding community, as well as in-service training for health care providers, are all part of health care today. The changing nature of health service delivery has stimulated greater emphasis on health education and provider-focused quality improvement strategies in physicians' offices, health maintenance organizations, public health clinics, and hospitals (Grol and others, 2007). Primary care settings, in particular, provide an opportunity to reach a substantial number of people (Campbell and others, 1993; Glanz and others, 1990). Health education in these settings focuses on preventing and detecting disease, helping people make decisions about genetic testing, and managing acute and chronic illnesses.

Homes. Health behavior change interventions are delivered to people in their homes, both through traditional public health means, like home visits, and through a variety of communication channels and media such as Internet, telephone, and mail (Science Panel on Interactive Communication and Health, 1999; McBride and Rimer, 1999). Use of strategies such as mailed tailored messages (Skinner and others, 1999) and motivational interviewing by telephone (Emmons and Rollnick, 2001) makes it possible to reach larger groups and high-risk groups in a convenient way that reduces barriers to their receiving motivational messages.

The Consumer Marketplace. The advent of home health and self-care products, as well as use of "health" appeals to sell consumer goods, has created new opportunities for health education but also can mislead consumers about the potential health effects of items they can purchase (Glanz and others, 1995). Social marketing, with its roots in consumer behavior theory, is used increasingly by health educators to enhance the salience of health messages and to improve their persuasive impact (see Chapter Nineteen). Theories of Consumer Information Processing (CIP) provide a framework for understanding why people do or do not pay attention to, understand, and make use of consumer health information such as nutrient labels on packaged food products (Rudd and Glanz, 1990).

The Communications Environment. As noted earlier, there have been striking and rapid changes in the availability and use of new communications technologies, ranging from mass media changes (for example, online versions of newspapers, blogs of radio programs) to personalized and interactive media (for example, PDAs, interactive telephone and Internet exchanges) and a host of wireless tools in homes, businesses, and communities (Viswanath, 2005). These channels are not "settings" per se and can be used in any of the settings described earlier. Yet they are unique and increasingly specialized, providing opportunities for intervention; they also require evaluation of their reach and impact on health behaviors (Ahern and others, 2007).

Audiences for Health Education

For health education to be effective, it should be designed with an understanding of recipients'—target audiences'—health and social characteristics, beliefs, attitudes, values, skills, and past behaviors. These audiences consist of people who may be reached as individuals, in groups, through organizations, as communities or sociopolitical entities, or through some combination of these. They may be health professionals, clients, people at risk for disease, or patients. This section discusses four dimensions along which the potential audiences can be characterized: (1) sociodemographic characteristics, (2) ethnic or racial background, (3) life cycle stage, and (4) disease or at-risk status.

Sociodemographic Characteristics and Ethnic/Racial Background. Socioeconomic status has been linked with both health status and health behavior, with less affluent persons consistently experiencing higher morbidity and mortality (Berkman and Kawachi, 2000). Recognition of differences in disease and mortality rates across socioeconomic and ethnic or racial groups has led to increased efforts to reduce or eliminate health disparities (Smedley, Stith and Nelson, 2003; World Health Organization, 2007). For example, it has long been known that African Americans die at earlier ages than whites. Life expectancy for African American males is almost seven years less than for white males. The difference of five years for African American versus white women is smaller, but still alarmingly discrepant. The gaps have grown over the past three decades and are even greater for those with lower levels of education and income (Crimmins and Saito, 2001; Franks, Muennig, Lubetkin, and Jia, 2006).

A variety of sociodemographic characteristics, such as gender, age, race, marital status, place of residence, and employment characterize health education audiences. The United States has experienced a rapid influx of new immigrant populations, especially from Africa and Europe, and the proportion of non-white minority residents continues to climb. These factors, although generally not *modifiable* within the bounds of health education programs, are important in guiding the targeting of strategies and educational material, and identifying channels through which to reach consumers. Health education materials should be appropriate for, and ideally matched to, the educational and reading levels of particular target audiences and be compatible with their ethnic and cultural backgrounds (Resnicow, Braithwaite, DiIorio, and Glanz, 2002).

Life Cycle Stage. Health education is provided for people at every stage of the life cycle, from childbirth education, whose beneficiaries are not yet born, to self-care education and rehabilitation for the very old. Developmental perspectives help guide the choice of intervention and research methods. Children may have misperceptions about health and illness. For example, they may think that illnesses are punishment for bad behavior (Armsden and Lewis, 1993). Knowledge of children's cognitive development helps provide a framework for understanding these beliefs and ways to respond to them. Adolescents may feel invulnerable to accidents and chronic diseases. The Health Belief Model (HBM; see Chapter Three) is a useful framework for understanding the factors that may predispose youth to engage in unsafe sexual practices. Older adults and their health providers may attribute symptoms of cancer to the inexorable process of aging rather than the disease itself. Such beliefs should be considered in designing, implementing, and evaluating health education programs (Rimer and others, 1983; Keintz, Rimer, Fleisher, and Engstrom, 1988). Federal health protection goals stress reaching people in every stage of life, with a special focus on vulnerability that may affect people at various life cycle stages (http://www.cdc.gov/osi/goals/people.html).

Disease or At-Risk Status. People who are diagnosed with specific diseases often experience not only symptoms but also the distress associated with their prognosis and having to make decisions about medical care (see Chapter Ten). Thus, they may benefit from health education, but illness may compromise their ability to attend to new information at critical points. Because of this, timing, channels, and audiences for patient education should be carefully considered. Successful patient education depends on a sound understanding of the patient's view of the world (Glanz and Oldenburg, 2001). For individuals at high risk due to family history or identified risk factors, health behavior change interventions may have heightened salience when linked to strategies for reducing individual risk (see Chapter Six on the Precaution Adoption Process Model). Even so, strategies used to enable initial changes in behavior, such as quitting smoking, may be insufficient to maintain behavior change over the long term, even in these people. Models and theories of health behavior can suggest strategies to prevent relapse and enhance maintenance of recommended practices for high-risk individuals (Glanz and Oldenburg, 2001).

PROGRESS IN HEALTH PROMOTION AND HEALTH BEHAVIOR RESEARCH

Over the past two decades, research programs have been established to identify and test the most effective methods to achieve health behavior change. More precise quantification of personal health behaviors and improved health outcomes has grown from partnerships between behavioral scientists and biomedical experts. During this period, findings from some major health behavior intervention studies have become available and have provided important insights for the field.

In the late 1970s and early 1980s, three large community cardiovascular disease intervention studies were begun in California, Minnesota, and Rhode Island (Winkleby, 1994). Each study addressed smoking, hypertension, high-fat diets, obesity, and physical inactivity—all widespread risk factors that many practitioners were tackling. The multicomponent risk-reduction programs in these trials used mass media, interpersonal education programs for the public, professionals, and those at high risk. Community organization strategies were used to create institutional and environmental support for the programs, and theoretically derived program planning strategies emphasized community participation (Winkleby, 1994). In the 1990s, all three studies reported their findings on risk-factor changes. They each found favorable secular trends in control sites and modest or nonsignificant intervention effects on risk-factor reduction (Farquhar and others, 1990; Luepker and others, 1994; Carleton and others, 1995). Two large worksite trials of multicomponent nutrition and smoking interventions yielded similar findings (Glasgow and others, 1995; Sorensen and others, 1996).

These studies produced a wealth of knowledge about health behavior, and many of the short-term, targeted interventions within the larger studies were found to be effective (Winkleby, 1994). Nonetheless, the results cast doubt on the presumed effectiveness of population-based intervention strategies over the long term, especially against the backdrop of a dynamic, changing environment. Still, the lack of significant communitywide effects in these studies should not be assumed to "disprove" the conceptual foundations of the intervention methods. An alternative view is to regard the interventions used in these studies as contributors to the substantial secular trend in chronic disease prevention (Winkleby, 1994). At the same time, several campaigns were effective in producing behavior changes conducive to health (Hornik, 2002). These experiences suggest that health education interventions must be carefully planned, developed from strong formative research, and theory-based (Randolph and Viswanath, 2004). Although randomized, controlled trials provide the most rigorous test of health behavior interventions, the past two decades have been marked by an increase in carefully designed evaluation research in health education, which combines quantitative and qualitative methods. Evaluations of community-based AIDS-prevention projects (Janz and others, 1996) and coalitions for prevention of alcohol, tobacco, and other drug abuse (Butterfoss, Goodman, and Wandersman, 1996) exemplify newer applications of community research methodologies that offer in-depth process information across multiple programs in diverse settings.

Overall, there has been a growing trend toward evidence-based health education and health behavior (HEHB), as the findings of numerous large health behavior intervention studies have been published (Rimer, Glanz, and Rasband, 2001). One review of research in health education from 1994 to 2003 observed a significant increase in the use of quantitative statistics, finding that the most common types of articles are from cross-sectional studies and review articles (Merrill, Lindsay, Shields, and Stoddard, 2007). That review was limited to three "health education" journals. However, other reviews of research design and statistics also found a preponderance of correlational and descriptive studies (Noar and Zimmerman, 2005; Weinstein, 2007; Painter and others, forthcoming).

As the research literature grows, it is increasingly important that the evidence base become accessible to both researchers and practitioners (Von Elm and others, 2007). Evidence reviews are defined as those using formalized methods to collect, prioritize, and weigh the findings of intervention research. Important progress has been made over the past ten to fifteen years to improve the process of systematic reviews and meta-analysis (Mulrow, Cook, and Davidoff, 1997). In reality, literature reviews cut across a continuum of scientific rigor in their methodologies for selecting, evaluating, and reporting the evidence. They may exclude all but the most rigorous studies or be all-inclusive, may provide detailed information on methodology or only report on findings, or may be highly quantitative in drawing conclusions or rely heavily on expert judgment (Rimer, Glanz, and Rasband, 2001; Lipsey, 2005). An important effort has been under way in the United States since the late 1990s and should continue to advance the evidence base in HEHB in the next few years. The U.S. Task Force on Community Preventive Services is defining, categorizing, summarizing, and rating the quality of evidence on the effectiveness of population-based interventions for disease prevention and control; providing recommendations on these interventions and methods for their delivery based on the evidence, and identifying and summarizing research gaps (Briss and others, 2000; http://www.thecommunityguide.org). Parallel efforts are under way in other countries as well, such as the National Institute for Health and Clinical Excellence (NICE) efforts in England (http://www.nice.org.uk).

The challenge of understanding and improving health behavior is central for health policy today and is "one of the most complex tasks yet confronted by science. To competently address that challenge, the . . . research community must simply do more and do it better" in certain key areas of behavioral research (McGinnis, 1994). A coordinated and focused effort will be essential to resolving many of the most vexing health issues facing our society (Smedley and Syme, 2000). Integration of the best available knowledge from theory, research, and health promotion and education practice can advance that agenda in the next decade.

SUMMARY

This chapter has discussed the dynamic nature of health education and health behavior today in the context of changing patterns of disease and trends in health care, health education, and disease prevention in the United States and globally. It has provided definitions of *health education, health promotion,* and *health behavior* and described the broad and diverse parameters of this maturing field. Health behavior research has experienced great progress, but mixed findings raise new questions and pose methodological, theoretical, and substantive challenges. The interrelationships and importance of theory, research, and practice are set against a backdrop of the important, growing, and complex challenges in health education and health behavior.

REFERENCES

Abegunde, D. O., and others. "The Burden and Costs of Chronic Diseases in Low-Income and Middle-Income Countries." *Lancet,* 2007, *370*(9603), 1929–1938.

Ahern, D. K., Phalen, J. M., Le, L. X., and Goldman, R. (eds.). *Childhood Obesity Prevention and Reduction: Role of eHealth.* Boston: Health e-Technologies Initiative, 2007.

Ammerman, A. S., Lindquist, C. H., Lohr, K. N., and Hersey, J. "The Efficacy of Behavioral Interventions to Modify Dietary Fat and Fruit and Vegetable Intake: A Review of the Evidence." *Preventive Medicine,* 2002, *35*(1), 25–41.

Armsden, G., and Lewis, F. "The Child's Adaptation to Parental Medical Illness: Theory and Clinical Implications." *Patient Education and Counseling,* 1993, *22,* 153–165.

Arora, N. K. "Interacting with Cancer Patients: The Significance of Physicians' Communication Behavior." *Social Science & Medicine,* 2003, *57*(5), 791–806.

Berkman, L. F., and Kawachi, I. *Social Epidemiology.* New York: Oxford University Press, 2000.

Breen, N., and others. "Reported Drop in Mammography: Is This Cause for Concern?" *Cancer,* 2007, *109*(12), 2405–2409.

Briss, P., and others. "Developing an Evidence-Based Guide to Community Preventive Services—Methods." *American Journal of Preventive Medicine,* 2000, *18*(1 Suppl), 35–43.

Bukachi, F., and Pakenham-Walsh, N. "Information Technology for Health in Developing Countries." *Chest,* 2007, *132*(5), 1624–1630.

Butterfoss, F. D., Goodman, R., and Wandersman, A. "Community Coalitions for Prevention and Health Promotion: Factors Predicting Satisfaction, Participation, and Planning." *Health Education Quarterly,* 1996, *23*(1), 65–79.

Campbell, M., and others. "The Impact of Message Tailoring on Dietary Behavior Change for Disease Prevention in Primary Care Settings." *American Journal of Public Health,* 1993, *84*(5), 783–787.

Carleton, R., and others. "The Pawtucket Heart Health Program: Community Changes in Cardiovascular Risk Factors and Projected Disease Risk." *American Journal of Public Health,* 1995, *85*(6), 777–785.

Centers for Disease Control and Prevention (CDC). "Use of Mammograms Among Women Aged≥40 Years—United States, 2000–2005." *MMWR Morbidity and Mortality Weekly Reports,* 2007a, *56*(3), 49–51.

Centers for Disease Control and Prevention (CDC). "Cigarette Smoking Among Adults—United States, 2006." *MMWR Morbidity and Mortality Weekly Reports,* 2007b, *56*(44), 1157–1161.

Crimmins, E. M., and Saito, Y. "Trends in Healthy Life Expectancy in the United States, 1970–1990: Gender, Racial, and Educational Differences." *Social Science & Medicine,* 2001, *52*(11), 1629–1641.

Derryberry, M. "Health Education: Its Objectives and Methods." *Health Education Monographs,* 1960, *8,* 5–11.

Edwards, A., and Elwyn, G. "How Should Effectiveness of Risk Communication to Aid Patients' Decisions Be Judged? A Review of the Literature." *Medical Decision Making,* 1999, *19,* 428–434.

Emmons, K. M., and Rollnick, S. "Motivational Interviewing in Health Care Settings: Opportunities and Limitations." *American Journal of Preventive Medicine,* 2001, *20,* 68–74.

Epp, L. *Achieving Health For All: A Framework for Health Promotion in Canada.* Toronto: Health and Welfare, Canada, 1986.

Epstein, R. M., and Street, R. L. Jr. "Patient-Centered Communication in Cancer Care: Promoting Healing and Reducing Suffering." NIH Publication No. 07–6225. Bethesda, Md.: National Cancer Institute, 2007.

Farquhar, J. W., and others. "Effect of Communitywide Education on Cardiovascular Disease Risk Factors: The Stanford Five-City Project." *Journal of the American Medical Association,* 1990, *264,* 359–365.

Fotheringham, M. J., Owies, D., Leslie, E., and Owen, N. "Interactive Health Communication in Preventive Medicine: Internet-Based Strategies in Teaching and Research." *American Journal of Preventive Medicine,* 2000, *19,* 113–120.

Franks, A., and others. "School-Based Programs: Lessons Learned from CATCH, Planet Health, and Not-On-Tobacco." *Preventing Chronic Disease,* 2007, *4*(2), A33.

Franks, P., Muennig, P., Lubetkin, E., and Jia, H. "The Burden of Disease Associated with Being African-American in the United States and the Contribution of Socioeconomic Status." *Social Science & Medicine,* 2006, *62*(10), 2469–2478.

Glanz, K., and Oldenburg, B. "Utilizing Theories and Constructs Across Models of Behavior Change." In R. Patterson (ed.), *Changing Patient Behavior: Improving Outcomes in Health and Disease Management.* San Francisco: Jossey-Bass, 2001.

Glanz, K., and Rimer, B. K. *Theory at a Glance: A Guide to Health Promotion Practice.* Bethesda, Md.: National Cancer Institute, 1995.

Glanz, K., and others. "Patient Reactions to Nutrition Education for Cholesterol Reduction." *American Journal of Preventive Medicine,* 1990, *60*(6), 311–317.

Glanz, K., and others. "Environmental and Policy Approaches to Cardiovascular Disease Prevention Through Nutrition: Opportunities for State and Local Action." *Health Education Quarterly,* 1995, *22*(4), 512–527.

Glanz, K., and others. "Reducing Minors' Access to Tobacco: Eight Years' Experience In Hawaii." *Preventive Medicine,* 2007, *44*(1), 55–58.

Glasgow, R. E., and Emmons, K. M. "How Can We Increase Translation of Research into Practice? Types of Evidence Needed." *Annual Review of Public Health,* 2007, *28,* 413–433.

Glasgow, R., and others. "Take Heart: Results from the Initial Phase of a Work-Site Wellness Program." *American Journal of Public Health,* 1995, *85*(2), 209–216.

Gochman, D. S. "Health Behavior Research: Definitions and Diversity." In D. S. Gochman (ed.), *Handbook of Health Behavior Research, Vol. I. Personal and Social Determinants.* New York: Plenum Press, 1997.

Gochman, D. S. "Labels, Systems, and Motives: Some Perspectives on Future Research." *Health Education Quarterly,* 1982, *9,* 167–174.

Gostin, L. O., and Powers, M. "What Does Social Justice Require for the Public's Health? Public Health Ethics and Policy Imperatives." *Health Affairs,* 2006, *25*(4), 1053–1060.

Green, L. W., and Kreuter, M. W. *Health Promotion Planning: An Educational and Environmental Approach.* (2nd Edition). Mountain View, Calif.: Mayfield, 1991.

Green, L. W., and Kreuter, M. W. *Health Promotion Planning: An Educational and Ecological Approach.* (4th Edition). New York: McGraw-Hill, 2005.

Green, L. W., Kreuter, M. W., Deeds, S., and Partridge, K., *Health Education Planning: A Diagnostic Approach.* Mountain View, Calif.: Mayfield, 1980.

Griffiths, W. "Health Education Definitions, Problems, and Philosophies." *Health Education Monographs,* 1972, *31,* 12–14.

Grol, R., and others. "Planning and Studying Improvement in Patient Care: The Use of Theoretical Perspectives." *The Milbank Quarterly,* 2007, *85*(1), 93–138.

Hawe, P., Degeling, D., and Hall, J. *Evaluating Health Promotion: A Health Worker's Guide.* Sydney, Australia: MacLennan and Petty, 1990.

Hesse, B. W., and others. "Trust and Sources of Health Information: The Impact of the Internet and Its Implications for Health Care Providers: Findings from the First Health Information National Trends Survey." *Archives of Internal Medicine,* 2005, *165*(22), 2618–2624.

Hochbaum, G. *Public Participation in Medical Screening Programs: A Sociopsychological Study.* Public Health Service Publication no. 572, 1958.

Hornik, R. "Public Health Communication: Making Sense of Contradictory Evidence." In R. Hornik (ed.), *Public Health Communication: Evidence For Behavior Change.* New York: Erlbaum, 2002.

Israel, B., and Schurman, S. "Social Support, Control, and the Stress Process." In K. Glanz, F. M. Lewis, and B. K. Rimer (eds.), *Health Behavior and Health Education: Theory, Research, and Practice.* San Francisco: Jossey-Bass, 1990.

Janz, N. K., and others. "Evaluation of 37 AIDS Prevention Projects: Successful Approaches and Barriers to Program Effectiveness." *Health Education Quarterly,* 1996, *23*(1), 80–97.

Kanfer, F. H., and Schefft, B. *Guiding the Process of Therapeutic Change.* Champaign, Ill.: Research Press, 1988.

Kasl, S. V., and Cobb, S. "Health Behavior, Illness Behavior, and Sick-Role Behavior: I. Health and Illness Behavior." *Archives of Environmental Health,* 1966a, *12,* 246–266.

Kasl, S. V., and Cobb, S. "Health Behavior, Illness Behavior, and Sick-Role Behavior: II. Sick-Role Behavior." *Archives of Environmental Health,* 1966b, *12,* 531–541.

Keintz, M., Rimer, B., Fleisher, L., and Engstrom, P. "Educating Older Adults About Their Increased Cancer Risk." *Gerontologist,* 1988, *28,* 487–490.

Kolbe, L. J. "The Application of Health Behavior Research: Health Education and Health Promotion." In D. S. Gochman (ed.), *Health Behavior: Emerging Research Perspectives.* New York: Plenum Press, 1988.

Lalonde, M. *A New Perspective on the Health of Canadians: A Working Document.* Toronto: Health and Welfare Canada, 1974.

Legler, J., and others. "The Effectiveness of Interventions to Promote Mammography Among Women with Historically Lower Rates of Screening." *Cancer, Epidemiology, Biomarkers and Prevention,* 2002, *11*(1), 59–71.

Levinsky, N. "Social, Institutional, and Economic Barriers to the Exercise of Patients' Rights." *New England Journal of Medicine,* 1996, *334*(8), 532–534.

Lipsey, M. W. "The Challenges of Interpreting Research for Use by Practitioners: Comments on the Latest Products from the Task Force on Community Preventive Services." *American Journal of Preventive Medicine,* 2005, *28*(2, Suppl1), 1–3.

Luepker, R. V., and others. "Community Education for Cardiovascular Disease Prevention: Risk Factor Changes in the Minnesota Heart Health Program." *American Journal of Public Health,* 1994, *84,* 1383–1393.

Luepker, R. V., and others. "Outcomes of a Trial to Improve Children's Dietary Patterns and Physical Activity: The Child and Adolescent Trial for Cardiovascular Health (CATCH)." *Journal of the American Medical Association,* 1996, *275,* 768–776.

Matarazzo, J. D., and others (eds.). *Behavioral Health: A Handbook of Health Enhancement and Disease Prevention.* New York: Wiley, 1984.

Mathers, C. D., and Loncar, D. "Projections of Global Mortality and Burden of Disease from 2002 to 2030." *PLoS Medicine,* 2006, *3*(11), 2011–2030.

McBride, C. M., and Rimer, B. K. "Using the Telephone to Improve Health Behavior and Health Service Delivery." *Patient Education and Counseling,* 1999, *37,* 3–18.

McGinnis, J. M. "The Role of Behavioral Research in National Health Policy." In S. Blumenthal, K. Matthews, and S. Weiss (eds.), *New Research Frontiers in Behavioral Medicine: Proceedings of the National Conference.* Bethesda, Md.: NIH Health and Behavior Coordinating Committee, 1994.

McKinlay, J. B., and Marceau, L. D. "Upstream Healthy Public Policy: Lessons from the Battle of Tobacco." *International Journal of Health Services,* 2000, *30*(1), 49–69.

McLeroy, K. R., Bibeau, D., Steckler, A., and Glanz, K. "An Ecological Perspective on Health Promotion Programs." *Health Education Quarterly,* 1988, *15,* 351–377.

Merrill, R. M., Lindsay, C. A., Shields, E. D., and Stoddard, J. "Have the Focus and Sophistication of Research in Health Education Changed?" *Health Education and Behavior,* 2007, *34*(1), 10–25.

Minkler, M. "Health Education, Health Promotion, and the Open Society: A Historical Perspective." *Health Education Quarterly,* 1989, *16,* 17–30.

Mokdad, A. H., Marks, J. S., Stroup, D. F., and Gerberding, J. L. "Actual Causes of Death in the United States, 2000." *Journal of the American Medical Association,* 2004, *291*(19), 1238–1245.

Mokdad, A. H., Marks, J. S., Stroup, D. F., and Gerberding, J. L. "Correction: Actual Causes of Death in the United States, 2000." *Journal of the American Medical Association,* 2005, *293*(3), 293–294.

Mullen, P. D., and others. "Settings as an Important Dimension in Health Education/Promotion Policy, Programs, and Research." *Health Education Quarterly,* 1995, *22,* 329–345.

Mulrow, C. D., Cook, D. J., and Davidoff, F. "Systematic Reviews: Critical Links in the Great Chain of Evidence." *Annals of Internal Medicine,* 1997, *126,* 389–391.

National Center for Health Statistics. *Healthy People 2000: Final Review.* DHHS Publication No. 01–0256. Hyattsville, Md.: Public Health Service, 2001.

National Commission on Prevention Priorities. *Preventive Care: A National Profile on Use, Disparities, and Health Benefits.* Washington, D.C.: Partnership for Prevention, 2007.

National Task Force on the Preparation and Practice of Health Educators, Inc. *A Framework for the Development of Competency-Based Curricula.* New York: National Task Force, Inc., 1985.

Noar, S. M, and Zimmerman, R. S. "Health Behavior Theory and Cumulative Knowledge Regarding Health Behaviors: Are We Moving in the Right Direction?" *Health Education Research,* 2005, *20,* 275–290.

Noell, J., and Glasgow, R. E. "Interactive Technology Applications for Behavioral Counseling: Issues and Opportunities for Health Care Settings." *American Journal of Preventive Medicine,* 1999, *17,* 269–274.

Nyswander, D. "The Open Society: Its Implications for Health Educators." *Health Education Monographs,* 1966, *1,* 3–13.

O'Donnell, M. P. "Definition of Health Promotion: Part III: Expanding the Definition." *American Journal of Health Promotion,* 1989, *3,* 5.

Painter, J. E., and others. "The Use of Theory in Health Behavior Research from 2000 to 2005: A Systematic Review." *Annals of Behavioral Medicine,* forthcoming.

Parkerson, G., and others. "Disease-Specific Versus Generic Measurement of Health-Related Quality of Life in Insulin Dependent Diabetic Patients." *Medical Care,* 1993, *31,* 629–637.

Paulussen, T. G., Kok, G., Schaalma, H. P., and Parcel, G. S. "Diffusion of AIDS Curricula Among Dutch Secondary School Teachers." *Health Education Quarterly,* 1995, *22,* 227–243.

PLoS Medicine Editors. "Thirty Ways to Improve the Health of the World's Poorest People." *PLoS Medicine,* 2007, *4*(10), e310. doi:10.1371/journal.pmed.0040310.

Popkin, B. M. "The World Is Fat." *Scientific American,* 2007, *297*(3), 88–95.

Ramanadhan, S., and Viswanath, K. "Health and the Information Non-seekers: A Profile." *Health Communication,* 2006, *20*(2), 131–139.

Randolph, W., and Viswanath, K. "Lessons from Mass Media Public Health Campaigns." *Annual Review of Public Health,* 2004, *25,* 419–437.

Resnicow, K. K., Braithwaite, R. L., DiIorio, C., and Glanz, K. "Applying Theory to Culturally Diverse and Unique Populations." In K. Glanz, B. K. Rimer, and F. M. Lewis (eds.), *Health Behavior and Health Education: Theory, Research, and Practice.* (3rd ed.) San Francisco: Jossey-Bass, 2002.

Rimer, B., and others. "Planning a Cancer Control Program for Older Citizens." *Gerontologist,* 1983, *23,* 384–389.

Rimer, B. K., Glanz, K., and Rasband, G. "Searching for Evidence About Health Education and Health Behavior Interventions." *Health Education and Behavior,* 2001, *28,* 231–248.

Rimer, B. K., and others. "Informed Decision Making: What is Its Role in Cancer Screening?" *Cancer,* 2004, *101*(5 Suppl), 1214–1228.

Rimer, B. K., and others. "How New Subscribers Use Cancer-Related Online Mailing Lists." *Journal of Medical Internet Research,* 2005, *7,* e32.

Rudd, J., and Glanz, K. "How Individuals Use Information for Health Action: Consumer Information Processing." In K. Glanz, F. M. Lewis, and B. K. Rimer (eds.), *Health Behavior and Health Education: Theory, Research, and Practice.* San Francisco: Jossey-Bass, 1990.

Schroeder, S. A. "We Can Do Better—Improving the Health of the American People." *New England Journal of Medicine,* 2007, *357,* 1221–1228.

Science Panel on Interactive Communication and Health. *Wired for Health and Well-Being: The Emergence of Interactive Health Communication.* Washington, D.C.: U.S. Department of Health and Human Services, U.S. Government Printing Office, April 1999.

Simonds, S. "Health Education in the Mid-1970s: State of the Art." In *Preventive Medicine USA.* New York: Prodist, 1976.

Skinner, C. S., and others. "How Effective is Tailored Print Communication?" *Annals of Behavioral Medicine,* 1999, *21,* 290–298.

Smedley, B. D., Stith, A. Y., and Nelson, A. R. (eds.). "Committee on Understanding and Eliminating Racial and Ethnic Disparities in Health Care." In *Unequal Treatment: Confronting Racial and Ethnic Disparities in Health Care.* Washington, D.C.: National Academy Press, 2003.

Smedley, B. D., and Syme, S. L. (eds.). *Promoting Health: Intervention Strategies from Social and Behavioral Research.* Washington, D.C.: National Academy Press, 2000.

Sorensen, G., and Barbeau, E. M. "Integrating Occupational Health, Safety and Worksite Health Promotion: Opportunities for Research and Practice." *La Medicina de Lavoro,* 2006, *97*(2), 240–257.

Sorensen, G., and others. "Working Well: Results From a Worksite-Based Cancer Prevention Trial." *American Journal of Public Health,* 1996, *86,* 939–947.

Stokols, D., Grzywacz, J. G., McMahan, S., and Phillips, K. "Increasing the Health Promotive Capacity of Human Environments." *American Journal of Health Promotion,* 2003, *18*(1), 4–13.

Story, M., Kaphingst, K., Robinson-O'Brien, R., and Glanz, K. "Creating Healthy Food and Eating Environments: Policy and Environmental Approaches." *Annual Review of Public Health,* 2008, *29,* 253–272.

Tilley, B., and others. "Nutrition Intervention for High-Risk Auto Workers: Results of the Next Step Trial." *Preventive Medicine,* 1999a, *28,* 284–292.

Tilley, B., and others. "The Next Step Trial: Impact of a Worksite Colorectal Cancer Screening Promotion Program." *Preventive Medicine,* 1999b, *28,* 276–283.

Turkkan, J. S., Kaufman, N. J., and Rimer, B. K. "Transdisciplinary Tobacco Use Research Centers: A Model Collaboration Between Public and Private Sectors." *Nicotine and Tobacco Research,* 2000, *2,* 9–13.

U.S. Department of Health, Education, and Welfare. *Healthy People: The Surgeon General's Report on Health Promotion and Disease Prevention.* Public Health Service Publication No. 79-55071. Washington, D.C.: U.S. Government Printing Office, 1979.

U.S. Department of Health and Human Services. *Promoting Health and Preventing Disease: Health Objectives for the Nation.* Washington, D.C.: U.S. Government Printing Office, 1980.

U.S. Department of Health and Human Services. *Healthy People 2000: National Health Promotion and Disease Prevention Objectives.* DHHS Publication No. PHS 91-50213. Washington, D.C.: U.S. Government Printing Office, 1991.

U.S. Department of Health and Human Services. *Healthy People 2010: Understanding and Improving Health.* Washington, D.C.: U.S. Department of Health and Human Services, Government Printing Office, 2000.

Viswanath, K. "The Communications Revolution and Cancer Control." *Nature Reviews: Cancer,* 2005, *5,* 828–835.

Viswanath, K. "Public Communications and its Role in Reducing and Eliminating Health Disparities." In G. E. Thomson, F. Mitchell, and M. B. Williams (eds.), *Examining the Health Disparities Research Plan of the National Institutes of Health: Unfinished Business.* Washington, D.C.: Institute of Medicine, 2006.

Von Elm, E., and others, for the STROBE Initiative. "The Strengthening of Reporting of Observational Studies in Epidemiology (STROBE) Statement: Guidelines for Reporting Observational Studies. *Annals of Internal Medicine,* 2007, *147,* 573–577.

Weinstein, N. D. "Misleading Tests of Health Behavior Theories." *Annals of Behavioral Medicine,* 2007, *33,* 1–10.

Winkleby, M. A. "The Future of Community-Based Cardiovascular Disease Intervention Studies." *American Journal of Public Health,* 1994, *84,* 1369–1372.

World Health Organization, Commission on Social Determinants of Health. *Interim Report.* [http://whqlibdoc.who.int/publications/2007/interim_statement_eng.pdf]. 2007.

Yach, D., Hawkes, C., Gould, C. L., and Hofman, K. J. "The Global Burden of Chronic Diseases: Overcoming Impediments to Prevention and Control." *Journal of the American Medical Association,* 2004, *291*(21), 2616–2622.

CHAPTER

2

THEORY, RESEARCH, AND PRACTICE IN HEALTH BEHAVIOR AND HEALTH EDUCATION

The Editors

KEY POINTS

This chapter will

- Discuss the interrelationships between theory, research, and practice.
- Define *theory* and the key characteristics and features of theories.
- Describe and provide examples of the building blocks of theory (concepts, constructs, variables) and related terms (models and principles).
- Provide a historical review of key paradigms for theory and research in health promotion and education.
- Summarize trends in the use of health behavior theories and models.
- Explain the selection of theories for inclusion in this book, as well as the related limitations.
- Introduce key considerations in fitting a theory or theories to research and practice.

THEORY, RESEARCH, AND PRACTICE: INTERRELATIONSHIPS

Aristotle distinguished between *theoria* and *praxis*. *Theoria* signifies those sciences and activities concerned with knowing for its own sake, whereas *praxis* corresponds to action or doing. This contrast between theory and practice (Bernstein, 1971) permeates Western philosophical and scientific thought from Aristotle to Marx and on to Dewey and other contemporary twentieth-century philosophers. Theory and practice long have been regarded as opposites with irreconcilable differences. Dewey attempted to resolve the dichotomy by focusing on similarities and continuities between theoretical and practical judgments and inquiries. He described "experimental knowing" essentially as an art that involves a conscious, directed manipulation of objects and situations. "The craftsman perfects his art, not by comparing his product to some 'ideal' model, but by the cumulative results of experience—experience which benefits from tried and tested procedures but always involves risk and novelty" (Bernstein, 1971). Dewey thus described empirical investigation—research—as the ground between theory and practice and the testing of theory in action.

Although the perception of theory and practice as a dichotomy has a long tradition in intellectual thought, we follow in Dewey's tradition and focus on the similarities and continuities rather than on the differences. Theory, research, and practice are a continuum along which the skilled professional should move with ease. Not only are they related, but they are each essential to health education and health behavior. Theory and research should not be solely the province of academics, just as practice is not solely the concern of practitioners. The best theory is informed by practice; the best practice should be grounded in theory. There is a tension between them that one must navigate continually, but they are not in opposition. Theory and practice enrich one another by their dynamic interaction. Researchers and practitioners may differ in their priorities, but the relationship between research and its application can and should move in both directions (D'Onofrio, 1992; Freudenberg and others, 1995). Professional fields like health education are ideal for "reflective practitioners," who can ensure that theories and practice build on each other (Schön, 1983).

The recognition that science and humanistic endeavors like public health are convergent is increasing. This view was articulated by the Dalai Lama (2005), who wrote, "Perhaps the most important point is to ensure that science never becomes divorced from the basic human feeling of empathy with our fellow beings."

The task of health behavior and health education is both to understand health behavior and to transform knowledge about behavior into effective strategies for health enhancement. Research in health education and health behavior ultimately will be judged by its contributions to improving the health of populations. Although basic behavioral research is important in developing theories, we must ultimately test our theories iteratively in real-world contexts (Rosenstock, 1990). When we do so, theory, research, and practice begin to converge. The authors of this book examine theories in light of their applicability. By including an explanation of theories and their application in each chapter, we are trying to break down the dichotomy between theory and practice.

Relationships among theory, research, and practice are not simple or linear. The larger picture of health improvement and disease reduction is better described as a cycle of interacting types of endeavors, including fundamental research (research into determinants, as well as development of methodologies), intervention research (research aimed toward change), surveillance research (tracking populationwide trends, including maintenance of change), and application and program delivery (Hiatt and Rimer, 1999; Sallis, Owen, and Fotheringham, 2000). At the heart of this cycle is knowledge synthesis. Continually updated critical appraisals of the available literature are central to identifying interventions that should be disseminated in order to reduce the burden of disease (Rimer, Glanz, and Rasband, 2001). There is increasing recognition that, as Larry Green has stated, "if we want more evidence-based practice, we need more practice-based evidence" (Green and Glasgow, 2006).

Health Behavior and Health Education aims to help educators—writ large—whatever their backgrounds or disciplines, understand some of the most important theoretical underpinnings of health education and health behavior and use theory to inform research and practice. The authors of *Health Behavior and Health Education* believe that "there is nothing so useful as a good theory" (Lewin, 1935). Each chapter demonstrates the practical value of theory; each summarizes what was learned through conceptually sound research and practice, and each draws the linkages among theory, research, and practice.

Professionals charged with responsibility for health education and health behavior are, by and large, interventionists. They are action-oriented. They use their knowledge to design and implement programs to improve health. This is true, whether they are working to encourage health-enhancing changes in individual or community behavior or conditions. It is equally true of most health education and health behavior research. Often, in the process of attempting to change behavior, environments, or policies, researchers must do precisely what practitioners do—develop and deliver interventions. At some level, both practitioners and researchers are accountable for results, whether these are measured in terms of participants' satisfaction with programs, or changes in their awareness, knowledge, attitudes, beliefs, or health behaviors, or in their improved decision making; institutional norms; community integration; or more distal results, including morbidity, mortality, and quality of life. Health educators may assess these results anecdotally, complete in-depth qualitative assessments, or conduct rigorous empirical evaluations.

The design of interventions that yield desirable changes can best be done with an understanding of theories of behavior change and an ability to use them skillfully in research and practice (Grol and others, 2007). Most health educators work in situations in which resources are limited. This makes it essential that they reach evidence-informed judgments about the choice of interventions, both in the interest of efficiency and to improve the odds of success. There may be no second chance to reach a critical target audience.

A synthesis of theory, research, and practice will advance what is known about health behavior. A health educator without a theory is like a mechanic or a technician, whereas the professional who understands theory and research comprehends the "why" and can design and craft well-tailored interventions. He or she does not blindly follow a cookbook recipe but constantly creates the recipe anew, depending on the circumstances, based, preferably, on evidence about the intended audience and previous interventions. In health education, the circumstances include the nature of the target audience, the setting, resources, goals, and constraints (Bartholomew, Parcel, Kok, and Gottlieb, 2006). Many good planning models are available to help professionals and communities decide which problems and variables to focus on and to help them understand key elements of the background situation (see Chapter Eighteen for examples).

An understanding of theory may guide users to measure more carefully and astutely in order to assess the impact of interventions (Grol and others, 2007). Learning from successive interventions and from published evidence strengthens the knowledge base of individual health professionals. Over time, such cumulative learning also contributes to the knowledge base of all.

The health professional in a health maintenance organization who understands the relevance of The Transtheoretical Model (TTM) or Social Cognitive Theory (SCT) may be able to design better interventions to help patients lose weight or stop smoking. The community health educator who understands principles of social marketing and media communication can make far better use of the mass media than one who does not. The nurse who recognizes that observational learning is important to how people learn, as postulated in SCT, may do a better job of teaching diabetics how to administer their injections. A working knowledge of community organization can help the educator identify and mobilize key individuals and groups to develop or maintain a health promotion program. The physician who understands interpersonal influence can communicate more effectively with patients. The health psychologist who understands TTM will know how to design better smoking cessation and exercise interventions and how to tailor them to the needs of his or her patients.

WHAT IS THEORY?

A theory is a set of interrelated concepts, definitions, and propositions that present a *systematic* view of events or situations by specifying relations among variables, in order to *explain* and *predict* the events or situations. The notion of *generality,* or broad application, is important, as is *testability* (van Ryn and Heaney, 1992). Theories are by their nature *abstract;* that is, they do not have a specified content or topic area. Like an empty coffee cup, they have a shape and boundaries but nothing concrete inside. They only come alive in public health and health behavior when they are filled with practical topics, goals, and problems.

A formal theory—more an ideal than a reality—is a completely closed, deductive system of propositions that identifies the interrelationships among the concepts and is a systematic view of the phenomena (Kerlinger, 1986; Blalock, 1969). In reality, there is no such system in the social sciences or health promotion and education; it can only be approximated (Blalock, 1969). Theory has been defined in a variety of ways, each consistent with Kerlinger's definition. Table 2.1 summarizes several definitions of theory. These definitions, put forth in the 1970s and 1980s, have stood the test of time. They have been articulated in more recent works without substantive changes (Isaac and Michael, 1995; Sussman, 2001).

Theories are useful during the various stages of planning, implementing, and evaluating interventions. Program planners can use theories to shape the pursuit of answers to *Why? What? How?* In other words, theories can be used to guide the search for *why* people are not following public health and medical advice or not caring for themselves in healthy ways. They can help pinpoint *what* one needs to know before developing and organizing an intervention program. They can provide insight into *how* to shape program strategies to reach people and organizations and make an impact on them. They also help to identify *what* should be monitored, measured, and compared in a program evaluation (Glanz, Lewis, and Rimer, 1996; Glanz, Rimer, and Lewis, 2002).

Thus, theories and models *explain* behavior and suggest ways to achieve behavior *change.* An explanatory theory (often called a *theory of the problem*) helps describe and identify why a problem exists. Such theories also predict behaviors under defined conditions and guide the search for modifiable factors like knowledge, attitudes, self-efficacy, social support, and lack of resources. Change theories, or *theories of action,* guide the development of interventions. They also form the basis for evaluation, pushing the evaluator to make explicit her or his assumptions about how a program should work. Implementation theories are change theories that link theory

TABLE 2.1. Definitions of Theory.

Definition	Source
A set of interrelated constructs (concepts), definitions, and propositions that present a systematic view of phenomena by specifying relations among variables, with the purpose of explaining and predicting phenomena	Kerlinger, 1986, p. 9
A systematic explanation for the observed facts and laws that relate to a particular aspect of life	Babbie, 1989, p. 46
Knowledge writ large in the form of generalized abstractions applicable to a wide range of experiences	McGuire, 1983, p. 2
A set of relatively abstract and general statements which collectively purport to explain some aspect of the empirical world	Chafetz, 1978, p. 2
An abstract, symbolic representation of what is conceived to be reality—a set of abstract statements designed to "fit" some portion of the real world	Zimbardo, Ebbesen, and Maslach, 1977, p. 53

specifically to a given problem, audience, and context (Institute of Medicine, 2002). These two types of theories often have different foci but are complementary.

Even though various theoretical models of health behavior may reflect the same general ideas, each theory employs a unique vocabulary to articulate the specific factors considered important. The *why* tells us about the processes by which changes occur in target variables. Theories vary in the extent to which they have been conceptually developed and empirically tested. Bandura (1986) stressed that "theories are interpreted in different ways depending on the stage of development of the field of study. In advanced disciplines, theories integrate laws; in less advanced fields, theories specify the determinants governing the phenomena of interest." The term *theory* is used in the latter sense in *Health Behavior and Health Education,* because the field is still relatively young.

As we discuss later in this chapter, many new "theories" or models have been and continue to be proposed in health behavior. The proliferation of theories in health behavior poses a challenge: When do we accept a theory as truly advancing our understanding of a phenomenon? Lakatos and Musgrave (1970), though referring to theories in physics, offer some rules of thumb. A new theory can be considered acceptable if it explains everything that the prior theories explain, provides explanation for phenomena that could *not* be explained by prior theories, and identifies conditions under which the theory could be falsified. Although this is a high standard for theories in social sciences, it provides a rough guidance on heuristic evaluation of theories in health behavior. Another expectation of an established theory is that there should be a body of research testing and supporting it—research that has been conducted by multiple scientists beyond the original developer or developers.

Concepts, Constructs, and Variables

Concepts are the major components of a theory; they are its building blocks or primary elements. Concepts can vary in the extent to which they have meaning or can be understood outside the context of a specific theory. When concepts are developed or adopted for use in a particular theory, they are called *constructs* (Kerlinger, 1986). The term *subjective normative belief* is an example of a construct within Ajzen and Fishbein's (1980) Theory of Reasoned Action (TRA; see Chapter Four); the specific construct has a precise definition in the context of that theory. Another example of a construct is *perceived susceptibility* in the Health Belief Model (HBM; see Chapter Three).

Variables are the empirical counterparts or operational forms of constructs. They specify how a construct is to be measured in a specific situation. *Variables* should be matched to *constructs* when identifying what should be assessed in the evaluation of a theory-driven program.

Principles

Theories go beyond principles. Principles are general guidelines for action. They are broad and nonspecific and may actually distort realities or results based on research.

Principles may be based on precedent or history *or* on research. At their worst, principles are so broad that they invite multiple interpretations and are therefore unreliable. In their weakest form, principles are like horoscopes: anyone can derive whatever meaning he or she wants from them. At their best, principles are based on accumulated research. In their best form, principles are the basis for hypotheses—"leading ideas," in the words of Dewey—and serve as our most informed hunches about how or what we should do to obtain a desired outcome in a target population.

Models

Health behavior and the guiding concepts for influencing it are far too complex to be explained by a single, unified theory. *Models* draw on a number of theories to help understand a specific problem in a particular setting or context. They are often informed by more than one theory, as well as by empirical findings (Earp and Ennett, 1991). Several models that support program planning processes are widely used in health promotion and education: Green and Kreuter's PRECEDE-PROCEED model (2005; see Chapter Eighteen), social marketing (see Chapter Nineteen), and ecological models (McLeroy, Bibeau, Steckler, and Glanz, 1988; see Chapter Twenty).

PARADIGMS FOR THEORY AND RESEARCH IN HEALTH PROMOTION AND EDUCATION

A paradigm is a basic schema that organizes our broadly based view of something (Babbie, 1989). Paradigms are widely recognized scientific achievements that, for a time, provide model problem-solving approaches to a community of practitioners and scientists. They include theory, application, and instrumentation and comprise models that represent coherent traditions of scientific research (Kuhn, 1962). Paradigms gain status because they are more successful than their competitors at solving pressing problems (Kuhn, 1962), but they also can impede scientific progress by protecting inconsistent findings until a crisis point is reached; these crisis points lead to scientific revolutions.

Paradigms create boundaries within which the search for answers occurs. They do not answer particular questions, but they do direct the search for answers (Babbie, 1989). Paradigms circumscribe or delimit what is important to examine in a given field of inquiry. The collective judgments of scientists define the dominant paradigm that constitutes the body of science (Wilson, 1952).

In health education and health behavior (and in this text), the dominant paradigm that supports the largest body of theory and research is that of *logical positivism,* or *logical empiricism.* This basic view, developed in the Vienna Circle from 1924 to 1936, has two central features: (1) an emphasis on the use of induction, or sensory experience, feelings, and personal judgments as the source of knowledge, and (2) the view that deduction is the standard for verification or confirmation of theory, so that theory must be tested through empirical methods and systematic observation of phenomena (Runes, 1984). Logical empiricism reconciles the deductive and inductive extremes;

it prescribes that the researcher begin with a hypothesis deduced from a theory and then test it, subjecting it to the jeopardy of disconfirmation through empirical test (McGuire, 1983).

An alternative worldview that is also important in health promotion and education relies more heavily on induction and is often identified as a predominantly constructivist paradigm. This perspective argues that the organization and explanation of events must be revealed through a process of discovery rather than organized into prescribed conceptual categories before a study begins (Lewis, 1996). In this paradigm, data collection methods such as standardized questionnaires and predetermined response categories have a limited place. Ethnography, phenomenology, and grounded theory are examples of approaches using a constructivist paradigm (Strauss, 1987; Kendler, 2005). It has become increasingly common in the field for work to originate within a constructivist paradigm and shift toward a focus on answering specific research questions using methodologies from the logical positivist paradigm. This approach has also gained traction in psychological research (Caciopo, Semin, and Berntson, 2004).

Lewin's meta-theory stipulates the rules to be followed for building good theory; it is consistent with logical positivism but focuses on his view that the function of social psychology is to further the understanding of the interrelationships between the individual and the social environment (Gold, 1992). This meta-theory is an orientation or approach, distinct from Lewin's specific field theory (Gold, 1992), and has been influential in health behavior theory since the earliest attempts to use social science to solve public health problems (Rosenstock, 1990). Key rules of Lewin's meta-theory include (1) analysis that starts with the situation as a whole, (2) contemporaneity, (3) a dynamic approach, (4) constructive method, (5) mathematical representation of constructs and variables, and (6) a psychological approach that explains both inner experiences and overt actions from the actor's perspective (Lewin, [1942] 1951). The last of these rules implies a single level of analysis requiring "closed theory" and poses a serious limitation to solving the problems of contemporary health promotion. It raises the issue—one that those concerned with health behavior often grapple with—that we must often trade off theoretical elegance in favor of relevance (Gold, 1992).

Although the paradigms described here focus on the basic schema for development and application of knowledge, health education and health behavior are also concerned with approaches to solving social problems—in other words, how to bring about change. Considerable scholarly and practitioner effort have been devoted to developing techniques that change behavior. Although these grew out of a desire to produce a better world, techniques that "push" people to change were experienced by many as manipulative, reducing freedom of choice and sustaining a balance of power in favor of the "change agent" (Kipnis, 1994). A paradigm shift occurred, and most behavioral techniques today (for example, social support, empowerment, and personal growth) are based on *reducing obstacles to change* and promoting informed decision making, rather than on pushing people to change.

New paradigms for understanding, studying, and applying knowledge about human behavior continue to arise and may be influential in the future of applied social sciences in health behavior and education. The Institute of Medicine's Committee on Capitalizing on Social Science and Behavioral Research to Improve the Public's Health recommended strongly that "interventions on social and behavioral factors should link multiple levels of influence" rather than focusing on a single or limited number of health determinants (Smedley and Syme, 2000). Today, this recommendation is echoed as health educators and social scientists struggle with some of the most challenging health behavior issues, such as tobacco control and obesity prevention, at a time when ecological models begin to be more clearly articulated and studied (see Chapter Twenty).

TRENDS IN USE OF HEALTH BEHAVIOR THEORIES AND MODELS

Theories that gain recognition in a discipline shape the field, help define the scope of practice, and influence the training and socialization of its professionals. Today, no single theory or conceptual framework dominates research or practice in health promotion and education. Instead, one can choose from a multitude of theories. For each edition of this book, we reviewed a sample of publications to identify the most often used theories (see Table 2.2). In a review of 116 theory-based articles published between 1986 and 1988 in two major health education journals, conducted during planning for the first edition of this book, we found fifty-one distinct theoretical formulations. At that time, the three most frequently mentioned theories were social learning theory, the TRA, and the HBM (Glanz, Lewis, and Rimer, 1990).

To plan for the second edition of this book, we reviewed 526 articles from twenty-four different journals in health education, medicine, and behavioral sciences, published from mid-1992 to mid-1994. Sixty-six different theories and models were identified, and twenty-one of these were mentioned eight times or more. Two-thirds of the total instances of theory use in the 497 articles involving one or more of the twenty-one most common theories and models were accounted for by the first eight: HBM, SCT, self-efficacy (Bandura, 1997), the TRA/TPB, community organization, TTM/Stages of Change, social marketing, and social support/social networks (Glanz, Lewis, and Rimer, 1996).

In our review of all issues of twelve journals in health education, health behavior, and preventive medicine published in 1999 and 2000, conducted for the third edition of this book (Glanz, Rimer, and Lewis, 2002), ten theories or models clearly emerged as the most often used. The first two, and by far the most dominant, were SCT and TTM/Stages of Change. The remainder of the top ten theories and models were the HBM, social support and social networks, patient-provider communication, the TRA and TPB, stress and coping, community organization, ecological models/social ecology, and diffusion of innovations.

In a recent, updated review of theory use in published research between 2000 and 2005, we found that the most often used theories were TTM, SCT, and the HBM (Painter and others, forthcoming). Overall, the same theories dominate as did in 1999 and 2000. As in previous reviews, this review revealed dozens of theories and models that were used, though only a few of them were used in multiple publications and by several authors. Several key constructs cut across the most often cited models for understanding behavior and behavior change: the importance of the individual's view of the world; multiple levels of influence; behavior change as a process; motivation versus intention; intention versus action; and changing behavior versus maintaining behavior change (Glanz and Oldenburg, 2001).

TABLE 2.2. **Trends in the Most Commonly Used Health Behavior Theories and Models.**

Theory/Model (# of theories identified)	1986–1988 (51)	1992–1994 (66)	1999–2000 (na)	2000–2005 (55)
Health Belief Model	✓	✓	✓	✓
Social Learning Theory				
Social Cognitive Theory	✓	✓	✓	✓
Theory of Reasoned Action				
Theory of Planned Behavior	✓	✓	✓	✓
The Transtheoretical Model/ Stages of Change		✓	✓	✓
Social Support and Social Networks		✓	✓	✓
Community Organization		✓	✓	
Social Marketing		✓		✓
Diffusion of Innovations		✓	✓	✓
Stress and Coping		✓	✓	✓
Patient-Provider Interaction		✓	✓	
Ecological Models/Social Ecology			✓	✓

Note: Definition as "theory/model" by authors of published articles; some reflect areas of study informed by multiple theories. See chapter for additional information.

Source: Based on reviews conducted for, and described in, first through fourth editions of this book (Glanz and others, 1990; Glanz and others, 1996; Glanz and others, 2002; and the current edition). Samples varied, but methods to identify "theory use" were comparable.

Along with the published observations about *which* theories are being used, concerns have been raised about *how* the theories are used (or not used) in research and practice. A common refrain is that researchers may not understand how to measure and analyze constructs of health behavior theories (Rejeski, Brawley, McAuley, and Rapp, 2000; Marsh, Johnson, and Carey, 2001) or that they may pick and choose variables from different theories in a way that makes it difficult to ascertain the role of theory in intervention development and evaluation. Considerable conceptual confusion among both researchers and practitioners about interrelationships between related theories and variables has also been observed (Rosenstock, Strecher, and Becker, 1988; Weinstein, 1993). Others have cautioned about the limitations of theory testing because of overreliance on correlational designs (Weinstein, 2007) and the paucity of studies that empirically compare more than one theory (Noar and Zimmerman, 2005; Weinstein and Rothman, 2005). The difficulty of reliably translating theory into interventions to improve clinical effectiveness has led to calls for more "pragmatic trials" (Bhattacharyya, Reeves, Garfinkel, and Zwarenstein, 2006), and increasing attention to the generalizability and translation of interventions into real-world clinical practice (Rothwell, 2005) and community settings (Rohrbach, Grana, Sussman, and Valente, 2006). These are reasonable questions that should encourage us to question how we use theory, how we test theory, how we turn theories into interventions, and what conclusions we draw from research.

Building on our distinctions among the type and degree of theory use (Glanz, 2002), our updated review of theory use from 2000 to 2005 classified articles that employed health behavior theory along a continuum:

- *Informed by theory*: in which a theoretical framework was identified, but no or limited application of the theory was used in specific study components and measures
- *Applied theory*: in which a theoretical framework was specified, and several of the constructs were applied in components of the study
- *Tested theory*: in which a theoretical framework was specified, and more than half the theoretical constructs were measured and explicitly tested, or two or more theories were compared to one another in a study
- *Building/creating theory*: in which new or revised/expanded theory was developed using constructs specified, measured, and analyzed in a study

Of all the theories used in the sample of articles (n = 69 articles using 139 theories), 69.1 percent used theory to inform a study; 17.9 percent of theories were "applied;" 3.6 percent were tested; and 9.4 percent involved building/creating theory (Painter and others, forthcoming). These findings lead us to reaffirm calls by Noar and Zimmerman (2005) and Weinstein and Rothman (2005) for thorough application and testing of health behavior theories to advance science and move the field forward.

SELECTION OF THEORIES FOR THIS BOOK

Our selection of theories and models for inclusion in the fourth edition of *Health Behavior and Health Education* was based on the published information summarized here, including an updated analysis of a sample of articles in the health behavior literature. An additional source of data regarding frequently used theories of health behavior is an evidence review on dietary behavior change interventions for cancer prevention (Ammerman and others, 2001). In what appears to be an emerging trend, the evidence tables reported on theories and models used in the 104 intervention studies included in the review. Although nearly two dozen theories were listed, only three were used in more than three studies: SCT, TTM/Stages of Change, and the HBM (Ammerman and others, 2001).

Each one of the most often cited theories and models is the focus of a chapter in this fourth edition of *Health Behavior and Health Education*. These have been selected to provide readers with a range of theories representing different units of intervention (for example, individuals, groups, and communities). They were also chosen because they represent, as with SCT, TTM, and the HBM—dominant theories of health behavior and health education. Others, like social marketing, the PRECEDE/ PROCEED Model, and community organization, were chosen for their practical value in applying theoretical formulations in a way that has demonstrated usefulness to professionals concerned with health behavior change. The perspectives chapters at the end of each section point to new directions in theory and highlight emerging theories, where appropriate.

Our selection of theories resulted from our review and also reflects some difficult editorial decisions. Three criteria, consistent with and confirming our review, also helped to define selection of material. First, we determined that, to be included, a theory must meet basic standards of adequacy for research and practice, thus having the potential for effective use by health education practitioners. Second, there must be evidence that the theory is being used in *current* health behavior and health education research. (That is why, for example, we include the HBM rather than Lewin's field theory.) The third criterion is that, there must be at least promising, if not substantial, empirical evidence supporting the theory's validity in predicting or changing health behaviors. This does not preclude the possibility of mixed findings and critiques of the evidence, which we believe are increasingly important to bring to light.

In some cases, a purpose rather than the theory is the identifying title for a chapter, as in the case of Chapter Eleven on Interpersonal Communication, which describes theories of interpersonal communication and social influence and illustrates their utility for health education. Chapter Thirteen on Community Organization is named for the resultant intervention strategies rather than for the convergent theoretical bases that form the foundation for community organization work. Chapters in Part Five present the PRECEDE-PROCEED Model for program planning, social marketing, and ecological models, each of which draws on multiple theories to understand health behavior and assist in development of effective intervention programs and strategies.

We recognize the lack of consensus regarding the definition and classification of theories, so we have taken a liberal, ecumenical stance toward theory. We concede that the lowest common denominator of the theoretical models herein might be that they are all *conceptual or theoretical frameworks,* or broadly conceived perspectives used to organize ideas. Nevertheless, we have not abandoned the term *theory,* because it accurately describes the spirit of this book and describes the goal to be attained for developing frameworks and tools for refining health education research and practice.

FITTING A THEORY OR THEORIES TO RESEARCH AND PRACTICE

Effective health education depends on marshaling the most appropriate theory and practice strategies for a given situation. Different theories are best suited to different units of practice, such as individuals, groups, and organizations. For example, when one is attempting to overcome women's personal barriers to obtaining mammograms, the HBM may be useful. TTM may be especially useful in developing smoking cessation interventions. The PAPM may be appropriate when trying to explain how people respond to risk communications. When trying to change physicians' mammography practices by instituting reminder systems, organizational change theories are more suitable. At the same time, physicians might use TTM to inform their discussions with individual patients about getting a first mammogram or annual screening. The choice of a suitable theory should begin with identifying the problem, goal, and units of practice (van Ryn and Heaney, 1992; Sussman and Sussman, 2001), *not* with selecting a theoretical framework because it is intriguing, familiar, or in vogue. As Green and Kreuter (2005) have argued, one should start with a logic model of the problem and work backwards to identify potential solutions.

The adequacy of a theory most often is assessed in terms of three criteria: (1) its *logic,* or *internal consistency* in not yielding mutually contradictory derivations, (2) the extent to which it is *parsimonious,* or broadly relevant while using a manageable number of concepts, and (3) its *plausibility* in fitting with prevailing theories in the field (McGuire, 1983).

Theories also are judged in the context of activities of practitioners and researchers. Practitioners may apply the pragmatic criterion of *usefulness* to a theory and thus would be concerned with its consistency with everyday observations (Burdine and McLeroy, 1992). Researchers make scientific judgments of a theory's *ecological validity,* or the extent to which it conforms to observable reality when empirically tested (McGuire, 1983). We should test our theories iteratively in the field (Rosenstock, 1990), as well as in more controlled settings. When we do so, theory, research, and practice begin to converge.

Practitioners of health education at once benefit from and are challenged by the multitude of theoretical frameworks and models from the social sciences available for their use, because the best choices and direct translations may not be immediately evident. The inherent danger in a book like this is that one can begin to think that the links between theory, research, and health promotion practice are easily forged. They are not. For the unprepared, the choices can be overwhelming, but for those who understand the commonalities and differences among theories of health behavior and health education, the growing knowledge base can provide a firm foundation on which to build. We find that one of the most frequent questions students around the world ask is, *"What theory should I use?"* It is an important question, the answer to which, we believe, will be found not just in the readings contained in this book but also in the experience and judgment that equip readers to apply what is learned here: *theory into practice and research.* We hope that *Health Behavior and Health Education* will provide and strengthen that foundation for readers.

Science is by definition cumulative, with periods of paradigm shifts that come more rarely as a result of crises when current theories fail to explain some phenomena (Kuhn, 1962). The same applies to the science base that supports long-standing, as well as innovative, health behavior interventions. More research is needed at all points along the research continuum. We need more basic research to develop and test theories, more intervention research to develop and test evidence-based interventions, and more concerted, focused attention to dissemination of evidence-based interventions (Rimer, Glanz, and Rasband, 2001; Weinstein, 2007; Rohrbach, Grana, Sussman, and Valente, 2006; Institute of Medicine, 2002). Moreover, both the research and practice communities in health education and health behavior are sorely in need of more rigor and precision in theory development and testing—in measurements, assessment of mediating variables, and specification of theoretical elements (Rejeski, Brawley, McAuley, and Rapp, 2000). We encourage more care and attention to how theories are tested, especially to the way variables are measured and analyzed. Building a solid, cumulative base of theory development is very difficult when one researcher's findings cannot be compared to another's.

The gift of theory is that it provides the conceptual underpinnings to well-crafted research and informed practice. "The scientist values research by the size of its contribution to that huge, logically articulated structure of ideas which is already, though not half built, the most glorious accomplishment of mankind" (Medawar, 1967).

In this book, we aim to demystify theory and to communicate theory and theoretically inspired research alongside their implications for practice. We encourage informed criticism of theories. Only through rigorous scrutiny will our theories improve. The ultimate test of these ideas and this information rests on its use over time. Like any long-term behavior, this will require social support, supportive environments, and periodic reinforcement. The beneficiaries will be practitioners, researchers, and the participants in health education programs.

As this chapter and the preceding one demonstrate, health education and health behavior are concerns of ever-increasing importance to the well-being of humankind worldwide. As scholars, researchers, and practitioners, all of us grapple with the complexities of human beings and society. We press forward within the limits of current methodologies while striving to build a cumulative body of knowledge in a fast-changing world. Our efforts are not always successful, but this should motivate, not deter, us in pursuing high-quality work. Continual dialogue between theory, research, and practice involves compromise, creativity, healthy criticism, appreciation of others' skills, and a willingness to cooperate to learn and to set high standards. "We must learn to honor excellence in every socially accepted human activity, however humble the activity, and to scorn shoddiness, however exalted the activity. An excellent plumber is infinitely more admirable than an incompetent philosopher. The society that scorns excellence in plumbing because plumbing is a humble activity and tolerates shoddiness in philosophy because it is an exalted activity will have neither good plumbing nor good philosophy. Neither its pipes nor its theories will hold water" (Gardner, 1984).

LIMITATIONS OF THIS BOOK

No text can be all-inclusive. This is certainly true of *Health Behavior and Health Education*. Some theories and frameworks presented in previous editions of this book do not appear in this edition: Consumer Information Processing (Rudd and Glanz, 1990), Multiattribute Utility Theory (Carter, 1990), Attribution Theory (Lewis and Daltroy, 1990), and Media Advocacy (Wallack, 1990). These theories and frameworks remain important, but we found them to be less widely used than those included in this edition. We did not update the chapters in the third edition on communication technology and health behavior change (Owen, Fotheringham, and Marcus, 2002) and applying theory to culturally diverse and unique populations (Resnicow, Braithwaite, DiIorio, and Glanz, 2002). Rather, these issues are woven throughout various chapters in this edition. Interested readers should refer to the first and third editions of this book for coverage of these frameworks.

Other important theories and conceptual frameworks could not be included because of space limitations. These include Self-Regulation Theory (Leventhal, Zimmerman, and Gutmann, 1984), Protection Motivation Theory (Rogers, 1975), and more familiar classical theories such as field theory (Lewin, 1935) and cognitive consistency (Festinger, 1957). Some of these are described as part of the historical origins of the various theories discussed in this book. Others are discussed in the synthesis and perspectives chapters.

This book is not intended to be a how-to guide or manual for program planning and development in health education and health behavior. Other books in health education, nursing, medicine, psychology, and nutrition serve that purpose, and readers should seek out key sources in each discipline for more on the nuts and bolts of practice. This volume will be most useful when it is included as part of a problem-oriented learning program, whether in a formal professional education setting or through continuing education venues. For examples of intervention strategies that use theories, the readers may want to look at such Web sites as The Guide to Community Preventive Services (http://www.thecommunityguide.org). For specific programs and tools, the Cancer Control P.L.A.N.E.T. (http://cancercontrolplanet.cancer.gov) and Research-Tested Intervention Programs (http://rtips.cancer.gov/rtips/index.do) provide examples relevant to cancer prevention and control. The National Registry of Evidence-Based Programs and Practices (http://nrepp.samhsa.gov) is a searchable online registry of mental health and substance abuse interventions that have been scientifically tested and can be readily disseminated.

Neither is this volume intended to serve as an in-depth treatise on research methods in health behavior and health education. Instead, it demonstrates by example how theories are operationalized in a modest number of examples. The reader who wishes more guidance on applied research for studies of health behavior and education will find ample resources in books on social science research methodology and measurement in health behavior and education.

The editors intend that readers emerge with a critical appreciation of theory and with the curiosity to pursue not only the theories presented in this book but other promising theories as well. Thus, *Health Behavior and Health Education* should be regarded as a starting point, not an end.

SUMMARY

Theories—or conceptual frameworks—can be and *are* useful, because they enrich, inform, and complement the practical technologies of health promotion and education. Thus the readers of this book should "pass with relief from the tossing sea of Cause and Theory to the firm ground of Result and Fact" (Churchill, 1898). As the ocean meets the shore, so we hope you will find that theory, research, and practice in health promotion and education stretch out to converge in a single landscape.

REFERENCES

Ajzen, I., and Fishbein, M. *Understanding Attitudes and Predicting Social Behavior.* Englewood Cliffs, N.J.: Prentice Hall, 1980.

Ammerman, A., and others. "Efficacy of Interventions to Modify Dietary Behavior Related to Cancer Risk." Evidence Report/Technology Assessment No. 25 (Contract No. 290-97-0011 to the Research Triangle Institute-University of North Carolina at Chapel Hill Evidence-Based Practice Center). AHRQ Publication No. 01-E029. Rockville, Md.: Agency for Healthcare Research and Quality, February 2001.

Babbie, E. *The Practice of Social Research.* (5th ed.) Belmont, Calif.: Wadsworth, 1989.

Bandura, A. *Social Foundations of Thought and Action: A Social Cognitive Theory.* Englewood Cliffs, N.J.: Prentice Hall, 1986.

Bandura, A. *Self-Efficacy: The Exercise of Control.* New York: W. H. Freeman, 1997.

Bartholomew, L. K., Parcel, G. S., Kok, G., and Gottlieb, N. H. *Planning Health Promotion Programs: An Intervention Mapping Approach.* San Francisco: Jossey-Bass, 2006.

Bhattacharyya, O., Reeves, S., Garfinkel, S., and Zwarenstein, M. "Designing Theoretically Informed Implementation Interventions: Fine in Theory, but Evidence of Effectiveness in Practice is Needed." *Implementation Science,* 2006, *1,* 5.

Bernstein, R. *Praxis and Action.* Philadelphia: University of Pennsylvania Press, 1971.

Blalock, H. M., Jr. *Theory Construction, From Verbal to Mathematical Constructions.* Englewood Cliffs, N.J.: Prentice Hall, 1969.

Burdine, J. N., and McLeroy, K. R. "Practitioners' Use of Theory: Examples from a Workgroup." *Health Education Quarterly,* 1992, *19*(3), 315–330.

Cacioppo, J. T., Semin, G. R., and Berntson, G. G. "Realism, Instrumentalism, and Scientific Symbiosis: Psychological Theory as a Search for Truth and the Discovery of Solutions." *American Psychologist,* 2004, *59,* 214–223.

Carter, W. "Health Behavior as a Rational Process: Theory of Reasoned Action and Multiattribute Utility Theory." In K. Glanz, F. M. Lewis, and B. K. Rimer (eds.), *Health Behavior and Health Education: Theory, Research, and Practice.* San Francisco: Jossey-Bass, 1990.

Chafetz, J. *A Primer on the Construction of Theories in Sociology.* Itasca, Ill.: Peacock, 1978.

Churchill, W. *The Malakand Field Force.* London: Longmans, Green, 1898.

Dalai Lama, H. H. *The Universe in a Single Atom: The Convergence of Science and Spirituality.* New York: Morgan Road Books, 2005.

D'Onofrio, C. N. "Theory and the Empowerment of Health Education Practitioners." *Health Education Quarterly,* 1992, *19*(3), 385–403.

Earp, J. A., and Ennett, S. T. "Conceptual Models for Health Education Research and Practice." *Health Education Research,* 1991, *6*(2), 163–171.

Festinger, L. *A Theory of Cognitive Dissonance.* Stanford, Calif.: Stanford University Press, 1957.

Freudenberg, N., and others. "Strengthening Individual and Community Capacity to Prevent Disease and Promote Health: In Search of Relevant Theories and Principles." *Health Education Quarterly,* 1995, *22*(3), 290–306.

Gardner, J. W. *Excellence: Can We Be Equal and Excellent Too?* (rev. ed.) New York: W. W. Norton, 1984.

Glanz, K. "Perspectives on Using Theory." In K. Glanz, F. M. Lewis, and B. K. Rimer (eds.), *Health Behavior and Health Education: Theory, Research, and Practice.* (3rd ed.) San Francisco: Jossey-Bass, 2002.

Glanz, K., Lewis, F. M., and Rimer, B. K. (eds.). *Health Behavior and Health Education: Theory, Research, and Practice.* San Francisco: Jossey-Bass, 1990.

Glanz, K., Lewis, F. M., and Rimer, B. K. (eds.). *Health Behavior and Health Education: Theory, Research, and Practice.* (2nd ed.) San Francisco: Jossey-Bass, 1996.

Glanz, K., and Oldenburg, B. "Utilizing Theories and Constructs Across Models of Behavior Change." In R. Patterson (ed.), *Changing Patient Behavior: Improving Outcomes in Health and Disease Management.* San Francisco: Jossey-Bass, 2001.

Glanz, K., Rimer, B. K., and Lewis, F. M. (eds.). *Health Behavior and Health Education: Theory, Research, and Practice.* (3rd ed.) San Francisco: Jossey-Bass, 2002.

Gold, M. "Metatheory and Field Theory in Social Psychology: Relevance or Elegance?" *Journal of Social Issues,* 1992, *48*(2), 67–78.

Green, L. W., and Glasgow, R. E. "Evaluating the Relevance, Generalization, and Applicability of Research: Issues in External Validation and Translation Methodology." *Evaluation and the Health Professions,* 2006, *29,* 126–153.

Green, L. W., and Kreuter, M. W. *Health Promotion Planning: An Educational and Ecological Approach.* (4th ed.) New York: McGraw-Hill, 2005.

Grol, R., and others. "Planning and Studying Improvement in Patient Care: The Use of Theoretical Perspectives." *The Milbank Quarterly,* 2007, *85*(1), 93–138.

Hiatt, R. A., and Rimer, B. K. "A New Strategy for Cancer Control Research." *Cancer, Epidemiology, Biomarkers and Prevention,* 1999, *8,* 957–964.

Institute of Medicine, Committee on Communication for Behavior Change in the 21st Century: Improving the Health of Diverse Populations. *Speaking of Health: Assessing Health Communication Strategies for Diverse Populations.* Washington, D.C.: National Academies Press, 2002.

Isaac, S., and Michael, W. B. *Handbook of Research and Evaluation.* (3rd ed.) San Diego: Educational and Industrial Testing Services, 1995.

Kendler, H. H. "Psychology and Phenomenology: A Clarification." *American Psychologist,* 2005, *60,* 318–324.

Kerlinger, F. N. *Foundations of Behavioral Research.* (3rd ed.) New York: Holt, Rinehart & Winston, 1986.

Kipnis, D. "Accounting for the Use of Behavior Technologies in Social Psychology." *American Psychologist,* 1994, *49*(3), 165–172.

Kuhn, T. S. *The Structure of Scientific Revolutions.* Chicago: University of Chicago Press, 1962.

Lakatos, I., and Musgrave, A. (eds.). *Criticism and the Growth of Knowledge.* Cambridge: Cambridge University Press, 1970.

Leventhal, H., Zimmerman, R., and Gutmann, M. "Compliance: A Self-Regulation Perspective." In D. Gentry (ed.), *Handbook of Behavioral Medicine.* New York: Guilford Press, 1984.

Lewin, K. *A Dynamic Theory of Personality.* New York: McGraw-Hill, 1935.

Lewin, K. "Field Theory and Learning." In D. Cartwright (ed.), *Field Theory in Social Science.* New York: Harper, 1951. (Originally published 1942.)

Lewis, F. "Whom and From What Paradigm Should Health Promotion Serve?" *Health Education Quarterly,* 1996, *23,* 448–452.

Lewis, F. M., and Daltroy, L. "How Causal Explanations Influence Health Behavior: Attribution Theory." In K. Glanz, F. M. Lewis, and B. K. Rimer (eds.), *Health Behavior and Health Education: Theory, Research, and Practice.* San Francisco: Jossey-Bass, 1990.

Marsh, K. L., Johnson, B. T., and Carey, M. P. "Conducting Meta-Analyses of HIV Prevention Literatures from a Theory-Testing Perspective." *Evaluation and the Health Professions,* 2001, *24,* 255–276.

McGuire, W. J. "A Contextualist Theory of Knowledge: Its Implications for Innovation and Reform in Psychological Research." *Advances in Experimental Social Psychology,* 1983, *16,* 1–47.

McLeroy, K. R., Bibeau, D., Steckler, A., and Glanz, K. "An Ecological Perspective on Health Promotion Programs." *Health Education Quarterly,* 1988, *15,* 351–377.

Medawar, P. B. *The Art of the Soluble.* New York: Methuen, 1967.

Noar, S. M., and Zimmerman, R. S. "Health Behavior Theory and Cumulative Knowledge Regarding Health Behaviors: Are We Moving in the Right Direction?" *Health Education Research,* 2005, *20,* 275–290.

Owen, N., Fotheringham, M. J., and Marcus, B. H. "Communication Technology and Health Behavior Change." In K. Glanz, B. K. Rimer, and F. M. Lewis (eds.), *Health Behavior and Health Education: Theory, Research, and Practice.* (3rd ed.) San Francisco: Jossey-Bass, 2002.

Painter, J. E., and others. "The Use of Theory in Health Behavior Research from 2000 to 2005: A Systematic Review." *Annals of Behavioral Medicine,* forthcoming.

Rejeski, W. J., Brawley, L. R., McAuley, E., and Rapp, S. "An Examination of Theory and Behavior Change in Randomized Clinical Trials." *Controlled Clinical Trials,* 2000, *21*(5 Suppl), 164S-170S.

Resnicow, K., Braithwaite, R. L., DiIorio, C., and Glanz, K. "Applying Theory to Culturally Diverse and Unique Populations." In K. Glanz, B. K. Rimer, and F. M. Lewis (eds.), *Health Behavior and Health Education: Theory, Research, and Practice.* (3rd ed.) San Francisco: Jossey-Bass, 2002.

Rimer, B. K., Glanz, K., and Rasband, G. "Searching for Evidence About Health Education and Health Behavior Interventions." *Health Education and Behavior,* 2001, *28,* 231–248.

Rogers, R. "A Protection Motivation Theory of Fear Appeals and Attitude Change." *Journal of Psychology,* 1975, *91,* 93–114.

Rohrbach, L. A., Grana, R., Sussman, S., and Valente, T. W. "Type II Translation: Transporting Prevention Interventions from Research to Real-World Settings." *Evaluation and the Health Professions,* 2006, *29,* 302–333.

Rosenstock, I. M. "The Past, Present, and Future of Health Education." In K. Glanz, F. M. Lewis, and B. K. Rimer (eds.), *Health Behavior and Health Education: Theory, Research, and Practice.* San Francisco: Jossey-Bass, 1990.

Rosenstock, I. M., Strecher, V. J., and Becker, M. H. "Social Learning Theory and the Health Belief Model." *Health Education Quarterly,* 1988, *15*(2), 175–183.

Rothwell, P. M. "External Validity of Randomized Controlled Trials: 'To Whom Do The Results of This Trial Apply?'" *Lancet,* 2005, *365,* 82–93.

Rudd, J., and Glanz, K. "How Individuals Use Information for Health Action: Consumer Information Processing." In K. Glanz, F. M. Lewis, and B. K. Rimer (eds.), *Health Behavior and Health Education: Theory, Research, and Practice.* San Francisco: Jossey-Bass, 1990.

Runes, D. *Dictionary of Philosophy.* Totawa, N.J.: Rowman and Allanheld, 1984.

Sallis, J. F., Owen, N., and Fotheringham, M. J. "Behavioral Epidemiology: A Systematic Framework to Classify Phases of Research on Health Promotion and Disease Prevention." *Annals of Behavioral Medicine,* 2000, *22,* 294–298.

Schön, D. *The Reflective Practitioner: How Professionals Think in Action.* London: Temple Smith, 1983.

Smedley, B. D., and Syme, S. L (eds.). *Promoting Health: Intervention Strategies from Social and Behavioral Research.* Washington, D.C.: National Academy Press, 2000.

Strauss, A. L. *Qualitative Analysis for Social Scientists.* Cambridge, England: Cambridge University Press, 1987.

Sussman, S. (ed.). *Handbook of Program Development for Health Behavior Research and Practice.* Thousand Oaks, Calif.: Sage, 2001.

Sussman, S., and Sussman, A. N. "Praxis in Health Behavior Program Development." In S. Sussman (ed.), *Handbook of Program Development for Health Behavior Research and Practice.* Thousand Oaks, Calif.: Sage, 2001.

van Ryn, M., and Heaney, C. A. "What's the Use of Theory?" *Health Education Quarterly,* 1992, *19*(3), 315–330.

Wallack, L. "Media Advocacy: Promoting Health Through Mass Communication." In K. Glanz, F. M. Lewis, and B. K. Rimer (eds.), *Health Behavior and Health Education: Theory, Research, and Practice.* San Francisco: Jossey-Bass, 1990.

Weinstein, N. D. "Testing Four Competing Theories of Health-Protective Behavior." *Health Psychology,* 1993, *12*(4), 324–333.

Weinstein, N. D. "Misleading Tests of Health Behavior Theories." *Annals of Behavioral Medicine,* 2007, *33,* 1–10.

Weinstein, N. D., and Rothman, A. J. "Commentary: Revitalizing Research on Health Behavior Theories." *Health Education Research,* 2005, *20,* 294–297.

Wilson, E. B. *An Introduction to Scientific Research.* New York: McGraw-Hill, 1952.

Zimbardo, P. G., Ebbesen, E. B., and Maslach, C. *Influencing Attitudes and Changing Behavior.* (2nd ed.) Reading, Mass.: Addison-Wesley, 1977.

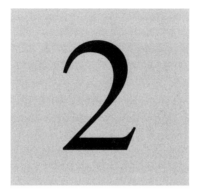

2

MODELS OF INDIVIDUAL HEALTH BEHAVIOR

Barbara K. Rimer

Individuals are essential units of health education and health behavior theory, research, and practice. This does not mean that the individual is the only or necessarily the most important unit of intervention. But all other units, whether they are groups, organizations, worksites, communities, or larger units, are composed of individuals.

A wide range of health professionals, including health educators, physicians, psychologists, dietitians, and nurses, focus all or most of their efforts on changing the health behavior of individuals. To intervene effectively and to make informed judgments about how to measure the success of such interventions, health professionals should understand the role of individuals in health behavior. This section of *Health*

Behavior and Health Education helps the reader achieve greater understanding of theories that focus primarily on individual health behavior. Ultimately, researchers and practitioners may combine some of these theories with theories that focus on other levels of intervention. Indeed, as discussed throughout this book, combinations of theories are becoming the norm in health behavior change interventions.

Lewin's seminal field theory (1935) was one of the early and most far-reaching theories of behavior, and most contemporary theories of health behavior owe a major intellectual debt to Lewin. Theories that focus on barriers and facilitators to behavior change and those that posit the existence of stages are rooted in the Lewinian tradition. During the 1940s and 1950s, researchers began to learn how individuals make decisions about health and what determines health behavior. In the 1950s, Rosenstock, Hochbaum, and others, from their vantage point at the U.S. Public Health Service, began their pioneering work to understand why individuals did or did not participate in screening programs for tuberculosis. This and related work led to the Health Belief Model (HBM). In the last twenty years, considerable progress has been made in understanding determinants of individuals' health-related behaviors and ways to stimulate positive behavior changes. Value expectancy theories, which include both the HBM and the Theory of Reasoned Action (TRA) and its companion, the Theory of Planned Behavior (TPB), matured during this time.

The Transtheoretical Model (TTM), also known as the Stages of Change (SOC) Model, which grew initially from the work of Prochaska, DiClemente, and colleagues, was developed in the late 1970s and 1980s and matured in the 1990s. Weinstein's Precaution Adoption Process Model (PAPM) is the final chapter in the section.

In Chapter Three, Champion and Skinner review the evolution of the HBM and the constructs that are part of its current formulation. The authors explain that the HBM is used to understand why people accept preventive health services and why they do or do not adhere to other kinds of health care regimens. The HBM has spawned thousands of health education and health behavior research studies and provided the conceptual basis for many interventions in the years since it was formulated. It has been used across the health continuum, including disease prevention, early disease detection, and illness and sick-role behavior (Becker and Maiman, 1975; Janz and Becker, 1984). It is among the most widely applied theoretical foundations for the study of health behavior change. The HBM is appealing and useful to a wide range of professionals concerned with behavioral change. Physicians, dentists, nurses, psychologists, and health educators have all used the HBM to design and evaluate interventions to alter health behavior.

In Chapter Four, Montaño and Kasprzyk discuss two value expectancy theories—the TRA and the TPB. This family of theories has had a major influence on both research and practice in health behavior and health education. The TRA, as developed by Fishbein and Ajzen (1975), and its extension by Ajzen to the TPB, propose that behavioral intentions and behaviors result from a rational process of decision making. Key constructs are subjective norms and intentions to perform specific actions. TPB also includes another construct—perceived behavioral control. These theories have been used to intervene in many health behaviors, including having mammo-grams, smoking, controlling weight, family planning, and using condoms to prevent AIDS (Jaccard and Davidson, 1972; Ajzen and Fishbein, 1980; McCarty, 1981; Lowe and Frey, 1983). The chapter also introduces and describes the Integrated Behavioral Model (IBM)—a further extension of the TRA and TPB, which grew out of increased interest in theory integration.

In Chapter Five, Prochaska, Redding, and Evers review TTM (or SOC), developed by Prochaska, DiClemente, and colleagues (Prochaska, DiClemente, Velicer, and Rossi, 1993). Over a relatively short time, this theory achieved widespread use and accept-ance by researchers and practitioners in health education and health behavior. The authors present the key components of the theory: concepts of stage, decisional bal-ance, pros and cons, and the processes of change that characterize people in different stages. They discuss the fact that to have a public health impact, increasingly it will be necessary for practitioners to use proactive strategies that reach out to people, rather than relying on reactive strategies that ultimately reach few individuals.

Chapter Six (the PAPM) is authored by Weinstein, who developed the PAPM, and his colleagues, Sandman and Blalock. Like the TTM (or SCM), PAPM is a stage model. As discussed in the Perspectives chapter (Chapter Seven), there are major dif-ferences between these two stage-based approaches. The building blocks of PAPM are the steps along a path from lack of awareness about a precaution (such as using condoms to protect against AIDS), to decision making, and then, in some cases, to adoption of the recommended precaution, initiation, and maintenance.

Taken together, these four chapters provide researchers and practitioners alike with an introduction to widely used theories of health education and health behavior. The different theories are suitable to different problems and populations. Some are more well-developed and easier to use and apply than others. But each has made an important contribution to our understanding of health behavior. Each deserves to be read, studied, and used. Further refinement of the theories will result from their use in research and practice. The distinguished authors have provided chapters that should be accessible to a wide range of health professionals.

Chapter Seven provides a review of the individual chapters, highlights similarities and differences, and identifies some important future challenges and new directions.

REFERENCES

Ajzen, I., and Fishbein, M. *Understanding Attitudes and Predicting Social Behavior.* Englewood Cliffs, N.J.: Prentice Hall, 1980.

Becker, M. H., and Maiman, L. A. "Sociobehavioral Determinants of Compliance with Health and Medical Care Recommendations." *Medical Care,* 1975, *13,* 10–24.

Fishbein, M., and Ajzen, I. *Belief, Attitude, Intention and Behavior: An Introduction to Theory and Research.* Reading, Mass.: Addison-Wesley, 1975.

Jaccard, J. J., and Davidson, A. R. "Toward an Understanding of Family Planning Behaviors: An Initial Inves-tigation." *Journal of Applied Social Psychology,* 1972, *2,* 228–235.

Janz, N. K., and Becker, M. H. "The Health Belief Model: A Decade Later." *Health Education Quarterly,* 1984, *11,* 1–47.

Lewin, K. *A Dynamic Theory of Personality.* New York: McGraw-Hill, 1935.

Lowe, R. H., and Frey, J. D. "Predicting Lamaze Childbirth Intentions and Outcomes: An Extension of the Theory of Reasoned Action to a Joint Outcome." *Basic and Applied Social Psychology,* 1983, *4,* 353–372.

McCarty, D. "Changing Contraceptive Usage Intention: A Test of the Fishbein Model of Intention." *Journal of Applied Social Psychology,* 1981, *11,* 192–211.

Prochaska, J. O., DiClemente, C. C., Velicer, W. F., and Rossi, J. S. "Standardized, Individualized, Interactive, and Personalized Self-Help Programs for Smoking Cessation." *Health Psychology,* 1993, *12,* 399–405.

Rosenstock, I. M. "Historical Origins of the Health Belief Model." *Health Education Monographs,* 1974, *2,* 328–335.

CHAPTER

3

THE HEALTH BELIEF MODEL

Victoria L. Champion
Celette Sugg Skinner

KEY POINTS

This chapter will

- Discuss the origins of the Health Belief Model (HBM) and its relationship to psychosocial theories.
- Present the key components of the HBM.
- Describe the measurement of HBM constructs.
- Give examples of applications of the HBM in breast cancer screening and AIDS-prevention behaviors.

Since the early 1950s, the Health Belief Model (HBM) has been one of the most widely used conceptual frameworks in health behavior research, both to explain change and maintenance of health-related behaviors and as a guiding framework for health behavior interventions. Over the past two decades, the HBM has been expanded, compared to other frameworks, and used to support interventions to change health behavior.

In this chapter, we review fundamental components of the HBM and examine other psychosocial constructs that further explain relationships within the model. First, origins of the HBM and the relationship of the HBM to psychosocial theories are explored. Second, we discuss issues related to the measurement of HBM constructs. Third, we give examples of applications of the HBM in breast cancer screening and AIDS-prevention behaviors. The applications describe how the HBM has been used to explain these behaviors and also as a basis for interventions. We use these examples because they represent two very different public health problems in our society, each with behavioral implications.

ORIGINS OF THE MODEL

The HBM was developed initially in the 1950s by social psychologists in the U.S. Public Health Service to explain the widespread failure of people to participate in programs to prevent and detect disease (Hochbaum, 1958; Rosenstock, 1960, 1974). Later, the model was extended to study people's responses to symptoms (Kirscht, 1974) and their behaviors in response to a diagnosed illness, particularly adherence to medical regimens (Becker, 1974). Although the model evolved gradually in response to very practical public health concerns, its basis in psychological theory is reviewed here to help readers understand its rationale for selected concepts and their relationships, as well as its strengths and weaknesses.

During the early 1950s, academic social psychologists were developing an approach to understanding behavior that grew from learning theories derived from two major sources: Stimulus Response (S-R) Theory (Watson, 1925) and Cognitive Theory (Lewin, 1951; Tolman, 1932). S-R theorists believed that learning results from events (termed *reinforcements*) that reduce physiological drives that activate behavior. Skinner (1938) formulated the widely accepted hypothesis that the frequency of a behavior is determined by its consequences or reinforcement. For Skinner, the mere temporal association between a behavior and an immediately following reward was regarded as sufficient to increase the probability that the behavior would be repeated. In this view, concepts such as *reasoning* or *thinking* are not required to explain behavior.

Cognitive theorists, however, emphasize the role of subjective hypotheses and expectations held by individuals, believing that behavior is a function of the subjective *value* of an outcome and of the subjective probability, or *expectation,* that a particular action will achieve that outcome. Such formulations are generally termed *value-expectancy* theories. Mental processes such as thinking, reasoning, hypothesizing, or expecting are critical components of all cognitive theories. Cognitive theorists believe that reinforcements operate by influencing expectations about the situation rather than by influencing behavior directly. When value-expectancy concepts were gradually reformulated in the context of health-related behaviors, it was assumed that individuals (1) *value* avoiding illnesses/getting well and (2) *expect* that a specific health action may prevent (or ameliorate) illness. The expectancy was further delineated in terms of the individual's estimates of personal susceptibility to and perceived severity of an illness, and of the likelihood of being able to reduce that threat through personal action.

DESCRIPTION OF HBM AND KEY CONSTRUCTS

The HBM contains several primary concepts that predict why people will take action to prevent, to screen for, or to control illness conditions; these include susceptibility, seriousness, benefits and barriers to a behavior, cues to action, and most recently, self-efficacy. Initially, Hochbaum (1958) studied perceptions about whether individuals believed they were susceptible to tuberculosis and their beliefs about the personal benefits of early detection (Hochbaum, 1958). Among individuals who exhibited beliefs both in their own susceptibility to tuberculosis and about the overall benefits from early detection, 82 percent had at least one voluntary chest X-ray. Of the group exhibiting neither of these beliefs, only 21 percent had obtained voluntary X-rays during the criterion period.

If individuals regard themselves as susceptible to a condition, believe that condition would have potentially serious consequences, believe that a course of action available to them would be beneficial in reducing either their susceptibility to or severity of the condition, and believe the anticipated benefits of taking action outweigh the barriers to (or costs of) action, they are likely to take action that they believe will reduce their risks.

In the case of medically established illness (rather than mere risk reduction), the dimension has been reformulated to include acceptance of the diagnosis, personal estimates of susceptibility to consequences of the illness, and susceptibility to illness in general. Definitions of the HBM constructs follow. Table 3.1 summarizes the constructs, definitions, and application examples, and Figure 3.1 illustrates the relationships among constructs.

Constructs

Perceived Susceptibility. Perceived susceptibility refers to beliefs about the likelihood of getting a disease or condition. For instance, a woman must believe there is a possibility of getting breast cancer before she will be interested in obtaining a mammogram.

Perceived Severity. Feelings about the seriousness of contracting an illness or of leaving it untreated include evaluations of both medical and clinical consequences (for example, death, disability, and pain) and possible social consequences (such as effects of the conditions on work, family life, and social relations). The combination of susceptibility and severity has been labeled as perceived *threat.*

Perceived Benefits. Even if a person perceives personal susceptibility to a serious health condition (perceived threat), whether this perception leads to behavior change will be influenced by the person's beliefs regarding perceived *benefits* of the various available actions for reducing the disease threat. Other non-health-related perceptions, such as the financial savings related to quitting smoking or pleasing a family member by having a mammogram, may also influence behavioral decisions. Thus, individuals exhibiting optimal beliefs in susceptibility and severity are not expected to accept any recommended health action unless they also perceive the action as potentially beneficial by reducing the threat.

Perceived Barriers. The potential negative aspects of a particular health action—perceived barriers—may act as impediments to undertaking recommended behaviors. A kind of nonconscious, cost-benefit analysis occurs wherein individuals weigh the action's expected benefits with perceived barriers—"It could help me, but it may be

TABLE 3.1. **Key Concepts and Definitions of the Health Belief Model.**

Concept	Definition	Application
Perceived susceptibility	Belief about the chances of experiencing a risk or getting a condition or disease	Define population(s) at risk, risk levels Personalize risk based on a person's characteristics or behavior Make perceived susceptibility more consistent with individual's actual risk
Perceived severity	Belief about how serious a condition and its sequelae are	Specify consequences of risks and conditions
Perceived benefits	Belief in efficacy of the advised action to reduce risk or seriousness of impact	Define action to take: how, where, when; clarify the positive effects to be expected
Perceived barriers	Belief about the tangible and psychological costs of the advised action	Identify and reduce perceived barriers through reassurance, correction of misinformation, incentives, assistance
Cues to action	Strategies to activate "readiness"	Provide how-to information, promote awareness, use appropriate reminder systems
Self-efficacy	Confidence in one's ability to take action	Provide training and guidance in performing recommended action Use progressive goal setting Give verbal reinforcement Demonstrate desired behaviors Reduce anxiety

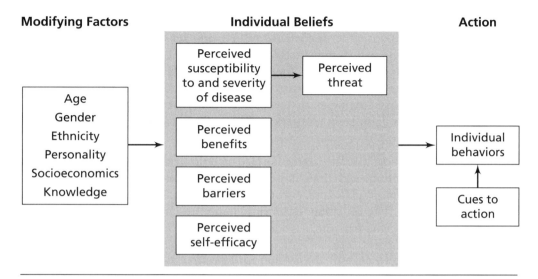

Modifying Factors   **Individual Beliefs**   **Action**

FIGURE 3.1. Health Belief Model Components and Linkages.

expensive, have negative side effects, be unpleasant, inconvenient, or time-consuming." Thus, "combined levels of susceptibility and severity provide the energy or force to act and the perception of benefits (minus barriers) provide a preferred path of action" (Rosenstock, 1974).

Cues to Action. Various early formulations of the HBM included the concept of cues that can trigger actions. Hochbaum (1958), for example, thought that readiness to take action (perceived susceptibility and perceived benefits) could only be potentiated by other factors, particularly by *cues* to instigate action, such as bodily events, or by environmental events, such as media publicity. He did not, however, study the role of cues empirically. Nor have cues to action been systematically studied. Indeed, although the concept of cues as triggering mechanisms is appealing, cues to action are difficult to study in explanatory surveys; a cue can be as fleeting as a sneeze or the barely conscious perception of a poster.

Self-Efficacy. *Self-efficacy* is defined as "the conviction that one can successfully execute the behavior required to produce the outcomes" (Bandura, 1997). Bandura distinguished *self-efficacy expectations* from *outcome expectations,* defined as a person's estimate that a given behavior will lead to certain outcomes. Outcome expectations are similar to but distinct from the HBM concept of *perceived benefits*. In 1988, Rosenstock, Strecher, and Becker suggested that self-efficacy be added to the HBM as a separate construct, while including original concepts of susceptibility, severity, benefits, and barriers.

 Self-efficacy was never explicitly incorporated into early formulations of the HBM. The original model was developed in the context of circumscribed preventive health actions (accepting a screening test or an immunization) that were not perceived to involve complex behaviors.

As discussed more thoroughly in Chapter Eight (on Social Cognitive Theory), a body of literature supports the importance of self-efficacy in initiation and maintenance of behavioral change (Bandura, 1997). For behavior change to succeed, people must (as the original HBM theorizes) feel threatened by their current behavioral patterns (perceived susceptibility and severity) and believe that change of a specific kind will result in a valued outcome at an acceptable cost (perceived benefit). They also must feel themselves competent (self-efficacious) to overcome perceived barriers to take action.

Other Variables. Diverse demographic, sociopsychological, and structural variables may influence perceptions and, thus, indirectly influence health-related behavior. For example, sociodemographic factors, particularly educational attainment, are believed to have an indirect effect on behavior by influencing the perception of susceptibility, severity, benefits, and barriers.

Relationships Among Health Belief Model Constructs

The HBM components are depicted in Figure 3.1. Arrows indicate relationships between constructs. Modifying factors include knowledge and sociodemographic factors that may influence health perceptions. Health beliefs include the major constructs of the HBM: susceptibility, severity, benefits, barriers, and self-efficacy. Modifying factors affect these perceptions, as do cues to action. The combination of beliefs leads to behavior. Within the "health belief" box, perceived susceptibility and severity are combined to identify threat.

Although the HBM identifies constructs that lead to outcome behaviors, relationships between and among these constructs are not defined. This ambiguity has led to variation in HBM applications. For example, whereas many studies have attempted to establish each of the major dimensions as independent, others have tried multiplicative approaches. Analytical approaches to identifying these relationships are needed to further the utility of the HBM in predicting behavior.

EVIDENCE FOR THE MODEL'S PERFORMANCE

A critical review of HBM studies conducted between 1974 and 1984 combined new results with earlier findings to permit an overall assessment of the model's performance (Becker, 1974; Janz and Becker, 1984). Summary results provided substantial empirical support for the model, with findings from prospective studies at least as favorable as those obtained from retrospective research. *Perceived barriers* were the most powerful single predictor across all studies and behaviors. Although both *perceived susceptibility* and *perceived benefits* were important overall, *perceived susceptibility* was a stronger predictor of preventive health behavior than sick-role behavior. The reverse was true for *perceived benefits*. Overall, *perceived severity* was the least powerful predictor; however, this dimension was strongly related to sick-role behavior. As there has not been an updated evidence review of HBM studies since 1984, this is the most current synthesis available. A new up-to-date review would help to confirm or modify these conclusions.

MEASUREMENT OF HBM CONSTRUCTS

One of the most important limitations in both descriptive and intervention research on the HBM has been variability in measurement of the central HBM constructs. Several important principles guide development of HBM measurement. Construct definitions need to be consistent with HBM theory as originally conceptualized, and measures need to be specific to the behavior being addressed (barriers to mammography may be quite different from barriers to colonoscopy) and relevant to the population among whom they will be used. To ensure content validity, it is important to measure the full range of factors that may influence the behavior. Using multiple items for each scale reduces measurement error and increases the probability of including all relative components of each construct. Finally, validity and reliability of measures need to be reexamined with each study. Cultural and population differences make applying scales without such examination prone to error. Only a few studies using the HBM that have developed or modified instruments to measure HBM constructs have conducted adequate reliability and validity testing prior to research.

HBM Scales for Breast Cancer Screening Behaviors

Assessments of HBM constructs relevant to breast cancer screening have been related to both the behaviors of breast self-examination (Champion, 1984; 1993) and mammography (Champion, 1999). In 1984, Champion developed and validated scales for perceived susceptibility, severity, benefits, and barriers to breast self-examination. A perceived severity scale was developed but dropped due to lack of variance and predictive power (Champion, 1984). These initial scales underwent revision in 1993, and a scale to measure self-efficacy was added. Champion revised the initial scales for benefits and barriers to be mammography-specific (Champion, 1999). Perception of benefits from breast self-examination and later mammography addressed the benefit the screening behavior (breast self-examination or mammography) would have in reducing the chance of death from breast cancer. Items included issues such as finding a lump early when breast cancer can be cured. Barriers were specific to the behavior being tested—originally, breast self-examination and later mammography. Barriers included such items as fear of finding a lump, time required for the test, forgetting to make or keep an appointment, and pain and fear of radiation associated with the mammography procedure. All revisions included testing for content and construct validity, as well as internal consistency and test-retest reliability. Cronbach's alpha—the measure used to assess reliability—was .75 for benefits and .88 for barriers. Perceived susceptibility has shown the highest internal consistency reliability across studies.

To achieve content validity, formative research is often required to identify the full range of factors that may be perceived as benefits or barriers for a particular behavior by members of a particular population. These particular identified benefits and barriers can be incorporated into scales, which must then be validated in the specific target population. For example, the Champion scales measuring HBM were adapted for an African American population in 1997 (Champion and Scott, 1997) and included several additional mammography-barrier items, based on focus groups' suggestions (for example, the potential barriers of not knowing how to schedule an appointment and not understanding the procedure). These revised scales were tested among 344 low-income African American women recruited into a mammography-promotion intervention study (Champion and others, forthcoming). Construct validity was confirmed through exploratory factor analysis. Cronbach's alphas ranged from .73 to .94.

In addition to their adaptation for African American populations, the original HBM scales developed by Champion have been translated into several languages and tested among a number of ethnic and cultural groups. Table 3.2 provides Cronbach's alphas for each scale, depending on cultural translation. Translation testing for all scales included construct validity testing through various modalities, such as exploratory and confirmatory factor analysis, and predictive validity of theoretical relationships. Samples included 500 students and employees in Jordan (Mikhail and Petro-Nustas, 2001), a Korean convenience sample of 264 women (Lee, Kim, and Song, 2002), a sample of first-generation Chinese American women (Wu and Yu, 2003), and 656 Turkish women from health centers (Secginli and Nahcivan, 2004). Taken together, findings from these studies support validity and reliability of these HBM scales when translated to different cultures.

Champion and colleagues also have developed scales to measure mammography-related self-efficacy—a woman's confidence in her ability to complete steps needed to obtain a mammogram. Ten items fit the conceptual definition of *self-efficacy*. Reliability and validity were tested among a sample of 1,233 women, of whom 54 percent were African American; Cronbach's alpha coefficient was .87, and confirmatory factor analysis supported construct validity. Self-efficacy significantly predicted mammography use and demonstrated change over time (Champion, Skinner, and Menon, 2005).

HBM Scales for Colorectal Cancer Screening Behaviors

Development of HBM scales for colorectal cancer (CRC) screening has been guided by the same measurement principles as those for mammography and breast self-examination. Formative research conducted by Rawl and colleagues (Rawl, Champion,

TABLE 3.2. **Cronbach's Alpha of Champion's HBM Scales Translated into Four Cultures.**

	Arabic (Mikhail)	Turkish (Secginli)	Korean (Lee)	Chinese (Wu)
Susceptibility	.85	.82	.92	.78
Seriousness	.81	.83	.85	.75
Benefits	.79	.82	.79	.87
Barriers	.77	.75	.74	.90

Menon, and Foster, 2000) used focus groups to identify specific benefits and barriers to CRC screening. Benefits identified by participants were similar to those for breast cancer screening and included finding cancer early, decreasing chances of dying from the cancer, freedom from worry, and reassurance when no cancer is found. Barriers identified included lack of knowledge, inconsistent recommendations from health care providers, and embarrassment associated with the tests. Reliability was measured by using Cronbach's alpha and was .65 for fecal occult blood test (FOBT), .67 for flexible sigmoidoscopy, and .70 for colonoscopy. Exploratory factor analysis identified dimensions for benefits of FOBT, sigmoidoscopy, and colonoscopy, with respective items loading at .54 to .78 for FOBT, .35 to .58 for flexible sigmoidoscopy, and .62 to .72 for colonoscopy.

Most recently, Wardle and colleagues developed a seven-item benefits scale specific to sigmoidoscopy (Wardle and others, 2003). Items demonstrated construct validity by loading at .40 or above; internal consistency reliability was .83. Constructs were salience and coherence, cancer worries, perceived susceptibility, response efficacy, and social influence. Perceived susceptibility was identical to that used in the original HBM definition. Response efficacy mirrored benefits, in that items related to decreasing the risk of disease threat. Cancer worries were identified as barriers to completing the behavior. Confirmatory factor analysis supported the identified constructs for males and females, as well as African Americans and Caucasians. Cronbach's alpha ranged from .60 to .64 (Marcus and others, 2005).

A major method of testing construct validity is to test theoretical relationships. Ambiguity about the relationships among theoretical constructs in the HBM makes tests of construct validity more difficult. HBM relationships between constructs have not been well described. It is possible that one of the variables may mediate relationships between the others. Temporality of relationships is also an issue. When health beliefs and behaviors are measured concurrently, apparent relationships between them might well turn out to be spurious. These factors may have contributed to the frequent lack of scientific rigor in measuring HBM constructs.

APPLICATIONS OF THE HBM TO MAMMOGRAPHY AND AIDS-RELATED BEHAVIORS

The HBM has been used extensively to determine relationships between health beliefs and health behaviors, as well as to inform interventions. A comprehensive review of all work using the HBM to address health behaviors is beyond the scope of this chapter. In this section, we discuss use of the HBM in two important areas: (1) breast cancer screening and (2) AIDS-related behaviors.

The HBM and Mammography

Association of HBM Constructs with Mammography Behavior. The HBM predicts that women will be more likely to adhere to screening mammography recommendations if they feel susceptible to breast cancer, think breast cancer is a severe disease, perceive barriers to screening as lower than perceived benefits, have higher self-efficacy for obtaining mammograms, and receive a cue to action. Indeed, many studies have found these expected relationships between HBM constructs and mammography adherence. Adherence has been significantly associated with greater perceived susceptibility, lower barriers, higher benefits, and cues in the form of recommendations from health care providers (Champion, 1984; Champion and Menon, 1997; Champion, Ray, Heilman, and Springston, 2000; Friedman, Neff, Webb, and Latham, 1998; Phillips and others, 1998). Because early studies found little variation in perceived severity, this construct has been less frequently measured in more recent mammography studies.

Studies conducted among diverse samples have found some differences in the specific types of beliefs about susceptibility, benefits, and barriers among different racial and ethnic groups. Different groups have different beliefs about the causes of breast cancer, which can affect perceived susceptibility. An example is the belief common among some groups of older African Americans that breast cancer is caused by an injury to the breast (Guidry, Matthews-Juarez, and Copeland, 2003; Skinner, Arfken, and Sykes, 1998); women who have not had such an injury may conclude that their susceptibility is quite low. Beliefs associated with lower perceived benefit from early detection, such as the notion that surgery causes cancer to spread and that cancer means death, are more common among African Americans than white women (Guidry, Matthews-Juarez, and Copeland, 2003; Skinner, Champion, Menon, and Seshadri, 2002). Certain types of barriers are more or less important for particular cultural or ethnic subgroups. Modesty is a special barrier associated with lack of adherence among Asian American women (Tang, Solomon, and McCracken, 2000). Fear, embarrassment, and cost are more likely to be barriers to adherence among African American women (Thompson and others, 1997). Finally, in addition to differences in specific perceptions about susceptibility, benefits, and barriers among racial or ethnic groups, researchers have found differences by race in explanatory power of HBM constructs. In 2004, Vadaparampil and colleagues used structural equation modeling to examine HBM constructs and differences in adherence for African American and Caucasian women, and found that HBM constructs explained only a small amount of variance in both groups—approximately 13 percent for Caucasians and 9 percent for African Americans (Vadaparampil and others, 2004). However, differences in some specific constructs had the greatest explanatory power. Whereas barriers were significantly related to adherence in both racial groups, higher perceived benefits were significantly related to adherence among African Americans and higher self-efficacy was significant only for whites.

Mammography-Promotion Interventions Based on the HBM.   A number of mammography-promotion interventions have addressed at least one HBM construct—usually perceived barriers—and have had significant effects on mammography outcomes (Allen and Bazargan-Hejazi, 2005; Carney, Harwood, Greene, and Goodrich, 2005; Costanza and others, 2000; Crane and others, 2000; Duan, Fox, Derose, and Carson, 2000; Lauver, Settersten, Kane, and Henriques, 2003; Lipkus, Rimer, Halabi, and Strigo, 2000; Rakowski and others, 2003; Valanis and others, 2003). This section summarizes findings from several different types of interventions based on the HBM.

Perhaps because constructs in the HBM are fairly intuitive, they have been used in a number of community-based interventions conducted among underserved groups with lower education levels. Lay health advisers have been equipped to assess their peers' HBM-related perceptions and then craft messages and plans to address those factors and facilitate mammography use (Earp and others, 2002). In the *Learn, Share and Live* intervention, Skinner and colleagues used the HBM to inform community-based education sessions for older, urban minority women (Skinner and others, 1998). The goal was to change perceptions and practices among the program participants and enable them, in turn, to address mammography-related perceptions and constructs effectively among their peers. Learning objectives guiding the three core education sessions are shown in Table 3.3, along with the HBM constructs each addressed.

To help women realize the benefits of early detection (Objective 1), program leaders distributed necklaces of wooden beads of graduated sizes (from 6 to 28 mm) so that women could actually see and feel differences in sizes of the average lump found by women in their own breasts versus the much smaller sizes of lumps that can be

TABLE 3.3. **Learning Objectives Used to Change Mammography Perceptions and Practices Among Urban Minority Women.**

Learning Objectives	Theoretical Constructs
1. Recognize that breast cancer screening is effective for finding early cancers.	Benefits (Health Belief Model) Response efficacy
2. Be aware of increased likelihood of favorable outcomes with early detected breast cancers.	Benefits (Health Belief Model)
3. Be aware that the risk of breast cancer increases with age.	Susceptibility (Health Belief Model)
4. Recognize that a number of factors may act as barriers to breast cancer screening.	Barriers (Health Belief Model)
5. Identify questions that can be used to determine women's perceived benefits and barriers to breast cancer screening.	Health education principles of behavioral diagnosis
6. Choose relevant messages for various perceptions.	Health education principles of message tailoring
7. Feel increased confidence that participant can encourage breast cancer screening among peers.	Self-efficacy (Social Cognitive Theory)

Source: Based on Skinner and others, 1998.

found via mammograms. To further communicate benefits of early detection, the program used a dandelion analogy, comparing the importance of pulling up dandelions before their seeds spread across a whole yard to the benefit of "taking care of the cancer before it can spread in your body and make you sick" (Skinner and others, 1998). To help the women understand how to assess and then address their peers' perceived benefits and barriers to screening, they participated in role-plays, in which they practiced asking about their friends' "reasons" for having or not having mammograms and then brainstormed ways to help their friends overcome these barriers. Whereas some barriers were related to beliefs (for example, that the radiation in mammograms actually caused cancer), others were logistical or structural (for example, costs associated with screening or not knowing how to arrange transportation to the mammography facility). To address these barriers, this intervention and others have put women in contact with community resources, such as mobile mammography units operated by local health systems or philanthropic organizations that cover costs of screening for uninsured women.

Some studies have compared the effectiveness of different media for delivering interventions addressing HBM constructs to women in clinic settings. In a longitudinal intervention study, Champion and colleagues compared HBM interventions delivered through (1) telephone counseling, (2) in-person counseling in the clinic, (3) physician letter only, (4) telephone counseling plus physician letter, or (5) in-person counseling plus letter. There were significant intervention effects on both HBM beliefs and mammography behavior. Adherence in all intervention groups, except the physician letter alone, was significantly different from standard care, with the combination of in-person and physician letter being the most significant (Champion and others, forthcoming).

Just as the HBM has guided community-based interventions to deliver information or persuasive messages to change perceptions and reduce barriers to screening, it has also guided interventions delivered through minimal contact with the intervention recipient. The most common and successful of these minimal-contact strategies have used printed materials and telephone calls to enhance perceived benefits for mammography screening and reduce perceived barriers. For example, a telephone counselor may ask, "What might keep you from having a mammogram?" and, depending on the woman's answer, deliver a message designed to reduce that barrier. Some of these intervention studies have resulted in mammography rates more than twice as large as those of a no-intervention comparison group (King and others, 1994).

Several studies have used HBM variables to tailor mammography interventions for particular recipients. In these tailored interventions, computer algorithms use women's interview data to select, from a library of potential messages, unique combinations for each individual recipient, based on her specific reported perceptions of susceptibility, benefits, barriers, and self-efficacy. In general, tailoring messages for breast cancer screening using the HBM constructs of susceptibility, benefits, and barriers has been found to increase mammography adherence.

In the first of these studies, 435 family practice patients were randomly assigned to receive mammography recommendation letters tailored to their specific HBM perceptions or a nontailored version of the letter (Skinner, Strecher, and Hospers, 1994). For example, tailored letters had paragraphs specifically addressing up to three barriers cited by women as holding them back from getting a mammogram; the nontailored version included messages about three common barriers but not the particular barriers mentioned by the recipient. Among subgroups with low adherence at baseline (African American and lower-income women), mammography adherence at follow-up was significantly higher among women who received letters tailored on HBM constructs.

Building on the tailored print mammography intervention findings, Champion and Skinner compared effects of letters with telephone counseling (Champion and others, 2007). Both were tailored on HBM constructs, meaning that women received messages about their susceptibility to breast cancer that mentioned their specific risk factors (for example, their current age and family history), and the messages about benefits and barriers were selected to address their specific concerns and to correct perceptions. For example, women whose survey responses indicated that they did not understand or appreciate the benefits of early detection got messages explaining and emphasizing these benefits. Telephone counseling plus mailings resulted in the highest adherence (40 percent), but telephone alone (36 percent) and mailed print alone (37 percent) also were significantly better than standard care. Similarly, Rimer and colleagues tested print and telephone interventions tailored on constructs from the HBM, as well as other models, and found superiority in the combination of phone and print (Rimer and others, 2002).

HBM variables have also formed the basis for tailoring interactive computer programs that include video segments. One of these—tailored on perceived susceptibility, benefits, and barriers—was testing among more than 300 low-income African American women. In the program, a narrator asked questions about HBM constructs, and women touched the screen to indicate their responses. The video clips that followed used narrative episodes, for example, to model a woman overcoming the barrier that had been selected by the user. Also included in the intervention was an in-person counseling session addressing each woman's perceived susceptibility, benefits, and barriers to mammography screening. For women who had never had mammograms, adherence was significantly higher in the HBM-based interactive intervention group (50 percent) than in the comparison group (18 percent) (Champion and others, 2006).

In summary, HBM constructs generally have been found to predict participation in breast cancer screening. In addition, a large number of intervention studies addressing HBM constructs have resulted in increased mammography use. This has been true for interventions delivered in community-based and minimal-contact settings. Finally, interventions tailored to address recipients' specific HBM beliefs have been found to be particularly effective. It is entirely consistent with the HBM that interventions will be more effective if they address a person's *specific* perceptions about susceptibility, benefits, barriers, and self-efficacy. Women who already believe they are at risk for developing breast cancer don't need messages trying to convince them of their susceptibility; those who know where to get a free mammogram but can't find a way to get there need interventions addressing transportation, not cost.

Just as it is important to be able to validly *measure* HBM constructs, tailoring technology has allowed interventions to *address* HBM constructs most relevant for particular individuals.

The HBM and Risky Sexual Behaviors

Association of HBM Constructs with Risky Sexual Behaviors. The HBM hypothesizes that AIDS-protective behavior decisions are a function of perceived risk of contracting the disease, perceived severity of the disease, and perceptions of benefits and barriers to specific AIDS-protective behaviors. The HBM suggests that, for individuals who exhibit high-risk behaviors, perceived susceptibility is necessary before commitment to changing these risky behaviors can occur. For individuals who do not believe they are at risk, the benefits or barriers to an action are irrelevant. Self-efficacy has been studied in relation to HIV-protective behaviors and defines an individual's perceived ability to carry out a behavior believed to be necessary to prevent infection with HIV (Janz and Becker, 1984). Studies addressing relationships between HBM constructs and risky sexual behaviors have focused on adolescents and young adults in the United States and on more general populations in Africa, where AIDS is a significant health problem.

The relationship between perceived susceptibility to negative outcomes of risky sexual behavior, such as becoming HIV-positive or contracting sexually transmitted diseases (STDs), varies across studies. Some researchers have found a significant relationship between condom use and perceived susceptibility (Basen-Engquist, 1992; Hounton, Carabin, and Henderson, 2005; Mahoney, Thombs, and Ford, 1995; Steers and others, 1996), whereas others haven't found the relationship (Hounton, Carabin, and Henderson, 2005; Volk and Koopman, 2001). Measurement issues may explain some of the discrepancy. Research by Ronis (1992) suggests that susceptibility questions should be clearly conditional on action or inaction. Some articles used a behavioral anchor in their susceptibility measures, for example, asking the question, "*If you do not practice safer sex, how likely are you to become infected with the AIDS virus?*" as opposed to simply, "How likely are you to become infected with the AIDS virus?" Not specifying conditions of action versus inaction could lead to a personalized interpretation (for example, respondents who indicate that their risk of infection is great, largely *because* they are not practicing safer sex). Therefore, comparisons of the predictive ability of perceived susceptibility across studies may be inconsistent.

Perceptions of AIDS severity address the perceived costs of being HIV-positive. Perceived seriousness, in this case, refers to personal evaluations of the probable biomedical, financial, and social consequences of contracting HIV and developing AIDS. Some might argue that asking about AIDS severity would be a waste of respondents' time, as it might be assumed that everyone would report AIDS to be an extremely severe disease. Most studies in the research literature have not included measures on HIV/AIDS perceived severity (Rosenstock, Strecher, and Becker, 1994).

Associations of perceived benefits and barriers to AIDS are identified, but results with behaviors are inconsistent. Reported condom use among Central Harlem youth was motivated by the perceived value of condoms to avoid pregnancy, as well as avoidance of HIV/AIDS, but the strongest motivation was avoiding pregnancy (Laraque and others, 1997). In a study of gay men's safer sex behavior, Wulfert, Wan, and Backus (1996) found that most men were convinced about the benefits of using condoms, but these perceived benefits were not associated with behavior. Several researchers have found a significant relationship between barriers and condom use (Hounton, Carabin, and Henderson, 2005; Volk and Koopman, 2001). As perceived barriers increased, condom use decreased. Barriers such as reduction of sensation and pleasure were associated with condom use, as well as worry about negative reactions from sexual partners (Wulfert, Wan, and Backus, 1996).

Self-efficacy has been one of the stronger predictors of condom use or safe sex behaviors (Lin, Simoni, and Zemon, 2005; Steers and others, 1996; Zak-Place and Stern, 2004). Self-efficacy was a significant predictor of sexual behaviors that included increased condom use, decreased number of sex partners, and decreased number of sexual encounters. Self-efficacy has also been found to have cultural differences in that it was significantly lower in Asian Americans than in whites, African Americans, or Hispanics (Hounton, Carabin, and Henderson, 2005; Lin, Simoni, and Zemon, 2005). Further, self-efficacy can vary between men and women because, in the case of condom use, the behavior is not under the woman's direct control (Wight, Abraham, and Scott, 1998).

In summary, many research studies have identified relationships of HBM constructs with safe sex behaviors. Although results have varied, support for significant relationships between perceived susceptibility, perceived benefits and barriers, and perceived self-efficacy are apparent. These concepts have been used in interventions developed to decrease risky sexual behaviors and are reviewed next.

Interventions Based on the HBM for Risky Sexual Behaviors. Booth, Zhang, and Kwiatkowski (1999) evaluated a peer-based intervention for runaway and homeless adolescents using principles derived from the HBM. The intervention was developed to reduce drug- and sex-related HIV-risk behaviors. Peer leaders were trained to have discussions with individual participants about their perceived susceptibility to HIV. Potential barriers were addressed by increasing skills in negotiating safer sex, avoiding situations where sexual intercourse was likely, and practicing refusal skills when drugs were offered. The authors found that those who perceived a greater chance of HIV infection were more likely to have used drugs and to have had a higher number of sex partners in the previous three months. Consistent with the HBM, lower concern with HIV infection was independently associated with the use of heroin and cocaine, as well as the overall number of drugs used among the runaway and homeless adolescents. There was not a significant association between HIV concern and risky sexual behavior.

Behavioral interventions targeting Indonesian sex workers included an education program based on the HBM and Social Cognitive Theory. One intervention arm included only the educational session, while the second arm included the educational session plus free condoms. The intervention was designed to increase knowledge, perceived susceptibility, and self-efficacy. A three-session series of interactive lectures was developed. Two community areas were used for intervention and one for control. The intervention included an educational program that sought to dispel the myth that AIDS is a tourist disease and increase perceived susceptibility that Indonesians themselves can become infected—that is, it sought to reduce the false stereotype that "people who get this disease are very different from me" (Wight, Abraham, and Scott, 1998). To increase perceived severity of AIDS, the program also included information about the terminal nature of HIV infection. Self-efficacy was increased by identifying prevention strategies, including negotiating condom use. Condom use increased significantly in the two intervention areas and, to a smaller extent, in the control community (Ford and others, 1996).

Self-efficacy training for condom use has been the target of several other interventions. Siegel and colleagues (2001) used a quasi-experimental design in an urban, ethnically mixed neighborhood. The intensive ten- to twelve-session intervention was incorporated into health classes and focused on decision-making and skill-based activities to increase self-efficacy. Self-efficacy was higher in the intervention group, as was intention to remain safe. In 2004, DiClemente and colleagues reported a significant decrease in risky behaviors among young female adolescents who received an intervention focusing on self-efficacy for condom application and communication skills.

In summary, behavioral interventions to reduce risky sexual behaviors have evolved during the last decade. Although results have varied, most attempted to use interventions to increase perceived risk and self-efficacy and targeted condom use. The common thread that seems to increase intervention effectiveness is skills training (self-efficacy). Interventions also have focused on relationship skills and perceived risk perceptions. Several successful interventions addressed communication and negotiation skills as necessary components of safer sexual behaviors. With a behavior that involves other individuals, peer or social influence must be considered, and interventions have evolved around increasing self-efficacy in negotiating condom use.

COMPARISON OF HBM TO OTHER THEORIES

A common direction in research involving the HBM is to determine its usefulness in combination with other models and frameworks. For instance, HBM constructs have been combined with The Transtheoretical Model's (TTM) component of staging outcome behavior. Saywell and others (2003) found that a more intensive intervention is needed for women who are not considering mammograms (classified by the TTM as "precontemplators") than for women who are considering being screened. Research also indicates that women who are contemplating being screened have an increased perception of threats and benefits to action, compared to precontemplators. Similarly, women in contemplation have fewer barriers to action than women in precontemplation. Identifying subgroups of women who are in precontemplation or contemplation for mammography allowed greater tailoring of interventions (Saywell and others, 2003).

Weinstein compared four commonly used models of health-protective behavior, including the HBM, the Theory of Reasoned Action (TRA), Protection Motivation Theory, and Subjective Expected Utility theory (Weinstein, 1993). Although published more than a decade ago, many of the issues raised are relevant today. First, models may identify different constructs, but the conceptualization of these constructs across theories is similar. The TRA identifies intention as preceding behavior changes. The TTM conceptualization of stages of behavior is a combination of actual behavior and intention. We need to identify the core conceptual definitions inherent in a model's constructs prior to attempting to combine constructs across theories.

Investigators should recognize that the combination of theories holds promise in further understanding health-related behaviors, but it is critical to consider relationships and independence between constructs. Although there are differences among models of health behavior change, especially with respect to how many different constructs are combined and used to predict behavioral outcomes, the theories are largely complimentary, with significant degrees of overlap (Weinstein, 1993). Therefore, the central issue is not which model is superior to other models or which variables may be more important but the relative utility and changes in relative utility with different behaviors and situations over time (Maddux, Ingram, and Desmond, 1995).

CHALLENGES IN FUTURE HBM RESEARCH

The HBM has been used for over half a century to predict health-related behaviors and to frame interventions to change behaviors. As indicated by the reviewed research, it has been useful in predicting and framing cancer screening and HIV-protective behaviors. Its simplicity has enabled researchers to identify constructs that may be important, thus increasing the probability that a theoretical base will be used to frame research interventions. Its simplicity, however, also creates some of its major limitations.

Several challenges remain when considering the HBM as a theory to predict health-related behaviors. First, perceived threat is a construct that has great relevance in health-related behaviors. The HBM couples severity with perceived susceptibility—a strength, compared with models that conceptualize threat as perceived risk alone. However, the relationship between risk and severity in forming threat is not always clear. A heightened state of severity is required before perceived susceptibility becomes a powerful predictor. It may be that perceived susceptibility is a stronger predictor of engagement if severity in health-related behaviors is perceived as higher versus lower. If this is true, a multiplicative variable should be computed that combines perceived susceptibility and severity, rather than considering each alone.

Relationships among other constructs in the HBM also should be tested more thoroughly. For instance, perceived benefits and barriers may be stronger predictors of behavior change when perceived threat (perceived severity × perceived susceptibility) is high than when it is low. Under conditions of low perceived threat, benefits of and barriers to engaging in health-related behaviors should not be salient. This relationship, however, may be altered in situations where benefits are perceived to be very high and barriers very low. Threat may not need to be high if perceived barriers are very low (for example, if flu shots are available at very convenient locations, like grocery stores). Therefore, the predictive power of one concept may depend on values of another.

The HBM is limited, in that it is a cognitively based model and does not consider the emotional component of behavior. Witte considered fear an essential part of a health-related behavior, defined as a negative emotion accompanied by a high state of arousal (Witte, 1992). We have experimented with adding fear to a model that predicts mammography behavior and have found relationships between HBM constructs and fear that might be useful predictors (Champion, Skinner, and Menon, 2005; Champion, Menon, Rawl, and Skinner, 2004). Fear was significantly predicted by perceived risk, benefits, and self-efficacy; fear, together with barriers, then predicted actual behavior. These findings are consistent with the Protection Motivation Theory (Rogers and Prentice-Dunn, 1997). The most persuasive communications are those that arouse fear while enhancing perceptions central to the HBM—the severity of an event, the likelihood of exposure to that event, the benefits of responses to that threat, and self-efficacy for accessing those benefits (Rogers and Prentice-Dunn, 1997). Inclusion of an emotional construct might help explain relationships among HBM constructs (Rogers and Prentice-Dunn, 1997).

Finally, cues to action are one component of the HBM often missing from research. Cues to action will have a greater influence on behavior in situations where perceived threat and benefits are high and perceived barriers are low. We know little about cues to action or their relative impact because this construct has not been identified clearly in research. Cancer screening studies have used reminder letters or postcards as an intervention and found that, for many participants, this intervention is significant. A reminder postcard may be a cue to action, but it is seldom labeled as such. Researchers have found that simple reminders may be all that is needed for women who have already had a mammogram or are contemplating getting another (Saywell and others, 2003).

SUMMARY

In this chapter we described the origins of the Health Belief Model (HBM), reviewed and defined its key components and their hypothesized relationships, described issues related to measuring HBM constructs, and gave examples of carefully developed measures. This chapter also gave examples of applications of the HBM in descriptive and intervention studies of breast cancer screening and AIDS-related risky sexual behaviors.

The concept of perceived threat, defined as a combination of perceived susceptibility and severity in the HBM, has great relevance for many health-related behaviors. Future challenges to HBM research include more thorough testing of the relationships among constructs beyond perceived thereat. The HBM is a cognitively based model that does not consider the emotional component of behavior—this component, as well as cues to action, should be added to or better incorporated in HBM research. Finally, an updated critical review of the research and findings based on the HBM is warranted and would help to map future directions for researchers and practitioners.

REFERENCES

Allen, B., Jr., and Bazargan-Hejazi, S. "Evaluating a Tailored Intervention To Increase Screening Mammography In An Urban Area." *Journal of the National Medical Association,* 2005, *97*(10), 1350–1360.

Bandura, A. *Self-efficacy: The Exercise of Control.* New York: W. H. Freeman, 1997.

Basen-Engquist, K. "Psychosocial Predictors of 'Safer Sex' Behaviors in Young Adults." *AIDS Education and Prevention,* 1992, *4,* 120–134.

Becker, M. H. "The Health Belief Model and Personal Health Behavior." *Health Education Monographs,* 1974, *2,* 324–473.

Booth, R. E., Zhang, Y., and Kwiatkowski, C. F. "The Challenge of Changing Drug and Sex Risk Behaviors of Runaway and Homeless Adolescents." *Child Abuse and Neglect,* 1999, *3*(12), 1295–1306.

Carney, P. A., Harwood, B. G., Greene, M. A., and Goodrich, M. E. "Impact of a Telephone Counseling Intervention on Transitions in Stage of Change and Adherence to Interval Mammography Screening." *Cancer Causes and Control,* 2005, *16*(7), 799–807.

Champion, V. "Instrument Development for Health Belief Model Constructs." *Advances in Nursing Science,* 1984, *6*(3), 73–85.

Champion, V. L. "Instrument Refinement for Breast Cancer Screening Behaviors." *Nursing Research,* 1993, *42*(3), 139–143.

Champion, V. L. "Revised Susceptibility, Benefits, and Barriers Scale for Mammography Screening." *Research in Nursing and Health,* 1999, *22*(4), 341–348.

Champion, V. L., and Menon, U. "Predicting Mammography and Breast Self-Examination in African American Women." *Cancer Nursing,* 1997, *20*(5), 315–322.

Champion, V. L., Menon, U., Rawl, S., and Skinner, C. S. "A Breast Cancer Fear Scale: Psychometric Development." *Journal of Health Psychology,* 2004, *9*(6), 769–778.

Champion, V. L., Ray, D. W., Heilman, D. K., and Springston, J. K. "A Tailored Intervention for Mammography Among Low-Income African-American Women." *Journal of Psychosocial Oncology,* 2000, *18*(4), 1–13.

Champion, V. L., and Scott, C. R. "Reliability and Validity of Breast Cancer Screening Belief Scales in African American Women." *Nursing Research,* 1997, *46*(6), 331–337.

Champion, V., Skinner, C. S., and Menon, U. "Development of a Self-Efficacy Scale for Mammography." *Research in Nursing and Health,* 2005, *28*(4), 329–336.

Champion, V. L., and others. "Comparison of Three Interventions to Increase Mammography Screening in Low Income African American Women." *Cancer Detection and Prevention,* 2006, *30*(6), 535–544.

Champion, V., and others. "The Effect of Telephone Versus Print Tailoring for Mammography Adherence." *Patient Education and Counseling,* 2007, *65*(3), 416–423.

Champion, V. L., and others "Measuring mammography and breast cancer beliefs in African American Women." *Journal of Health Psychology,* forthcoming.

Costanza, M. E., and others. "Promoting Mammography: Results of a Randomized Trial of Telephone Counseling and a Medical Practice Intervention." *American Journal of Preventive Medicine,* 2000, *19*(1), 39–46.

Crane, L., and others. "Effectiveness and Cost-Effectiveness of Multiple Outcalls to Promote Mammography Among Low-Income Women." *Cancer Epidemiology, Biomarkers and Prevention,* 2000, *9,* 923–931.

DiClemente, R. J., and others. "Efficacy of an HIV Prevention Intervention for African American Adolescent Girls: A Randomized Controlled Trial." *The Journal of The American Medical Association,* 2004, *292*(2), 171–179.

Duan, N., Fox, S. A., Derose, K. P., and Carson, S. "Maintaining Mammography Adherence Through Telephone Counseling in a Church-Based Trial." *American Journal of Public Health,* 2000, *90*(9), 1468–1471.

Earp, J. A., and others. "Increasing Use of Mammography Among Older, Rural African American Women: Results From a Community Trial." *American Journal of Public Health,* 2002, *92*(4), 646–654.

Ford, K., and others. "Behavioral Interventions for Reduction of Sexually Transmitted Disease/HIV Transmission Among Female Commercial Sex Workers and Clients in Bali, Indonesia." *AIDS,* 1996, *10*(2), 213–222.

Friedman, L. C., Neff, N. E., Webb, J. A., and Latham, C. K. "Age-Related Differences in Mammography Use and in Breast Cancer Knowledge, Attitudes, and Behaviors." *Journal of Cancer Education,* 1998, *13,* 26–30.

Guidry, J. J., Matthews-Juarez, P., and Copeland, V. A. "Barriers to Breast Cancer Control for African-American Women: The Interdependence of Culture and Psychosocial Issues." *Cancer,* 2003, *97*(1 Suppl), 318–323.

Hochbaum, G. M. *Public Participation in Medical Screening Programs: A Socio-Psychological Study.* Washington, D.C.: U.S. Dept. of Health, Education, and Welfare, 1958.

Hounton, S. H., Carabin, H., and Henderson, N. J. "Towards an Understanding of Barriers to Condom Use in Rural Benin Using the Health Belief Model: A Cross Sectional Survey." *BMC Public Health,* 2005, *5,* 8.

Janz, N. K., and Becker, M. H. "The Health Belief Model: A Decade Later." *Health Education Quarterly,* 1984, *11*(1), 1–47.

King, E. S., and others. "Promoting Mammography Use Through Progressive Interventions: Is It Effective?" *American Journal of Public Health,* 1994, *84*(1), 104–106.

Kirscht, J. P. "The Health Belief Model and Illness Behavior." *Health Education Monographs,* 1974, *2,* 2387–2408.

Laraque, D., and others. "Predictors of Reported Condom Use in Central Harlem Youth as Conceptualized by The Health Belief Model." *Journal of Adolescent Health,* 1997, *21*(5), 318–327.

Lauver, D. R., Settersten, L., Kane, J. H., and Henriques, J. B. "Tailored Messages, External Barriers, and Women's Utilization of Professional Breast Cancer Screening Over Time." *Cancer,* 2003, *97*(11), 2724–2735.

Lee, E. H., Kim, J. S., and Song, M. S. "Translation and Validation of Champion's Health Belief Model Scale with Korean Women." *Cancer Nursing,* 2002, *25*(5), 391–395.

Lewin, K. "The Nature of Field Theory." In M. H. Marx (ed.), *Psychological Theory, Contemporary Readings.* New York: Macmillan, 1951.

Lin, P., Simoni, J., and Zemon, V. "The Health Belief Model, Sexual Behaviors, and HIV Risk among Taiwanese Immigrants." *AIDS Education and Prevention,* 2005, *17,* 469–483.

Lipkus, I., Rimer, B., Halabi, S., and Strigo, T. "Can Tailored Interventions Increase Mammography Use Among HMO Women?" *American Journal of Preventive Medicine,* 2000, *18*(1), 1–10.

Maddux, J. F., Ingram, J. M., and Desmond, D. P. "Reliability of Two Brief Questionnaires for Drug Abuse Treatment Evaluation." *American Journal of Drug and Alcohol Abuse,* 1995, *21*(2), 209–221.

Mahoney, C. A., Thombs, D. L., and Ford, O. J. "Health Belief and Self-Efficacy Models: Their Utility in Explaining College Student Condom Use." *AIDS Education and Prevention,* 1995, *7,* 32–49.

Marcus, A. C., and others. "The Efficacy Of Tailored Print Materials in Promoting Colorectal Cancer Screening: Results from a Randomized Trial Involving Callers to the National Cancer Institute's Cancer Information Service." *Journal of Health Communication,* 2005, *10*(Suppl 1), 83–104.

Mikhail, B.I., and Petro-Nustas, W.I. "Transcultural Adaptation of Champion's Health Belief Model Scales." *Journal of Nursing Scholarship,* 2001, *33,* 159–165.

Phillips, K. A., and others. "Factors Associated with Women's Adherence to Mammography Screening Guidelines." *Health Services Research,* 1998, *33*(1), 29–53.

Rakowski, W., and others. "Reminder Letter, Tailored Stepped-Care, and Self-Choice Comparison for Repeat Mammography." *American Journal of Preventive Medicine,* 2003, *25*(4), 308–314.

Rawl, S., Champion, V., Menon, U., and Foster, J. "The Impact of Age and Race on Mammography Practices." *Health Care for Women International,* 2000, *21,* 583–597.

Rimer, B. K., and others. "Effects of a Mammography Decision-Making Intervention at 12 and 24 Months." *American Journal of Preventive Medicine,* 2002, *22*(4), 247–257.

Rogers, R. W., and Prentice-Dunn, S. *Protection Motivation Theory.* New York: Plenum, 1997.

Ronis, D. L. "Conditional Health Threats: Health Beliefs, Decisions, and Behaviors Among Adults." *Health Psychology,* 1992, *11*(2), 127–134.

Rosenstock, I. M. "What Research in Motivation Suggests for Public Health." *American Journal of Public Health,* 1960, *50,* 295–302.

Rosenstock, I. M. "The Health Belief Model and Preventive Health Behavior." *Health Education Monographs,* 1974, *2*(4), 354–386.

Rosenstock, I. M., Strecher, V. J., and Becker, M. H. "Social Learning Theory and the Health Belief Model." *Health Education Quarterly,* 1988, *15*(2), 175–183.

Rosenstock, I. M., Strecher, V. J., and Becker, M. H. "The Health Belief Model and HIV Risk Behavior Change." In J. Peterson and R. DiClemente (eds.), *Preventing AIDS: Theory and Practice of Behavioral Interventions.* New York: Plenum, 1994.

Saywell, R. M., Jr., and others. "The Cost Effectiveness of 5 Interventions to Increase Mammography Adherence in a Managed Care Population." *The American Journal of Managed Care,* 2003, *9,* 33–44.

Secginli, S., and Nahcivan, N. O. "Reliability and Validity of the Breast Cancer Screening Belief Scale Among Turkish Women." *Cancer Nursing,* 2004, *27,* 287–294.

Siegel, D. M., Aten, M. J., and Enaharo, M. "Long-term Effects of a Middle School- and High School-Based Human Immunodeficiency Virus Sexual Risk Prevention Intervention." *Archive of Pediatric and Adolescent Medicine,* 2001, *155*(10), 1117–1126.

Skinner, B. F. *The Behavior of Organisms.* Englewood Cliffs, N.J.: Appleton-Century-Crofts, 1938.

Skinner, C. S., Arfken, C. L., and Sykes, R. K. "Knowledge, Perceptions, and Mammography Stage of Adoption Among Older Urban Women." *American Journal of Preventive Medicine,* 1998, *14*(1), 54–63.

Skinner, C. S., Champion, V. L., Menon, U., and Seshadri, R. "Racial and Educational Differences in Mammography-Related Perceptions Among 1,336 Nonadherent Women." *Journal of Psychosocial Oncology,* 2002, *20,* 1–18.

Skinner, C. S., Strecher, V. J., and Hospers, H. "Physicians' Recommendations for Mammography: Do Tailored Messages Make a Difference?" *American Journal of Public Health,* 1994, *84,* 43–49.

Skinner, C. S., and others. "Learn, Share, and Live: Breast Cancer Education for Older, Urban Minority Women." *Health Education and Behavior,* 1998, *25*(1), 60–78.

Steers, W. N., and others. "Health Beliefs as Predictors of HIV-Preventive Behavior and Ethnic Differences in Prediction." *Journal of Social Psychology,* 1996, *136*(1), 99–110.

Tang, T. S., Solomon, L. J., and McCracken, L. M. "Cultural Barriers to Mammography, Clinical Breast Exam, and Breast Self-Exam Among Chinese-American Women 60 and Older." *Preventive Medicine,* 2000, *31*(5), 575–583.

Thompson, B., and others. "Attitudes and Beliefs Toward Mammography Among Women Using an Urban Public Hospital." *Journal of Health Care for the Poor and Underserved,* 1997, *8*(2), 186–201.

Tolman, E. C. *Purposive Behavior in Animals and Men.* New York: Appleton-Century-Crofts, 1932.

Vadaparampil, S. T., and others. "Using the Health Belief Model to Examine Differences in Adherence to Mammography Among African-American and Caucasian Women." *Journal of Psychosocial Oncology,* 2004, *21*(4), 61–81.

Valanis, B., and others. "Screening Rarely Screened Women: Time-To-Service and 24-Month Outcomes of Tailored Interventions." *Preventive Medicine,* 2003, *37*(5), 442–450.

Volk, J. E., and Koopman, C. "Factors Associated with Condom Use in Kenya: A Test of the Health Belief Model." *The AIDS Education and Prevention Journal,* 2001, *13,* 495–508.

Wardle, J., and others. "Increasing Attendance at Colorectal Cancer Screening: Testing the Efficacy of a Mailed, Psychoeducational Intervention in a Community Sample of Older Adults." *Health Psychology,* 2003, *22*(1), 99–105.

Watson, J. B. *Behaviorism.* New York: Norton, 1925.

Weinstein, N. D. "Testing Four Competing Theories of Health-Protective Behavior." *Health Psychology,* 1993, *12*(4), 324–333.

Wight, D., Abraham, C., and Scott, S. "Towards a Psycho-Social Theoretical Framework for Sexual Health Promotion." *Health Education Research,* 1998, *13*(3), 317–330.

Witte, K. "Putting the Fear Back Into Fear Appeals: The Extended Parallel Process Model." *Communication Monographs,* 1992, *59*(4), 329–349.

Wu, T. Y., and Yu, M. Y. "Reliability and Validity of the Mammography Screening Beliefs Questionnaire Among Chinese American Women." *Cancer Nursing,* 2003, *26,* 131–142.

Wulfert, E., Wan, C. K., and Backus, C. A. "Gay Men's Safer Sex Behavior: An Integration of Three Models." *Journal of Behavioral Medicine,* 1996, *19*(4), 345–366.

Zak-Place, J., and Stern, M. "Health Belief Factors and Dispositional Optimism as Predictors of STD and HIV Preventive Behavior." *Journal of College Health,* 2004, *52,* 229–236.

CHAPTER

4

THEORY OF REASONED ACTION, THEORY OF PLANNED BEHAVIOR, AND THE INTEGRATED BEHAVIORAL MODEL

Daniel E. Montaño

Danuta Kasprzyk

KEY POINTS

This chapter will

- Describe the historical development of the Theory of Reasoned Action (TRA), Theory of Planned Behavior (TPB), and Integrated Behavioral Model (IBM).
- Describe and explain the main constructs in the TRA, TPB, and IBM.
- Explain the similarity between these theories' key constructs and constructs from other behavioral theories.
- Describe measurement of the key constructs of TRA, TPB, and IBM.
- Explain how and why elicitation should be conducted to identify and select the content for the model construct measures for the health behavior and population studied.

■ Provide a cross-cultural application to understand condom use behavior among rural Zimbabweans, and to use the findings to design messages for behavior change interventions.

The Theory of Reasoned Action (TRA) and the Theory of Planned Behavior (TPB) focus on theoretical constructs concerned with individual motivational factors as determinants of the likelihood of performing a specific behavior. TRA and TPB both assume the best predictor of a behavior is behavioral intention, which in turn is determined by attitude toward the behavior and social normative perceptions regarding it. TPB is an extension of the TRA and includes an additional construct: perceived control over performance of the behavior. In recent years, Fishbein and colleagues have further expanded TRA and TPB to include components from other major behavioral theories and have proposed use of an Integrated Behavioral Model (IBM).

The TRA and TPB, which focus on the constructs of attitude, subjective norm, and perceived control, explain a large proportion of the variance in behavioral intention and predict a number of different behaviors, including health behaviors. Evidence comes from hundreds of studies that have been summarized in several meta-analyses and reviews (Armitage and Conner, 2001; Albarracin, Johnson, Fishbein, and Muellerleile, 2001; Albarracin and others, 2003; Albarracin, Kumkale, and Johnson, 2004; Albarracin and others, 2005; Downs and Hausenblas, 2005; Durantini and others, 2006; Hardeman and others, 2002; Sheeran and Taylor, 1999; Webb and Sheeran, 2006). Although TRA and TPB have been criticized, based on whether correlational results can explain behavior (Weinstein, 2007), many published intervention study reports show that changing TRA or TPB constructs leads to subsequent change in behaviors (Albarracin and others, 2003, 2005; Jemmott, Jemmott, and Fong, 1992; Kamb and others, 1998; Rhodes and others, 2007; Kalichman, 2007). TRA and TPB have been used successfully to predict and explain a wide range of health behaviors and intentions, including smoking, drinking, health services utilization, exercise, sun protection, breastfeeding, substance use, HIV/STD-prevention behaviors and use of contraceptives, mammography, safety helmets, and seatbelts (Albarracin, Fishbein, and Goldestein de Muchinik, 1997; Albarracin, Johnson, Fishbein, and Muellerleile, 2001; Bandawe and Foster, 1996; Bosompra, 2001; Bogart, Cecil, and Pinkerton, 2000; Fishbein, 1993; Montaño and Taplin, 1991; Morrison, Spencer, and Gillmore, 1998; Steen, Peay, and Owen, 1998; Trafimow, 1996). Findings have been used to develop many effective behavior change interventions (Fishbein, 1990; Fisher, Fisher, and Rye, 1995; Gastil, 2000; Hardeman and others, 2005; Jemmott, Jemmott, and Fong, 1992; Jemmott and Jemmott, 2000).

ORIGINS AND HISTORICAL DEVELOPMENT

TRA was developed to better understand relationships between attitudes, intentions, and behaviors (Fishbein, 1967). Many previous studies of these relationships found relatively low correspondence between attitudes and behavior, and some theorists proposed eliminating attitude as a factor underlying behavior (Fishbein, 1993; see, for example, Abelson, 1972; Wicker, 1969). In the work that led to development of the TRA, Fishbein distinguished between attitude toward an object and attitude toward a behavior with respect to that object. For example, most attitude theorists were measuring attitude toward an object (such as an attitude toward cancer) in trying to predict a behavior (such as mammography or breast cancer screening). Fishbein demonstrated that attitude toward the behavior (for example, attitude toward mammography) is a much better predictor of that behavior (obtaining mammography) than attitude toward the object (cancer) at which the behavior is directed (Fishbein and Ajzen, 1975).

Fishbein and Ajzen (Fishbein and Ajzen,1975; Ajzen and Fishbein,1980; Ajzen, 1991) clearly defined underlying beliefs (behavioral and normative), intentions, and behavior and their measurement. They have shown that it is critical to have a high degree of correspondence between measures of attitude, norm, perceived control, intention, and behavior in terms of action (for example, go get), target (for example, a mammogram), context (for example, at the breast screening center), and time (for example, in the next twelve months). A change in any of these factors results in a different behavior being explained. Low correspondence between model construct measures on any of these factors will result in low correlations between TRA/TPB variables, while high correspondence will result in high correlations (Ajzen and Albarracin, 2007; Trafimow, 2007).

Operationalization of TRA constructs was developed from a long history of attitude measurement theory rooted in the concept that an attitude (toward an object or an action) is determined by expectations or beliefs concerning attributes of the object or action and evaluations of those attributes. This expectancy-value conceptualization has been applied extensively in psychology in many areas, including learning theories, attitude theories, and decision-making theories (Rotter, 1954; Rosenberg, 1956; Edwards, 1954).

In addition to TRA and TPB, a modest number of behavioral theories and models have been used most often to investigate health behaviors (Glanz, Rimer, and Lewis, 2002), including Social Cognitive Theory (see Chapter Eight), Health Belief Model (HBM; see Chapter Three), theory of subjective culture (Triandis, 1972), and The Transtheoretical Model (TTM; see Chapter Five). Though many constructs in these theories are similar or complementary, too much attention has been paid to their differences (Weinstein, 1993). Thus, the National Institutes of Mental Health (NIMH) sponsored a workshop with the primary architects of several of these theories, to develop a theoretical framework to integrate their constructs (Fishbein and others, 1992).

At the same time, we carried out a longitudinal study of HIV-prevention behaviors in collaboration with Fishbein, in which we developed an integrated model that coincided substantially with the recommendations resulting from the NIMH theorists' workshop (Kasprzyk, Montaño, and Fishbein, 1998). With increased interest in theory integration, Fishbein and colleagues have described an integrative model focusing primarily on the determinants of behavioral intention (Fishbein, 2000; Fishbein and Cappella, 2006). The 2002 Institute of Medicine (IOM) report, *Speaking of Health,* recommended an integrated model for using communication strategies to change health behavior (IOM, 2002). Based on this work and on our experience with several studies over the past ten years, we propose use of the Integrated Behavioral Model (IBM) as a further extension of the TRA and TPB and describe it in this chapter.

THEORY OF REASONED ACTION AND THEORY OF PLANNED BEHAVIOR

TRA asserts that the most important determinant of *behavior* is *behavioral intention* (see unshaded boxes in Figure 4.1). Direct determinants of individuals' behavioral intention are their *attitude* toward performing the behavior and their *subjective norm* associated with the behavior. TPB adds *perceived control* over the behavior, taking into account situations where one may not have complete volitional control over a behavior (see shaded boxes in Figure 4.1).

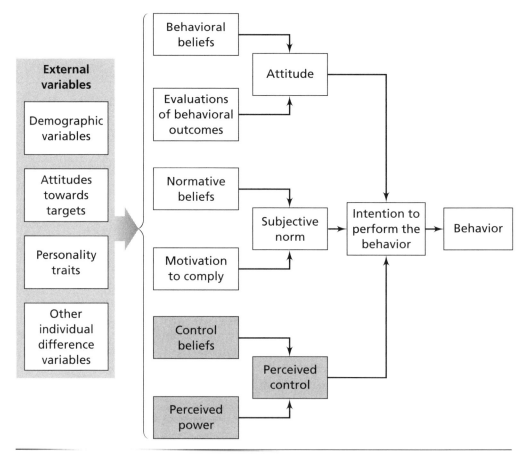

FIGURE 4.1. Theory of Reasoned Action and Theory of Planned Behavior.*

*Note: Upper light area shows the Theory of Reasoned Action; entire figure shows the Theory of Planned Behavior.

Attitude is determined by the individual's beliefs about outcomes or attributes of performing the behavior (*behavioral beliefs*), weighted by evaluations of those outcomes or attributes. Thus, a person who holds strong beliefs that positively valued outcomes will result from performing the behavior will have a positive attitude toward the behavior. Conversely, a person who holds strong beliefs that negatively valued outcomes will result from the behavior will have a negative attitude.

Similarly, a person's subjective norm is determined by his or her *normative beliefs,* that is, whether important referent individuals approve or disapprove of performing the behavior, weighted by his or her motivation to comply with those referents. A person who believes that certain referents think she should perform a behavior and is motivated to meet expectations of those referents will hold a positive subjective norm. Conversely, a person who believes these referents think she should *not* perform the behavior will have a negative subjective norm, and a person who is less motivated to comply with those referents will have a relatively neutral subjective norm.

TRA assumes that the most important direct determinant of behavior is behavioral intention. Success of the theory in explaining behavior depends on the degree to which the behavior is under volitional control (that is, individuals can exercise a large degree of control over the behavior). It is not clear that the TRA components are sufficient to predict behaviors in which volitional control is reduced. Thus, Ajzen and colleagues (Ajzen, 1991; Ajzen and Driver, 1991; Ajzen and Madden, 1986) added *perceived behavioral control* to TRA to account for factors outside individual control that may affect intentions and behaviors. With this addition, they created the Theory of Planned Behavior (TPB; see shaded boxes in Figure 4.1). Perceived control is determined by *control beliefs* concerning the presence or absence of facilitators and barriers to behavioral performance, weighted by their perceived power or the impact of each control factor to facilitate or inhibit the behavior.

Ajzen's inclusion of perceived control (Ajzen, 1991) was based in part on the idea that behavioral performance is determined jointly by motivation (intention) and ability (behavioral control). A person's perception of control over behavioral performance, together with intention, is expected to have a direct effect on behavior, particularly when perceived control is an accurate assessment of actual control over the behavior and when volitional control is not high. The effect of perceived control declines, and intention is a sufficient behavioral predictor in situations in which volitional control over the behavior is high (Madden, Ellen, and Ajzen, 1992). Thus, similar to Triandis's (1980) conceptualization of facilitating conditions, perceived control is expected to moderate the effect of intention on behavior. However, this interaction hypothesis has received very little empirical support (Ajzen, 1991; Yzer, 2007).

TPB also postulates that perceived control is an independent determinant of behavioral intention, along with attitude toward the behavior and subjective norm. Holding attitude and subjective norm constant, a person's perception of the ease or difficulty of behavioral performance will affect his behavioral intention. Relative weights of these three factors in determining intentions should vary for different behaviors and populations. Few studies have operationalized perceived control using the underlying measures of control beliefs and perceived power; instead, researchers have mostly used the direct measure of perceived control (Ajzen, 2002).

TRA and TPB assume a causal chain that links behavioral beliefs, normative beliefs, and control beliefs to behavioral intentions and behaviors via attitudes, subjective norms, and perceived control. Hypothesized causal relationships among model components are clearly specified, and measurement and computation are delineated by Ajzen and Fishbein (Ajzen and Fishbein, 1980; Ajzen, 1991; Ajzen, 2006). This is one of the major strengths of the TRA/TPB approach. Other factors, including demographic and environmental characteristics, are assumed to operate through model constructs and do not independently contribute to explain the likelihood of performing a behavior.

Measures of TRA and TPB Constructs

TRA and TPB measures can use either 5- or 7-point scales. A person's behavioral beliefs about the likelihood that performance of the behavior will result in certain outcomes are measured on bipolar "unlikely-likely" or "disagree-agree" scales. Evaluations of each outcome are measured on bipolar "good-bad" scales. For example, one outcome of "my quitting smoking" may be that this "will cause me to gain weight." A person's behavioral belief about this outcome is measured by having him rate the likelihood that "my quitting smoking will cause me to gain weight." The person's evaluation of this outcome is measured by having him rate the degree to which "my gaining weight" is good versus bad. These behavioral belief and evaluation ratings are usually scored from −3 to +3, capturing the psychology of double negatives, where a belief that a behavior will *not* result in a negative outcome contributes positively to the person's attitude. An "indirect measure" of the person's attitude toward performing the behavior is computed by first multiplying her behavioral belief concerning each outcome by her corresponding outcome evaluation ratings and then summing these product scores across all outcomes of the behavior.

In the example, a person may believe that "quitting smoking" is very unlikely to result in "gaining weight" (belief scored as −3), and may evaluate gaining weight as very bad (evaluation scored as −3), resulting in a belief-evaluation product score of +9. Thus, the strong belief that performing the behavior will *not* result in (will avoid) a negatively valued outcome contributes just as positively to the person's attitude as would a strong belief that the action will result (+3) in a positively valued (+3) outcome (product = +9). Conversely, a strong belief that the behavior will *not* result (−3) in a positively valued outcome (+3) contributes negatively (product = −9) to the person's attitude, because performance of the behavior will *not* achieve a highly valued outcome. In the example of "quitting smoking," beliefs and evaluations of *all* salient outcomes of this behavior will enter into the computation of an indirect measure of the person's attitude.

Similarly, a person's normative beliefs about whether each referent thinks he should perform the behavior are measured on bipolar scales scored −3 to +3, while the person's motivation to comply with each referent is measured on unipolar scales scored 1 to 7. For example, one potential referent with regard to "quitting smoking" might be the person's best friend. A person's normative belief concerning his best friend is measured by asking him to rate the degree to which he believes his best friend thinks he should versus should not quit smoking. Motivation to comply is measured by having the person rate his agreement versus disagreement with the statement: "Generally, I want to do what my best friend thinks I should do." An indirect measure of the person's subjective norm is computed by multiplying his normative belief about each referent by his motivation to comply with that referent and then summing these product scores across all referents.

Applications of TPB suggest that control beliefs regarding each factor should be measured on a bipolar likelihood of occurrence scale scored −3 to +3. Perceived power of each factor is measured on a bipolar "easy-difficult" scale (Terry, Gallois, and McCamish, 1993; Ajzen, 1991). For example, some individuals might identify "restaurant smoking restrictions" as a factor that affects their perceived behavioral control over quitting smoking. A person's control belief regarding this factor is measured by having her rate her likelihood of encountering "a restaurant smoking restriction," while perceived power is measured by having the person rate her perception of the effect of "restaurant smoking restrictions" in making it easier versus more difficult to quit smoking. These measures are obtained for all factors identified as facilitating or impeding the behavior. An "indirect measure" of the person's perceived behavioral control is then computed by multiplying each control belief by the corresponding perceived power (impact) rating, and then summing these product scores across all control factors (Ajzen and Driver, 1991).

In addition to the indirect measures computed from behavioral, normative, and control beliefs, it is important to obtain a "direct measure" of each model component. Table 4.1 summarizes the direct and indirect measures of attitudes, subjective norms, and perceived behavioral control. A direct measure of attitude toward performing the behavior is obtained using semantic differential scale items, such as "good-bad" and "pleasant-unpleasant," and summing them. A direct measure of subjective norm uses a single item, asking the person to rate "Most people important to me think I should" perform the behavior. This rating is made on a bipolar "unlikely-likely" or "agree-disagree" scale. The direct measure of perceived behavioral control generally uses semantic differential scale items such as "under my control–not under my control" and "easy-difficult."

These direct measures are important for two reasons. First, direct measures are usually more strongly associated with intentions and behaviors than indirect measures. The associations between the "direct" measures and behavioral intention indicate the relative importance of attitude, subjective norm, and perceived control in explaining or predicting a given behavior. It is important to demonstrate these associations before analyzing indirect measures. Second, indirect measures should be associated strongly with direct measures to be assured that appropriate beliefs were included in the indirect measures and that the composite beliefs (behavioral, normative, and control) are adequate measures of respective TRA/TPB constructs. Once this is demonstrated, indirect measures are of most interest. Behavioral, normative, and control beliefs help us understand what drives behaviors and provide a focus for intervention messages (von Haeften, Fishbein, Kasprzyk, and Montaño, 2001; Fishbein and Cappella, 2006). The process of assessing which construct is most closely related to behavioral intention and deciding which behavioral, normative, and control

TABLE 4.1. **TRA, TPB, and IBM Constructs and Definitions.**

	Construct	Definition	Measure
	Behavioral Intention	Perceived likelihood of performing the behavior	Bipolar unlikely-likely scale; scored −3 to +3
Attitude	*Experiential Attitude (Affect)* Direct Measure:	Overall affective evaluation of the behavior	Semantic differential scales: for example, pleasant-unpleasant; enjoyable-unenjoyable
	Indirect Measure: Behavioral belief	Belief that behavioral performance is associated with certain positive or negative feelings	Bipolar unlikely-likely scale; scored −3 to +3
	Instrumental Attitude Direct Measure:	Overall evaluation of the behavior	Semantic differential scales: for example, good-bad; wise-foolish
	Indirect Measure: Behavioral belief	Belief that behavioral performance is associated with certain attributes or outcomes	Bipolar unlikely-likely scale; scored −3 to +3
	Evaluation	Value attached to a behavioral outcome or attribute	Bipolar bad-good scale; scored −3 to +3
Perceived Norm	*Subjective (Injunctive) Norm* Direct Measure:	Belief about whether most people approve or disapprove of the behavior	Bipolar disagree-agree scale; scored −3 to +3
	Indirect Measure: Normative belief	Belief about whether each referent approves or disapproves of the behavior	Bipolar disagree-agree scale; scored −3 to +3
	Motivation to comply	Motivation to do what each referent thinks	Unipolar unlikely-likely scale; scored 1 to 7
	Descriptive Norm Direct Measure:	Belief about whether most people perform the behavior	Bipolar disagree-agree scale; scored −3 to +3
	Indirect Measure: Normative belief	Belief about whether each referent performs the behavior	Bipolar disagree-agree scale; scored −3 to +3

TABLE 4.1. TRA, TPB, and IBM Constructs and Definitions, Cont'd.

	Construct	Definition	Measure
Personal Agency	*Perceived Behavioral Control*		
	Direct Measure:	Overall measure of perceived control over the behavior	Semantic differential scales: for example, under my control–not under my control; easy-difficult
	Indirect Measure: Control belief	Perceived likelihood of occurrence of each facilitating or constraining condition	Unlikely-likely scale; scored –3 to +3 or 1 to 7
	Perceived power	Perceived effect of each condition in making behavioral performance difficult or easy	Bipolar difficult-easy scale; scored –3 to +3
	Self-Efficacy		
	Direct Measure:	Overall measure of ability to perform behavior	Certain I could not–certain I could scale for overall behavior; scored –3 to +3 or 1 to 7
	Indirect Measure: Self-efficacy belief	Perceived ability to overcome each facilitating or constraining condition	Certain I could not–certain I could scale; scored –3 to +3 or 1 to 7

Note: TRA/TPB constructs are shaded.

beliefs should be used to focus intervention messages is illustrated in the theory application example that follows.

Research Designs and Analytical Approaches to Testing TRA/TPB

A prospective study design is recommended to discern relationships between constructs, with attitudes, subjective norms, perceived control, and intentions measured at one time point and behavior measured following a time interval. Cross-sectional studies are often used to test the TRA/TPB, but they may provide poor prediction and understanding of previous behavior because the time order of motivations and behavior cannot be discerned. Regression and structural equation analytic methods are usually used to test relationships in the TRA/TPB (Rhodes and others, 2007; Bryan, Schmiege, and Broaddus, 2007). Relative weights of model constructs are determined empirically for the particular behavior and population under investigation. This information provides guidance as to which constructs are most important to target for behavior change effort. Some behaviors are entirely under attitudinal control (Albarracin and others, 2003), while others are under normative control (Albarracin, Kumkale, and Johnson, 2004; Durantini and others, 2006) or perceived control (Albarracin and others, 2005; Yzer, 2007). For example, in a study of adults over age forty, McLallen and Fishbein found colonoscopy intention to be almost completely under normative control, whereas exercise intention was influenced by both attitudes and perceived control (Fishbein and Cappella, 2006). Similarly, a behavior may be under attitudinal control in one population but under normative control in another population (Fishbein, 1990, Fishbein, von Haeften, and Appleyard, 2001). Our research found that condom use with a main partner is primarily under normative control for female injecting drug users but influenced by attitude, norm, and perceived control for females who do not inject drugs (von Haeften and Kenski, 2001; Kenski and others, 2001). Once the significant constructs are identified, analyses of the beliefs underlying those constructs can determine which specific behavioral, normative, or control beliefs are most strongly associated with intention and behavior, thus providing empirically identified targets for intervention efforts.

Uses for and Evidence to Support TRA/TPB

The name *Theory of Reasoned Action* has often led to the misrepresentation that the focus is purely on "rational behavior" (for example, St. Lawrence and Fortenberry, 2007). This is far from correct. A fundamental assumption of TRA is that individuals are "rational actors" who process information and that underlying reasons determine motivation to perform a behavior. These reasons, made up of a person's behavioral, normative, and control beliefs, determine his attitudes, subjective norms, and perceived control, regardless of whether those beliefs are rational, logical, or correct by some objective standard. (See Fishbein, 2007, for additional discussion regarding this aspect of the TRA/TPB.) A strength of TRA/TPB is that they provide a framework to discern those reasons and to decipher individuals' actions by identifying, measuring, and combining beliefs relevant to individuals or groups, allowing us to understand their own reasons that motivate the behavior of interest. TRA and TPB do not specify particular beliefs about behavioral outcomes, normative referents, or control beliefs that should be measured. As noted in the examples, relevant behavioral outcomes, referents, and control beliefs will likely be different for different populations and behaviors.

TRA and TPB provide a framework to identify key behavioral, normative, and control beliefs affecting behaviors. Interventions can then be designed to target and change these beliefs or the value placed on them, thereby affecting attitude, subjective norm, or perceived control and leading to changes in intentions and behaviors.

TRA/TPB has been applied to explain a variety of health behaviors, including exercise, smoking and drug use, HIV/STD-prevention behaviors, mammography use, clinicians' recommendation of and provision of preventive services, and oral hygiene behaviors. These studies generally have supported perceived control as a direct predictor of both intentions and behaviors (Albarracin, Johnson, Fishbein, and Mueller-leile, 2001; Ajzen, 1991; Blue, 1995; Craig, Goldberg, and Dietz, 1996; Godin and Kok, 1996; Millstein, 1996; Montaño, Phillips, and Kasprzyk, 2000; Montaño, Thompson, Taylor, and Mahloch, 1997). However, most studies have used direct measures of perceived control, rather than computing perceived control from measures of control beliefs and perceived power concerning specific facilitators and constraints. The few studies that have measured control beliefs (indirect measure) found them to be important predictors of intentions and behaviors (Ajzen and Driver, 1991; Kasprzyk, Montaño, and Fishbein, 1998). Clearly, if perceived behavioral control is an important determinant of intentions or behaviors, knowledge of the effects of control beliefs concerning each facilitator or constraint would be useful in the development of interventions.

AN INTEGRATED BEHAVIORAL MODEL

As noted previously, we recommend use of an integrated behavioral model that includes constructs from TRA/TPB, as well as from other influential theories (Figure 4.2). As in TRA/TPB, the most important determinant of behavior in the IBM is intention to

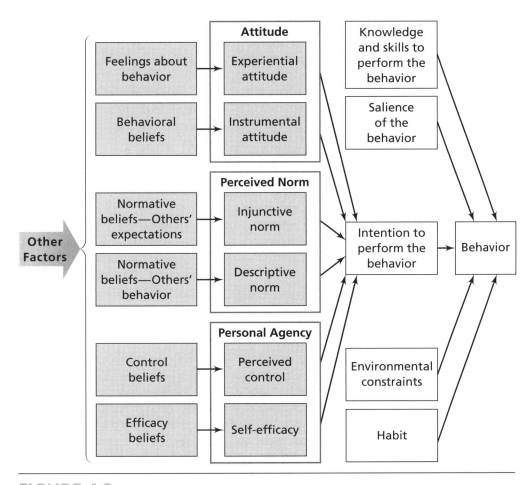

FIGURE 4.2. Integrated Behavior Model.

perform the behavior. Without motivation, a person is unlikely to carry out a recommended behavior. Four other components directly affect behavior (Jaccard, Dodge, and Dittus, 2002). Three of these are important in determining whether behavioral intentions can result in behavioral performance. First, even if a person has a strong behavioral intention, she needs knowledge and skill to carry out the behavior. Second, there should be no or few environmental constraints that make behavioral performance very difficult or impossible (Triandis, 1980). Third, behavior should be salient to the person (Becker, 1974). Finally, experience performing the behavior may make it habitual, so that intention becomes less important in determining behavioral performance for that individual (Triandis, 1980).

Thus, a particular behavior is most likely to occur if (1) a person has a strong intention to perform it and the knowledge and skill to do so, (2) there is no serious environmental constraint preventing performance, (3) the behavior is salient, and (4) the person has performed the behavior previously. All these components and their interactions are important to consider when designing interventions to promote health behaviors. For example, if a woman has a strong intention to get a mammogram, it is important to ensure that she has sufficient knowledge of her health care system to act on this intention and that no serious environmental constraints, such as lack of transportation or limited clinic hours, may prevent her from getting the mammogram. For an action that is carried out between long intervals, such as mammography, the behavior must also be made salient, or cued, so that she will remember to carry out her intention. For other behaviors that are to be performed more often and that may be under habitual control, environmental constraints must similarly be removed to promote behavioral performance. A careful analysis should be conducted of the behavior and population studied to determine which of these components are most important to target to promote the behavior. Very different strategies may be needed for different behaviors, as well as for the same behavior in different settings or populations.

Clearly, strong behavioral intentions are required for an intervention addressing model components, such as skills or environmental constraints, to affect behavioral performance. According to the model, behavioral intention is determined by three construct categories listed in Table 4.1. The first is *attitude toward the behavior,* defined as a person's overall favorableness or unfavorableness toward performing the behavior. Many theorists have described attitude as composed of affective and cognitive dimensions (Triandis, 1980; Fishbein, 2007; French and others, 2005). Experiential attitude or affect (Fishbein, 2007) is the individual's emotional response to the idea of performing a recommended behavior. Individuals with a strong negative emotional response to the behavior are unlikely to perform it, whereas those with a strong positive emotional reaction are more likely to engage in it. Instrumental attitude is cognitively based, determined by beliefs about outcomes of behavioral performance, as in the TRA/TPB. Conceptualization of experiential attitude (affect) is different from "mood or arousal," which Fishbein (2007) argues may affect intention indirectly by influencing perceptions of behavioral outcome likelihood or evaluation of outcomes.

Second, *perceived norm* reflects the social pressure one feels to perform or not perform a particular behavior. Fishbein (2007) indicates that subjective norm, as defined in TRA/TPB as an injunctive norm (normative beliefs about what others think one should do and motivation to comply), may not fully capture normative influence. In addition, perceptions about what others in one's social or personal networks are doing (descriptive norm) may also be an important part of normative influence. This construct captures the strong social identity in certain cultures which, according to some theorists, is an indicator of normative influence (Bagozzi and Lee, 2002; Triandis, 1980; Triandis and others, 1988). Both injunctive and descriptive norm components are included in Figure 4.2.

Finally, *personal agency,* described by Bandura (2006) as bringing one's influence to bear on one's own functioning and environmental events, was proposed in the IOM report, *Speaking of Health,* as a major factor influencing behavioral intention (IOM, 2002). In IBM, personal agency consists of two constructs—self-efficacy and perceived control. Perceived control, as described previously, is one's perceived amount of control over behavioral performance, determined by one's perception of the degree to which various environmental factors make it easy versus difficult to carry out the behavior. In contrast, self-efficacy is one's degree of confidence in the ability to perform the behavior in the face of various obstacles or challenges. This is measured by having respondents rate their behavioral confidence on bipolar "certain I could not–certain I could" scales (see Table 4.1). Although only a few studies have discussed the similarities and differences between these two constructs (Ajzen, 2002; Fishbein, 2007), our studies suggest the utility of including both measures.

The relative importance of the three categories of theoretical constructs (attitude, perceived norm, personal agency) in determining behavioral intention may vary for different behaviors and for different populations. For example, intention to perform one behavior may be primarily determined by attitude toward the behavior, while another behavioral intention may be determined largely by normative influence. Similarly, intention to perform a particular behavior may be primarily under attitudinal influence in one population, while more influenced by normative influence or personal agency in another population. Thus, to design effective interventions to influence behavioral intentions, it is important first to determine the degree to which that intention is influenced by attitude (experiential and instrumental), perceived norm (injunctive and descriptive), and personal agency (self-efficacy and perceived control). Once this is understood for a particular behavior and population, an understanding of the determinants of those constructs also is essential.

Instrumental and experiential attitudes, injunctive and descriptive norms, self-efficacy, and perceived control are all functions of underlying beliefs. As seen in Figure 4.2, instrumental attitudes are a function of beliefs about outcomes of performing the behavior, as described earlier in the TRA and TPB. The stronger one's beliefs that performing the behavior will lead to positive outcomes and prevent negative outcomes, the more favorable one's attitude will be toward performing the behavior in question. In contrast to TRA and TPB, evaluation of outcomes is not specified in this model. Research suggests that, for many health behaviors, there is very little variance in people's evaluations of behavioral outcomes (von Haeften, Fishbein, Kasprzyk, and Montaño, 2001; von Haeften and Kenski, 2001; Fishbein, von Haeften, and Appleyard,

2001; Kasprzyk and Montaño, 2007). If most people agree in their evaluations of the various behavioral outcomes, there is little benefit in measuring outcome evaluations. However, if preliminary study of a behavior indicates individual variation in outcome evaluations, this measure should be assessed.

Perceived norms are a function of normative beliefs, as in the TRA and TPB. The stronger one's beliefs that specific individuals or groups think one should perform the behavior or that others are performing the behavior, the stronger one's perception of social pressure to carry out the behavior. Again, in contrast to TRA/TPB, motivation to comply with individuals or groups is not specified in the IBM because, as with outcome evaluations, we have found that there is often little variance in these measures. However, if variance is found in motivation to comply, this should also be measured. Perceived control, as described earlier in the TPB, is a function of control beliefs about the likelihood of occurrence of various facilitating or constraining conditions, weighted by the perceived effect of those conditions in making behavioral performance easy or difficult. Finally, the stronger one's beliefs that one can perform the behavior despite various specific barriers, the greater one's self-efficacy about carrying out the behavior.

Most important in the application of the IBM as a framework to identify specific belief targets for behavior change interventions is the conceptualization of experiential and instrumental attitudes, injunctive and descriptive norms, and perceived control and self-efficacy being determined by specific underlying beliefs. This is described in detail in the application that follows. Interventions built on one model construct may have effects that further affect the same or other model constructs. For example, by changing normative beliefs, one may be sufficiently motivated to engage in the behavior once. If this is a positive experience, it may result in more positive behavioral beliefs, as well as positive emotional feelings about the behavior, leading to stronger future intention with respect to the behavior.

Application of the IBM and TRA/TPB to Diverse Behaviors and Populations

Often, very different behavioral, normative, efficacy, and control beliefs affect one's intention to engage in different behaviors. For example, behavioral beliefs about getting a mammogram (such as the belief that it will be painful) are likely to be very different from the relevant behavioral beliefs about using a condom with one's partner (such as the belief that it will cause my partner to think I don't trust her or him). These relevant underlying beliefs may also be very different for similar behaviors, such as using condoms with one's main partner versus using condoms with a commercial sex partner. Just as important, the relevant underlying beliefs for a particular behavior may be very different for different populations. For this reason, Fishbein has emphasized repeatedly that although an investigator can sit in an office and develop measures of attitudes, perceived norms, self-efficacy, and perceived control, this process may not identify the correct beliefs relevant to the behavior or the population (Fishbein, 2000; Fishbein and Cappella, 2006). One must go to the population to identify salient behavioral, normative, efficacy, and control beliefs associated with the behavior.

Thus, an essential step in the application of this model is to conduct interviews with the population being studied to elicit information about the behavioral, normative, efficacy, and control beliefs for that behavior and population. Once these are identified, appropriate measures of the IBM constructs can be designed for that particular behavior and population, a quantitative survey using those measures conducted, and analyses carried out to identify the specific beliefs that best explain behavioral intention. These steps are described in the application that follows.

Although TRA, TPB, and IBM are sometimes denigrated as being "Western" and not applicable to other cultures (Airhihenbuwa and Obregon, 2000), the elicitation process is exactly what makes the model applicable to all cultures. The theoretical constructs in Figure 4.2 are relevant to behaviors across cultures, having been studied in over fifty countries in both the developed and developing world (Fishbein, 2000). It is the specific beliefs underlying these constructs that must be specific to the behavior and population being investigated. Failure to elicit these beliefs from the population, with investigators often measuring beliefs that *they* think should be relevant, is the reason that some investigators have concluded that the model is Western and not appropriate cross-culturally. In applying the models, it is critical to investigate and understand the behavior from the perspective of the study population (Fishbein, 2000).

Finally, as noted in the descriptions of TRA and TPB, other demographic, personality, attitudinal, and individual difference variables may be associated with behaviors, but their influence is indirect, through the theoretical constructs. They are considered distal variables. Thus, certain demographic groups may be more likely than others to engage in the behavior, because there are demographic differences on the proximal variables. For example, individuals in certain demographic groups may be more likely than other demographic groups to hold beliefs about positive outcomes of the behavior, and thus hold more positive attitudes and stronger intention to carry out the behavior. Therefore, these variables are shown in Figure 4.2 as external variables, because they are not considered to have a direct effect on intention or behavior. It is important to investigate and understand how belief patterns may differ among various groups, based on these external variables, as it may be useful to segment the population on such distal variables and to design different interventions for different segments if there are clear differences in belief patterns.

IBM has been used to understand behavioral intention and behavior for condom use and other HIV/STD-prevention behaviors (Kasprzyk, Montaño, and Fishbein, 1998; Kenski and others, 2001; von Haeften, Fishbein, Kasprzyk, and Montaño, 2001; Kasprzyk and Montaño, 2007). The model also has served as the theoretical framework for two large multi-site intervention studies, the AIDS Community Demonstration Projects (CDC, 1999) and Project Respect (Kamb and others, 1998; Rhodes and others, 2007). The model was used to identify issues to target by these interventions, while the two interventions themselves were delivered in very different ways. This differentiation is important in designing interventions. The IBM provides a theoretical basis from which to understand behavior and identify specific beliefs to target. Other communication and behavior change theories should be used to guide strategies to change those target beliefs.

Elicitation

We said that a critical step in applying TRA/TPB/IBM is to conduct open-ended elicitation interviews to identify relevant behavioral outcomes, referents, and environmental facilitators and barriers for each particular behavior and population under investigation. The formative phase of intervention projects is a good time to conduct these interviews. Elicitation interviews should be conducted with a sample of at least fifteen to twenty individuals from each target group, about half of whom have performed or intend to perform the behavior under investigation and half of whom have not performed the behavior.

When interviewed, people should be asked to provide four types of information:

1. Positive or negative feelings about performing the behavior (experiential attitude or affect)
2. Positive or negative attributes or outcomes of performing the behavior (behavioral beliefs)
3. Individuals or groups to whom they might listen who are in favor of or opposed to their performing the behavior (normative referents)
4. Situational or environmental facilitators and barriers that make the behavior easy or difficult to perform (control beliefs and self-efficacy)

Table 4.2 provides examples of questions that should systematically be asked of all individuals interviewed. It is important to probe for both negative and positive responses to each question. Interviewing fifteen to twenty individuals is a minimum. Ideally, elicitation interviews should be continued until "saturation," when no new responses are elicited. The process is described in detail by Middlestadt and colleagues (1996) and in a special supplement issue of the journal, *AIDS,* that summarizes formative research including elicitation interviews done in Zimbabwe prior to the National Institute of Mental Health HIV/STD Prevention Trial (NIMH, 2007a).

Elicitation interviews, then, are content-analyzed to identify relevant behavioral attributes or outcomes, normative referents, and facilitators and barriers. This information then provides questionnaire content, and TRA/TPB/IBM measures are developed. Measures should capture interviewees' language as much as possible so that questions resonate with the issues raised. A poorly conducted elicitation phase will likely result in inadequate identification of the relevant issues, poor IBM measures, and thus poor behavioral prediction, ultimately providing inadequate information for the development of effective behavior change interventions.

APPLICATION OF IBM TO HIV PREVENTION IN ZIMBABWE

In the past several years, we have been conducting intervention research in Zimbabwe to increase safe sex behaviors. Here we provide an example to show how we applied IBM in a developing world setting to examine cross-cultural applicability of the model. In this example, we illustrate several important steps in applying the model, including the elicitation phase to identify salient issues, design of a questionnaire to measure model constructs with attention to cultural issues, analysis of data to

TABLE 4.2. **Table of Elicitation Questions.**

Construct	Elicitation Questions
Experiential Attitude	How do you feel about the idea of *behavior X*? What do you like/dislike about *behavior X*? What do you enjoy/hate about *behavior X*?
Instrumental Attitude	What are the plusses of your doing *behavior X*? (What are some advantages of doing *behavior X*? What are the benefits that might result from doing *behavior X*?)
	What are the minuses of your doing *behavior X*? (What are some disadvantages of doing *behavior X*? What are the negative effects that might result from doing *behavior X*?)
Normative Influence	Who would support your doing *behavior X*?
	Who would be against your doing *behavior X*?
Perceived Control	What things make it easy for you to do *behavior X*?
	What things make it hard for you to do *behavior X*?
Self-Efficacy	If you want to do *behavior X*, how certain are you that you can?
	What kinds of things would help you overcome any barriers to do *behavior X*?

identify targets for intervention, and plans to incorporate findings into a behavior change intervention.

Elicitation Phase to Identify Salient Issues

The behavioral focus is *using condoms all the time with steady partners in the next three months*. This behavior is clear in terms of action (using), target (condoms), context (all the time with steady partners), and time (next three months). This behavior was studied, along with several other HIV-prevention behaviors (such as using condoms with other partners, sticking to one partner, avoiding commercial sex workers, and so on) among rural residents in Zimbabwe. Because this work was part of a larger study that followed individuals at one-year intervals, a three-month behavioral measure could not be collected. Thus, this application focuses on the determinants of behavioral intention. Twelve- and twenty-four-month data also were collected and will be used ultimately to determine how IBM constructs predict behavior and behavior change.

Elicitation interviews were conducted in conjunction with preparation for a large intervention trial in thirty-two rural villages in Zimbabwe. Individual interviews, structured by IBM components, were conducted in either Shona or Ndebele (local languages of Zimbabwe), with about eight randomly selected people aged eighteen to thirty in each village. Half were males and half were females. Participants were asked to think about using condoms with their steady partners and then to describe their feelings and beliefs about outcomes, sources of normative influence, and barriers and facilitators with respect to this behavior, using questions similar to the ones in Table 4.2.

Interviews were audio recorded, transcribed, and translated into English. They were then content-analyzed to extract all statements made with respect to each of the IBM constructs that determine behavioral intention. The content analysis process resulted in lists of feelings, behavioral outcomes, normative referents in favor and opposed, and barriers and facilitators with respect to using condoms with steady partners.

Questionnaire Development

Lists of beliefs resulting from this content analysis were used to construct items to measure each of the key psychosocial constructs in Figure 4.2. These included direct and indirect measures of instrumental attitude, affect (experiential attitude), injunctive norm, perceived control, and self-efficacy. Measures used verbatim comments from elicitation interviews as much as possible to reflect actual wording used by participants to capture the issues. These measures were extensively tested in two rural villages in Zimbabwe that represented the two main ethnic groups (Shona and Ndebele). Measures were revised on the basis of these results.

Pilot results led to improved clarity of questions and exclusion of some questions. The direct measure of subjective norm was excluded because we found no variance in the measure. Similarly, we excluded measures of behavioral outcome evaluations and motivation to comply with various referents, as there was little variance in those measures. Thus, the indirect measures of instrumental attitude and injunctive norm consisted of unweighted behavioral and normative beliefs, as noted in the earlier IBM description. The pilot also found little variance in the indirect perceived control measures (easy-difficult measures); thus, we relied on a single direct perceived control measure. This elicitation and questionnaire design process is described in more detail elsewhere (Kasprzyk and Montaño, 2007).

Final model construct measures were as follows. Behavioral intention was measured with a bipolar 5-point scale with endpoints "strongly disagree" and "strongly agree." Direct measures of experiential (affect) and instrumental attitude were measured with 5-point semantic differential scales, as in Table 4.1. Similarly, a direct measure of perceived control was measured on a single 5-point scale, with endpoints "extremely difficult" and "extremely easy." A direct measure of self-efficacy was obtained by asking respondents to rate their level of certainty that they could carry out the behavior on a 5-point scale, with endpoints "extremely certain I could not" and "extremely certain I could." Behavioral belief and normative belief measures used 5-point scales with endpoints "strongly disagree" and "strongly agree," as described in Table 4.1. Efficacy beliefs were measured by asking respondents to rate their level of certainty that they could carry out the behavior under various conditions identified by elicitation phase participants.

The final survey instrument, which included sections about several safe sex behaviors, was translated from English to Shona and Ndebele and back-translated to ensure that the meaning of questions did not change. Surveys were administered to about 185 residents aged eighteen to thirty in each of thirty rural sites in Zimbabwe (N = 5,546), through personal interviews in their preferred languages; 2,212 respondents who said they had steady partners within the previous year completed the survey section about IBM constructs.

Confirmation of Model Component Determinants of Intention

Prior to carrying out analyses to identify targets for interventions, it is important to confirm that the indirect measures assess the constructs they were designed to measure, and that the model constructs explain behavioral intention. Indirect measures of attitude, perceived norm, and self-efficacy first were computed as the mean of the respective underlying beliefs. Attitude was computed from thirteen beliefs about outcomes of using condoms with steady partners, perceived norm was computed from four normative beliefs, and self-efficacy was computed from eleven beliefs concerning certainty of behavioral performance under different conditions. Attitude ($r = .42$, $p < .001$) and self-efficacy ($r = .71$, $p < .001$) scales computed from underlying beliefs each were highly correlated with direct measures (not assessed for perceived norm since a direct measure was not obtained). Intention to use condoms all the time with steady partners was explained significantly ($r = .69$, $p < .001$) by attitude ($r = .46$, $p < .001$), perceived norm ($r = .49$, $p < .001$), self-efficacy ($r = .65$, $p < .001$), and perceived control ($r = .42$, $p < .001$).

Identification of Beliefs to Change Intention

Though self-efficacy had the highest correlation with intention, attitude, perceived norm, and perceived control were also correlated highly with intention. Based on these zero-order correlations, all four model constructs were considered potentially important targets for an intervention among the population of rural Zimbabweans to increase intention to use condoms with steady partners. Since these findings were nearly identical when data were analyzed separately for males and females, we present results combined for males and females.

Conceptualization of the IBM constructs as being determined by underlying beliefs is most important in identifying specific targets for intervention communications. The next analytical step was to determine which behavioral, normative, and efficacy beliefs best predict behavioral intention (this analysis did not include perceived control because control beliefs were not measured).

Table 4.3 presents correlations of behavioral, normative, and efficacy beliefs with intention to use condoms with steady partners. All beliefs underlying these three model constructs were correlated significantly with behavioral intention, confirming that the elicitation phase identified salient beliefs important in determining attitude, perceived norm, and self-efficacy with respect to this behavior. Survey respondents also were divided into those who intended (marked "somewhat" or "strongly agree") and those who did not intend to use condoms with steady partners. Table 4.3 presents the mean belief scores for these two groups. All behavioral, normative, and efficacy beliefs significantly discriminated between intenders and non-intenders.

TABLE 4.3. **Strength of Association of Behavioral, Normative, and Efficacy Beliefs with Intention to Use Condoms with Steady Partners.**

Behavioral Beliefs:	Correlation	Mean Belief		% Strongly Disagree	
	r	Non-Intend	Intend	Non-Intend	Intend
Make your partner angry	−0.37	3.0	1.7	42.4	78.0
Show lack of respect for your partner	−0.40	3.0	1.6	43.7	80.5
Show that you think your partner is unclean/diseased	−0.37	3.3	1.9	36.1	72.3
Show that you are unclean/diseased	−0.37	3.1	1.8	41.3	76.5
Be embarrassing	−0.29	1.9	1.2	73.1	92.4
Make your partner think you don't love her/him	−0.37	3.2	1.9	38.0	74.6
Spoil the relationship	−0.36	2.7	1.5	52.2	83.3
Show your partner you don't trust him/her	−0.38	3.3	1.8	38.2	75.8
Mean you would get less pleasure	−0.21	2.5	1.8	53.7	73.1
Make your partner think you are having other partners	−0.39	3.5	2.0	33.5	70.3
Be unnecessary, because your steady partner does not have other partners	−0.31	2.7	1.7	47.5	75.7
Mean you will not have physical or sexual release	−0.24	2.3	1.6	60.3	81.3
Encourage promiscuity in your steady partner	−0.29	2.8	1.8	51.0	76.9
Multiple Correlation—R	0.47				

TABLE 4.3. **Strength of Association of Behavioral, Normative, and Efficacy Beliefs with Intention to Use Condoms with Steady Partners, Cont'd.**

	Correlation	Mean Belief		% Strongly Disagree	
Normative Beliefs:	**r**	**Non-Intend**	**Intend**	**Non-Intend**	**Intend**
Your family	0.25	3.4	4.2	49.9	69.2
Your closest friends	0.29	3.9	4.7	66.7	85.9
Radio shows or radio dramas	0.20	4.5	4.8	80.5	91.9
Your partner	0.56	2.3	4.3	24.1	74.7
Multiple Correlation—R	0.58				

	Correlation	Mean Belief		% Strongly Disagree	
Efficacy Beliefs:	**r**	**Non-Intend**	**Intend**	**Non-Intend**	**Intend**
If you or your steady partner gets carried away and can't wait to have sex, how certain are you that you could always use condoms?	0.57	2.5	4.4	25.6	74.7
If you have been drinking before you have sex, how certain are you that you could always use condoms?	0.52	2.5	4.2	21.7	64.9
If your steady partner has been drinking before sex, how certain are you that you could always use condoms?	0.53	2.6	4.4	24.3	70.1
If you or your steady partner is using another method of birth control, how certain are you that you could always use condoms?	0.59	2.5	4.5	23.6	76.3

TABLE 4.3. **Strength of Association of Behavioral, Normative, and Efficacy Beliefs with Intention to Use Condoms with Steady Partners, Cont'd.**

Efficacy Beliefs:	Correlation r	Mean Belief		% Strongly Disagree	
		Non-Intend	Intend	Non-Intend	Intend
If your steady partner doesn't want to, how certain are you that you could always use condoms?	0.56	2.2	4.2	17.7	70.1
If you believe AIDS will affect you, how certain are you that you could always use condoms?	0.43	3.8	4.8	59.4	90.8
If you or your steady partner has a condom with you, how certain are you that you could always use condoms?	0.57	3.0	4.7	38.2	84.6
If you or your steady partner knows how to use a condom, how certain are you that you could always use condoms?	0.59	3.0	4.8	37.6	86.3
If condoms are available in your community, how certain are you that you could always use condoms?	0.60	3.0	4.8	36.9	86.3
If you had to talk about it with your steady partner, how certain are you that you could always use condoms?	0.56	3.1	4.8	40.9	86.3
If you thought your steady partner had other partners, how certain are you that you could always use condoms?	0.45	3.6	4.8	55.7	88.2
Multiple Correlation—R	0.67				

Note: All correlations significant $p < .001$.

All differences between means significant $p < .001$.

Because it is not always feasible to address a large number of beliefs in an intervention, it is important to determine which beliefs may be most important and are likely to have the greatest impact on intention, if targeted. It was clear, and logical, that the normative belief about one's partner had far more impact than any other source of influence on intention to use condoms with steady partners. Selecting the most important behavioral and efficacy beliefs was not as simple, since multiple beliefs had similarly high correlations with behavioral intention. After identifying beliefs significantly associated with intention, Fishbein and Cappella (2006) recommend using additional criteria suggested by Hornik and Woolf (1999) to select beliefs for intervention targets. There should be enough people who do not already hold the belief to make intervention worthwhile, and it should be possible to change the belief through persuasive arguments.

To further evaluate beliefs based on the first of these criteria, the "behavioral beliefs" section of Table 4.3 includes percentages of intenders and non-intenders who "strongly disagree" with each behavioral belief (these are all negative outcomes). The "normative beliefs" and "efficacy beliefs" sections of the table include percentages of intenders and non-intenders who "strongly agree" with each normative and efficacy belief. Less than 40 percent of non-intenders strongly disagreed with four behavioral beliefs: *show you think your partner is unclean*; *make partner think you don't love him/her*; *show partner you don't trust him/her*; and *make partner think you are having other partners.* These relatively low percentages, compared to intenders, make these beliefs potentially important for intervention targets because of the large potential to increase percentages among non-intenders. Substantially higher percent disagreement by non-intenders, along with relatively small differences with intenders, indicated that beliefs about embarrassment and lack of sexual release are probably not useful targets for change. Similarly, five efficacy beliefs were endorsed by less than 30 percent of non-intenders: *perception of ability to use condoms when carried away*; *respondent had been drinking*; *partner had been drinking*; *using another method of birth control*; and *partner doesn't want to.* As with behavioral beliefs, there is considerable room to change non-intender beliefs to be like intender beliefs on these five efficacy issues. With respect to perceived norm, the greatest room for change is the normative belief about one's steady partner, with only 24 percent of non-intenders believing that the steady partner wants to use condoms.

After identifying potential target beliefs, the next step is to consider whether each of these beliefs can be changed through persuasive communications. The normative belief about steady partners may be the most difficult to change through persuasive arguments, unless the intervention also involves or targets the steady partner. The four behavioral beliefs identified earlier appear to be reasonable targets for change through persuasive arguments. For example, an argument may recommend that a person talk to the steady partner about using condoms until they are both tested, and that this will show enough love for the partner enough to protect him or her. This will help to counter beliefs about *showing you don't love or trust the partner, thinking the partner is unclean,* and *making the partner think you are having other partners.* The five efficacy beliefs also seem reasonable to target through persuasive arguments that would provide strategies for a person to use to enhance the ability to use condoms in spite of *drinking, being carried away, using another birth control method,* and *the partner being against using condoms.*

Summary and Use of Findings to Inform Behavior Change Intervention

To summarize, this application provides a cross-cultural example to demonstrate the following steps to apply the IBM as a framework to identify specific targets for an intervention:

■ Clearly specify the behavior in terms of action, target, context, and time.
■ Conduct qualitative interviews with members of the study population to elicit from them the salient behavioral outcomes, affective response, sources of normative influence, and barriers and facilitators associated with the target behavior. This step is necessary and critical. These salient issues often are different for different behaviors and population groups.
■ Use elicitation findings to design a culturally appropriate survey instrument to measure IBM constructs. Questions were designed to measure beliefs with respect to the specific salient issues identified in the elicitation study. Pilot testing ensured that question wording and response scale format were reliable, valid, and culturally appropriate.
■ Confirm that IBM measures explain behavioral intention, and determine which constructs best explain intention and should serve as the focus for intervention efforts.
■ Use findings to analyze and identify specific behavioral, normative, and efficacy beliefs that may be the best targets for persuasive communications in an intervention to strengthen behavioral intention and lead to greater likelihood of behavior performance.

Once critical belief targets are identified, the next steps in designing an intervention are to develop persuasive arguments to change those beliefs and then to select channels by which to deliver persuasive communications to target populations. TRA, TPB, and IBM are theories to explain behavioral intentions and behaviors and to identify intervention targets. They are *not* theories of communication. Available theories of communication are not as clear in guiding how best to design and deliver persuasive messages to target the issues identified through application of behavioral theory (Fishbein and Cappella, 2006; IOM, 2002).

One communication approach that has been found to be successful in changing safe sex behaviors in communities is the Community Popular Opinion Leader (CPOL) model, based on the theory of Diffusion of Innovations (NIMH, 2007b; see also Chapter Fourteen). This intervention identifies and trains popular opinion leaders (POLs) to have conversations with peers and to model themselves as having adopted the behaviors that are being promoted. We have demonstrated that the CPOL intervention method is feasible and well accepted by POLs and by community members in Zimbabwe (NIMH, 2007c). Thus, we are using the CPOL model as the communication method to design and deliver persuasive messages concerning target beliefs identified earlier. This includes training POLs to understand the IBM conceptualization, educating them about the beliefs identified in this study as important targets for behavior change, and role-playing to develop and rehearse persuasive arguments with respect to each of those beliefs. POLs are trained to have structured conversations with friends and to use the IBM as a framework to elicit issues that are salient to the person they are conversing with, and respond by (1) reinforcing positive behavioral beliefs and countering negative beliefs, (2) reinforcing beliefs about behavioral support from important referents, and (3) suggesting or modeling strategies to overcome barriers in order to increase confidence about behavioral performance, despite those barriers. Thus, POL conversations include persuasive communications designed by the POLs to address the key issues identified in IBM research, and specifically target issues brought up by people with whom they speak. Evaluation involves surveys of community members over multiple time points to assess whether the intervention results in change in the targeted behavioral, normative, and efficacy beliefs, and whether there is corresponding change in behavioral intention and behavior.

Value of the TRA, TPB, and IBM Frameworks

Theoretical frameworks help to organize thought and planning of research, intervention, and analysis. TRA, TPB, and IBM provide excellent frameworks to conceptualize, measure, and identify factors that affect behavior. TRA focuses on cognitive factors (beliefs and values) that determine motivation (behavioral intention). The theory has been useful in explaining behaviors, particularly behaviors under volitional control. In applying behavioral theories, it is important to continually reassess them and consider other theory-driven constructs that may enhance explanatory power. TPB extends TRA by adding perceived behavioral control, concerned with facilitating or constraining conditions that affect intention and behavior. This is particularly important for behaviors over which people have less volitional control. IBM includes constructs from both TPB and TRA, as well as constructs from other excellent theories of behavior. IBM was developed through discussions and consensus among major behavioral theorists and has been modified through empirical work over the past decade.

We cannot stress enough the importance of conducting in-depth, open-ended elicitation interviews with audiences who are studied with TRA/TPB/IBM and for whom interventions will be designed. Elicitation interviews identify the behavioral outcomes, normative referents, and barriers and facilitators that are relevant to the particular behavior and population under investigation. This ensures that TRA/TPB/IBM measures are empirically grounded.

For theory to drive interventions, it must provide a framework to select important factors that can be influenced from among many factors associated with behaviors. TRA, TPB, and IBM are particularly useful in this regard. Application of IBM to understand a particular behavior will identify underlying beliefs that determine one's attitude (instrumental and experiential), perceived norm (injunctive and descriptive), perceived control, and self-efficacy, and thereby affect the likelihood of performing the behavior. Often, important beliefs affecting behavior are different for different behaviors and different populations.

TRA, TPB, and IBM provide frameworks to guide research that can empirically identify factors on which intervention efforts should focus. However, selection of specific beliefs to change through interventions must be done carefully. Targeting a few beliefs may not be effective if they represent a small proportion of the total set of beliefs affecting intentions. Similarly, targeting beliefs that comprise a model component not strongly associated with behavioral intention may be ineffective. It is also important to consider the effect of intervention messages on the entire set of beliefs underlying behavior. An intervention communication may change one targeted belief in the desired direction but could adversely affect other important beliefs. Further, intervention development should pay attention to all model components simultaneously. For example, attempting to modify efficacy or control beliefs may be effective only if a person is sufficiently motivated to perform the behavior in the first place. Conversely, changing attitude may not result in behavior change if the person holds strong control or self-efficacy beliefs about conditions that constrain the behavior.

It is important to assess the effect of interventions on the beliefs targeted and on other components of the model. TRA, TPB, and IBM provide a basis to evaluate behavior change interventions because they lead to hypotheses about how an intervention targeting a set of beliefs will affect the model component to which those items belong (for example, attitude) and thereby affect intention and behavior. The evaluation design should make it possible to measure model components as intermediate outcomes, both before and after intervention, to assess how they are influenced by the intervention and whether change in model components is associated with behavior change. These theories should be applied in conjunction with communication theories to design and deliver behavior change interventions. In this way, the IBM can complement the use of other theories of change and thereby improve health behavior research and practice.

SUMMARY

In this chapter we described the Theory of Reasoned Action (TRA), the Theory of Planned Behavior (TPB), and the Integrated Behavioral Model (IBM), as well as how the IBM emerged from efforts to integrate constructs from TRA/TPB with constructs from other important theories of behavior. We provided detailed descriptions of how to measure the constructs in these theories. We emphasized that while TRA, TPB, and IBM provide a structure to understand how behavioral, normative, control, and efficacy beliefs determine the respective model constructs and affect behavioral intention, it is essential to elicit the specific content for the measures from the study population with respect to the behavior under investigation. Finally, we described a cross-cultural application of the IBM in Zimbabwe to demonstrate development of IBM measures, analyses to confirm that model constructs explain behavioral intention, and most important, analyses to identify specific key beliefs that should be targeted by behavior change interventions.

REFERENCES

Abelson, R. P. "Are Attitudes Necessary?" In B. T. King and E. McGinnies (eds.), *Attitudes, Conflict, and Social Change.* New York: Academic Press, 1972.

Airhihenbuwa, C. O., and Obregon, R. "A Critical Assessment of Theories/Models Used in Health Communication for HIV/AIDS." *Journal of Health Communication,* 2000, *5*(Suppl), 5–15.

Ajzen, I. "The Theory of Planned Behavior." *Organizational Behavior and Human Decision Processes,* 1991, *50,* 179–211.

Ajzen, I. "Perceived Behavioral Control, Self-Efficacy, Locus of Control, and the Theory of Planned Behavior." *Journal of Applied Social Psychology,* 2002, *32,* 1–20.

Ajzen, I. "Constructing a TPB Questionnaire: Conceptual and Methodological Considerations." [http://www.people.umass.edu/aizen/pdf/tpb.measurement.pdf]. 2006.

Ajzen, I., and Albarracin, D. "Predicting and Changing Behavior." In I. Ajzen, D. Albarracin, and R. Hornik (eds.), *Prediction and Change of Health Behavior: Applying the Reasoned Action Approach.* Hillsdale, N.J.: Erlbaum, 2007.

Ajzen, I., and Driver, B. L. "Prediction of Leisure Participation from Behavioral, Normative, and Control Beliefs: An Application of the Theory of Planned Behavior." *Leisure Sciences,* 1991, *13,* 185–204.

Ajzen, I., and Fishbein, M. *Understanding Attitudes and Predicting Social Behavior.* Englewood Cliffs, N.J.: Prentice Hall, 1980.

Ajzen I., and Madden, T. J. "Prediction of Goal-Directed Behavior: Attitudes, Intentions, and Perceived Behavioral Control." *Journal of Experimental Social Psychology,* 1986, *22,* 453–474.

Albarracin, D., Fishbein, M., and Goldestein de Muchinik, E. "Seeking Social Support in Old Age as Reasoned Action: Structural and Volitional Determinants in a Middle-Aged Sample of Argentinean Women." *Journal of Applied Social Psychology,* 1997, *27*(6), 463–476.

Albarracin, D., Johnson, B. T., Fishbein, M., and Muellerleile, P. A. "Theories of Reasoned Action and Planned Behavior as Models of Condom Use: A Meta-analysis." *Psychological Bulletin,* 2001, *127*(1), 142–161.

Albarracin, D., and others. "Persuasive Communications to Change Actions: An Analysis of Behavioral and Cognitive Impact in HIV Prevention." *Health Psychology,* 2003, *22,* 166–177.

Albarracin, D., Kumkale, G. T., and Johnson, B. T. "Influences of Social Power and Normative Support on Condom Use Decision: A Research Synthesis." *AIDS Care,* 2004, *16*(6), 700–723.

Albarracin, D., and others. "A Test of Major Assumptions About Behavior Change: A Comprehensive Look at the Effects of Passive and Active HIV-Prevention Interventions Since the Beginning of the Epidemic." *Psychological Bulletin,* 2005, *131*(6), 856–897.

Armitage, C. J., and Conner, M. "Efficacy of the Theory of Planned Behaviour: A Meta-Analytic Review." *British Journal of Social Psychology*, 2001, *40*(Pt 4), 471–499.

Bagozzi, R. P., and Lee, K-H. "Multiple Routes for Social Influence: The Role of Compliance, Internalization, and Social Identity." *Social Psychology Quarterly,* 2002, *65*(3), 226–247.

Bandawe, C. R., and Foster, D. "AIDS-Related Beliefs, Attitudes and Intentions Among Malawian Students in Three Secondary Schools." *AIDS Care,* 1996, *8*(2), 223–232.

Bandura, A. "Toward a Psychology of Human Agency." *Perspectives on Psychological Science,* 2006, *1*(2), 164–180.

Becker, M. H. "The Health Belief Model and Personal Health Behavior." *Health Education Monographs, 1974, 2,* 324–473.

Blue, C. L. "The Predictive Capacity of the Theory of Reasoned Action and the Theory of Planned Behavior in Exercise Research: An Integrated Literature Review." *Research in Nursing and Health,* 1995, *18*(2), 105–121.

Bogart, L. M., Cecil, H., and Pinkerton, S. D. "Intentions to Use the Female Condom Among African American Adults." *Journal of Applied Social Psychology,* 2000, *30*(9), 1923–1953.

Bosompra, K. "Determinants of Condom Use Intentions of University Students in Ghana: An Application of the Theory of Reasoned Action." *Social Science and Medicine,* 2001, *52,* 1057–1069.

Bryan, A., Schmiege, S. J., and Broaddus, M. R. "Mediational Analysis in HIV/AIDS Research: Estimating Multivariate Path Analytic Models in a Structural Equation Modeling Framework." *AIDS and Behavior,* 2007, *11*(3), 365–383.

Centers for Disease Control and Prevention (CDC), and AIDS Community Demonstration Project (ACDP) Research Group. "Community-Level HIV Intervention in 5 Cities: Final Outcome Data for the CDC AIDS Community Demonstration Projects." *American Journal of Public Health,* 1999, *89*(3), 336–345.

Craig, S., Goldberg, J., and Dietz, W. H. "Psychosocial Correlates of Physical Activity Among Fifth and Eighth Graders." *Preventive Medicine,* 1996, *25*(5), 506–513.

Downs, D. S., and Hausenblas, H. A. "Elicitation Studies and the Theory of Planned Behavior: A Systematic Review of Exercise Beliefs." *Psychology of Sport and Exercise,* 2005, *6,* 1–31.

Durantini, M. R., and others. "Conceptualizing the Influence of Social Agents of Change: A Meta-Analysis of HIV Prevention Interventions for Different Groups." *Psychological Bulletin,* 2006, *132,* 212–248.

Edwards, W. "The Theory of Decision Making." *Psychological Bulletin,* 1954, *51,* 380–417.

Fishbein, M. (ed.). *Readings in Attitude Theory and Measurement.* New York: Wiley, 1967.

Fishbein, M. "AIDS and Behavior Change: An Analysis Based on the Theory of Reasoned Action." *Interamerican Journal of Psychology,* 1990, *24,* 37–56.

Fishbein, M. "Introduction." In D. J. Terry, C. Gallois, and M. McCamish (eds.), *The Theory of Reasoned Action: Its Application to AIDS Preventive Behaviour.* Oxford, Great Britain: Pergamon Press, 1993.

Fishbein, M. "The Role of Theory in HIV Prevention." *AIDS Care,* 2000, *12*(3), 273–278.

Fishbein, M. "A Reasoned Action Approach: Some Issues, Questions, and Clarifications." In I. Ajzen, D. Albarracin, and R. Hornik (eds.), *Prediction and Change of Health Behavior: Applying the Reasoned Action Approach.* Hillsdale, N.J.: Erlbaum, 2007.

Fishbein, M., and Ajzen I. *Belief, Attitude, Intention, and Behavior: An Introduction to Theory and Research.* Reading, Mass.: Addison-Wesley, 1975.

Fishbein, M., and Cappella, J. N. "The Role of Theory in Developing Effective Health Communications." *Journal of Communication,* 2006, *56,* S1–S17.

Fishbein, M., and others. *Factors Influencing Behavior and Behavior Change.* Final Report, Theorists' Workshop. Bethesda, Md.: National Institute of Mental Health, 1992.

Fishbein, M., von Haeften, I., and Appleyard, J. "The Role of Theory in Developing Effective Interventions: Implications From Project SAFER." *Psychology, Health & Medicine,* 2001, *6*(2), 223–238.

Fisher, W. A., Fisher, J. D., and Rye, B. J. "Understanding and Promoting AIDS Preventive Behavior: Insights From the Theory of Reasoned Action." *Health Psychology,* 1995, *14,* 255–264.

French, D. P., and others. "The Importance of Affective Beliefs and Attitudes in the Theory of Planned Behavior: Predicting Intention to Increase Physical Activity." *Journal of Applied Social Psychology.* 2005, *35*(9), 1824–1848.

Gastil, J. "Thinking, Drinking, and Driving: Application of the Theory of Reasoned Action to DWI Prevention." *Journal of Applied Social Psychology,* 2000, *30*(11), 2217–2232.

Glanz, K., Rimer, B. K., and Lewis, F. M. "Theory, Research, and Practice in Health Behavior and Health Education." In K. Glanz, B. K. Rimer, and F. M. Lewis (eds.), *Health Behavior and Health Education: Theory, Research, and Practice.* (3rd ed.) San Francisco: Jossey-Bass, 2002.

Godin, G., and Kok, G. "The Theory of Planned Behavior: A Review of its Applications to Health-related Behaviors." *American Journal of Public Health,* 1996, *11*(2), 87–98.

Hardeman, W., and others. "Application of the Theory of Planned Behaviour in Behaviour Change Interventions: A Systematic Review." *Psychology and Health,* 2002, *17*(2), 123–158.

Hardeman, W., and others. "A Causal Modelling Approach to the Development of Theory-Based Behaviour Change Programmes for Trial Evaluation." *Health Education Research,* 2005, *20*(6), 676–687.

Hornik, R., and Woolf, K. D. "Using Cross-sectional Surveys to Plan Message Strategies." *Social Marketing Quarterly,* 1999, *5*(1), 34–41.

Institute of Medicine (U.S.), Committee on Communication for Behavior Change in the 21st Century: Improving the Health of Diverse Populations. *Speaking of Health: Assessing Health Communication Strategies for Diverse Populations.* Washington, D.C.: National Academies Press, 2002.

Jaccard, J., Dodge, T., and Dittus, P. "Parent-Adolescent Communication About Sex and Birth Control: A Conceptual Framework." In S. Feldman and D. A. Rosenthal (eds.), *Talking Sexuality: Parent-Adolescent Communication.* New Directions in Child and Adolescent Development, No. 97, W. Damon, Editor-in-Chief. San Francisco: Jossey-Bass, 2002.

Jemmott, J. B., Jemmott, L. S., and Fong, G. T. "Reductions in HIV Risk—Associated Sexual Behaviors among Black Male Adolescents: Effects of an AIDS Prevention Intervention." *American Journal of Public Health,* 1992, *82*(3), 372–377.

Jemmott, J. B. 3rd, and Jemmott, L. S. "HIV Risk Reduction Behavioral Interventions with Heterosexual Adolescents." *AIDS,* 2000, *14*(Suppl 2), S40–S52.

Kalichman, S. C. "The Theory of Reasoned Action and Advances in HIV/AIDS." In I. Ajzen, D. Albarracin, and R. Hornik (eds.), *Prediction and Change of Health Behavior: Applying the Reasoned Action Approach.* Hillsdale, N.J.: Erlbaum, 2007.

Kamb, M., and others. "Efficacy of Risk-Reduction Counseling to Prevent Human Immunodeficiency Virus And Sexually Transmitted Diseases." *Journal of the American Medical Association, 1988, 280,* 1161–1167.

Kasprzyk, D., Montaño, D. E., and Fishbein, M. "Application of an Integrated Behavioral Model to Predict Condom Use: A Prospective Study Among High HIV Risk Groups." *Journal of Applied Social Psychology,* 1998, *28*(17), 1557–1583.

Kasprzyk, D., and Montaño, D. E. "Application of an Integrated Behavioral Model to Understand HIV Prevention Behavior of High Risk Men in Rural Zimbabwe." In I. Ajzen, D. Albarracin, and R. Hornik (eds.), *Prediction and Change of Health Behavior: Applying the Reasoned Action Approach.* Hillsdale, N.J.: Erlbaum, 2007.

Kenski, K., and others. "Theoretical Determinants of Condom Use Intentions for Vaginal Sex with a Regular Partner Among Male and Female Injecting Drug Users." *Psychology, Health & Medicine,* 2001, 6(2), 179–190.

Madden, T. J., Ellen, P. S., and Ajzen, I. "A Comparison of the Theory of Planned Behavior and the Theory of Reasoned Action." *Personality and Social Psychology Bulletin,* 1992, *18,* 3–9.

Middlestadt, S. E., and others. "The Use of Theory Based Semistructured Elicitation Questionnaires: Formative Research for CDC's Prevention Marketing Initiative." *Public Health Reports,* 1996, *3*(Suppl 1), 18–27.

Millstein, S. G. "Utility of the Theories of Reasoned Action and Planned Behavior for Predicting Physician Behavior: A Prospective Analysis." *Health Psychology,* 1996, *15*(5), 398–402.

Montaño, D., Phillips, W., and Kasprzyk, D. "Explaining Physician Rates of Providing Flexible Sigmoidoscopy." *Cancer Epidemiology, Biomarkers & Prevention, 2000, 9,* 665–669.

Montaño, D., and Taplin, S. "A Test of an Expanded Theory of Reasoned Action to Predict Mammography Participation." *Social Science and Medicine, 1991, 32,* 733–741.

Montaño, D., Thompson, B., Taylor, V. M., and Mahloch, J. "Understanding Mammography Intention and Utilization among Women in an Inner City Public Hospital Clinic." *Preventive Medicine, 1997, 26,* 817–824.

Morrison, D. M., Spencer, M. S., and Gillmore, M. R. "Beliefs about Substance Use Among Pregnant and Parenting Adolescents." *Journal of Research on Adolescence, 1998, 8,* 69–95.

NIMH Collaborative HIV/STD Prevention Trial Group. "Design and Integration of Ethnography Within an International Behavior Change HIV/Sexually Transmitted Disease Prevention Trial." *AIDS,* 2007a, *21*(Suppl 2), S37–S48.

NIMH Collaborative HIV/STD Prevention Trial Group. "The Community Popular Opinion Leader HIV Prevention Programme: Conceptual Basis and Intervention Procedures." *AIDS,* 2007b, *21*(Suppl 2), S59–S68.

NIMH Collaborative HIV/STD Prevention Trial Group. "Formative Study Conducted in Five Countries to Adapt the Community Popular Opinion Leader Intervention." *AIDS,* 2007c, *21*(Suppl 2), S91–S98.

Rhodes F., and others. "Using Theory to Understand How Interventions Work: Project RESPECT, Condom Use, and the Integrative Model." *AIDS and Behavior,* 2007, *11*(3), 393–407.

Rosenberg, M. J. "Cognitive Structure and Attitudinal Affect." *Journal of Abnormal and Social Psychology,* 1956, *53,* 367–372.

Rotter, J. B. *Social Learning and Clinical Psychology.* Englewood Cliffs, N.J.: Prentice Hall, 1954.

Sheeran, P., and Taylor, S. "Predicting Intentions to Use Condoms: A Meta-Analysis and Comparison of the Theories of Reasoned Action and Planned Behavior." *Journal of Applied Social Psychology,* 1999, *29,* 1624–1675.

St. Lawrence, J. S., and Fortenberry, J. D. "Behavioral Interventions for STDs: Theoretical Models and Intervention Methods." In S. O. Aral and J. M. Douglas (eds.), *Behavioral Interventions for Prevention and Control of Sexually Transmitted Diseases.* New York: Springer, 2007.

Steen, D. M., Peay, M. Y., and Owen, N. "Predicting Australian Adolescents' Intentions to Minimize Sun Exposure." *Psychology and Health,* 1998, *13*(1), 111–119.

Terry, D., Gallois, C., and McCamish, M. "The Theory of Reasoned Action and Health Care Behaviour." In D. J. Terry, C. Gallois, and M. McCamish (eds.), *The Theory of Reasoned Action: Its Application to AIDS Preventive Behaviour.* Oxford, Great Britain: Pergamon Press, 1993.

Trafimow, D. "The Importance of Attitudes in the Prediction of College Students' Intentions to Drink." *Journal of Applied Social Psychology,* 1996, *26*(24), 2167–2188.

Trafimow, D. "Distinctions Pertaining to Fishbein and Ajzen's Theory of Reasoned Action." In I. Ajzen, D. Albarracin, and R. Hornik (eds.), *Prediction and Change of Health Behavior: Applying the Reasoned Action Approach.* Hillsdale, N.J.: Erlbaum, 2007.

Triandis, H. C. *The Analysis of Subjective Culture.* New York: Wiley, 1972.

Triandis, H. C. "Values, Attitudes, and Interpersonal Behavior." In H. E. Howe and M. Page (eds.), *Nebraska Symposium on Motivation, 1979.* Lincoln: University of Nebraska Press, 1980.

Triandis, H. C., and others. "Individualism and Collectivism: Cross-Cultural Perspectives on Self-In Group Relationships." *Journal of Personality and Social Psychology,* 1988, *54*(2), 323–338.

von Haeften, I., Fishbein, M., Kasprzyk, D., and Montaño, D. "Analyzing Data to Obtain Information to Design Targeted Interventions." *Psychology, Health & Medicine,* 2001, *6*(2), 151–164.

von Haeften, I., and Kenski, K. "Multi-Partnered Heterosexual's Condom Use for Vaginal Sex With Their Main Partner as a Function of Attitude, Subjective Norm, Partner Norm, Perceived Behavioural Control, and Weighted Control Beliefs." *Psychology, Health & Medicine,* 2001, *6*(2), 165–178.

Webb, T. L., and Sheeran, P. "Does Changing Behavioral Intentions Engender Behavior Change? A Meta-Analysis of the Experimental Evidence." *Psychological Bulletin,* 2006, *132,* 249–268.

Weinstein, N. D. "Testing Four Competing Theories of Health-Protective Behavior." *Health Psychology,* 1993, *12*(4), 324–333.

Weinstein, N. D. "Misleading Tests of Health Behavior Theories." *Annals of Behavioral Medicine*, 2007, *33*(1), 1–10

Wicker, A. W. "Attitudes vs. Actions: The Relationship of Verbal and Overt Behavioral Responses to Attitude Objects." *Journal of Social Issues,* 1969, *25,* 41–78.

Yzer, M. "Does Perceived Control Moderate Attitudinal and Normative Effects on Intention? A Review of Conceptual and Methodological Issues." In I. Ajzen, D. Albarracin, and R. Hornik (eds.), *Prediction and Change of Health Behavior: Applying the Reasoned Action Approach.* Hillsdale, N.J.: Erlbaum, 2007.

CHAPTER

5

THE TRANSTHEORETICAL MODEL AND STAGES OF CHANGE

James O. Prochaska

Colleen A. Redding

Kerry E. Evers

KEY POINTS

This chapter will

- Explain the stages of change and the other core Transtheoretical Model (TTM) constructs.
- Explore empirical support for and challenges to TTM.
- Examine how TTM interventions can be tailored to the needs of individuals while treating entire populations for smoking cessation.
- Expand on how such TTM interventions can be applied to changing multiple health risk behaviors in high-risk populations.

The Transtheoretical Model (TTM) uses stages of change to integrate processes and principles of change across major theories of intervention, hence the name *Transtheoretical*. The TTM emerged from a comparative analysis of leading theories of psychotherapy and behavior change in an effort to integrate a field that had fragmented into more than 300 theories of psychotherapy (Prochaska, 1984). The impetus for the model arose when Prochaska and colleagues conducted a comparative analysis of self-changers compared to smokers in professional treatments. Across these study populations, we identified ten processes of change that were predictive of successful quitting (DiClemente and Prochaska, 1982). These included consciousness raising from the Freudian tradition (Freud, 1959), contingency management from the Skinnerian tradition (Skinner, 1971), and helping relationships from the Rogerian tradition (Rogers, 1951).

We assessed how frequently each group used each of ten processes (DiClemente and Prochaska, 1982). Participants used different processes at different times in their struggles with smoking. These naïve subjects taught researchers about a phenomenon that was not then a formal part of any therapy theories. They revealed that behavior change unfolds through a series of stages (Prochaska and DiClemente, 1983). This profound insight changed the course of our research and led to development of the TTM.

From initial studies of smoking, the stage model rapidly was expanded to include investigations and applications to a broad range of health and mental health behaviors, including alcohol and substance abuse, anxiety and panic disorders, bullying, delinquency, depression, eating disorders and obesity, high-fat diets, HIV/AIDS prevention, mammography and other cancer screening, medication compliance, unplanned pregnancy prevention, pregnancy and smoking, radon testing, sedentary lifestyles, sun exposure, and physicians practicing preventive medicine. Over time, researchers across the world have expanded, validated, applied, and challenged core constructs of the TTM (Hall and Rossi, 2008; Noar, Benac, and Harris, 2007; Prochaska, Wright, and Velicer, in press).

CORE CONSTRUCTS

Table 5.1 briefly describes core constructs of the TTM.

TABLE 5.1. **Transtheoretical Model Constructs.**

Constructs	Description
Stages of Change	
Precontemplation	No intention to take action within the next 6 months
Contemplation	Intends to take action within the next 6 months
Preparation	Intends to take action within the next 30 days and has taken some behavioral steps in this direction
Action	Changed overt behavior for less than 6 months
Maintenance	Changed overt behavior for more than 6 months
Termination	No temptation to relapse and 100% confidence

TABLE 5.1. **Transtheoretical Model Constructs.**

Constructs	Description
Processes of Change	
Consciousness raising	Finding and learning new facts, ideas, and tips that support the healthy behavior change
Dramatic relief	Experiencing the negative emotions (fear, anxiety, worry) that go along with unhealthy behavioral risks
Self-reevaluation	Realizing that the behavior change is an important part of one's identity as a person
Environmental reevaluation	Realizing the negative impact of the unhealthy behavior or the positive impact of the healthy behavior on one's proximal social and/or physical environment
Self-liberation	Making a firm commitment to change
Helping relationships	Seeking and using social support for the healthy behavior change
Counterconditioning	Substitution of healthier alternative behaviors and cognitions for the unhealthy behavior
Reinforcement management	Increasing the rewards for the positive behavior change and decreasing the rewards of the unhealthy behavior
Stimulus control	Removing reminders or cues to engage in the unhealthy behavior and adding cues or reminders to engage in the healthy behavior
Social liberation	Realizing that the social norms are changing in the direction of supporting the healthy behavior change
Decisional Balance	
Pros	Benefits of changing
Cons	Costs of changing
Self-Efficacy	
Confidence	Confidence that one can engage in the healthy behavior across different challenging situations
Temptation	Temptation to engage in the unhealthy behavior across different challenging situations

Stages of Change

The stage construct is important, in part, because it represents a temporal dimension. In the past, behavior change often was construed as a discrete event, such as quitting smoking, drinking, or overeating. The TTM posits change as a process that unfolds over time, with progress through a series of six stages, although frequently not in a linear manner.

Precontemplation is the stage in which people do not intend to take action in the near term, usually measured as the next six months. The outcome interval may vary, depending on the behavior. People may be in this stage because they are uninformed or under-informed about the consequences of their behavior. Or they may have tried to change a number of times and become demoralized about their abilities to change. Both groups tend to avoid reading, talking, or thinking about their high-risk behaviors. They are often characterized as resistant or unmotivated clients or as not ready for therapy or health promotion programs. An alternative explanation is that traditional health promotion programs were not ready for such individuals and were not motivated to match their needs.

In *contemplation,* people intend to change their behaviors in the next six months. They are more aware than precontemplators of the pros of changing but are also acutely aware of the cons. This balance between the costs and benefits of changing can produce profound ambivalence and keeps people stuck in contemplation for long periods of time. This phenomenon is often characterized as chronic contemplation or behavioral procrastination. These folks also are not ready for traditional action-oriented programs that expect participants to take action immediately.

In *preparation,* people intend to take action soon, usually measured as the next month. Typically, they already have taken some significant step toward the behavior in the past year. They have a plan of action, such as joining a health education class, consulting a counselor, talking to their physician, buying a self-help book, or relying on a self-change approach. These are the people who should be recruited for action-oriented programs, such as traditional smoking-cessation or weight-loss clinics.

People in the *action* stage have made specific, overt modifications in their lifestyles within the past six months. Because action is observable, behavior change often has been equated with action. In the TTM, action is only one of six stages. Typically, not all modifications of behavior count as action in this model. In most applications, people have to attain a criterion that scientists and professionals agree is sufficient to reduce risks for disease. In smoking, for example, the field used to count reduction in number of cigarettes or switching to low tar and nicotine cigarettes as action. Now, the consensus is clear—only total abstinence counts as action, as these other changes do not necessarily lead to quitting and do not lower risks associated with smoking to zero.

Maintenance is the stage in which people have made specific, overt modifications in their lifestyles and are working to prevent relapse, but they do not apply change processes as frequently as people in action. They are less tempted to relapse and are increasingly more confident that they can continue their changes. Based on temptation and self-efficacy data, it was estimated that maintenance lasts from six months to about five years. Longitudinal data from the 1990 Surgeon General's Report (U.S. Department of Health and Human Services, 1990) supported this temporal estimate. After twelve months of continuous abstinence, 43 percent of individuals returned to regular smoking. It was not until five years of continuous abstinence that the risk for relapse dropped to 7 percent.

People in the *termination* stage have zero temptation and 100 percent self-efficacy. Whether they are depressed, anxious, bored, lonely, angry, or stressed, they are sure they will not return to their old unhealthy behaviors. It is as if they never acquired the behavior in the first place or their new behavior has become automatic. Examples are adults who buckle their seatbelts as soon as they get in their cars or automatically take their antihypertensive medications at the same time and place each day. In a study of former smokers and alcoholics, we found that less than 20 percent of each group had reached the criterion of zero temptation and total self-efficacy (Snow, Prochaska, and Rossi, 1992). The criterion may be too strict, or this stage may be an ideal goal for the majority of people. In other areas, like exercise, consistent condom use, and weight control, the realistic goal may be a lifetime of maintenance, because relapse temptations are so prevalent and strong. Termination has received much less research attention than other stages.

Processes of Change

Processes of change are the covert and overt activities people use to progress through stages. Processes of change provide important guides for intervention programs, as processes are like independent variables that people need to apply to move from stage to stage. Ten processes have received the most empirical support in research to date (see Table 5.1).

1. *Consciousness raising* involves increased awareness about the causes, consequences, and cures for a particular problem behavior. Interventions that can increase awareness include feedback, confrontations, interpretations, bibliotherapy, and media campaigns.

2. *Dramatic relief* initially produces increased emotional experiences, followed by reduced affect or anticipated relief if appropriate action is taken. Role-playing, grieving, personal testimonies, health risk feedback, and media campaigns are examples of techniques that can move people emotionally.

3. *Self-reevaluation* combines both cognitive and affective assessments of one's self-image with and without an unhealthy behavior, such as one's image as a couch potato and an active person. Values clarification, healthy role models, and imagery are techniques that can move people evaluatively.

4. *Environmental reevaluation* combines both affective and cognitive assessments of how the presence or absence of a personal behavior affects one's social environment, such as the impact of one's smoking on others. It can also include awareness that one can serve as a positive or negative role model for others. Empathy training, documentaries, testimonials, and family interventions can lead to such reassessments.

5. *Self-liberation* is both the belief that one can change and the commitment and re-commitment to act on that belief. New Year's resolutions, public testimonies, and multiple rather than single choices can enhance what the public calls willpower.

6. *Social liberation* requires an increase in social opportunities or alternatives, especially for people who are relatively deprived or oppressed. Advocacy, empowerment procedures, and appropriate policies can produce increased opportunities for minority health promotion, gay health promotion, and health promotion for impoverished people. These same procedures can be used to help all people change, as is the case with smoke-free zones, salad bars in school lunchrooms, and easy access to condoms and other contraceptives.

7. *Counterconditioning* requires learning healthier behaviors that can substitute for problem behaviors. Relaxation, assertion, desensitization, nicotine replacement, and positive self-statements are strategies for safer substitutes.

8. *Stimulus control* removes cues for unhealthy habits and adds prompts for healthier alternatives. Avoidance, environmental re-engineering, and self-help groups can provide stimuli that support change and reduce risks for relapse.

9. *Contingency management* provides consequences for taking steps in a particular direction. Although contingency management can include the use of punishment, we found that self-changers rely on reward much more than punishment. Reinforcements are emphasized, since a philosophy of the stage model is to work in harmony with how people change naturally. Contingency contracts, overt and covert reinforcements, incentives, and group recognition are procedures for increasing reinforcement and the probability that healthier responses will be repeated.

10. *Helping relationships* combine caring, trust, openness, and acceptance, as well as support for healthy behavior change. Rapport building, therapeutic alliances, counselor calls, and buddy systems can be sources of social support.

Decisional Balance

Decisional balance reflects an individual's relative weighing of the pros and cons of changing. Originally, TTM relied on Janis and Mann's (1977) model of decision making that included four categories of pros (instrumental gains for self and others and approval from self and others) and four categories of cons (instrumental costs to self and others and disapproval from self and others). Over many studies attempting to produce this structure of eight factors, a much simpler two-factor structure was almost always found—pros and cons of changing.

Self-Efficacy

Self-efficacy is the situation-specific confidence that people can cope with high-risk situations without relapsing to their former behaviors. This construct was integrated from Bandura's (1982) self-efficacy theory.

Temptation

Temptation reflects the converse of self efficacy   the intensity of urges to engage in a specific behavior when in difficult situations. Typically, three factors reflect most common types of temptations: negative affect or emotional distress, positive social situations, and craving.

Critical Assumptions

The TTM has concentrated on five stages of change, ten processes of change, pros and cons of changing, self-efficacy, and temptation. It is also based on critical assumptions about the nature of behavior change and interventions that can best facilitate such change. The following set of assumptions drive theory, research, and practice related to the TTM:

1. No single theory can account for all complexities of behavior change. A more comprehensive model is most likely to emerge from integration across major theories.
2. Behavior change is a process that unfolds over time through a sequence of stages.
3. Stages are both stable and open to change, just as chronic behavioral risk factors are stable and open to change.
4. The majority of at-risk populations are not prepared for action and will not be served effectively by traditional action-oriented behavior change programs.
5. Specific processes and principles of change should be emphasized at specific stages to maximize efficacy.

Empirical Support and Challenges

Each of the core constructs has been subjected to a wide variety of studies across a broad range of behaviors and populations. Early in the process of applying TTM to new behaviors, formative research and measurement work begins (Redding, Maddock, and Rossi, 2006), followed by intervention development and refinement, leading to formal efficacy and effectiveness trials. Ideally, cohorts of individuals should be followed over time to determine how they respond. Only a sampling of these studies can be reviewed here.

Stage Distribution. If interventions are to match needs of entire populations, we should know the stage distributions for specific high-risk behaviors. A series of studies on smoking in the United States (for example, Velicer and others, 1995; Wewers, Stillman, Hartman, and Shopland, 2003) clearly demonstrated that less than 20 percent of smokers were in preparation. Approximately 40 percent of smokers were in contemplation, and another 40 percent were in precontemplation. In countries without a long history of tobacco control campaigns, stage distributions were even more challenging. In Germany, about 70 percent of smokers were in precontemplation, and about 10 percent of smokers were in preparation (Etter, Perneger, and Ronchi, 1997); in China, more than 70 percent were in precontemplation and about 5 percent in preparation (Yang and others, 2001). In a sample of 20,000 members of an HMO across fifteen health-risk behaviors, only a small minority were ready for action (Rossi, 1992a).

Pros and Cons Structure Across Twelve Behaviors. Across studies of twelve different behaviors (smoking cessation, quitting cocaine, weight control, dietary fat reduction, safer sex, condom use, exercise acquisition, sunscreen use, radon testing, delinquency reduction, mammography screening, and physicians practicing preventive medicine), the two-factor structure was remarkably stable (Prochaska and others, 1994).

Integration of Pros and Cons and Stages of Change Across Twelve Health Behaviors. *Stage* is a construct, not a theory. A theory requires systematic relationships between a set of constructs, ideally culminating in mathematical relationships. Systematic relationships have been found between stage and pros and cons of changing for twelve health behaviors.

In all twelve studies, cons of changing were higher than pros for people in precontemplation (Prochaska and others, 1994), and pros increased between precontemplation and contemplation. From contemplation to action for all twelve behaviors, cons of changing were lower in action than in contemplation. In eleven of the twelve studies, pros of changing were higher than cons for people in action. These relationships suggest that to progress from precontemplation to later stages, pros of changing should increase. To progress from contemplation, cons should decrease. To move to action, pros should be higher than cons.

Strong and Weak Principles of Progress Across Forty-Eight Behaviors. Across these same twelve studies, mathematical relationships were found between pros and cons of changing and progress across the stages (Prochaska, 1994).

The Strong Principle is

$$PC \rightarrow A \cong 1 \; SD \uparrow PROS$$

Progress from precontemplation to action involves about one standard deviation (SD) increase in the pros of changing. On intelligence tests, a one SD increase would be 15 points, which is a substantial increase.

In a recent meta-analysis of forty-eight health behaviors and 120 data sets from ten countries, it was predicted that the pros of changing would increase one SD. The Strong Principle was confirmed to the second decimal with the increase being 1.00 SD (Hall and Rossi, 2008).

The Weak Principle is

$$PC \rightarrow A \cong 0.5 \; SD \downarrow CONS$$

Progress from precontemplation to action involves ~0.5 SD decrease in the cons of changing.

Evidence from the recent meta-analysis for the Weak Principle was not as precise: 0.56 SD (Hall and Rossi, in press). Nevertheless, the multitude of data on forty-eight behaviors from 120 datasets could be integrated in a single graph that supported two mathematical principles.

Practical implications of these principles are that pros of changing must increase about twice as much as cons must decrease. Perhaps twice as much emphasis should be placed on raising benefits as on reducing costs or barriers to enact recommended behaviors. For example, if couch potatoes in precontemplation can only list five pros of exercise, then being too busy will be a big barrier to change. But if program participants come to appreciate that there can be more than fifty benefits for exercising most days of the week, being too busy may become a relatively small barrier.

Processes of Change Across Behaviors. One of the assumptions of TTM is that people can apply a common set of change processes across a broad range of behaviors. The higher-order measurement structure of the processes (experiential and behavioral) has been replicated across problem behaviors better than have specific processes (Rossi, 1992b). Typically, support has been found for the standard set of ten processes across such behaviors as smoking, diet, cocaine use, exercise, condom use, and sun exposure. But the measurement structure of the processes across studies has not been as consistent as the mathematical relationships between the stages and the pros and cons of changing. In some studies, fewer processes are found. Occasionally, evidence for one or two additional processes is found. It is also very possible that for some behaviors, fewer change processes may be used. With a regular but infrequent behavior like yearly mammograms, for example, fewer processes may be required to progress to long-term maintenance (Rakowski and others, 1998).

Relationships Between Stages and Processes of Change. One of the earliest empirical integrations was the discovery of systematic relationships between people's stages and the processes they were applying. Table 5.2 presents the empirical integration (Prochaska, DiClemente, and Norcross, 1992). This integration suggests that, in early stages, people apply cognitive, affective, and evaluative processes to progress through stages. In later stages, people rely more on commitments, conditioning, contingencies, environmental controls, and support for progressing toward maintenance or termination.

TABLE 5.2. **Processes of Change That Mediate Progression Between the Stages of Change.**

	Precontemplation	Contemplation	Preparation	Action	Maintenance
Processes	Consciousness raising				
	Dramatic relief				
	Environmental reevaluation				
		Self-reevaluation			
			Self-liberation		
				Counterconditioning	
				Helping relationships	
				Reinforcement management	
				Stimulus control	

Note: Social liberation was omitted due to its unclear relationship to the stages.

Table 5.2 has important practical implications. To help people progress from precontemplation to contemplation, such processes as consciousness raising and dramatic relief should be applied. Applying processes like contingency management, counterconditioning, and stimulus control to people in precontemplation would represent a theoretical, empirical, and practical mistake. But for people in action, such strategies would represent optimal matching.

As with the structure of processes, relationships between the processes and stages have not been as consistent as relationships between stages and pros and cons of changing. Although part of the problem may be due to the greater complexity of integrating ten processes across five stages, processes of change need more basic research and may be more specific to each problem behavior.

Applied Studies.   Across a large, diverse body of applied studies that used TTM, several trends are clear. The most common application involves TTM-tailored expert system communications, which match intervention messages to an individual's needs across TTM constructs. For example, people in precontemplation could receive feedback designed to increase pros of changing to help them progress to contemplation. In the past, these interventions were usually printed either on-site (for example, at a worksite or doctor's office) or mailed to participants at home. With growth of the Internet, multimedia expert system programs (Redding and others, 1999) can be delivered in this manner, potentially reaching many more people than programs delivered in fixed sites.

The largest number of TTM-related intervention studies have focused on smoking cessation (Aveyard and others, 1999; Curry and others, 1995; Dijkstra, DeVries, and Roijackers, 1999; Dijkstra, Conijm, and DeVries, 2006; Hall and others, 2006; Hollis and others, 2005; O'Neill, Gillespie, and Slobin, 2000; Pallonen and others, 1998; Prochaska, DiClemente, Velicer, and Rossi, 1993; Prochaska and others, 2001a, 2001b; Strecher and others, 1994; Velicer and others, 1999); diet (Beresford and others, 1997; Brug and others, 1998; Campbell and others, 1994; Glanz and others, 1998; Horwath, 1999); and exercise (Cardinal and Sachs, 1996; Marcus and others, 1998; Rossi and others, 2005). Recent randomized controlled trial outcome studies include stress management (Evers and others, 2006), medication adherence (Johnson and others, 2006a, 2006b), and bullying prevention (Prochaska and others, 2007). The number of applications is growing, from alcohol abuse (Project Match, 1997; Carbonari and DiClemente, 2000), to condom use (CDC, 1999; Parsons and others, 2000; Redding, Morokoff, Rossi, and Meier, 2007), to domestic violence offenders (Levesque, Driskell, Prochaska, and Prochaska, forthcoming), to organ donation (Robbins and others, 2001) and multiple behavior changes (Gold, Anderson, and Serxner, 2000; Kreuter and Strecher, 1996; Steptoe, Kerry, Rink, and Hilton, 2001).

TTM has been applied in many settings, including primary care (Goldstein and others, 1999; Hollis and others, 2005), home (Curry and others, 1995; Gold, Anderson, and Serxner, 2000), churches (Voorhees and others, 1996), schools (Aveyard and others, 1999), campuses (J. M. Prochaska and others, 2004), communities (Centers for Disease Control and Prevention, 1999), and worksites (Prochaska and others, 2008). Although many of these applications have been effective, some have not (for example, Aveyard and others, 1999). A recent meta-analysis of tailored print communications found that TTM was the most commonly used theory across a broad range of behaviors (Noar, Benac, and Harris, 2007). TTM or Stage of Change Models were used in thirty-five of the fifty-three studies. Significantly greater effect sizes were found when tailored communications included each of the following TTM constructs: stages of change, pros and cons of changing, self-efficacy, and processes of change (Noar, Benac, and Harris, 2007). In contrast, interventions that included the non-TTM construct of perceived susceptibility had significantly worse outcomes. Tailoring on non-TTM constructs like social norms and behavioral intentions did not produce significantly greater effect sizes (Noar, Benac, and Harris, 2007).

Although each of the major TTM constructs (stage, pros and cons, self-efficacy, and processes) produced greater effect sizes when included in tailored communications, what happens when only some of constructs are used? Spencer and colleagues (2002) systematically reviewed twenty-three interventions that used one or more TTM variables for smoking cessation. Most studies used just stage of change; of these, only about 40 percent produced significant effects. Five used stage plus pros and cons or self-efficacy; 60 percent produced significant effects. Another five used all TTM variables; 80 percent found significant effects. This analysis raises the important dissemination question of what it means for practice and applied research to be theory-driven. Most studies were variable-driven (for example, using the "stage" variable) rather than theory-driven. Future research should determine whether applied research is most effective when a full theory, like TTM, is applied or whether there is an optimal number of theoretical variables that can produce the same effect sizes, while placing fewer demands on participants and practitioners.

Challenging Studies. As with any model, not all research is supportive. Farkas and colleagues (1996) and Abrams and colleagues (2000) compared addiction variables to TTM variables as predictors of cessation over twelve to twenty-four months. Addiction variables, like number of cigarettes smoked and duration of prior quits (for example, more than 100 days) out-predicted TTM variables, suggesting that addiction models were preferable to TTM. Responses to these comparative studies included concerns that Farkas and colleagues (1996) compared fourteen addiction type variables to just the single stage variable from TTM (Prochaska and Velicer, 1996; Prochaska, 2006). The Abrams and colleagues (2000) study included self-efficacy and the contemplation ladder—an alternative measure of readiness or stage, as part of their addiction model, but these are part of TTM. Also, from an intervention perspective, amount of variance accounted for by predictor variables is less important than amount of variance that can be controlled or changed. Although duration of previous quits (for example, 100 days) may be more predictive than stage, little can be done to change this historical variable, whereas a dynamic variable like stage is amenable to intervention.

In the first of a series of studies, Herzog and colleagues (1999) found that six processes of change were not adequate predictors of stage progress over a twelve-month period. In a second report, processes predicted stage progress but only when the contemplation ladder was used (Herzog and others, 2000). In the third report,

TTM measures predicted twelve-month outcomes, but self-efficacy and the contemplation ladder were not counted as TTM variables (Abrams, Herzog, Emmons, and Linnan, 2000). Other research has found that change processes and other TTM variables predict stage progress (for example, Prochaska and others, 1985; Prochaska and others, 1991; Prochaska, Velicer, Prochaska, and Johnson, 2004; Prochaska and others, 2008; DiClemente and others, 1991; Dijkstra, Conijm, and De Vries, 2006; Johnson and others, 2000; Sun, Prochaska, Velicer, and Laforge, 2007; Velicer, Redding, Sun, and Prochaska, 2007). Johnson and colleagues (2000) explained some of the inconsistencies in previous research by demonstrating better predictions over six months versus twelve months, and better predictions using all ten processes of change instead of just a subset.

One productive response to studies critical of the TTM is to conduct further research. In response to the criticism that addiction levels are better predictors of long-term outcomes than stage of change, a series of studies was conducted to determine which types of effects predict long-term outcomes across multiple behaviors. To date, four such effects have been found (Prochaska, 2008). The first is a severity effect, in which individuals with less severe behavior risks at baseline are more likely to progress to action or maintenance at twenty-four-month follow-up for smoking, diet, and sun exposure. This effect includes the level of addiction that Farkas and colleagues (1996) and Abrams and colleagues (2000) preferred. The second is a stage effect in which participants in preparation at baseline have better twenty-four-month outcomes for smoking, diet, and sun exposure than those in contemplation, who do better than those in precontemplation. This stage effect is what Farkas and colleagues (1996) and Abrams and colleagues (2000) criticized. The third is a treatment effect in which participants in treatment do better at twenty-four months than those randomly assigned to control groups for smoking, diet, and sun exposure. The fourth is an effort effect, in which participants in both treatment and control groups who progressed to action and maintenance at twenty-four months were making better efforts with TTM variables like pros and cons, self-efficacy, and processes at baseline. There were no consistent demographic effects across the three behaviors, indicating that no single demographic group did better across these multiple behaviors. What these results indicate is that either-or thinking (such as either severity or stage) is not as helpful as a more inclusive approach that seeks to identify the most important effects, whether they are based on TTM or on an addiction or severity model.

APPLICATIONS OF THE TRANSTHEORETICAL MODEL TO SMOKING CESSATION

Applying a theory like TTM to an entire at-risk population, like smokers, requires a systematic approach that begins with recruiting and retaining a high percentage of the eligible population. The program should help participants progress through the stages of change by applying a process that matches or tailors interventions to the needs of each individual at each stage of change. Such systematic applications can then be evaluated in terms of outcomes by assessing impacts on reducing the prevalence of smoking in the target population.

Smoking is costly to individual smokers and to society. In the United States, approximately 47,000,000 Americans continue to smoke. Over 500,000 preventable deaths per year are attributable to smoking (U.S. Department of Health and Human Services, 2000). Globally, the consequences are likely to be catastrophic. Of the people alive in the world today, 500,000,000 are expected to die from this single behavior, losing approximately 5 billion years of life to tobacco use. Providing smoking cessation to entire populations could prevent millions of premature deaths and help preserve billions of years of life.

Recruitment

Population cessation requires interventions that reach or recruit high percentages of smokers. In two home-based programs with about 5,000 smokers in each study, we reached out either by telephone alone or by personal letters, followed by telephone calls if needed, and recruited smokers to stage-matched interventions. For each of five stages, interventions included self-help manuals; individualized computer feedback reports based on assessments of pros and cons, processes, self-efficacy and temptations; and/or counselor protocols based on computer reports. Using proactive recruitment methods and stage-matched interventions resulted in rates of 80 percent to 85 percent, respectively (Prochaska and others, 2001a, 2001b). Such high recruitment rates provide the potential to generate unprecedented impacts with entire populations of smokers.

Population impact has been defined as participation rate × the rate of efficacy or action (Velicer and DiClemente, 1993). If a program produced 30 percent efficacy (for example, long-term abstinence), historically it was judged to be better than a program that produced 25 percent abstinence. A program that generates 30 percent efficacy but only 5 percent participation has an impact of only 1.5 percent (30 percent × 5 percent). A program that produces only 25 percent efficacy but 60 percent participation has an impact of 15 percent. With health promotion programs, the impact on a high-risk population would be ten times greater.

TTM programs shift outcomes from efficacy alone to impact. To achieve such high impact, we need to shift from reactive recruitment, where we advertise or announce programs and react when people reach us, to proactive recruitments, where we reach out to interact with all potential participants, including those not yet ready to change behaviors.

Proactive recruitment alone will not work. In the most intensive recruitment protocol to date (Lichtenstein and Hollis, 1992), physicians spent up to five minutes with smokers to get them to sign up for an action-oriented cessation clinic. If that didn't work, a nurse spent ten minutes to persuade each smoker to sign up, followed by twelve minutes with a videotape and health educator and even a proactive counselor call, if necessary. This resulted in 1 percent initial participation. The proactive protocol resulted in 35 percent of smokers in precontemplation enrolling; only 3 percent showed up, and 2 percent completed. With a combination of smokers in contemplation and preparation, 65 percent signed up, 15 percent showed up, and 11 percent completed the program.

To optimize impacts, proactive protocols are used to recruit participants to programs that match their stages. Once high recruitment rates are achieved, the next practical concern is to generate high retention rates, lest many of the initial participants drop out.

Retention

One of the skeletons in the closet of psychotherapy and behavior change interventions is their relatively poor retention rates. Across 125 studies, the average retention rate was only about 50 percent (Wierzbicki and Pekarik, 1993). Furthermore, this meta-analysis found few consistent predictors of who would drop out prematurely and who would continue in therapy. In studies on smoking, weight control, substance abuse, and a mixture of mental health problems, stage of change measures proved to be the best predictors of premature termination. In a study of psychotherapy for mental health problems, the pre-treatment stage profile of the entire 40 percent who dropped out prematurely, as judged by their therapists, was that of patients in precontemplation. The 20 percent who terminated quickly but appropriately had a profile of patients in action. Pre-treatment stage-related measures correctly classified 93 percent of the three groups (Brogan, Prochaska, and Prochaska, 1999).

Therapists cannot treat people in precontemplation as if they were ready for action interventions and expect them to stay in treatment or to succeed as a consequence of treatment. Relapse prevention strategies would be indicated for smokers who are taking action. But those in precontemplation are more likely to need drop-out prevention strategies.

The best strategy to promote retention is to match interventions to stage of change. In three smoking cessation studies using such matching strategies, smokers in precontemplation were retained at the same high levels as those who started in the preparation stage (Prochaska, DiClemente, Velicer, and Rossi, 1993; Prochaska and others, 2001a, 2001b).

Progress

The amount of progress participants make following health promotion programs is directly related to their stage at the start of interventions. Across sixty-six different predictions of progress, smokers starting in contemplation were about two-thirds more successful than those in precontemplation at six-, twelve-, and eighteen-month follow-ups. Similarly, those in preparation were about two-thirds more successful than those in contemplation at the same follow-ups (Prochaska and others, 2001a).

These results can be used in practice. A reasonable goal for each therapeutic intervention with smokers is to help them progress one stage. If over the course of brief therapy they progress two stages, they will be about 2.66 times more successful at longer-term follow-ups (Prochaska and others, 2001a).

This strategy was taught to more than 6,000 primary care physicians, nurses, and physicians' assistants in Britain's National Health System. With stage-matched counseling, the strategic goal is to help each patient progress one stage following one brief intervention. One of the first reports was a marked improvement in the morale of such health promoters intervening with all patients who smoke, abuse substances, and have unhealthy diets. These professionals now have strategies that match the needs of all of their patients, not just the minority prepared to take action. Furthermore, practitioners can assess progress across stages in the majority of these patients, where previously they experienced mostly failure when taking action was their only measure of movement (Steptoe, Kerry, Rink, and Hilton, 2001).

Processes

Different processes of change need to be applied at different stages of change. Classic conditioning processes like counterconditioning, stimulus control, and contingency control can be highly successful strategies for participants taking action, but using them can produce resistance with individuals in precontemplation. With these individuals, more experiential processes, like consciousness raising and dramatic relief, can move people cognitively and affectively and help them shift to contemplation (Prochaska, Norcross, and DiClemente, 1994).

After fifteen years of research, fourteen variables have been identified on which to intervene to accelerate progress across the first five stages of change (Prochaska, Norcross, and DiClemente, 1994). At any particular stage, a maximum of six variables should be intervened upon. To help guide people at each stage of change, computer-based expert systems have been developed to deliver individualized, interactive, TTM-tailored interventions to entire populations (Redding and others, 1999). These computer programs can be used alone or in conjunction with counselors.

Outcomes

In our first large-scale clinical trial, we compared four treatments: (1) one of the best home-based action-oriented cessation programs (standardized); (2) stage-matched manuals (individualized); (3) expert system computer reports plus manuals (interactive); and (4) counselors plus computers and manuals (personalized). We randomly assigned by stage 739 smokers to one of the four treatments (Prochaska, DiClemente, Velicer, and Rossi, 1993).

In the computer condition, participants completed by mail or telephone forty questions that were entered in our central computers and used as the basis for computer-generated feedback reports. These reports informed participants about their stage of change, their pros and cons of changing, and their use of change processes appropriate to their stages. At baseline, participants were given positive feedback on what they were doing correctly and guidance on which principles and processes they should apply to progress. In two progress reports delivered over the next six months, they also received positive feedback on any improvement they made on any of the variables relevant to progressing. Therefore, demoralized and defensive smokers could begin progressing without having to quit and without having to work too hard. Smokers in

the contemplation stage could begin taking small steps (like delaying their first cigarette in the morning for an extra thirty minutes) that would increase their self-efficacy
and help them become better prepared for quitting. In the personalized condition, smokers received four proactive counselor calls over the six-month intervention period.

The two self-help manual conditions paralleled each other for twelve months. At
eighteen months, the stage-matched manuals moved ahead. This is an example of a
delayed action effect, which is often observed with stage-matched programs specifically and others have observed with self-help programs generally (Glynn, Anderson,
and Schwarz, 1992). It takes time for participants in early stages to progress to action. Therefore, some treatment effects, measured by action, will be observed only
after considerable delay. It is encouraging to find treatments producing therapeutic
effects months and even years after treatment ended.

Computer alone and computer plus counselor conditions paralleled each other
for twelve months. Then, effects of the counselor condition flattened out while the
computer condition effects continued to increase. Participants in the personalized
condition may have become somewhat dependent on the social support and social
control of the counselor calling. The last call was after the six-months assessment,
and benefits would be observed at twelve months. Termination of counselors could
result in no further progress because of the loss of social support and control. The
classic pattern in smoking cessation clinics is rapid relapse beginning as soon as the
treatment is terminated. Some of this rapid relapse could well be due to the sudden
loss of social support or social control provided by the counselors and other participants in the clinic.

In this clinical trial, smokers were recruited reactively. They called us in response
to advertisements, announcements, and articles. How would their results compare to
the smokers proactively recruited to our programs? Most people would predict that
smokers who call us for help would succeed more than smokers we called to help.

Figure 5.1 shows remarkable results comparing smokers in a study whom we
called (reactive) (Prochaska, DiClemente, Velicer, and Rossi, 1993) to those in a study
whom we called (proactive) (Prochaska and others, 2001a). Both groups received the
same home-based expert system computer reports delivered over a six-month period.
Although the reactively recruited subjects were slightly more successful at each follow-up, what is striking is the similarity of results.

Outcomes with Diverse Groups

Outcomes with diverse groups were part of an analysis that combined data from five
effectiveness trials where 2,972 smokers were proactively recruited; all received the
same TTM-tailored intervention plus stage-matched manuals. The intervention produced a consistent 22 percent to 26 percent long-term cessation rate across the five
studies, with a mean of about 24 percent (Velicer, Redding, Sun, and Prochaska, 2007).
There were no significant differences in abstinence rates between females (24.6 percent) and males (23.6 percent). There were no significant differences between African
Americans (30.2 percent) and Caucasians (23.9 percent) or between Hispanics and

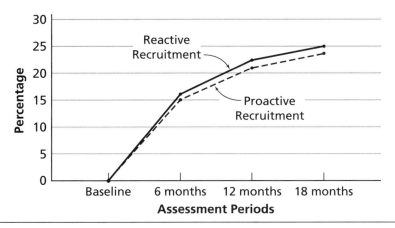

FIGURE 5.1. Point Prevalence Abstinence Rates Over Time for Smokers Recruited by Reactive Versus Proactive Strategies and Treated with TTM-Tailored Home-Based Expert System Interventions.

non-Hispanics. Older smokers (65 and older) had abstinence rates (35.2 percent) that were 45 percent higher than the mean. College graduates had abstinence rates (30.1 percent) that were significantly higher than average.

The Surgeon General's Report on Adolescent Smoking (U.S. Department of Health and Human Services, 1994) concluded that teenage smokers would not participate in treatments, and if they did, they would not quit. Hollis and colleagues (2005) proactively recruited 65 percent of teens in primary care to a smoking cessation program based on TTM-tailored communications. At long-term follow-up, regular smokers receiving treatment had significantly higher cessation rates (23.9 percent) than the randomized control group (11.4 percent). Furthermore, their quit rate of 23.9 percent was essentially the same as the average quit rate in our adult treatment groups (Hollis and others, 2005).

Working with smokers who have co-morbidities (other diseases or conditions, such as diabetes or hypertension) presents important challenges. The Clinical Guidelines for the Treatment of Tobacco (Fiore and others, 2000) identified no evidence-based treatments for smokers with mental illnesses, even though such smokers consume nearly 50 percent of all cigarettes in the United States. Hall and colleagues (2006) reached out to smokers who were being treated for depression in clinics at the University of California at San Francisco. Those randomized to treatment received our TTM-tailored program plus counseling and nicotine replacement therapy. At twenty-four-month follow-up, the treatment group had significantly higher abstinence rates (24.6 percent) than the controls (19.1 percent), and their quit rates were remarkably similar to those of treated adults in other studies (Hall and others, 2006).

These outcomes with diverse groups receiving similar TTM-tailored treatments challenge stereotypes that assume some groups do not have the ability to change. Minorities, older adults, adolescents, and mentally ill groups may be assumed to have less ability to change. These results suggest that the issue may not be their ability to change. The issue may be their access to quality change programs.

If these results are replicated, health promotion programs could produce unprecedented impacts on major risk behaviors like smoking among entire populations. We believe that such unprecedented impacts require scientific and professional shifts from

- An action paradigm to a stage paradigm
- Reactive to proactive recruitment
- Expecting participants to match the needs of our programs to having our programs match their needs
- Clinic-based to community-based behavioral health programs that still apply the field's most powerful individualized and interactive intervention strategies
- Assuming some groups do not have the ability to change to making sure that all groups have easy accessibility to evidence-based programs

MULTIPLE-BEHAVIOR CHANGE PROGRAMS

One of the greatest challenges for the application of any theory is to keep raising the bar, to increase impacts the theory has on enhancing health. The original impact equation was Impact = Reach × Efficacy. With TTM clinical trials having recruited 80 percent or more of eligible smokers in a population, any produced increase in impacts would have to come from increasing efficacy, such as the abstinence rate with smokers. Across a series of enhancement studies, we have been unable to increase cessation efficacy by using counselors (Prochaska and others, 2001b, increasing number of contacts (Velicer and others, 1999), adding a hand-held computer (Prochaska and others, 2001), adding nicotine replacement therapy (Velicer and others, 2006), or adding telecounseling (Velicer and others, 2006).

One potential alternative to increase the impact of TTM interventions was to treat multiple behaviors in a population, because populations with multiple-behavior risks are at greatest risk for chronic disease and premature death. These populations also account for a disproportionate percentage of health care costs. The best estimates are that about 60 percent of health care costs are due to about 15 percent of the population, all of whom have multiple-behavior risks (Edington, 2001).

From a TTM perspective, applying an action paradigm to multiple behaviors could overwhelm populations, as action is the most demanding stage; taking action on two or more behaviors at once could be daunting. But in individuals with four health behavior risks, like smoking, diet, sun exposure, and sedentary lifestyles, less than 10 percent of the population was ready to take action on two or more behaviors (Prochaska and Velicer, 1997). The same thing was true for populations with diabetes who needed to change four behaviors (Ruggiero and others, 1997).

The DISC (Diabetes Stages of Change) study was implemented with (N = 1,029) type 1 and type 2 diabetes patients randomized to TTM-tailored treatment or standard care comparison group (Jones and others, 2003). The treatment group received interventions for three risk behaviors: smoking, healthy diet, and blood glucose self-monitoring, if they were at risk for any one of these behaviors. The TTM-tailored group demonstrated greater progress at final outcome measurement than the comparison group on all targeted risk behaviors, as well as a significant reduction in Hemoglobin A1C—a biomarker for diabetes control (Jones and others, 2003).

The *SENIOR Project* was a randomized community intervention that included manuals, newsletters, TTM-tailored feedback reports, and telephone coaching delivered to 1,276 older adults (mean age was 75.4 years) over twelve months, designed to increase exercise and fruit and vegetable consumption. Final twenty-four-month outcomes showed progression to action/maintenance for exercise was greater for all treatment groups (44 percent) relative to controls (26 percent) (Rossi and others, 2005). Servings of fruit and vegetables for those who received the diet intervention increased, compared to those who did not (Greene and others, in press; Rossi and others, 2005).

Applying best practices of a stage-based multiple behavior manual and expert system TTM-tailored feedback reports over twelve months, we proactively intervened on a population of parents of teens who were participating in parallel projects at school (J. O. Prochaska and others, 2004). First, we had to demonstrate that we could proactively recruit a high percentage of parents if impacts were to be high. We recruited 83.6 percent of available parents. The treatment group received up to three expert system reports at zero, six, and twelve months. At twenty-four-month follow-up, the smoking cessation rate was significantly greater in the treatment group (22 percent abstinent) than the controls (17 percent). The parents did even better on diet, with 33.5 percent progressing to the action or maintenance stage and going from high-fat to low-fat diets, compared to 25.9 percent of the controls. With sun exposure, 29.7 percent of baseline at-risk parents had reached action or maintenance stages in the treatment group, compared to 18.1 percent of the controls.

With a population of 5,545 patients from primary care practices, we recruited 65 percent for a second multiple behavior change project (Prochaska and others, 2005). This represents the lowest recruitment rates to date and appeared to be due to patient concerns that we had received their names and phone numbers from their managed care company, which many did not trust.

With this population, mammography screening was also targeted. Significant treatment effects were found for all four target behaviors. At twenty-four months, 25.4 percent of the treatment group, compared to 18 percent for the controls, had quit smoking, and 28.8 percent of the treatment group had progressed from high-fat to low-fat diets, compared to 19.5 percent of the control group. With sun exposure, 23.4 percent of the treatment group was in action or maintenance, compared to 14.4 percent of the controls. And, with mammography screening, twice as many in the control group relapsed (6 percent), compared to the treatment group (3 percent).

Comparison across three multiple-risk behavior studies shows that efficacy rates for smoking of 22 percent and 25 percent abstinent fall within the narrow range of 22 percent to 25 percent efficacy that we had consistently found when targeting only the single behavior of smoking (Prochaska and others, 2006). Further, smokers with a single risk were no more successful in quitting than smokers who were treated for two or three risk behaviors. The same was found for participants with a single risk of diet or sun exposure, compared with those with two or three risk behaviors. Taken together, these results indicate that TTM-tailored interventions may be producing unprecedented impacts on multiple behaviors for disease prevention and health promotion.

LIMITATIONS OF THE MODEL

Although TTM has been applied across at least forty-eight behaviors and populations from many countries, the model still has limitations. The problem area that has produced the most disappointment has been primary prevention of substance abuse in children. To date, population trials based on TTM have not produced significant prevention effects (see, for example, Aveyard and others, 1999; Hollis and others, 2005). Unfortunately, little can be concluded from nonsignificant results. For example, Peterson and colleagues (2000) also reported that sixteen out of seventeen such trials failed and suggested that the field should move beyond social influence models. Prevention trials have proved challenging across theories.

Part of the challenge from a TTM perspective is that almost all young people who have not yet used substances like tobacco, alcohol, or other drugs are in the precontemplation stage for acquisition of such use. One promising approach was to identify subgroups based on pros, cons, and temptation to try using. Those with a profile of low pros for using, high cons, and low temptations were clearly the most protected. This profile showed the best effort effects at baseline and the least acquisition at twelve, twenty-four, and thirty-six months (Velicer, Redding, Sun, and Prochaska, 2007). The first trials applying such profiles did not produce significant effects, but new trials can learn from such experiences and apply more creative and effective interventions. It remains to be seen whether effective TTM-tailored prevention programs can be developed that build on both theoretical and empirical insights.

It might be assumed that TTM does not apply very well to children and adolescents. There is a basic question as to the age at which intentional behavior change begins. But applied studies in bullying prevention in elementary, middle, and high schools have all produced impressive results (Prochaska and others, 2007). Similarly, early intervention with adolescent smokers using TTM-tailored treatments produced significant abstinence rates at twenty-four months that were almost identical to rates found with treated adult smokers (Hollis and others, 2005). This was also true of TTM-tailored interventions targeting sun-protective behaviors in adolescents (Norman and others, 2007). One problem is that there has been much more research applying TTM to reducing risks than to preventing risks.

Given the global application of TTM, it will be important to determine in which cultures TTM can be applied effectively and in which cultures it may require major adaptations. In basic meta-analysis research on the relationships between stages and pros and cons of changing in ten countries, there was no significant effect by country (Hall and Rossi, 2008). But this was only in ten of the many countries in the world.

FUTURE RESEARCH

Although research results to date are encouraging, much still needs to be done to advance TTM. Basic research should be done with other theoretical variables, such as processes of resistance, framing, and problem severity, to determine if such variables relate systematically to the stages and predict progress across particular stages. More research is needed on the structure or integration of processes and stages of change across a broad range of behaviors, such as acquisition behaviors, like exercise, and extinction behaviors, like smoking cessation (Rosen, 2000). It is important to examine what modifications are needed for specific types of behaviors, such as fewer processes perhaps for infrequent behaviors, like mammography screening, or behaviors that may relapse less often, such as sunscreen use.

Since tailored communications represent the most promising interventions for applying TTM to entire populations, more research is needed to compare effectiveness, cost-effectiveness, and impacts of alternative technologies. The Internet is excellent for delivering individualized interactions at low cost, but it cannot produce the high participation rates generated by person-to-person outreach via telephone or primary care practitioners (Prochaska and others, 2008; Prochaska, Velicer, Prochaska, and Johnson, 2004; Prochaska and others, 2005).

Although application of TTM-tailored interventions with diverse populations has been promising, more research needs to be done comparing alternative modalities for reaching and helping these populations. Perhaps menus of alternative intervention modalities (such as telephone, Internet, neighborhood or church leaders, person-to-person, or community programs) could empower diverse populations to best match health-enhancing programs to their particular needs.

Changing multiple behaviors represents special challenges, such as the demands placed on participants and providers. Alternative strategies need to be tried beyond the sequential (one at a time) and simultaneous (each treated intensely at the same time). Integrative approaches are promising. With bullying prevention, multiple behaviors (for example, hitting, stealing, ostracizing, mean gossiping and labeling, damaging personal belongings) and multiple roles (bully, victim, and passive bystander) required treatment. Available classroom intervention time was only thirty minutes. If behavior change is construct-driven (for example, by stage or self-efficacy), what is a higher-order construct that could integrate all of these more concrete behaviors and roles? "Relating with respect" was used and, as indicated earlier, significant and important improvements across roles and behaviors were found for elementary, middle, and high school students (Prochaska and others, 2007). As with any theory, effective applications may be limited more by our creativity and resources for testing than by the ability of the theory to drive significant research and effective interventions. The Transtheoretical Model is a dynamic theory of change, and it should remain open to modifications and enhancements as more students, scientists, and practitioners apply the stage paradigm to a growing number and diversity of theoretical issues, public health problems, and at-risk populations.

SUMMARY

In this chapter, we described the fifteen core constructs of TTM and how these constructs can be integrated across the stages of change. Empirical support for the basic constructs of TTM and for applied research was presented, along with conceptual and empirical challenges from critics of TTM. Applications of TTM-tailored interventions with entire populations were explored with examples for the single behavior of smoking and for multiple-health-risk behaviors. A major theme is that programmatically building and applying the core constructs of TTM at the individual level can ultimately lead to high-impact programs for enhancing health at the population level.

REFERENCES

Abrams, D. B., Herzog, T. A., Emmons, K. M., and Linnan, L. "Stages of Change Versus Addiction: A Replication and Extension." *Nicotine & Tobacco Research,* 2000, *2,* 223–229.

Aveyard, P., and others. "Cluster Randomised Controlled Trial of Expert System Based on the Transtheoretical ('Stages Of Change') Model for Smoking Prevention and Cessation in Schools." *British Medical Journal,* 1999, *319,* 948–953.

Bandura, A. "Self-Efficacy Mechanism in Human Agency." *American Psychologist,* 1982, *37,* 122–147.

Beresford, S.A.A., and others. "A Dietary Intervention in Primary Care Practice: The Eating Patterns Study." *American Journal of Public Health,* 1997, *87,* 610–616.

Brogan, M. M., Prochaska, J. O., and Prochaska, J. M. "Predicting Termination and Continuation Status In Psychotherapy Using The Transtheoretical Model." *Psychotherapy,* 1999, *36,* 105–113.

Brug, J., and others. "The Impact of Computer-Tailored Feedback and Iterative Feedback on Fat, Fruit, and Vegetable Intake." *Health Education & Behavior,* 1998, *25,* 517–531.

Campbell, M. K., and others. "Improving Dietary Behavior: The Effectiveness of Tailored Messages in Primary Care Settings." *American Journal of Public Health,* 1994, *84,* 783–787.

Carbonari, J. P., and DiClemente, C. C. "Using Transtheoretical Model Profiles to Differentiate Levels of Alcohol Abstinence Success." *Journal of Consulting and Clinical Psychology,* 2000, *68,* 810–817.

Cardinal, B. J., and Sachs, M. L. "Effects of Mail-Mediated, Stage-Matched Exercise Behavior Change Strategies on Female Adults Leisure-Time Exercise Behavior." *Journal of Sports Medicine and Physical Fitness,* 1996, *36,* 100–107.

CDC AIDS Community Demonstration Projects Research Group. "Community-Level HIV Intervention in 5 Cities: Final Outcome Data from the CDC AIDS Community Demonstration Projects." *American Journal of Public Health,* 1999, *89*(3), 336–345.

Curry, S. J., and others. "A Randomized Trial of Self-Help Materials, Personalized Feedback, and Telephone Counseling with Nonvolunteer Smokers." *Journal of Consulting and Clinical Psychology,* 1995, *63,* 175–180.

DiClemente, C. C., and Prochaska, J. O. "Self Change and Therapy Change of Smoking Behavior. A Comparison of Processes of Change in Cessation and Maintenance." *Addictive Behavior,* 1982, *7,* 133–142.

DiClemente, C. C., and others. "The Processes of Smoking Cessation: An Analysis of Precontemplation, Contemplation, and Preparation Stages of Change." *Journal of Consulting and Clinical Psychology,* 1991, *59,* 295–304.

Dijkstra, A., DeVries, H., and Roijackers, J. "Targeting Smokers with Low Readiness to Change with Tailored and Non-tailored Self-help Materials." *Preventive Medicine,* 1999, *28,* 203–211.

Dijkstra, A., Conijm, B., and DeVries, H. "A Match-Mismatch Test of a Stage Model of Behavior Change in Tobacco Smoking." *Addiction,* 2006, *101,* 1035–1043.

Edington, D. W. "Emerging Research: A View from One Research Center." *American Journal of Health Promotion,* 2001, *15*(5), 341–349.

Etter, J. F., Perneger, T. V., and Ronchi, A. "Distributions of Smokers by Stage: International Comparison and Association with Smoking Prevalence." *Preventive Medicine,* 1997, *26,* 580–585.

Evers, K. E., and others. "A Randomized Clinical Trial of a Population and Transtheoretical-Based Stress Management Intervention." *Health Psychology,* 2006, *25*(4), 521–529.

Farkas, A. J., and others. "Addiction Versus Stages of Change Models in Predicting Smoking Cessation." *Addiction,* 1996, *91,* 1271–1280.

Fiore, M. C., and others. "Clinical Practice Guideline: Treating Tobacco Use and Dependence." Washington, D. C.: U.S. Department of Health and Human Services, Public Health Service, 2000.

Freud, S. "The Question of Lay Analysis." In J. Strachey (ed.), *The Standard Edition of the Complete Psychological Works of Sigmund Freud.* Vol. 20. London: Hogarth Press, 1959.

Glanz, K., and others. "Impact of Work Site Health Promotion on Stages of Dietary Change: The Working Well Trial." *Health Education & Behavior,* 1998, *25,* 448–463.

Glynn, T. J., Anderson, D. M., and Schwarz, L. "Tobacco Use Reduction among High Risk Youth: Recommendations of a National Cancer Institute Expert Advisory Panel." *Preventive Medicine,* 1992, *24,* 354–362.

Gold, D. B., Anderson, D. R., and Serxner, S. A. "Impact of Telephone-based Intervention on the Reduction of Health Risks." *American Journal of Health Promotion,* 2000, *15*(2), 97–106.

Goldstein, M. G., and others. "Physician-Based Physical Activity Counseling for Middle-Aged and Older Adults: A Randomized Trial." *Annals of Behavioral Medicine,* 1999, *21,* 40–47.

Greene, G. W., and others. "Change in Fruit and Vegetable Intake over 24 Months in Older Adults: Results of the SENIOR Project Intervention." *The Gerontologist,* forthcoming.

Hall, K. L., and Rossi, J. S. "Meta-Analytic Examination of the Strong and Weak Principles across 48 Health Behaviors." *Preventive Medicine,* 2008, *46,* 266–274.

Hall, S. M., and others. "Treatment of Depressed Mental Health Outpatients for Cigarette Smoking: A Randomized Clinical Trial." *American Journal of Public Health,* 2006, *96*(10), 1808–1814.

Herzog, T. A., Abrams, D. B., Emmons, K. M., and Linnan, L. "Predicting Increases in Readiness to Quit Smoking: A Prospective Analysis Using the Contemplation Ladder." *Psychology & Health,* 2000, *15,* 369–381.

Herzog, T. A., and others. "Do Processes of Change Predict Stage Movements? A Prospective Analysis of the Transtheoretical Model." *Health Psychology,* 1999, *18,* 369–375.

Hollis, J. F., and others. "Teen REACH: Outcomes from a Randomized Controlled Trial of a Tobacco Reduction Program for Teens Seen in Primary Medical Care." *Pediatrics,* 2005, *115*(4), 981–989.

Horwath, C. C. "Applying the Transtheoretical Model to Eating Behaviour Change: Challenges and Opportunities." *Nutrition Research Review,* 1999, *12,* 281–317.

Janis, I. L., and Mann, L. *Decision Making*: *A Psychological Analysis of Conflict, Chance and Commitment.* London: Cassil & Collier Macmillan, 1977.

Johnson, J. L., and others. "What Predicts Stage of Change for Smoking Cessation?" *Annals of Behavioral Medicine,* 2000, *22,* S173. (Abstract).

Johnson, S. S., and others. "Transtheoretical Model Intervention for Adherence to Lipid-Lowering Drugs." *Disease Management,* 2006a, *9*(2), 102–114.

Johnson, S. S., and others. "Efficacy of a Transtheoretical Model Based Expert System for Antihypertensive Adherence." *Disease Management,* 2006b, *9*(5), 291–301.

Jones, H., and others. "Changes in Diabetes Self-Care Behaviors Make a Difference in Glycemic Control: The Diabetes Stages of Change (DISC) Study." *Diabetes Care,* 2003, *26,* 732–737.

Kreuter, M., and Strecher, V. J. "Do Tailored Behavior Change Messages Enhance the Effectiveness of Health Risk Appraisal? Results From a Randomized Trial." *Health Education Research,* 1996, *11,* 97–105.

Levesque, D. A., Driskell, M., Prochaska, J. M., and Prochaska, J. O. "Acceptability of a Stage-Matched Expert System Intervention for Domestic Violence Offenders." *Violence and Victims,* forthcoming.

Lichtenstein, E., and Hollis, J. "Patient Referral to Smoking Cessation Programs: Who Follows Through?" *The Journal of Family Practice,* 1992, *34,* 739–744.

Marcus, B. H., and others. "Efficacy of an Individualized, Motivationally-Tailored Physical Activity Intervention." *Annals of Behavioral Medicine,* 1998, *20,* 174–180.

Noar, S. M., Benac, C., and Harris, M. "Does Tailoring Matter? Meta-Analytic Review of Tailored Print Health Behavior Change Interventions." *Psychological Bulletin,* 2007, *133,* 673–693.

Norman, G. J., and others. "A Randomized Controlled Trial of a Multicomponent Intervention for Adolescent Sun Protection Behaviors." *Archives of Pediatric & Adolescent Medicine,* 2007, *161,* 146–152.

O'Neill, H. K., Gillespie, M. A., and Slobin, K. "Stages of Change and Smoking Cessation: A Computer Administered Intervention Program for Young Adults." *American Journal of Health Promotion,* 2000, *15*(2), 93–96.

Pallonen, U. E., and others. "Computer-Based Smoking Cessation Interventions in Adolescents: Description, Feasibility, and Six-Month Follow-up Findings." *Substance Use & Misuse,* 1998, *33,* 935–965.

Parsons, J. T., and others. "Maintenance of Safer Sexual Behaviours: Evaluation of a Theory-Based Intervention for HIV Seropositive Men with Haemophilia and Their Female Partners." *Haemophilia,* 2000, *6,* 181–190.

Peterson, A. V., Jr., and others. (2000). "Hutchinson Smoking Prevention Project: Long-Term Randomized Trial in School-Based Tobacco Use Prevention—Results on Smoking." *Journal of the National Cancer Institute,* 2000, *92,* 1979–1991.

Prochaska, J. J., and others. "Comparing Intervention Outcomes in Smokers Treated for Single Versus Multiple Behavioral Risks." *Health Psychology,* 2006, *25*(3), 380–388.

Prochaska, J. M., and others. "The Transtheoretical Model of Change for Multi-Level Interventions for Alcohol Abuse on Campus." *Journal of Alcohol and Drug Education,* 2004, *47*(3), 34–50.

Prochaska, J. O. *Systems of Psychotherapy: A Transtheoretical Analysis.* (2nd ed.) Pacific Grove, Calif.: Brooks-Cole, 1984.

Prochaska, J. O. "Strong and Weak Principles for Progressing from Precontemplation to Action Based on Twelve Problem Behaviors." *Health Psychology,* 1994, *13,* 47–5l.

Prochaska, J. O. "Moving Beyond the Transtheoretical Model." *Addiction,* 2006, *101,* 768–778.

Prochaska, J. O. "Multiple Health Behavior Research Represents the Future of Preventive Medicine." *Preventive Medicine,* 2008, *46,* 281–285.

Prochaska, J. O., and DiClemente, C. C. "Stages and Processes of Self-Change of Smoking: Toward an Integrative Model of Change." *Journal of Consulting and Clinical Psychology,* 1983, *51,* 390–395.

Prochaska, J. O., DiClemente, C. C., and Norcross, J. C. "In Search of How People Change: Applications to the Addictive Behaviors." *American Psychologist,* 1992, *47,* 1102–1114.

Prochaska, J. O., DiClemente, C. C., Velicer, W. F., and Rossi, J. S. "Standardized, Individualized, Interactive, and Personalized Self-Help Programs for Smoking Cessation." *Health Psychology,* 1993, *12,* 399–405.

Prochaska, J. O., Norcross, J. C., and DiClemente, C. C. *Changing for Good.* New York: William Morrow, 1994.

Prochaska, J. O, and Velicer, W. F. "On Models, Methods and Premature Conclusions." *Addictions,* 1996, *91,* 1281–1283.

Prochaska, J. O., and Velicer, W. F. "The Transtheoretical Model of Health Behavior Change." *American Journal of Health Promotion,* 1997, *12*(1), 38–48.

Prochaska, J. O., Velicer, W. F., Prochaska, J. M., and Johnson, J. L. "Size, Consistency and Stability of Stage Effects for Smoking Cessation." *Addictive Behaviors,* 2004, *29,* 207–213.

Prochaska, J. O, Wright, J., and Velicer, W. F. "Evaluating Theories of Health Behavior Change: A Hierarchy of Criteria Applied to the Transtheoretical Model." *Applied Psychology: An International Review,* forthcoming.

Prochaska, J. O., and others. "Predicting Change in Smoking Status for Self-Changers." *Addictive Behaviors,* 1985, *10,* 395–406.

Prochaska, J. O., and others. "Patterns of Change: Dynamic Typology Applied to Smoking Cessation." *Multivariate Behavioral Research,* 1991, *26,* 83–107.

Prochaska, J. O., and others. "Stages of Change and Decisional Balance for Twelve Problem Behaviors." *Health Psychology,* 1994, *13,* 39–46.

Prochaska, J. O., and others. "Evaluating a Population-based Recruitment Approach and a Stage-Based Expert System Intervention for Smoking." *Addictive Behaviors,* 2001a, *26,* 583–602.

Prochaska, J. O., and others. "Counselor and Stimulus Control Enhancements of a Stage-Matched Expert System Intervention for Smokers in a Managed Care Setting." *Preventive Medicine,* 2001b, *32,* 23–32.

Prochaska, J. O., and others. "Impact of Simultaneous Stage-matched Expert System Interventions for Smoking, High Fat Diet and Sun Exposure in a Population of Parents." *Health Psychology,* 2004, *23*(5), 503–516.

Prochaska, J. O., and others. "Stage-Based Expert Systems to Guide a Population of Primary Care Patients to Quit Smoking, Eat Healthier, Prevent Skin Cancer and Receive Regular Mammograms." *Preventive Medicine,* 2005, *41,* 406–416.

Prochaska, J. O., and others. "Efficacy and Effectiveness Trials: Examples from Smoking Cessation and Bullying Prevention." *Journal of Health Psychology,* 2007, *12*(1), 170–178.

Prochaska, J. O., and others. "Initial Efficacy of MI, TTM Tailoring and HRI's with Multiple Behaviors for Employee Health Promotion." *Preventive Medicine,* 2008, *46,* 226–231.

Project Match Research Group. "Matching Alcoholism Treatments to Client Heterogeneity: Project MATCH Post Treatment Drinking Outcomes." *Journal of Studies on Alcohol,* 1997, *58,* 7–29.

Rakowski, W. R., and others. "Increasing Mammography Among Women Aged 40–74 by Use of a Stage-Matched, Tailored Intervention." *Preventive Medicine,* 1998, *27,* 748–756.

Redding, C. A., Maddock, J. E., and Rossi, J. S. "The Sequential Approach to Measurement of Health Behavior Constructs: Issues in Selecting and Developing Measures." *Californian Journal of Health Promotion,* 2006, *4*(1), 83–101.

Redding, C. A., Morokoff, P. J., Rossi, J. S., and Meier, K. S. "A TTM-Tailored Condom Use Intervention for At-risk Women and Men." In T. Edgar, S. M. Noar, and V. Freimuth (eds.), *Communication Perspectives on HIV/AIDS for the 21st Century.* Hillsdale, N.J.: Erlbaum, 2007.

Redding, C. A., and others. "Transtheoretical Individualized Multimedia Expert Systems Targeting Adolescents' Health Behaviors." *Cognitive & Behavioral Practice,* 1999, *6*(2), 144–153.

Robbins, M. L., and others. "Assessing Family Members' Motivational Readiness and Decision Making for Consenting to Cadaveric Organ Donation." *Journal of Health Psychology,* 2001, *6,* 523–536.

Rogers, C. *Client-Centered Therapy.* Boston: Houghton-Mifflin, 1951.

Rosen, C. S. "Is the Sequencing of Change Processes by Stage Consistent Across Health Problems? A Meta-Analysis." *Health Psychology,* 2000, *19,* 593–604.

Rossi, J. S. "Stages of Change for 15 Health Risk Behaviors in an HMO Population." Paper presented at 13th meeting of the Society for Behavioral Medicine, New York, 1992a.

Rossi, J. S. "Common Processes of Change Across Nine Problem Behaviors." Paper presented at 100th meeting of American Psychological Association, Washington, D.C., 1992b.

Rossi, J. S., and others. "Effectiveness of Transtheoretical Model-Based Interventions on Exercise and Fruit and Vegetable Consumption in Older Adults." *Annals of Behavioral Medicine,* 2005, *29,* S134.

Ruggiero, L., and others. "Diabetes Self-management. Self-reported Recommendations and Patterns in a Large Population." *Diabetes Care,* 1997, *20*(4), 568–576.

Skinner, B. F. *Beyond Freedom and Dignity.* New York: Bantam/Vintage, 1971.

Snow, M. G., Prochaska, J. O., and Rossi, J. S. "Stages of Change for Smoking Cessation Among Former Problem Drinkers: A Cross-Sectional Analysis." *Journal of Substance Abuse,* 1992, *4,* 107–116.

Spencer, L., Pagell, F., Hallion, M. E., and Adams, T. B. "Applying the Transtheoretical Model to Tobacco Cessation and Prevention: A Review of the Literature." *American Journal of Health Promotion,* 2002, *17*(1), 7–71.

Steptoe, A., Kerry, S., Rink, E., and Hilton, S. "The Impact of Behavioral Counseling on Stages of Change in Fat Intake, Physical Activity, and Cigarette Smoking in Adults at Increased Risk of Coronary Heart Disease." *American Journal of Public Health,* 2001, *91*(2), 26.

Strecher, V. J., and others. "The Effects of Computer Tailored Smoking Cessation Messages in Family Practice Settings." *The Journal of Family Practice,* 1994, *39,* 262–270.

Sun, X., Prochaska, J. O., Velicer, W. F., and Laforge, R. G. "Transtheoretical Principles and Processes for Quitting Smoking: A 24-month Comparison of a Representative Sample of Quitters, Relapsers and Non-Quitters." *Addictive Behaviors,* 2007, *32,* 2707–2726.

U.S. Department of Health and Human Services. "The Health Benefits of Smoking Cessation. A Report of the Surgeon General." Rockville, Md.: U.S. Department of Health and Human Services, Public Health Service, Centers for Disease Control, Office on Smoking and Health, 1990.

U.S. Department of Health and Human Services. "Preventing Tobacco Use Among Young People. A Report of the Surgeon General." Atlanta: U.S. Department of Health and Human Services, Public Health Service, Centers for Disease Control and Prevention, Office on Smoking and Health, 1994.

U.S. Department of Health and Human Services. *Healthy People 2010: Understanding and Improving Health.* (2nd ed.) Washington, D.C.: U.S. Government Printing Office, 2000.

Velicer, W. F., and DiClemente, C. C. "Understanding and Intervening with the Total Population of Smokers." *Tobacco Control,* 1993, *2,* 95–96.

Velicer, W. F., and others. "Interactive Versus Non-Interactive Interventions and Dose-Response Relationships for Stage Matched Smoking Cessation Programs in a Managed Care Setting." *Health Psychology,* 1999, *18,* 21–28.

Velicer, W. F., Redding, C. A., Sun, X., and Prochaska, J. O. "Demographic Variables, Smoking Variables, and Outcome Across Five Studies." *Health Psychology,* 2007, *26*(3), 278–287.

Velicer, W. F., and others. "Distribution of Smokers by Stage in Three Representative Samples." *Preventive Medicine,* 1995, *24,* 401–411.

Velicer, W. F., and others. "Evaluating Nicotine Replacement Therapy and Stage-Based Therapies in a Population-Based Effectiveness Trial." *Journal of Consulting and Clinical Psychology,* 2006, *74*(6), 1162–1172.

Voorhees, C. C., and others. "Heart, Body, and Soul: Impact of Church-Based Smoking Cessation Interventions on Readiness to Quit." *Preventive Medicine,* 1996, *25,* 277–285.

Wewers, M. E., Stillman, F. A., Hartman, A. M., and Shopland, D. R. "Distribution of Daily Smokers by Stage of Change: Current Population Survey Results." *Preventive Medicine,* 2003, *36,* 710–720.

Wierzbicki, M., and Pekarik, G. "A Meta-Analysis of Psychotherapy Dropout." *Professional Psychology: Research and Practice,* 1993, *29,* 190–195.

Yang G., and others. "Smoking Cessation in China: Findings from the 1996 National Prevalence Survey." *Tobacco Control,* 2001, *10*(2), 170–174.

CHAPTER

6

THE PRECAUTION ADOPTION PROCESS MODEL

Neil D. Weinstein
Peter M. Sandman
Susan J. Blalock

KEY POINTS

This chapter will

- Explain the differences between stage theories and other decision-oriented health behavior theories.
- Describe and justify the Precaution Adoption Process Model (PAPM).
- Show how to use the PAPM to understand and change behavior: the example of osteoporosis prevention.
- Describe how to test stage theories: general issues and the example of home radon testing.
- Review research using the PAPM.
- Identify the criteria for using stage-based interventions.

To understand why many young adults put themselves at risk for AIDS, it seems logical to investigate their beliefs about HIV and AIDS. A questionnaire based on popular theories of health behavior might ask a sample of young adults about the likelihood that they will have sexual contact with someone who is HIV-positive, their chance of becoming infected by this person, the effectiveness of various precautions, the social consequences of taking such precautions, the behavior of their peers, and other topics like these.

This research strategy makes sense today. But what if the year were 1987, when the public was first learning about AIDS? At that time, some young adults might have been aware that AIDS is a fatal disease, but few would have known anything more. In fact, they would have been unable to answer most of your questions. The riskiness of their behavior would vary. Some young adults would have had many sexual partners, and others would have had few or none; some would have used condoms, and others would not. Yet neither their current behavior nor subsequent changes in their behavior would have been explained or predicted by their beliefs about AIDS. They had not yet formed such beliefs.

As this example shows, theories that try to explain health behavior by focusing on beliefs about costs and benefits of particular actions are relevant only to people who have been engaged sufficiently by the health threat to have formed such beliefs. Since this does not include everyone—and, with respect to HIV, included hardly anyone in 1987—there must be other stages (or phases) to precaution taking (that is, actions taken with the goal of reducing the threat of illness or injury or of increasing the prospects for recovery). The Precaution Adoption Process Model (PAPM) seeks to identify all the stages involved when people commence health-protective behaviors and to determine the factors that lead people to move from one stage to the next.

HOW STAGE THEORIES APPROACH THE ISSUE OF EXPLAINING AND CHANGING BEHAVIOR

Many theories of individual health behavior, such as those focusing on perceived pros and cons of action, specify a single equation that they use to predict behavior. These theories acknowledge *quantitative* differences among people in their positions on different variables, and consequently, in their likelihood of action. The goal of interventions is to maximize the variables that increase the value of the prediction equation. Any action-promoting variable that has not already reached its maximum value is an appropriate goal for an intervention.

Advocates of stage theories like PAPM claim that there are *qualitative* differences among people and question whether changes in health behaviors can be de-

The authors are indebted to Alexander Rothman and Stephen Sutton for their assistance in clarifying the characteristics and testing of stage theories and to Cara L. Cuite, Mary Lou Klotz, Judith E. Lyon, Paul Miller, Nancy E. Roberts, Brenda M. DeVellis, Robert F. DeVellis, Deborah T. Gold, John J. B. Anderson, Mary Anne Dooley, Karen B. Giorgino, Shannon Smith Currey, Carol C. Patterson, Marci K. Campbell, Diane R. Orenstein, Kate Queen, Jane Lesesne, and Jeannie Shaffer for their contributions to the radon and osteoporosis research described here.

scribed by a single prediction equation. They suggest, in effect, that we must develop a series of explanatory equations, one for each stage transition. This is a much more complicated goal than finding a single prediction rule, but it offers the possibility of greater accuracy, greater intervention effectiveness, and greater intervention efficiency.

Stage theories have four principal elements and assumptions (Weinstein, Rothman, and Sutton, 1998):

1. *A category system to define the stages.* Stages are theoretical constructs. An ideal or "prototype" must be defined for each stage, even if few people match this ideal. Stages can be useful, even if the actual boundaries between stages are not as clear-cut as the theories suggest.

2. *An ordering of the stages.* Stage theories assume that before people act, they usually pass through all the stages in order. However, forward progression is neither inevitable nor irreversible (compare with Bandura, 1995). There is no minimum length of time people must spend in a particular stage. In fact, people may sometimes progress so rapidly that, for practical purposes, they can be said to skip stages (for example, when a doctor recommends a new screening test and the patient agrees without any further deliberation). Some stages may lie on side paths that are not on the route to action. An example would be a stage representing people who have decided not to act. Obviously, people do not need to pass through stages on paths that do not lead to action.

3. *Common barriers to change facing people in the same stage.* Knowing the stage of an individual or group is helpful in designing an intervention program only if people at that stage have to address similar types of issues before they can progress to the next stage. Thus, interventions can be tailored on the basis of stage, without having to investigate a wide range of potential tailoring variables.

4. *Different barriers to change facing people in different stages.* If factors producing movement toward action were the same regardless of a person's stage, the same intervention could be used for everyone, and the concept of stages would be superfluous.

A completely specified stage theory includes both criteria that define stages and factors that govern movement between adjacent stages. Although its stage definitions are meant to apply across behaviors, particular issues that constitute barriers to progress may be behavior- or hazard-specific. Factors that enter into decisions to lose weight, for example, may be quite different from those that affect decisions to use condoms. A model that proposes a particular sequence of stages in the change process could be correct about these stages, even if it has not identified all the determinants of each transition from one stage to the next. At present, the PAPM does not provide detailed information about barriers at each stage. It is a conceptual framework or skeleton that needs to be fleshed out for each behavior with information about how stage transitions occur.

THE PRECAUTION ADOPTION PROCESS MODEL

Description of the Model

The PAPM attempts to explain how a person comes to decisions to take action and how he or she translates that decision into action. Adoption of a new precaution or cessation of a risky behavior requires deliberate steps unlikely to occur outside of conscious awareness. The PAPM applies to these types of actions, not to the gradual development of habitual patterns of behavior, such as exercise and diet, in which health considerations may play some role (though it would apply to the initiation of a new exercise program or a new diet). Nor does the PAPM explain the commencement of risky behaviors, such as a teenager accepting his first cigarette, which seem to be better explained in terms of a "willingness" to act rather than in terms of any plan to act (Gibbons, Gerrard, Blanton, and Russell, 1998).

Initial work on the PAPM was stimulated by Irving Janis and Leon Mann (1977), who tried to explain responses to threats by proposing discrete categories determined by people's beliefs about their capacity to cope with the threats. Like their work, the PAPM describes a set of categories (stages), defined in terms of psychological processes within individuals. All PAPM stages prior to action are defined in terms of mental states, rather than in terms of factors external to the person, such as current or past behaviors. PAPM stages are also not defined in terms of criteria that are salient only to health professionals. PAPM stages refer to behaviors that are salient to laypeople, such as how often they eat red meat, rather than to criteria salient mainly to professionals, such as percentage of fat in a person's diet.

Although several aspects of the PAPM were first discussed in 1988 (Weinstein, 1988), the present formulation, published in 1992 (Weinstein and Sandman, 1992), differs in some respects from the initial version. The current PAPM identifies seven stages along the path from lack of awareness to action (see Figure 6.1). At some initial point in time, people are unaware of the health issue (Stage 1). When they first learn something about the issue, they are no longer unaware, but they are not yet engaged by it either (Stage 2). People who reach the decision-making stage (Stage 3) have become engaged by the issue and are considering their response. This decision-making process can result in one of three outcomes: they may suspend judgment, remaining in Stage 3 for the moment; they may decide to take no action, moving to Stage 4 and halting the precaution adoption process, at least for the time being; or they may decide to adopt the precaution, moving to Stage 5. For those who decide to adopt the precaution, the next step is to initiate the behavior (Stage 6). A seventh stage, if relevant, indicates that the behavior has been maintained over time (Stage 7).

The stages have been labeled with numbers, but these numbers have no more than ordinal values. They would not even have ordinal value if Stage 4 were included, because it is not a stage on the path to action. The numbers should never be used to calculate correlation coefficients, calculate the mean stage for a sample, or conduct regression analyses with "stage" treated as a continuous, independent variable. All such calculations assume that the stages represent equal-spaced intervals along a single underlying dimension, which violates a fundamental assumption of stage theory. Although not shown in Figure 6.1, movement backward toward an earlier stage can

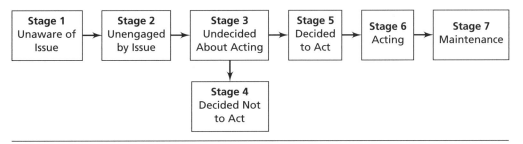

FIGURE 6.1. Stages of the Precaution Adoption Process Model.

also occur, without necessarily going back through all the intermediate stages, although obviously it is not possible to go from later stages to Stage 1.

Two concrete examples—the stages relevant to home radon testing and to taking calcium for osteoporosis prevention—are shown in Figure 6.2.

On the surface, the PAPM resembles another stage theory—The Transtheoretical Model (TTM), developed by Prochaska, DiClemente, Velicer, and their colleagues

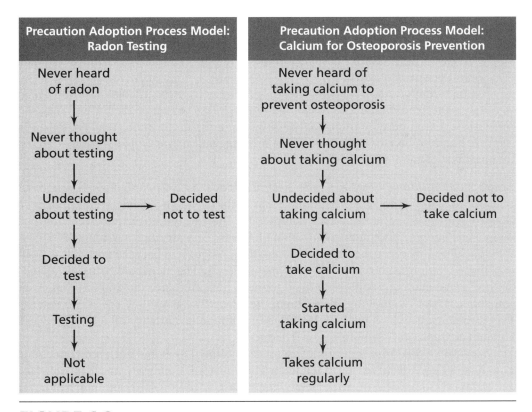

FIGURE 6.2. Two Examples of the Stages of the Precaution Adoption Process Model: Home Radon Testing and Taking Calcium to Prevent Osteoporosis.

(see Chapter Five). However, the main similarity lies in the names given to the stages. The number of stages is not the same in the two theories, and even those stages with similar names are defined according to quite different criteria. For example, the PAPM refers primarily to mental states, whereas TTM emphasizes days or months until intended action. We are not aware of any research directly comparing the two theories' predictions.

Justification for the PAPM Stages

There should be good reasons to propose the separate stages that make up a stage theory. What is the justification for the stages in the PAPM?

Stage 1 (Unaware). Much health research deals with well-known hazards, like smoking, AIDS, and high-fat diets. In such cases, asking someone about his or her beliefs and plans is quite reasonable; most people have considered the relevance of these threats to their own lives. But if people have never heard of a hazard or a potential precaution, they cannot have formed opinions about it. The reluctance of respondents to answer survey questions about less familiar issues suggests that investigators ought to allow people to say that they "don't know" or have "no opinion" rather than forcing them to state a position. Participants in many health behavior investigations are not given this opportunity. Even when participants are permitted to say that they "don't know," these responses are often coded as missing or are collapsed into another category. To say "I don't know" indicates something important and constitutes real data that should not be discarded.

Media often have a major influence in getting people from Stage 1 of the PAPM to Stage 2 and from Stage 2 to Stage 3, and much less influence thereafter. This and other factors that may be important in producing different transitions are given in Table 6.1 and in Weinstein (1988). These are suggestions for consideration, not core assumptions of the PAPM.

Stage 2 (Unengaged) Versus Stage 3 (Undecided). Once people have heard about a health precaution and have begun to form opinions about it, they are no longer in Stage 1. However, so many issues compete for their limited time and attention that people can know a moderate amount about a hazard or a precaution without ever having considered whether they need to do anything about it. This idea parallels a well-established finding with respect to mass media effects. The media are better at "agenda setting"—persuading people that they ought to consider an issue and have an opinion about it (that is, moving from Stage 2 to Stage 3)—than they are at influencing the opinion itself, which tends to require more individual sorts of influences (see also Chapter Sixteen on Communication Theory).

We believe that this condition of awareness without personal engagement is quite common. In a 1986 survey of radon testing (Weinstein, Sandman, and Klotz, 1987), for example, 50 percent of respondents in a high-risk region said that they had never thought about testing their own homes, even though all had indicated that they knew what radon was, and most had correctly answered more than half of the questions on a knowledge test.

TABLE 6.1. **Examples of Factors Likely to Determine Progress Between Stages.**

Stage Transition	Factor
Stage 1 to Stage 2	Media messages about the hazard and precaution
Stage 2 to Stage 3	Media messages about the hazard and precaution
	Communications from significant others
	Personal experience with hazard
Stage 3 to Stage 4 or Stage 5	Beliefs about hazard likelihood and severity
	Beliefs about personal susceptibility
	Beliefs about precaution effectiveness and difficulty
	Behaviors and recommendations of others
	Perceived social norms
	Fear and worry
Stage 5 to Stage 6	Time, effort, and resources needed to act
	Detailed "how-to" information
	Reminders and other cues to action
	Assistance in carrying out action

The PAPM suggests further that it is important to distinguish between the people who have never thought about an action and those who have given the action some consideration but are undecided. There are several reasons for making this distinction. First, people who have thought about acting are likely to be more knowledgeable. Also, getting people to think about an issue may require different sorts of communications (and entail different sorts of obstacles) than getting them to adopt a particular conclusion. Thus, whether a person has or has not thought about taking action appears to be an important distinction.

Stage 3 (Undecided) Versus Stage 4 (Decided Not to Act) and Stage 5 (Decided to Act). Research reveals important differences between people who have not yet formed opinions and those who have made decisions. People who have come to a definite position on an issue, even if they have not yet acted on their opinions, have different responses to information and are more resistant to persuasion than people who have not formed opinions (Anderson, 1983; Brockner and Rubin, 1985; Cialdini, 1988; Ditto and Lopez, 1992; Jelalian and Miller, 1984; Nisbett and Ross, 1980, Chapter 8). This widely recognized tendency to adhere to one's own position has been termed "confirmation bias," "perseverance of beliefs," and "hypothesis preservation." It manifests itself in a variety of ways. According to Klayman (1995), these include overconfidence in one's beliefs; searches for new evidence that are biased to favor one's beliefs; biased interpretations of new data; and insufficient adjustment of one's beliefs in light of new evidence. For these reasons, the PAPM holds that it is significant when people say they have decided to act or have decided not to act, and that the implications of people saying that they have decided not to act are not the same as saying it is "unlikely" they will act.

We believe that cost-benefit theories of health behavior, such as the Health Belief Model, the Theory of Reasoned Action, Protection Motivation Theory, and Subjective Expected Utility Theory, are dealing mainly with the factors that govern how people who get to Stage 3 decide what to do. The factors these theories focus on are certainly important, but they relate mostly to this one phase of the precaution adoption process. These theories also overlook another possibility: that people faced with a difficult decision might get stuck and quit trying to make up their minds, moving back to Stage 2. Determinants of this regression to an earlier stage might be different from the factors that lead people toward Stages 4 or 5.

Perceived susceptibility (or, equivalently, "perceived personal likelihood") is one factor that can influence what people decide and is included in most theories of health behavior (Connor and Norman, 1995). People are reluctant to acknowledge personal susceptibility to harm, even when they acknowledge risks faced by others (Weinstein, 1987). Consequently, overcoming this reluctance is a major barrier to getting people to decide to act.

Stage 5 (Decided to Act) Versus Stage 6 (Acting). The distinction between decision and action is common to most stage theories. For example, Schwarzer's Health Action Process Approach (Schwarzer, 1992; Schwarzer and Fuchs, 1996) distinguishes between an initial, motivation phase, during which people develop an intention to act, based on beliefs about risk, outcomes, and self-efficacy, and the volition phase in which they plan the details of action, initiate action, and deal with the difficulties of carrying out that action successfully.

Even Ajzen's (Ajzen, 1985; Ajzen and Madden, 1986) Theory of Planned Behavior, which is not a stage theory, separates intentions from actions. Protection Motivation Theory is not a stage theory either, but its developers implicitly recognize the need for sequencing interventions. According to Rogers and Prentice-Dunn, "PMT experiments always present information in the same order, threatening information followed by coping information" (Rogers and Prentice-Dunn, 1997). These researchers also speak of first developing motivation and then developing coping skills.

A growing body of research (Gollwitzer, 1999) suggests that there are important gaps between intending to act and carrying out this intention, and that helping people develop specific implementation plans can reduce these barriers. The PAPM suggests that detailed implementation information would be uninteresting to people in early stages. Yet, for people who have decided to act, such information is often essential to produce the transition from decision to action. This claim is echoed by temporal construal theory (Trope and Liberman, 2003), which asserts that decisions about action are based initially on abstract construals of the options but become more focused on concrete event details when the actual choice comes near.

Stage 6 (Acting) Versus Stage 7 (Maintenance). For any health behavior that is more than a one-time action, adopting the behavior for the first time is different from repeating the behavior at intervals or developing a habitual pattern of response. Once a woman gets her first mammogram, for example, she will have acquired both more information in general and personal experience (perhaps positive as well as negative). These will play a part in the decision to be re-screened. Similarly, a man who stops smoking or loses weight must deal with the acute withdrawal experience and the glow of success in the early stage of taking action, but must address different challenges in the maintenance stage. The distinction between action and maintenance is widely recognized (for example, Dishman, 1988; Marlatt and Gordon, 1985; Meichenbaum and Turk, 1987).

Stages of Inaction. One value of the PAPM is its recognition of differences among the people who are neither acting nor intending to act. People in Stage 1 (unaware), Stage 2 (unengaged), Stage 3 (undecided), and Stage 4 (decided not to act) all fit in this broad category. Those in Stage 1 need basic information about the hazard and the recommended precaution. People in Stage 2 need something that makes the threat and action seem personally relevant. Individualized messages and contact with friends and neighbors who have considered action should help these individuals move to the next stage. Another powerful influence on the transition from Stage 2 to Stage 3 is probably the awareness that others are making up their minds, that one is obliged to have some opinion on this current issue of the day.

As stated earlier, people who have thought about and rejected action (Stage 4) are a particularly difficult group. Evidence shows that they can be quite well informed (Blalock and others, 1996; Weinstein and Sandman, 1992), and, as noted earlier, they will tend to dispute or ignore information that challenges their decision not to act.

USING THE PAPM TO DEVELOP AND EVALUATE BEHAVIOR CHANGE INTERVENTIONS

Blalock and colleagues used the PAPM in three studies conducted from 1994–2000 that focused on osteoporosis prevention (Blalock, 2005, 2007; Blalock and others, 1996, 2000, 2002). Osteoporosis is a metabolic bone disorder that results in decreased bone density and increased susceptibility to fractures (Riggs and Melton, 1986). Precautions recommended to reduce the risk of developing osteoporosis vary across the lifespan. However, adequate calcium intake and weight-bearing exercise are recommended for individuals of all ages ("Osteoporosis Prevention, Diagnosis, and Therapy," 2000). The research was designed to better understand the factors that (1) discriminate among women in different stages with respect to calcium intake and exercise and (2) predict different types of stage transitions (Blalock and others, 1996; Blalock, 2007). This information was used to develop stage-based educational interventions (Blalock and others, 2000, 2002). These studies provide examples of the necessary steps in using the PAPM to develop and evaluate behavior change interventions. These steps are outlined next.

The first step involves identifying and clearly defining the behavior of interest. Although the PAPM focuses on the adoption of specific health behaviors (for example, "daily walking for at least 30 minutes"), it may also be used to intervene at a broader, behavioral category level (for example, "increasing exercise"). In either case, care should be taken to define the target behavior(s) in terms that are meaningful to laypeople. Calcium intake is best considered a behavioral category (Blalock and others, 1996) because adequate intake may be achieved by a variety of specific behaviors (for example, by the use of dietary supplements or by increased intake of dairy products). Although Blalock and colleagues defined the target behavior in terms of a specific daily calcium intake—a value that has little meaning to most laypeople—they overcame this problem by providing study participants with feedback that informed them of their current calcium intake. This step would not have been needed if the behavior criterion had been simpler, such as "using a calcium supplement."

Second, a system must be developed to classify individuals according to their current stage. Especially if the target is a category of behaviors, it is necessary to decide what will constitute "acting" and what will constitute "maintenance." Either or both may require a complex algorithm (doing A, or doing both B and C, or doing D at least three times). Most research using the PAPM has defined these two stages dichotomously, so that a person either is or is not "acting." Figure 6.2 provides examples that can help in the development of appropriate questions when the criterion is a simple dichotomy.

The stage classification system allows health professionals to assess the distribution of stages within a target population at a particular point in time, guiding the design of both individual and community-level interventions. As described in the AIDS example at the beginning of this chapter, if awareness and knowledge of a health threat change over time, the effectiveness of different types of interventions is likely to change as well. Thus, monitoring temporal changes in the distribution of people across stages makes it possible to design dynamic interventions that accommodate the dynamic nature of the behavior change process.

Third, it is necessary to have at least a preliminary understanding of the factors that influence different types of stage transitions. This understanding is needed to tailor interventions to people, or groups of people, who are in different stages of change. Early work by Blalock and colleagues (Blalock and others, 1996) suggested that to move people, or groups of people, from Stages 1 and 2 (unaware, unengaged) to Stage 3 (undecided), interventions should focus on increasing awareness of the health problem of interest; behavioral recommendations to minimize risk, and potential benefits associated with adopting the behavioral recommendations, including the effectiveness of the recommended behaviors in terms of risk reduction (that is, precaution effectiveness). In addition, the PAPM suggests that information must be presented in a manner that maximizes its personal relevance to the target group. Otherwise, awareness of an issue may increase, but engagement may remain low. As described earlier, many theories provide insight into the factors that influence transitions from Stage 3 (undecided) to either Stage 4 (decided not to act) or Stage 5 (decided to act). Interventions that focus on these types of beliefs may facilitate the transition from Stage 3 to Stage 5.

To increase the likelihood that individuals will be able to act on their decisions (that is, move into Stages 6 and 7), the work by Blalock and colleagues highlights the importance of reducing factors such as lack of skills or resources that may make it difficult to adopt the behavior of interest.

The cross-sectional and prospective research carried out by Blalock and colleagues searched for between-stage differences. Significant differences between stages on particular variables suggest that these variables are worthy of additional attention, as well as of inclusion in interventions at early stages of research, but they are not proof of causation. Furthermore, if interventions succeed in altering these variables but fail to move people to stages closer to action, this does not prove that the stages themselves are invalid. The variables that actually cause each stage transition must be identified empirically.

Fourth, intervention strategies are needed to address variables associated with different stage transitions. For example, media campaigns and informational materials may be able to increase awareness of a health problem, behavioral recommendations, and the benefits associated with action. However, more intensive interventions are often needed to help individuals acquire the skills and resources needed to support behavior change efforts. The intensity of the intervention required will depend on the behavior of interest and what barriers need to be overcome. For example, Blalock and colleagues used a combination of written materials and telephone counseling focused on helping women identify potential barriers to action and develop strategies to overcome those barriers. This approach led to a significant increase in calcium intake among women who were thinking about or trying to increase their calcium intake at baseline. However, a similar intervention focused on exercise had no effect on exercise level. These findings may not be surprising, because calcium intake is likely much easier to change than exercise level. Nonetheless, the findings underscore the importance of considering carefully the skills and resources needed to adopt the recommended behavior, and of including intervention components that address these needs.

Obviously, interventions should emphasize those barriers most relevant to the population of interest. Among smokers already interested in quitting, for instance, the early stages of the PAPM can be ignored. Yet, when a hazard is very new, such as West Nile virus or avian influenza, few people will be ready to act. In such cases, interventions should focus on the earliest stages of the model.

Fifth, health educators must specify how the effectiveness of the intervention will be determined. Will it be considered effective if it results in stage progression, even if the proportion of people in the action and maintenance stages remains the same? Or is success contingent on behavior change in the target group? If a behavior is difficult to change and people are in early stages, the PAPM suggests that a single, one-shot intervention—especially an intervention that focuses on movement to the next stage—should not be judged solely by whether it changes behavior.

Finally, educators and evaluators must determine the timeframe for follow-up assessments. The PAPM and other stage theories suggest that the behavior change process is dynamic. Intervention-induced changes in beliefs and behavior may be transient, so intervention effects may be missed if only long-term follow-up assessments are used. Although long-term behavior change generally is desired, a stage model perspective raises the possibility that even transient changes may be steps in the right direction, helping us to understand the barriers at different stages and increasing the success of subsequent behavior change attempts.

HOW STAGE THEORIES, INCLUDING THE PAPM, CAN BE TESTED

A variety of approaches have been used to determine whether a particular behavior change passes through the sequence of stages proposed by a stage theory (Weinstein, Rothman, and Sutton, 1998). Many of these approaches have serious limitations. For example, a common but weak strategy is to use cross-sectional data from interviews or questionnaires to look for differences among people thought to be in different stages. Simply finding differences among people at different stages tells us little, however, as non-stage processes will also produce such differences. To reflect a stage process, the variables that distinguish between people who are not in the same stage must differ, depending on what stages are compared (for example, the variables that differentiate between people in Stages 1 and 2 must not be the same ones that differentiate between people in Stages 2 and 3). A somewhat stronger approach would be prospective, measuring the stages that people are in and following up to determine which variables predict whether they took action or not.

Intervention research provides a much stronger test of theory. Experimental studies using matched and mismatched interventions are perhaps the best strategy for testing stage theories. If it is true that different variables influence movement at different stages, individuals in a given stage should respond better to an intervention that is *correctly matched* to their stage than to one that is *mismatched* (that is, matched to a different stage). At the conclusion of the experiment, researchers employing such designs should consider providing full information about the precaution to participants in all conditions.

Stage models also predict that the sequencing of treatments is important. For maximum effectiveness, order of interventions should follow the hypothesized order of stages. Consequently, sequence effects provide further evidence of a stage process. Unfortunately, because testing for sequence effects requires sequential interventions, such tests are very difficult to carry out.

AN EXAMPLE USING MATCHED AND MISMATCHED TREATMENTS TO TEST THE PAPM

A field experiment focusing on home radon testing (Weinstein, Lyon, Sandman, and Cuite, 1998) was designed to examine several aspects of the PAPM. Radon is an invisible, odorless, radioactive gas produced by the decay of small amounts of naturally occurring uranium in soil. Radiation from the decay of radon can damage cells in the lungs, and radon is the second leading cause of lung cancer after smoking (National Academy of Sciences, 1988; U.S. Environmental Protection Agency [EPA], 1992). Radon tests can be carried out by homeowners with a modest degree of effort; a single do-it-yourself test typically costs between $10 and $50.

The experiment focused on two stage transitions: from being undecided about testing one's home for radon (Stage 3) to deciding to test (Stage 5), and from deciding to test (Stage 5) to actually ordering a test (Stage 6). The study did not examine the transition from being unaware of the radon issue (Stage 1) to being aware but not engaged (Stage 2), or from being unengaged (Stage 2) to thinking about testing (Stage 3), because merely agreeing to participate in a radon study and answering questions about testing would probably be sufficient to move people to Stage 3. People who had already decided not to test (Stage 4) were excluded, because a brief intervention would have difficulty reversing that decision. Thus, although this example does not examine all features of the PAPM, it is a realistic example of how critical stages and stage transitions can be studied.

To determine whether the two transitions studied involve different barriers, as the theory claims, two interventions were used—one matched to each transition. Based on previous surveys and experiments (Sandman and Weinstein, 1993; Weinstein, Sandman, and Roberts, 1990), information about the local radon risk and rebuttals to myths of invulnerability were chosen as the focus of the intervention aimed at helping move people from Stage 3 to Stage 5. Interventions focusing mainly on risk had not been effective, however, in getting people to actually order tests (Weinstein, Sandman, and Roberts, 1990, 1991). Instead, several studies had found that test orders could be increased by increasing the ease of testing (Doyle, McClelland, and Schulze, 1991; Weinstein, Sandman, and Roberts, 1990, 1991). Thus, to move people from Stage 5 to Stage 6, the second intervention aimed at lowering barriers to action by providing information about do-it-yourself test kits and an actual test order form.

Method

The study took place in Columbus, Ohio, a city with high radon levels. To refresh their memories of the issue, all participants viewed a general informational video about radon before receiving any experimental treatment. Their stage of testing was assessed after this first video (preintervention measurement) using the algorithm in Table 6.2.

After the first questionnaires had been returned, homeowners who were in Stage 3 or Stage 5 of radon testing were assigned at random to an experimental condition, and treatment videos were delivered to participants by mail. Participants in the High-Likelihood condition received a five-minute video, *Radon Risk in Columbus Area Homes,* and an accompanying cover letter. The video focused on evidence of high local radon levels, pictures of actual local homes with high levels, testimony by a local homeowner and a city health official, and refutations of common myths about radon. The cover letter mentioned that test kits could be ordered from the American Lung Association (ALA) but did not include an order form.

TABLE 6.2. Precaution Adoption Process Model: Stage Classification Algorithm.

1. Have you ever heard about {home radon testing}?	
No	Stage 1
Yes [go to 2]	
2. Have you {tested your own house for radon}?	
Yes	Stage 6
No [go to 3]	
3. Which of the following best describes your thoughts about {testing your home}?	
I've never thought about {testing}	Stage 2
I'm undecided about {testing}	Stage 3
I've decided I don't want to {test}	Stage 4
I've decided I do want to {test}	Stage 5

Note: The material in curly brackets can be replaced with other precautions to create a staging algorithm for these precautions.

Participants in the Low-Effort condition received a five-minute video, *How to Test Your Home for Radon,* an accompanying cover letter, and a form to order test kits through the ALA. The video described how to select a kit type (making an explicit recommendation in order to reduce uncertainty), locate and purchase a kit, and conduct a test. The process was described as simple and inexpensive.

Participants in the Combination condition received a ten-minute video that combined the two separate treatments, along with the same letter and order form as people in the Low-Effort condition. Participants in the Control condition received a letter stating that their further assistance was not needed and thanking them for their participation.

Follow-up telephone interviews were conducted 9–10 weeks after respondents returned the second video questionnaires (follow-up measurement). Interviews assessed whether participants had purchased radon test kits and, if not, determined their final stages. The final sample consisted of 1,897 homeowners.

Results

Predicting Progress Toward Action. Table 6.3 shows the percentage of people from each preintervention stage who progressed *one or more* stages toward testing. This criterion (rather than progress of only a single stage toward testing) was chosen because,

TABLE 6.3. **Progressed One or More Stage Toward Purchasing a Radon Test (percentage).**

| Preintervention Stage | Condition | | | |
	Control	High-Likelihood	Low-Effort	Combination
Undecided	18.8 (138)	41.7 (144)	36.4 (130)	54.5 (139)
Decided-to-test	8.0 (339)	10.4 (338)	32.5 (329)	35.8 (345)

Note: The group size in each cell is shown in parentheses.

although people who stopped at one stage were hypothesized to lack the requirements to get to the next stage, it seemed likely that some individuals would already possess the information or skills needed to overcome later barriers. The upper half of the table indicates the percentage of people at follow-up who had moved from the undecided stage to either the decided-to-test or the testing stage. The lower half of the table shows the percentage of decided-to-test people who had moved on to the testing stage.

Statistical analyses showed more people progressed from the undecided stage than from the decided-to-test stage, $F (1, 1886) = 61.6$, $p < .0001$. There also was more progress among those who received the High-Likelihood treatment than among those who did not, $F (1, 1886) = 31.5$, $p < .0001$. Most important, there was a significant stage by High-Likelihood treatment interaction, $F (1, 1886) = 18.5$, $p < .0001$, indicating that the High-Likelihood treatment was much more effective for undecided participants than for decided-to-act participants.

There was also a large main effect of the Low-Effort treatment, $F (1, 1886) = 89.4$, $p < .0001$. The stage by Low-Effort treatment interaction, $F (1, 1886) = 5.9$, $p < .02$, indicated that, as hypothesized, the Low-Effort treatment in the Low-Effort and Combination conditions had a relatively bigger effect on people already planning to test than on people who were undecided.

Predicting Test Orders. Radon tests were ordered by 342 study participants or 18 percent of the sample (Table 6.4). For people already planning to test at the preintervention

TABLE 6.4. **Radon Test Orders (percentage).**

| Preintervention Stage | Condition | | | |
	Control	High-Likelihood	Low-Effort	Combination
Undecided	(a) 5.1	(b) 3.5	(c) 10.1	(d) 18.7
Decided-to-test	(e) 8.0	(f) 10.4	(g) 32.5	(h) 35.8

assessments, planning to test, "progress," and testing are the same according to the PAPM, so the data in the lower half of Table 6.4 are identical to those in the lower half of Table 6.3. As expected, there was more testing from the decided-to-test stage than from the undecided stage, $F (1, 1887) = 42.3$, $p < .0001$, and much more testing among people exposed to a Low-Effort treatment than among those who did not receive this treatment, $F (1, 1887) = 87.9$, $p < .0001$. Most important was the highly significant interaction between stage and Low-Effort treatment, $F (1, 1887) = 18.2$, $p < .0001$.

Eight more specific tests concern predicted cell-by-cell contrasts. In subsequent paragraphs, predictions are presented in brackets. Experimental groups are labeled with letters that refer to the cells in Table 6.4.

Test order rates of both undecided and decided-to-test participants in the Control condition were expected to be quite low, because both groups were viewed as lacking information needed to progress to action [(a)≅(e), both small].

The Low-Effort treatment was expected to be much more helpful than the High-Likelihood treatment in getting people who had already decided to test to order tests [(g)>(f)]. In fact, it was predicted that the High-Likelihood treatment would be ineffective in eliciting testing from people planning to test [(f)≅(e)], and, more obviously, unable to elicit test orders from undecided people [(b)≅(a)]. Furthermore, since people in the decided-to-test stage should not need further information about risk, it was predicted that testing in the Combination condition would not be significantly greater than testing in the Low-Effort condition [(h)≅(g)].

According to the PAPM, people who are undecided have to decide to test before acting. Consequently, a Low-Effort intervention alone was not expected to produce test orders from this group [(c)≅(a)]. Since undecided people in the Combination condition received both high-likelihood information and low-effort assistance, some of these people might be able to make two stage transitions [(d)>(c)], but not as many as decided-to-test people in the Combination condition who needed to advance only one stage [(d)<(h)]. Theories based on a single equation would not make detailed predictions like these, especially predictions that vary with initial stage. Furthermore, such theories would predict that the more ingredients in an intervention, the greater the response.

T-tests comparing means of cells mentioned in the preceding eight hypotheses demonstrated that none of the pairs predicted to be approximately the same were significantly different (p's > .3). All pairs predicted to be different were significantly different (all p's < .0001 except for the hypothesis that (d) > (c), $p = .03$).

Radon Study Implications for Theory

The radon study has several theoretical implications. First, it provides support for our claim that being undecided and having decided to act represent distinct stages, with different barriers to moving to the next stage. Second, the data support the suggestion that information about risk is helpful in getting people to decide to act, even though this same information may have little value in producing action among those individuals who have already decided to act. Third, information that increases perceived and actual ease of action appears to greatly aid people who have decided to act, but it is less important among people who are still undecided. More research is needed to determine whether these same factors are important at the same stages for other health behaviors.

Acceptance of the idea that stages exist also has implications for theory development. If factors that facilitate movement toward action vary from stage to stage, few, if any, factors will be important at all stages. Thus, the standard approach of comparing people who have acted with everyone who has not will be a poor way to discover variables important for precaution adoption. In fact, when all who have not acted are simply lumped together in a single category, some stages may be missing or barely represented. In this case, it would be impossible to discover the role of a variable that might be crucial to people reaching or leaving this stage—and therefore crucial to the precaution process—but not relevant to other transitions. Stage theories suggest that we will be better able to identify important barriers if we compare people who are in adjacent stages.

If we had compared people who had tested for radon to all those who had not, we would have found many differences in beliefs and experiences, and we might have based our interventions on some of these. Yet, when we compared people who had tested with those who had decided to test but had not yet acted, we found almost no differences on these variables. This finding led us to explore the idea that factors external to individuals—especially matters of opportunity and effort—were responsible for getting people to move from intention to action. Much of our success in generating radon test purchases came from this idea.

Radon Study Implications for Practice

Effects produced by the radon testing experiment are large enough to have practical implications. Viewed in terms of radon test order ratios, the interventions created a three-fold difference in test orders between the undecided and decided-to-test stages in the Low-Effort condition and a ten-fold difference between cells with the highest and lowest testing rates.

Stage-targeted communications have never been used in actual radon testing promotions and, until relatively recently, had not been used for any health behaviors. The most widely disseminated radon communications—national television public service announcements—have focused on persuading viewers that the radon hazard is substantial for people in general. To the extent that a target audience stage can be inferred, these public service announcements appeared to be aimed primarily at viewers who are unaware of the radon problem (Stage 1) or had never thought about their own response (Stage 2). This was a defensible choice when the issue was new and the medium used (national television) was scattershot. But twenty years after radon first received substantial public attention, most radon communication campaigns have retained the same focus, even though there is reason to think that much of the audience is beyond Stages 1 and 2.

REVIEW OF RESEARCH USING THE PAPM

Types of Studies Conducted

The PAPM has been applied to many types of health behaviors, including osteoporosis prevention (Blalock and others, 1996, 2000, 2002; Blalock, 2005, 2007; Sharp and Thombs, 2003), cancer screening (Clemow and others, 2000; Costanza and others, 2005; Glanz, Steffen, and Taglialatela, 2007; Sifri and others, 2006), hepatitis B vaccination (Hammer, 1997), home radon testing (Weinstein, Lyon, Sandman, and Cuite, 1998; Weinstein and Sandman, 1992; Weinstein, Sandman, and Klotz, 1987; Weinstein, Sandman, and Roberts, 1990, 1991), smoking cessation (Borrelli and others, 2002), and red meat consumption (Sniehotta, Luszczynska, Scholz, and Lippke, 2005). As discussed earlier in this chapter, stage theories—with their numerous assumptions about stages and about the changing barriers between stages—are complex. Given the limited, though growing, number of studies relating to the PAPM and the variety of behaviors examined, it is not yet possible to reach firm conclusions about the model's validity or its helpfulness for designing interventions. Instead, this section reviews the ways in which the PAPM is being used and some of the problems researchers encounter in these investigations.

As is true for health behavior research in general, most articles reporting on the PAPM present cross-sectional data (for example, Blalock and others, 1996; Clemow and others, 2000; Costanza and others, 2005; McClain, Bernhardt, and Beach, 2005; Sandman and Weinstein, 1993; Sniehotta, Luszczynska, Scholz, and Lippke, 2005), though a few describe longitudinal data (Blalock, 2007) or have conducted interventions with control groups (Blalock, 2000, 2002; Borrelli and others, 2002; Glanz, Steffen, and Taglialatela, 2007; Weinstein, Sandman, Lyon, and Cuite, 1998).

The degree to which these studies actually make use of ideas embodied in the PAPM varies tremendously. A few researchers (for example, Edwards, Iris, Ferkel, and Feinglass, 2006; Mauck and others, 2002; Sharp and Thombs, 2003) report the distribution of their study samples across the PAPM stages, but use neither stage ideas nor the PAPM in any other way. Other studies measure both people's stages and their standing on selected variables. Such studies compare values of these variables across stages—emphasizing pairs of stages that are adjacent in the PAPM—and look for significant differences. If the concern of such researchers is to test the validity of the theory, they search for variables that differentiate between some pairs of adjacent stages and not others (for example, Sniehotta, Luszczynska, Scholz, and Lippke, 2005; Sandman and Weinstein, 1993). Differences between stages are viewed as possible barriers to stage movement, and the analysis responds to the claim that at least some barriers to movement differ from transition to transition. Other researchers are less interested in theory testing than in using the model to develop behavior change interventions (Clemow and others, 2000; Blalock and others, 1996). For them, variables that differ between stages become potential components of programs to encourage precautionary action.

Stage comparisons based on the PAPM do find many differences (for example, Blalock and others, 1996; Clemow and others, 2000; Costanza and others, 2005;

Sniehotta, Luszczynska, Scholz, and Lippke, 2005; Hammer, 1997; Sandman and Weinstein, 1993) and, further, find that the variables that distinguish one stage from another vary, depending on which two stages are compared. These results support the claim that the PAPM stages are qualitatively different.

Intervention studies emphasizing behavior change base their treatments on variables that have differed across stages in prior research or variables mentioned as possible barriers in discussions of the PAPM (for example, Blalock and others, 2000, 2002; Borrelli and others, 2002; Glanz, Steffen, and Taglialatela, 2007). Because these studies typically deliver the same treatment to all participants, regardless of stage, they make only limited use of stage concepts. The question they address is whether variables suggested by the stage model produce greater changes in behavior than the control condition (which could be a no-intervention control condition; a nonspecific, healthy-living control condition, or a treatment focusing on variables specified by other theories).

A more complete use of the stage character of the PAPM would be to develop stage-specific treatments and match treatments to participants' stages. Any of the three types of control conditions just identified might be used. To test the value of stage matching per se, the control condition could be a composite of stage-specific treatments. The most rigorous test of the model is the radon testing experiment described earlier in this chapter (Weinstein, Lyon, Sandman, and Cuite, 1998).

Problems and Issues

Interpretation of the PAPM. Perhaps because the very first version of the PAPM (Weinstein, 1988) distinguished among certain stages on the basis of individuals' beliefs about personal vulnerability, some researchers have interpreted the model as primarily focused on risk perception. This is incorrect. All later versions of the PAPM defined stages in terms of mental states regarding the *health action* in question, not regarding personal vulnerability to harm. Another mistake is to view the variables in Table 6.1 as assumptions of the PAPM. Variables in the table are ones that the creators of the model believe may prove important. However, it is incumbent on researchers to decide for themselves—from their own or others' empirical research or from other theories—which variables may determine movement from one stage to the next.

Interpreting and Analyzing Data. Differences between stages—in the perceived pros and cons of action, perceived susceptibility, self-efficacy, or other variables—might indicate that such variables are determinants of behavior change. But the change in stage may have produced the change in the variable, rather than the other way around (Weinstein, 2007). For example, because preventive measures are designed to reduce risks, the worry and the perceived vulnerability of people who have taken these measures are likely to be lower than those for people who have not acted. This should not be misinterpreted to mean that low perceived risk increases the likelihood of action.

A different problem arises when investigators combine stages before analyzing their data. This often occurs when they find small numbers of individuals in particular stages. Yet the stages are claimed by the PAPM to be qualitatively different, so these composite categories contain mixtures of different types of individuals. To compare all the people who are not acting or intending to act (Stages 1–4) with all those who intend to act or are already acting (Stages 5–7), for example, ignores nearly everything that makes the PAPM different from non-stage theories, such as the theories of reasoned action, planned behavior, or protection motivation. It would be better to drop from analyses stages with few members.

Definitions of Stages When Health Behaviors Are Complex.   The PAPM, like most other theories of health behavior, maps most readily onto single health behaviors that are dichotomous, such as being vaccinated versus not being vaccinated. Many precautions, however, are more complicated. For example, sun protection and colorectal cancer screening can each be achieved by a variety of actions. Furthermore, some sun protection actions, such as wearing a hat, are dichotomous, but others, such as the amount of time one spends outdoors during peak sun hours, are continuous. Some precautions—such as wearing a hat and a long-sleeved shirt—complement one another, but others are mutually exclusive (if you stay out of the sun during high-risk times, you have little need to use sunscreen).

In general, we recommend that researchers define stages in terms of concrete behaviors, such as wearing a hat, rather than in terms of broad health goals, such as "protecting oneself from the sun" or "eating a healthy diet." However, there are undoubtedly instances where people do focus on the overall goal (for example, sun protection, low-fat diet, regular exercise) and treat the actions that can help them reach this goal as a menu from which they can make daily choices, rather than feeling that they have to make fixed decisions about whether or not to perform each separate action. In other words, people may decide to do *something,* or they may decide to do *specific things.* Thus, some people may decide to reduce their sun exposure and adopt actions that may change from day to day, whereas others may focus on one action and decide to apply sunscreen each morning.

Another difficult question for users of the PAPM is whether to add stages that differentiate people on the basis of their past actions. For example, a person who quit smoking temporarily and is undecided about trying to quit again is, according to the model, placed in the same stage as a smoker who is undecided about quitting and has never tried to stop. Yet the first person, having gotten to the point of making a quit attempt and having gained concrete experience from trying to quit, seems to be in a different position from the second. Do they need to be placed in different stages?

If someone has made only partial progress toward a goal—such as eating five servings a day of fruit and vegetables—should she be grouped with people who have made no dietary change or with people who consume the recommended five servings a day, or should there be a separate category of action that is under way but incomplete? And what of behaviors that need to be repeated, such as cancer screening, but at intervals that may range from a year to a decade? Because some of these behaviors may never become deeply engrained habits, perhaps the stage we have called maintenance will not apply.

Answers to questions about what stages provide the best explanation of precaution adoption cannot be derived from logic alone and must await the accumulated findings of careful empirical research.

CRITERIA FOR APPLYING STAGE-BASED INTERVENTIONS

A variety of issues should be considered to determine the practical utility of the PAPM or any other stage theory.

Superiority over Unstaged Messages

The practical utility of a stage theory depends on the extent to which it leads to interventions that are more effective than generic messages.

For the radon testing study described here, we had to develop two different interventions. Because the combination treatment in our experiment produced the greatest progress among both undecided and decided-to-test participants, one might be tempted to conclude that the PAPM did not provide any new treatment ideas. "Just use the combination treatment," someone might say. There are several flaws in this reasoning. First, the combination treatment was about twice as long as each of its two components. Media time is expensive; speakers usually have a fixed length of time for their presentations; some people will not attend an educational presentation; and audiences have a limited attention span. Thus, attempting to replace the Low-Effort or High-Likelihood interventions with their combination would involve substantial costs.

Second, people are most likely to be engaged by a treatment that matches their stage, and a mismatched treatment may lose their attention. Thus, members of the general public who have already decided to act may be put off by risk information and may fail to attend to the subsequent, detailed procedural information that they do need. Nevertheless, if only a single message can be given to a mixed-stage audience, the combination intervention would probably be the most appropriate.

Stage Assessment

A second relevant criterion is the ability to identify stages accurately and efficiently. The PAPM requires only a simple process to assess a person's stage, so it can be used easily in individual and small-group settings. Clinicians could integrate this assessment without disrupting their practices. Similarly, a filtering question on a Web site can easily assess stage and send visitors to the page most relevant to their stage. Even in a large audience, a show of hands might be used to quickly determine the distribution of stages present. However, if the audience is dispersed, the budget is small, or time is tight, efforts to measure stage may be impractical.

Delivery of Stage-Targeted Messages

The feasibility of delivering stage-targeted messages in different situations varies greatly. If communication is one-on-one, as in a doctor's office or counseling session, delivering the message appropriate for an individual is relatively easy. In group settings, such as public lectures, messages can be chosen to fit the overall audience, though not individual members. In mass communications, a stage approach is more often practicable with print than with broadcast media. Within print channels, pamphlets and magazines offer more opportunities for stage targeting than newspapers; within broadcasting, cable offers more opportunities for stage targeting than networks. The Internet makes it possible for individual users to choose different information pathways, depending on their self-perceived information needs. This should provide unprecedented opportunities for low-cost message targeting, though evidence on the cost of such tailored messaging is scanty. There is evidence, though, that people in different PAPM stages do perceive themselves as needing different types of information (Weinstein, Lyon, Sandman, and Cuite, 1998).

The ability to deliver targeted messages to members of a group also depends on the range of stages present in that group. The greater the range of stages, the more difficult it is to choose a single message. For a mass audience, the most efficient way to encourage a new health-protective action may be with a comprehensive broadcast message that ignores stage or assumes everyone to be at a very early stage. As the issue matures, however, distinctive audiences, separable by stage, merit distinctive messages, and print or "narrowcasting" becomes the medium of choice for mass communications.

The Difficulty of Behavior Change

A final criterion of importance concerns the difficulty of the action being advocated and the expected resistance of the audience to the behavior change recommendation. When a behavior is easy and resistance is low, stage may matter little. In such situations, interventions and messages needed to help people progress from stage to stage can be brief, and several may be combined into a single comprehensive treatment. In contrast, when change is difficult and resistance is high, there is a greater need to have separate messages for each stage. Note that although some precautions, such as changing to a fluoride-containing toothpaste, are clearly easy to carry out, the ease of others may vary greatly from one person to the next. Health professionals should never assume that a behavior is easy without considering carefully the obstacles that may exist.

Radon testing appears so easy and radon test kits so accessible, that it comes as a surprise to many professionals that there is any need for an effort-reducing intervention. Even apparently simple actions may raise questions that need to be answered before people feel confident that they can carry out the behavior successfully. Actions often seem much more difficult to the public than to professionals. Some types of lifestyle changes—exercise, smoking cessation, dietary change, cancer screening, and others—are genuinely difficult or frightening for many people, and it is hard to convince audiences that action is needed. In cases like these, matching interventions to stage would be expected to matter more.

FUTURE DIRECTIONS

Most other (non-stage) theories of individual health behavior regard adoption of new precautions as involving only one step: from inaction to action (or, perhaps, inaction to intention); the variables typically claimed to produce this step clearly characterize it as a judgment about the relative costs and benefits of action. The PAPM does not reject the variables identified by these theories. Rather, it sees the theories as describing just one part of the precaution adoption process—the stage when people are actively weighing options and deciding what to do. The PAPM, however, shows that other issues important to behavior change arise before people ever think seriously about action, and still different issues arise after people have decided to act.

Because the PAPM is not composed of a short list of variables, it does not offer a simple process for designing interventions. Rather, it is a framework that can be used to identify barriers that inhibit movement from one stage to the next. As additional research is conducted, we will learn more about barriers at each stage and will see how consistent these barriers are from one health behavior to the next.

SUMMARY

This chapter describes the Precaution Adoption Process Model (PAPM)—a stage theory that seeks to explain the adoption of new health-protective behaviors. The model asserts that progress toward behavior change is best explained in terms of a sequence of qualitatively different stages. These are called "unaware," "uninvolved," "undecided," "decided to act," "acting," and "maintaining action," plus a stage "decided not to act," that is a branch away from action. The barriers impeding progress toward action vary, depending on what stage people have reached. The characteristics of stage theories are explained, as well as ways they can be tested. The chapter contains a review summarizing the ways in which the PAPM has been used, and it includes detailed examples from osteoporosis prevention and home radon testing.

REFERENCES

Ajzen, I. "From Intentions to Actions: A Theory of Planned Behavior." In J. Kuhl and J. Beckmann (eds.), *Action Control: From Cognition to Behavior.* Heidelberg: Springer-Verlag, 1985.

Ajzen, I., and Madden, T. J. "Prediction of Goal-Directed Behavior: Attitudes, Intentions, and Perceived Behavioral Control." *Journal of Experimental Social Psychology,* 1986, *22,* 453–474.

Anderson, C. A. "Abstract and Concrete Data in the Perseverance of Social Theories: When Weak Data Lead to Unshakable Beliefs." *Journal of Experimental Social Psychology,* 1983, *19,* 93–108.

Bandura, A. "Moving into Forward Gear in Health Promotion and Disease Prevention." Address presented at the Annual Meeting of the Society of Behavioral Medicine, San Diego, Calif., March 1995.

Blalock, S. J. "Toward a Better Understanding of Calcium Intake: Behavioral Change Perspectives." *Journal of Reproductive Medicine,* 2005, *50*(11 Suppl), 901–906.

Blalock, S. J. "Predictors of Calcium Intake Patterns: A Longitudinal Analysis." *Health Psychology,* 2007, *26*(3), 251–258.

Blalock, S. J., and others. "Osteoporosis Prevention in Premenopausal Women: Using a Stage Model Approach to Examine the Predictors of Behavior." *Health Psychology,* 1996, *15,* 84–93.

Blalock, S. J., and others. "Effects of Educational Materials Concerning Osteoporosis on Women's Knowledge, Beliefs, and Behavior." *American Journal of Health Promotion,* 2000, *14,* 161–169.

Blalock, S. J., and others. "Effects of Osteoporosis Prevention Program Incorporating Tailored Educational Materials." *American Journal of Health Promotion,* 2002, *16,* 146–156.

Borrelli, B., and others. "Motivating Parents of Kids with Asthma to Quit Smoking: The PAQS Project." *Health Education Research,* 2002, *17,* 659–669.

Brockner, J., and Rubin, J. Z. *Entrapment in Escalating Conflicts: A Social Psychological Analysis.* New York: Springer-Verlag, 1985.

Cialdini, R. B. *Influence: Theory and Practice.* Glenview, Ill: Scott, Foresman, 1988.

Clemow, L., and others. "Underutilizers of Mammography Screening Today: Characteristics of Women Planning, Undecided About, and Not Planning a Mammogram." *Annals of Behavioral Medicine,* 2000, *22*(1), 80–88.

Connor, M., and Norman, P. *Predicting Health Behavior.* Philadelphia: Open University Press, 1995.

Costanza, M. E., and others. "Applying a Stage Model of Behavior Change to Colon Cancer Screening." *Preventive Medicine,* 2005, *41,* 707–719.

Dishman, R. K. *Exercise Adherence: Its Impact on Public Health.* Champaign, Ill: Human Kinetics, 1988.

Ditto, P. H., and Lopez, D. F. "Motivated Skepticism: Use of Differential Decision Criteria for Preferred and Nonpreferred Conclusions." *Journal of Personality and Social Psychology,* 1992, *63,* 568–584.

Doyle, J. K., McClelland, G. H., and Schulze, W. D. "Protective Responses to Household Risk: A Case Study of Radon Mitigation." *Risk Analysis,* 1991, *11,* 121–134.

Edwards, B. J., Iris, M., Ferkel, E., and Feinglass, J. "Postmenopausal Women with Minimal Trauma Fractures are Unapprised of the Existence of Low Bone Mass or Osteoporosis." *Maturitas,* 2006, *53,* 260–266.

Gibbons, F. X., Gerrard, M., Blanton, H., and Russell, D. W. "Reasoned Action and Social Reaction: Willingness and Intention as Independent Predictors of Health Risk." *Journal of Personality and Social Psychology,* 1998, *74,* 1164–1181.

Gollwitzer, P. "Implementation Intentions: Strong Effects of Simple Plans." *American Psychologist,* 1999, *54,* 493–503.

Glanz, K., Steffen, A. D., and Taglialatela, L. A. "Effects of Colon Cancer Risk Counseling for First-Degree Relatives." *Cancer, Epidemiology, Biomarkers and Prevention,* 2007, *16,* 1485–1491.

Hammer, G. P. "Hepatitis B Vaccine Acceptance Among Nursing Home Workers." Unpublished doctoral dissertation, Department of Health Policy and Management, Johns Hopkins University, 1997.

Janis, I. L., and Mann, L. *Decision Making: A Psychological Analysis of Conflict, Choice, and Commitment.* New York: Free Press, 1977.

Jelalian, E., and Miller, A. G. "The Perseverance of Beliefs: Conceptual Perspectives and Research Developments." *Journal of Social and Clinical Psychology,* 1984, *2,* 25–56.

Klayman, J. "Varieties of Confirmation Bias." In J. Busemeyer, R. Hastie (eds.), *The Psychology of Learning and Motivation.* Vol. 32: *Decision Making from a Cognitive Perspective.* New York: Academic Press, 1995.

Marlatt, G. A., and Gordon, J. R. *Relapse Prevention: Maintenance Strategies in the Treatment of Addictive Behaviors.* New York: Guilford, 1985.

Mauck, K. F., and others. "The Decision to Accept Treatment of Osteoporosis Following Hip Fracture: Exploring the Woman's Perspective Using a Stage-of-Change Model." *Osteoporosis International,* 2002, *13,* 560–564.

McClain, J., Bernhardt, J. M., and Beach, M. J. "Assessing Parents' Perception of Children's Risk for Recreational Water Illnesses." *Emerging Infectious Diseases,* 2005, *11,* 670–676.

Meichenbaum, D., and Turk, D. C. *Facilitating Treatment Adherence: A Practitioner's Handbook.* New York: Plenum, 1987.

National Academy of Sciences. *Health Effects of Radon and Other Internally Deposited Alpha-Emitters: BEIR IV.* Washington, D.C.: National Academy Press, 1988.

Nisbett, R., and Ross, L. *Human Inference: Strategies and Shortcomings of Social Judgment.* Englewood Cliffs, N.J.: Prentice Hall, 1980.

"Osteoporosis Prevention, Diagnosis, and Therapy." NIH Consensus Statement 2000 March 27–29; *17*(1): 1–36. [http://consensus.nih.gov/2000/2000Osteoporosis111html.htm].

Riggs, B. L., and Melton, L.J.I. "Involutional Osteoporosis." *New England Journal of Medicine,* 1986, *314,* 1676–1686.

Rogers, R. W., and Prentice-Dunn, S. "Protection Motivation Theory." In D. Gochman (ed.), *Handbook of Health Behavior Research.* Vol. 1. *Determinants of Health Behavior: Personal and Social.* New York: Plenum, 1997.

Sandman, P. M., and Weinstein, N. D. "Predictors of Home Radon Testing and Implications for Testing Promotion Programs." *Health Education Quarterly,* 1993, *20,* 1–17.

Schwarzer, R. "Self-Efficacy in the Adoption and Maintenance of Health Behaviors: Theoretical Approaches and a New Model." In R. Schwarzer (ed.), *Self-Efficacy: Thought Control of Action.* Washington, D.C.: Hemisphere, 1992.

Schwarzer, R., and Fuchs, R. "Self-Efficacy and Health Behaviors." In M. Conner and P. Norman (eds.), *Predicting Health Behavior: Research and Practice with Social Cognition Models.* Buckingham, England: Open University Press, 1996.

Sharp, K., and Thombs, D. L. "A Cluster Analytic Study of Osteoprotective Behavior in Undergraduates." *American Journal of Health Behavior,* 2003, *27,* 364–372.

Sifri, R., and others. "Decision Stage and Screening Preference in Colorectal Cancer Screening." Paper presented at the American Society of Preventive Oncology, Bethesda, Md., February 2006.

Sniehotta, F. F., Luszczynska, A., Scholz, U., and Lippke, S. "Discontinuity Patterns in Stages of the Precaution Adoption Process Model: Meat Consumption During a Livestock Epidemic." *British Journal of Health Psychology,* 2005, *10,* 221–235.

Trope, Y., and Liberman, N. "Temporal Construal Theory." *Psychological Review,* 2003, *100,* 403–421.

U.S. Environmental Protection Agency Office of Radiation Programs, and U.S. Department of Health and Human Services Centers for Disease Control. *A Citizen's Guide to Radon.* (2nd ed.) Washington, D.C.: Author, 1992.

Weinstein, N. D. "Unrealistic Optimism About Susceptibility to Health Problems: Conclusions from a Community Wide Sample." *Journal of Behavioral Medicine,* 1987, *10,* 481–500.

Weinstein, N. D. "The Precaution Adoption Process." *Health Psychology,* 1988, *7,* 355–386.

Weinstein N. D. "Misleading Tests of Health Behavior Theories." *Annals of Behavioral Medicine,* 2007, *33,* 1–10.

Weinstein, N. D., Lyon, J. E., Sandman, P. M., and Cuite, C. L. "Experimental Evidence for Stages of Precaution Adoption." *Health Psychology,* 1998, *17,* 445–453.

Weinstein, N. D., Rothman A., and Sutton, S. "Stage Theories of Health Behavior." *Health Psychology,* 1998, *17,* 290–299.

Weinstein, N. D., and Sandman, P. M. "A Model of the Precaution Adoption Process: Evidence from Home Radon Testing." *Health Psychology,* 1992, *11,* 170–180.

Weinstein, N. D., Sandman, P. M., and Klotz, M. L. *Public Response to the Risk from Radon, 1986.* New Brunswick, N.J.: Environmental Communications Research Program, Rutgers University, 1987.

Weinstein, N. D., Sandman, P. M., and Roberts, N. E. "Determinants of Self-Protective Behavior: Home Radon Testing." *Journal of Applied Social Psychology,* 1990, *20,* 783–801.

Weinstein, N. D., Sandman, P. M., and Roberts, N. E. "Perceived Susceptibility and Self-Protective Behavior: A Field Experiment to Encourage Home Radon Testing." *Health Psychology,* 1991, *10,* 25–33.

CHAPTER

7

PERSPECTIVES ON HEALTH BEHAVIOR THEORIES THAT FOCUS ON INDIVIDUALS

Noel T. Brewer

Barbara K. Rimer

KEY POINTS

This chapter will

- Comment on four theories introduced in Part Two of this book: Health Belief Model (HBM), Theory of Planned Behavior (TPB), the Transtheoretical Model (TTM), and Precaution Adoption Process Model (PAPM).
- Discuss why theory is needed.
- Examine some of the strengths and weaknesses of the four theories.
- Consider challenges and opportunities in the field.

We thank Seth Noar, Neil Weinstein, and the Editors for their ideas and feedback. Partial support for development of this chapter came from the American Cancer Society (MSRG-06-259-01-CPPB) and the National Cancer Institute (5R01 CA105786).

Theories that focus on beliefs and actions of individuals were among the first theories of health behavior to be developed and remain the most widely used today. In this chapter, we comment on four theories introduced in Part Two of this book: the Health Belief Model (HBM), Theory of Planned Behavior (TPB), the Transtheoretical Model (TTM), and the Precaution Adoption Process Model (PAPM). We discuss why theory is needed, examine some of the strengths and weaknesses of the four theories, and consider challenges and opportunities in the field.

WHY THEORY?

Most interventions to change health behavior are based on ideas about what will work. Some are guided by formally stated theories, such as those discussed in this book (see Chapters One and Two). Others are guided by less formally defined notions about behavior developed from personal experiences, intuition, and opinions. Which approach is better?

Theory provides a bridge from findings in one study to another. Using well-defined constructs allows researchers to compare findings across studies to identify "active ingredients." Using well-developed constructs can help to identify when findings from one population are likely to generalize to another population. For example, will a study of condom use among sex workers in Tanzania yield findings that apply to sex workers in China? Will it generalize to people who aren't sex workers? If studies and interventions are designed without theory, it will be more difficult to generalize findings to other populations, settings, and times.

Interventions informed by well-developed and tested theories also may be more effective in changing behavior than those not based on theory. Several reviews have compared interventions developed using theories to those developed without formal theoretical frameworks. Five of seven meta-analyses that analyzed whether using theory to design interventions to increase condom use improved their effectiveness found that theory-based interventions were somewhat or clearly superior (Noar, forthcoming). However, a meta-analysis of interventions to increase mammography use found that theory-based interventions were not more effective in increasing mammography uptake (Legler and others, 2002). A limitation of such systematic reviews is that the key factor (theory-based versus not) relies on whether investigators accurately reported their use of theory. The reviews may overstate the effectiveness of interventions that reported having used theory-based approaches, because they may have differed on many other correlated dimensions, including care with which the interventions were designed and implemented and fidelity to the theories. However, the benefits of using theory may be understated, because some investigators may have used constructs from theory in their interventions without necessarily reporting that they were using theory. In addition, theory may have been used, but the process of translating theory into interventions requires many discretionary judgments.

Another approach to understanding whether theory-based interventions are more effective in changing behavior is to examine interventions that emphasize constructs central to key theories. A meta-analysis of almost 200 intervention studies to increase condom use found that many constructs in commonly used theories of health behavior were changed successfully by interventions, and some of these constructs mediated changes in condom use (Albarracín and others, 2005). A systematic review of counseling interventions to increase healthy diets drew similar conclusions about the benefits of targeting theorized mediating variables (Pignone and others, 2003). These reviews provide modest support for the benefits of using theory-informed interventions.

Despite many potential benefits of using theory, one theory is unlikely to be enough for all or perhaps even most health behavior problems. While the theories we discuss in this chapter focus primarily on individual-level beliefs and processes, powerful influences occur at other levels, such as interpersonal relationships, neighborhoods, work settings, and policies. Later chapters in this book focus on these influences and relevant theories. Readers should consider integrating theories from more than one level and using these theories to design and evaluate health behavior interventions.

WHICH THEORY TO USE?

We encourage researchers and practitioners to be critical consumers of health behavior theories. Although this chapter focuses primarily on four theories, there are dozens of health behavior theories (see Chapter Two). Many are variations on others, sharing key constructs, such as self-efficacy, or assumptions, such as progressing through a series of stages before behaviors get adopted. Theories also differ in their focus on different variables or processes. This complexity has prompted students as close as Chapel Hill, North Carolina, and as far as Iran and China to pose versions of the same question to us about theory: *"How do you pick one theory over another?"* We address here how to choose among health behavior theories that focus on individuals.

Some theories are much more widely used than others, and the use of some has increased markedly over time. Three of the theories covered in Part Two (HBM, TPB, and TTM) are widely cited and used (see Chapter Two; Noar and Zimmerman, 2005). Some theories are more intuitively appealing than others, matching people's naïve theories of the motivators of health behavior. Other theories are quite complex, and their use in the health behavior field increases only after accessible measurement scales are developed (for example, the Revised Illness Perception Questionnaire for the Common Sense Model of Self-Regulation; Moss-Morris and others, 2002) or a specific application to the health domain is derived from a more general theory (for example, recommendations for when to use gain- and loss-framing, as derived from Prospect Theory (Rothman and Salovey, 1997). Although using theory in designing studies and interventions can be beneficial, little evidence suggests that any one theory is preferable to another. Of almost three thousand articles reporting studies guided by health behavior theories, only nineteen empirically compared multiple theories (Noar and Zimmerman, 2005). Of these, only three did so using rigorous methods that included longitudinal (as opposed to cross-sectional) designs and behavioral outcomes (Weinstein and Rothman, 2005). In the absence of good data on which theory is better, researchers and practitioners should select theories based on their assessments of the theories' merits and appropriateness to their specific questions, including empirical support for the theories' constructs in predicting (or changing) a specific behavior or the population of interest.

A CLOSER LOOK AT INDIVIDUAL-LEVEL THEORIES

In this section, we discuss the four theories presented in Chapters Three through Six to aid readers in evaluating the theories' merits and suitability for answering their research and practical questions.

Health Belief Model

The most appealing aspects of the Health Belief Model (HBM) are its intuitive logic and clearly stated central tenets (see Chapter Three). The HBM is based on the idea that value and expectancy beliefs guide behavior. In other words, people are more inclined to engage in a health behavior when they think doing so can reduce a threat that is likely and would have severe consequences if it occurred. Expectancy and value apply to the health threat (perceived likelihood and severity of harm) and the health behavior (perceived benefits of and barriers to taking action). Cues to action—a fifth HBM construct not based on expectancy or value—may be as diverse as medical symptoms, a doctor's recommendation, reminders from a health plan, or a media campaign. Self-efficacy—a sixth construct, proposed well after the model was initially formulated—is also not based in expectancy value, but if self-efficacy is construed as the perceived probability that an attempt to perform a behavior will be successful, it fits into the expectancy value framework. In HBM, self-efficacy applies especially to performance of repeated or habitual behaviors such as physical activity, eating, smoking, and sexual practices (Rosenstock, Strecher, and Becker, 1988), but it may not be needed for health behaviors that are relatively easy to accomplish.

Symptoms are central to patients' experiences of disease, and it is surprising that the HBM and one other long-standing health behavior theory (The Self-Regulation Model; Leventhal, Meyer, and Nerenz, 1980) are among the few to explicitly include them. This often under-appreciated dimension of the HBM, theorizing that medical symptoms are cues to action that prompt behavior, is as relevant today in studying AIDS, diabetes, and cancer prevention as it was in helping to explain tuberculosis screening behavior in the 1950s. These diseases are treated most successfully if diagnosed before a person develops symptoms. For some individuals, the belief that cancer always causes recognizable symptoms may be a critical variable in explaining nonparticipation in cancer screening. Some women feel they do not need mammograms because they do not have symptoms (Stoddard and others, 1998). Ironically, their not having symptoms is what makes the mammogram precisely the right test, and this applies to other screening tests as well.

Constructs in the HBM have received substantial empirical support for their ability to predict behavior based on correlational studies (Janz and Becker, 1984; Mullen, Hersey, and Iverson, 1987) and to a lesser extent in intervention studies (Albarracín and others, 2005). No systematic reviews or meta-analyses have been done yet of

HBM interventions across a range of health behaviors that allow us to know whether interventions designed using the model are more effective than those designed in some other way.

When the HBM is used as the theoretical basis for data collection, several important conceptual and statistical issues should be considered. Perceived threat—a central component of the HBM yielded by the combination of perceived susceptibility and severity—is tested by examining their statistical interactions (Strecher and Rosenstock, 1996; Weinstein, 1993). However, reviews of the model and of the effects of risk perception have looked only at the simple effects of perceived susceptibility and severity (Brewer and others, 2007; Janz and Becker, 1984; Mullen, Hersey, and Iverson, 1987), and few studies have found the predicted interaction (Weinstein, 1993). Another issue is that subtracting ratings of perceived barriers from ratings of perceived benefits can be limiting. Doing so prevents researchers from better understanding the roles that perceived barriers and benefits separately play in health behaviors. Careful attention to statistical tests of the HBM is warranted, as analyses too often examine each construct's relationship to the health behavior of interest without combining them.

Study design, especially the implied temporality among variables, affects the interpretability of data gathered using the HBM (and the other three models). Beliefs can motivate behavior as the model suggests, but behavior can also cause people to reassess their beliefs (Brewer, Weinstein, Cuite, and Herrington, 2004; Brewer and others, 2007). Cross-sectional studies may yield confusing and potentially incorrect information about the size and even the direction of belief-behavior relationships (Brewer, Weinstein, Cuite, and Herrington, 2004; Weinstein, 2007). This problem has been demonstrated empirically for perceived likelihood, but it may also apply to other HBM constructs. For example, a negative correlation of "vaccination" to "risk perception" does not necessarily mean that people at high risk were less likely to get vaccinated; it may simply be that people who got vaccinated correctly see themselves as less at risk. In other words people can align (and realign) their beliefs to match their behaviors.

In focusing on individuals' health-related perceptions, the HBM does not explicitly address important social, interpersonal, and contextual issues. This observation is relevant to most individually focused theories of health behavior. They also may miss important factors that are not intrinsically health-related but play an important role in shaping health behaviors.

The HBM can be a parsimonious model in terms of the number of questions needed to assess key constructs, requiring as few as six questions in total. HBM constructs can be measured by a variety of techniques, ranging from clinical interviews to population-based surveys. Although substantial HBM measurement work has occurred in select topic areas (see Chapter Three), the HBM never has had the kind of broad-based standardized measurement approaches called for in the Theory of Planned Behavior (see Chapter Four). Important work remains to be done with the HBM, especially in understanding better the effectiveness of HBM-based interventions, but the model is a proven way to identify correlates of health behavior.

Theory of Planned Behavior

The Theory of Planned Behavior (TPB) and the HBM share a foundation in the argument that behavior reflects expected value. TPB aims to explain rationally motivated, intentional health and non-health behaviors. The model applies as well to protecting oneself from infectious disease as it does to voting and consumer behaviors.

TPB assumes a causal chain that links attitudes, subjective norms, and perceived behavioral control to behavior through behavioral intentions. Several aspects of this claim merit additional discussion. First, the theory requires highly specific behavioral intentions measures that closely match the intended behaviors. Behavioral intentions measures can assess planning (for example, "Do you plan to use a mosquito net over your child's bed?"), desire (for example, "Would you like to use a mosquito net over your child's bed?"), and expectation (for example, "How likely is it that you will use a mosquito net over your child's bed?") (Conner and Sparks, 2001). Using multiple items increases statistical power by increasing measurement reliability. In recent years, researchers have proposed two new conceptualizations of intentions that go beyond the behavioral intentions conceptualization of the TPB. *Behavioral willingness* addresses behaviors that people may not necessarily intend to engage in (such as an adolescent trying marijuana or having unsafe sex) (Gibbons, Gerrard, Blanton, and Russell, 1998). *Implementation intention* interventions encourage people to specify exactly when and under what conditions they will engage in a behavior. Behavioral willingness can predict behavior above and beyond behavioral intentions, and implementation intentions are a potent intervention, stronger than only having people form more general intentions to act (Gollwitzer, 1999).

Second, TPB postulates that intentions lead to behavior, but the empirical data suggest a more qualified assessment. Although longitudinal studies suggest a very strong intention-behavior relationship (Sheeran, Trafimow, Finlay, and Norman, 2002), better designed, experimental studies show a much smaller effect (Webb and Sheeran, 2006). Furthermore, intentions often overstate but sometimes understate actual behavior. Many factors affect the relationship between change in intentions and change in behaviors. The relationship is substantially weaker for risk behaviors typically performed in a social context, for behaviors supported by habits, and when intentions were measured further away in time from behavior (Webb and Sheeran, 2006). Many other factors can weaken intention-behavior relationships to a lesser extent. The many uncertainties that accompany whether or not intentions will yield behavior change mean that behavioral intentions, while potentially useful in preliminary or pilot studies, are an inadequate primary outcome for studies and interventions intended to benefit the public's health. This same caveat applies equally to the idea of using stage change toward contemplation or preparation in the Transtheoretical Model (TTM) as a proxy for actual behavior change.

Third, TPB posits that attitudes can affect behavior only through intentions. Data from as far back as the 1970s lead us to question this assertion, showing that attitudes often directly predict behavior not mediated by intentions (for a review of the technical issues, see Liska, 1984). Intentions can change over time, as can attitudes, making their relationships to behavior something of a moving target. A related problem is that people do not form intentions for all behaviors, especially when the window of opportunity for action is a long time away. Analyses that control for past behavior often find that intention is no longer a significant predictor of behavior (Hagger, Chatzisarantis, and Biddle, 2002), but others question whether it is appropriate to control statistically for past behavior in examining these relationships (Weinstein, 2007).

The TPB provides a systematic method to identify those issues that are most important to a person's decisions about performing specific behaviors. Because many important beliefs and attitudes are changeable, they are ideal targets for subsequent interventions. Measurement methods stipulated by the TPB, though powerful for prediction are challenging in practice. They rely on extensive pilot work, including interviewer-administered personal interviews, and can require more items than many modern surveys can realistically accommodate. Although ultimately useful, this can be a demanding, costly process and can reduce participation rates. Collecting more intensive pilot data can be challenging when programs must be developed quickly. However, the emphasis on specificity of the intended behavior is both central to the TPB and one of the model's most important strengths.

Because the TPB is a theory of behavior that results from rational planning, some important health behaviors may not be explained by its principles. Although more experimental work remains to be done in testing the mediating relationships proposed in the model, the TPB is well supported by existing data from laboratory experiments, field studies, and health behavior interventions.

The Transtheoretical Model

Due in part to its intuitive appeal, the Transtheoretical Model (TTM; see Chapter Five) quickly became one of the most widely used models of health behavior. TTM departs substantially from many other individually oriented models of health behavior by focusing more on changes in behavior and less on cognitive variables (such as perceived risk or perceived barriers) believed to predict health behavior and behavior change. TTM argues that people are in different stages of readiness to make health behavior changes, and these stages are qualitatively different with respect to the constructs and processes that move people closer to behavior. TTM postulates that people should receive interventions appropriate for their stage in the behavior change process. If TTM assumptions are correct, treating people as though they are all the same inevitably dilutes the impact of interventions. For example, if a factory worker is unaware that chemical and particulate matter exposures at her worksite may be harmful to her, providing detailed information about protective behaviors is pointless. It would be far better to raise her awareness of the harms associated with the exposures and the benefits to be achieved from behavioral change. The fundamental underlying assumption is similar to the basic health education principle of "starting where the people are" (Green and Kreuter, 2005). Once stage of change is assessed, people can be provided with therapist-guided, self-initiated, or other interventions suited to their needs.

Researchers are vigorously debating several aspects of TTM. Several literature reviews have not found support for stage-based interventions as an effective way to change some behaviors, including physical activity and smoking (Bridle and others, 2005; van Sluijs, van Poppel, and van Mechelen, 2004; Riemsma and others, 2003), although Chapter Five provides several examples of effective interventions. An intriguing study that deliberately mismatched interventions for smokers concluded that matching did not increase the likelihood of quitting, and smokers who received the active intervention were most likely to quit, regardless of stage (Quinlan and McCaul, 2000). Reviews of TTM research may overstate empirical support for the model, because the control conditions in many studies lack the intensive personal contact of the interventions. Reviews also may also underestimate the power of the TTM, because many TTM-informed interventions did not use the full model (using, for example, only the stages of change). In sum, reviews provide mixed evidence and suggest that TTM-guided interventions do not always change health behaviors, but readers should also carefully analyze the reviews.

Another concern is that stages of change may be just another way of measuring behavioral intentions. Current measures of stages of change place people in categories ranging from inaction to action, and these measures share substantial similarity with intention measures that assess whether one is unlikely or likely to act (Sutton, 2001). Stages of change and behavioral intentions often are correlated highly, suggesting significant overlap in the two constructs (for example, de Vet, de Nooijer, de Vries, and Brug, 2007). In correlational studies, intention measures do as well at predicting subsequent behavior as stages of change (Abrams, Herzog, Emmons, and Linnan, 2000), a finding that makes the additional contribution of stages of change less clear.

Moving people from one early non-behavioral stage to another is not equivalent to behavior change, and interventions that alter stages of change (or intentions) may or may not yield behavior change (see also the earlier comments on TPB). It is also not clear whether people have to move through all the stages. Readers interested in other more detailed discussions of stage models and concerns that have been raised about the TTM should look at work by Sutton, Weinstein, and others (Sutton, 2001; Weinstein, Rothman, and Sutton, 1998; West, 2005).

Some apparent limitations of the TTM may result not from the model's deficiencies but instead from how researchers operationalize stages of change and design interventions. Stage definitions that are arbitrarily set at certain time points (for example, 30 days, 6 months) may be better defined using less arbitrary cut points and may vary by population and, certainly, by behavior. Measurement of stage can also be inaccurate, because people do not always correctly respond to questions that would put them in one or another stage, and they can move among stages during the time of a study or intervention, and between measurement occasions. Fewer or more stages may be appropriate, depending on the population and behavior. It is also unclear whether the *processes* of change must always be measured; in fact, they are often not assessed in TTM-based studies or practice applications. Important questions exist about the appropriate statistical analyses for assessing stage-related changes (for example, see Hedeker, Mermelstein, and Weeks, 1999). Many steps occur between theory and application, and it usually is not clear why an intervention designed using a particular theory is unsuccessful.

TTM has spawned a large body of research and lively debate. The many reviews of the TTM no doubt reflect the substantial enthusiasm and attention the model has received. TTM framework has a likeable simplicity, but researchers and practitioners who use it should do so wisely, comprehensively, and critically.

Precaution Adoption Process Model

The Precaution Adoption Process Model (PAPM) also assumes that people go through stages before modifying their behaviors (Chapter Six). Although bearing some similarity to TTM, PAPM stages differ somewhat both in their number and conceptualization. The PAPM explicitly recognizes a stage in which people may be unaware of a risk or precaution, and it includes a stage in which people have specifically decided not to act, which TTM does not include. The early stages of precaution adoption also focus more on increasing awareness of risk than similar TTM stages.

PAPM provides a framework of behavioral change that emphasizes the role of risk perceptions, an emphasis shared with the HBM. PAPM highlights processes not emphasized in other frameworks, such as consideration of costs and benefits over time and the competition between precautionary behaviors and other life demands. These considerations also can be found in the HBM, but the PAPM articulates them more precisely. Growing awareness of the threat posed by avian flu illustrates how quickly people may go from a state of unawareness to awareness and action (that is, travelers canceling trips to Asia and flight attendants wearing face masks). PAPM also provides a heuristic framework to categorize people at different stages of behavior change, and it includes mediating variables amenable to assessment in intervention programs.

PAPM has been studied most comprehensively by Weinstein and his collaborators and has received less critical attention than the other theories in this section. The model has not been used enough to provide a substantial body of data that either can affirm or refute its predictions. However, concerns about risk perception related to the HBM apply to this model as well. Although risk perception robustly predicts behavior in cross-sectional and longitudinal studies (Brewer and others, 2007), interventions focused on risk perception have had difficulty changing it and subsequently changing behavior, at least for HIV-prevention interventions (Albarracín and others, 2005).

PAPM is more of a conceptual framework than a completely specified theory (that is, providing detailed specification of the causes of change between stages). If the stages are valid, they should help in identifying causal factors (by comparing stages), but the model doesn't provide an a priori list of these factors. In this way, the PAPM is similar to the TPB, which calls for developmental work to identify the specific beliefs and attitudes of the target population.

COMMONALITIES AND DIFFERENCES ACROSS THE THEORIES

Theories in this section have much in common. Perceived barriers inhibit behavioral change explicitly in the HBM, TPB, and TTM and implicitly in the PAPM. Perceived risk is important in the HBM, PAPM, and, depending on the results of pilot work for a given study, may be important in the TPB. Self-efficacy is embodied in three of the theories (TTM and included in modifications of the HBM and TPB). Readiness is a central component of the TTM and the HBM.

The models differ in their intended scope. HBM grew out of research on disease prevention, initially focusing more on factors affecting people without diagnosed conditions (Rosenstock, 1974). TPB emerged from research to understand why attitudes did not always prompt behavior. This general focus persists today in the model's emphasis on rationally decided behaviors but explicitly excludes behaviors that are automatic (for example, habits). TTM places special emphasis on stages beyond action, including maintenance of the behavior, which may be especially important for behaviors such as dietary change in which the steps required for losing weight may differ from those involved in keeping it off. The same can be said for smoking cessation, maintenance of quitting, and physical activity. PAPM refers to adoption of precautions but not commencement of risky behaviors (such as drug use). It does not claim to explain the full range of health-affecting behaviors as do the other individually focused theories covered in Part Two.

Stage-based theories have a long tradition in behavioral research reaching back to Lewin's stage model (Lewin, 1935). Of the two stage theories we discussed, PAPM and TTM, only the former explicitly recognizes a distinct state in which one is unaware of a risk. In the TTM, people who are unaware generally would be classified as being in precontemplation. This puts those strongly opposed to the recommended behavior and those who simply have not heard of it in the same category. These groups are actually quite different (Greene and others, 1999). Although stage-based models are appealing, support for stage-matched interventions is equivocal.

Some theories are easier to use than others. Appropriable theories—those that can easily be adapted—are especially appealing to researchers and practitioners (Turkle, 1995). Part of the appeal of the HBM and TTM is undoubtedly that they are appropriable theories. PAPM and TPB are perhaps more challenging but worth the effort. Many people are attracted to the TTM because of its intuitive logic. We all know people who are precontemplators for a particular behavior, or we may have experienced the state of chronic contemplation with regard to a behavior we want to change but have not been able to achieve. The fact that one theory may appear to be harder to use and another a lot easier should not keep theory users from taking an informed second look.

Measurement of key variables in each of the theories requires careful attention. More attention is needed not only to the appropriate, consistent measurement (or manipulations) of independent and dependent variables in these models but also to understanding the mediators of behavior (Baron and Kenny, 1986; Sussman and Wills, 2000). Understanding mediators of behavior change is an important step in advancing theory and developing more effective interventions (Baranowski, Anderson, and Carmack, 1998; Sallis, 2001).

Following recommended measurement strategies can be resource-intensive. In practice, many who use the TPB probably do not do the extensive development work the authors recommend, and no literature of which we are aware demonstrates that questions developed through this process more powerfully predict behavior, although it certainly makes intuitive sense. Using the TTM as its developers intended can also be a daunting challenge. Many researchers and practitioners have used the decisional balance measures but not the processes of change. If theory users would make more of their questions openly available, theory testing would be enhanced, and it would facilitate using some of the less accessible theories.

Different theories in this part of the book have many similarities. Recognizing this fact, Fishbein (2000) recommended the use of an integrated model (see Chapter Four) that includes key variables from several of the theories in this section as well as Social Cognitive Theory. The Integrative Behavioral Model is appealing, because it incorporates intra-individual factors, including self-efficacy, as well as environmental factors known to influence health behaviors. More research is needed to determine the viability of this expanded model.

It is common for researchers and practitioners to combine or blend theories. Thoughtful combinations may result in more robust interventions. However, a potential downside is the practical limit to how many theories can be combined. If relevant constructs in the models are not measured or are not measured well, it may not be possible to really understand how an intervention exerted its impact. If our theories are to be refined, it is critical that some researchers continue to focus on rigorous tests of single theories and on studies that critically compare two or more theories.

Limitations

In the last several years, researchers and practitioners in health behavior and health education have paid increasing attention to the larger environment in which behavior occurs. Some groups have criticized the focus on individuals and their health-related beliefs as typified by the theories in Part Two (Smedley and Syme, 2000). For behaviors in which individual action is required, such as stopping smoking, individual-focused theories are usually appropriate, but even a very individual behavior such as getting mammograms can be strongly affected by policy or social context. Program developers should not ignore the array of higher-level influences that affect behavior. A recent review found that the combination of access-enhancing and individual-directed interventions were the most effective type of strategy for promoting mammography use (Legler and others, 2002). The recommendation also is supported by a systematic review of adult preventive behaviors that found benefits for educating individual patients but larger benefits for financial incentives and organizational change (Stone and others, 2002).

More attention in all the theories should be paid to maintenance of behavior change. The TTM and PAPM explicitly include maintenance of behavior changes, and the HBM and TPB do not exclude it. However, conceptualization and prediction of maintenance of behavior change may require refinement of constructs and measures or other theories altogether (Rothman, 2000). One study found that the TPB was useful in predicting attendance at health screenings, but the theory could not reliably differentiate people who delayed attending or initially attended and then relapsed

(Sheeran, Conner, and Norman, 2001). These apparent nuances are very important, not only in classifying and describing health behavior but also in developing new interventions.

New Directions

Health behavior theories that focus on individuals have remained remarkably similar for the past fifteen years (Chapter Two; Weinstein and Rothman, 2005). One issue is the paucity of studies comparing theories, and another is the relative absence of the developers of the main theories in these activities. Of nineteen studies comparing theories of health behavior, none involved the developers of the theories (Nigg and Jordan, 2005). The theories make specific, testable predictions about behavior, and, in time, some theories will be supported while others will not. We encourage researchers to design studies to test two or more theories.

Theories should be tested using stronger study designs. The broad health field is demanding higher-quality evidence to identify effective intervention techniques (Harris and others, 2001), and we should demand the same rigor of health behavior theory. Although many early studies using these theories were cross-sectional, and subsequently conducted longitudinal studies gave us better data, more experimental studies are needed to test these theories (Weinstein, 2007).

In many cases, intervention studies have used research designs that miss opportunities to identify "active ingredients." All four theories in this section can claim successful health behavior change interventions, indicating their potential value. However, factorial designs would more quickly advance our understanding of which components are most useful in predicting or changing behavior (Rimer and Glassman, 1999). These designs offer the option of testing an additional "free" research question, by nesting additional conditions within the existing ones.

Although the number of meta-analyses is increasing, allowing us to better assess what is known, meta-analyses provide definitive answers only when sufficient high-quality data exist. Meta-analyses of experiments provide very strong evidence of effectiveness. However, the results of meta-analyses that compare studies with different features cannot replace the results of true experiments that directly compare those features.

NEW CONSTRUCTS AND THEORIES

Many other theories of health behavior, in addition to those included in this section, emphasize the individual. Prospect Theory (Kahneman and Tversky, 1982) contributed to understanding message framing of the positive or negative consequences of a behavior. One prediction from Prospect Theory's tenets is that gain-framed messages should be more effective in increasing prevention (for example, sunscreen use) and recuperation behaviors (for example, medication use), whereas loss-framed messages should more effectively motivate detection (for example, HIV testing) (Rothman and Salovey, 1997). The benefits of gain-framing but not loss-framing are supported by recent meta-analyses (O'Keefe and Jensen, 2007).

The Common Sense Model of Self-Regulation was developed to address the health behaviors of medical patients (Leventhal, Meyer, and Nerenz, 1980). One unique characteristic of the theory is a substantive and nuanced description of the representation or beliefs about the disease, condition, or recommended action. These include the constructs of identity/symptoms, timeline, consequences, causes, and cure/control, which can be assessed using a standardized instrument (Moss-Morris and others, 2002). The model has been used in over twenty illness populations (Hagger and Orbell, 2003). However, because most evidence is from cross-sectional studies, data about the effectiveness of interventions based on the model constructs are insufficient.

Although emotions play a prominent role in several theories of health behavior, they deserve more attention than they receive in the four theories in this section of the book. For example, although TPB has called attitudes (the feeling that outcomes can be good or bad) a type of emotional response and locates other emotions as distant antecedents of attitudes, new findings call for a separate and more central role for affect (Fredrickson, 2003). Research suggests at least four ways that emotions affect decisions related to health, including focusing people's attention on a threat, helping people choose among several courses of action, facilitating decisions about dissimilar outcomes such as money and health, and prompting people to spring into action. Emotions can be negative (for example, fear, anticipated regret), but they can also be positive (for example, joy, hopefulness) (Frederickson, 2003; Salovey, Rothman, Detweiler, and Steward, 2000). Some constructs, such as worry, seem to mix emotion and cognition. Health behavior theories that place special emphasis on emotions include the Common Sense Model, Protection Motivation Theory (Prentice-Dunn and Rogers, 1986), the Extended Parallel Process Model, and theories of stress and coping (see Chapter Ten). Although specifics differ across models, they suggest that people cope with threats either by addressing the threat (see a doctor) or by addressing their emotional reactions to the threat (put it out of their minds).

Given the special role of fear communication in the history of health behavior interventions, it is surprising that none of the most commonly used theories can adequately explain key findings in this literature (Witte and Allen, 2000). Fear appeals in HIV-prevention interventions are more effective when they are of greater intensity (Albarracín and others, 2005). The hypothesis that fear appeals become less effective past a certain point is probably untrue. Fear communications generally are most effective when people are given clear guidance about how to take or plan action (Witte and Allen, 2000).

The models in Chapters Three through Six all emphasize rational decisions based on thoughts and feelings that people can report using interviews and surveys. Health behaviors are influenced by many other motivations and factors that may be unconscious or uncontrollable. Some theorists argue that most behavior is outside of conscious control and have impressive data to support their claims (Bargh and Chartrand, 1999; Gollwitzer, 1999). For example, recent work on goal states has shown that what people want depends on the situations they are in, or even whom they recently were thinking about (Shah, 2003). A similar issue is that much of our planning and intentional behavior requires that we have an accurate idea of what we will want in the future. Recent work on affective forecasting suggests that most people are not good at anticipating their future responses to health outcomes and other life changes (Wilson and Gilbert, 2005). Health behavior theories that take into account the effects of environmental and structural factors partially address some of these issues, but current theories that focus on the individual may need to be revised to consider processes that are outside of conscious awareness.

Disappointing outcomes for some health behavior interventions should drive us to consider, or reconsider, the use of persuasion strategies in combination with effective intervention (Cappella, 2006). Several well-tested theories of persuasion, including the Elaboration Likelihood Model (Petty and Cacioppo, 1986), Heuristic Systematic Model (Chaiken, Liberman, and Eagly, 1989), and the Unimodel (Kruglanski and Thompson, 1999), deserve more attention. These theories postulate that people process messages deliberately or through less effortful means (Rudd and Glanz, 1990).

SUMMARY

Some commentators have dismissed these theories, saying they do not take into account the complexity of factors that influence health behaviors. Focusing on individual acceptance of bed nets to prevent malaria use must account for the fact that many of the people we want to reach might want to use bed nets but might not be able to find places to buy them. We could spend months and years on bed net adoption and fail if we did not account for lack of availability. Theories that emphasize individual health behavior have an important role to play in our understanding of how to improve human health, but they are not the answer to all health problems. One must nearly always consider the social and community context to understand where beliefs come from and to find ways to change both beliefs and external constraints. We encourage students and health professionals to consider the nature of the health problem or condition on which they wish to intervene and select the appropriate theory, sometimes employing multiple theories to permit intervention at multiple levels.

REFERENCES

Abrams, D. B., Herzog, T. A., Emmons, K. M., and Linnan, L. "Stages of Change Versus Addiction: A Replication and Extension." *Nicotine Addiction Research,* 2000, *2,* 223–229.

Albarracín, D., and others. "A Test of Major Assumptions about Behavior Change: A Comprehensive Look at HIV Prevention Interventions since the Beginning of the Epidemic." *Psychological Bulletin,* 2005, *131,* 856–897.

Baranowski, T., Anderson, C., and Carmack, C. "Mediating Variable Framework in Physical Activity Interventions: How Are We Doing?" *American Journal of Preventive Medicine,* 1998, *15,* 266–297.

Bargh, J. A., and Chartrand, T. L. "The Unbearable Automaticity of Being." *American Psychologist,* 1999, *54,* 462–479.

Baron, R. M., and Kenny, D. A. "The Moderator-Mediator Variable Distinction in Social Psychological Research: Conceptual, Strategic, and Statistical Considerations." *Journal of Personality and Social Psychology,* 1986, *51,* 1173–1182.

Brewer, N. T., Weinstein, N. D., Cuite, C. L., and Herrington, J. E. "Risk Perceptions and Their Relation to Risk Behavior." *Annals of Behavioral Medicine,* 2004, *27*(2), 125–130.

Brewer, N. T., and others. "A Meta-Analysis of the Relationship between Risk Perception and Health Behavior: The Example of Vaccination." *Health Psychology,* 2007, *26,* 136–145.

Bridle, C., and others. "Systematic Review of the Effectiveness of Health Behavior Interventions Based on the Transtheoretical Model." *Psychology and Health,* 2005, *20,* 283–301.

Cappella, J. N. "Integrating Message Effects and Behavior Change Theories: Organizing Comments and Unanswered Questions." *Journal of Communication,* 2006, *56*(Suppl), S265–S279.

Chaiken, S., Liberman, A., and Eagly, A. H. "Heuristic and Systematic Processing Within and Beyond the Persuasion Context." In J. S. Uleman and J. A. Bargh (eds.), *Unintended Thought.* New York: Guilford, 1989.

Conner, M., and Sparks, P. "The Theory of Planned Behavior and Health Behaviors." In M. Conner and P. Norman (eds.), *Predicting Health Behavior.* Philadelphia: Open University Press, 2001.

de Vet, E., de Nooijer, J., de Vries, N. K., and Brug, J. "Comparing Stage of Change and Behavioral Intention to Understand Fruit Intake." *Health Education Research,* 2007, *22,* 599–608.

Fishbein, M. "The Role of Theory in HIV Prevention." *AIDS Care,* 2000, *12*(3), 273–278.

Fredrickson, B. L. "Cultivating Positive Emotions to Optimize Health and Well-Being." *Prevention and Treatment,* 2003, *3*(1). [http://content.apa.org/journals/pre/3/1/1].

Gibbons, F. X., Gerrard, M., Blanton, H., and Russell, D. W. "Reasoned Action and Social Reaction: Willingness and Intention as Independent Predictors of Health Risk." *Journal of Personality and Social Psychology,* 1998, *74,* 1164–1180.

Gollwitzer, P. M. "Implementation Intentions: Strong Effects of Simple Plans." *American Psychologist,* 1999, *54,* 493–503.

Greene, G. W., and others. "Dietary Applications of the Stages of Change Model." *Journal of the American Dietetic Association,* 1999, *99*(6), 673–678.

Green, L. W., and Kreuter, M. W. *Health Promotion Planning: An Educational and Ecological Approach.* (4th ed.) New York: McGraw-Hill, 2005.

Hagger, M., and Orbell, S. "A Meta-Analytic Review of the Common-Sense Model of Illness Representations." *Psychology and Health,* 2003, *18,* 141–184.

Hagger, M. S., Chatzisarantis, N.L.D., and Biddle, S.J.H. "A Meta-Analytic Review of the Theories of Reasoned Action and Planned Behavior in Physical Activity: Predictive Validity and the Contribution of Additional Variables." *Journal of Sport & Exercise Psychology,* 2002, *24,* 3–32.

Harris, R. P., and others, for the Methods Work Group, Third U.S. Preventive Services Task Force. "Current Methods of the U.S. Preventive Services Task Force: A Review of the Process." *American Journal of Preventive Medicine,* 2001, *20,* 21–35.

Hedeker, D., Mermelstein, R. J., and Weeks, K. "The Thresholds of Change Model: An Approach to Analyzing Stages of Change Data." *Annals of Behavioral Medicine,* 1999, *21,* 61–70.

Janz, N. K., and Becker, M. H. "The Health Belief Model: A Decade Later." *Health Education Quarterly,* 1984, *11,* 1–47.

Kahneman, D., and Tversky, A. "The Psychology of Preferences." *Scientific American,* 1982, *247,* 160–173.

Kruglanski, A. W., and Thompson, E. P. "Persuasion by a Single Route: A View from the Unimodel." *Psychological Inquiry,* 1999, *10,* 83–109.

Legler, J., and others. "The Effectiveness of Interventions to Promote Mammography Among Women with Historically Lower Rates of Screening." *Cancer, Epidemiology, Biomarkers, and Prevention,* 2002, *11*(1), 59–71.

Leventhal, H., Meyer, D., and Nerenz, D. R. "The Common Sense Representation of Illness Danger." In S. Rachman (ed.), *Contributions to Medical Psychology.* New York: Pergamon Press, 1980.

Lewin, K. *A Dynamic Theory of Personality.* New York: McGraw-Hill, 1935.

Liska, A. E. "A Critical Examination of the Causal Structure of the Fishbein/Ajzen Attitude-Behavior Model." *Social Psychology Quarterly,* 1984, *47,* 61–74.

Moss-Morris, R., and others. "The Revised Illness Perception Questionnaire (IPQ-R)." *Psychology and Health,* 2002, *17,* 1–16.

Mullen, P. D., Hersey, J. C., and Iverson, D. C. "Health Behavior Models Compared." *Social Science and Medicine,* 1987, *24,* 973–981.

Nigg, C. R., and Jordan, P. J. "Commentary: It's a Difference of Opinion That Makes a Horserace. . . ." *Health Education Research,* 2005, *20,* 291–293.

Noar, S. M. "Behavioral Interventions to Reduce HIV-Related Sexual Risk Behavior: Review and Synthesis of Meta-Analytic Evidence." *AIDS and Behavior,* forthcoming.

Noar, S. M., and Zimmerman, R. S. "Health Behavior Theory and Cumulative Knowledge Regarding Health Behaviors: Are We Moving in the Right Direction?" *Health Education Research,* 2005, *20,* 275–290.

O'Keefe, D. J., and Jensen, J. D. "The Relative Persuasiveness of Gain-Framed Loss-Framed Messages for Encouraging Disease Prevention Behaviors: A Meta-Analytic Review." *Journal of Health Communication,* 2007, *12,* 623–644.

Petty, R. E., and Cacioppo, J. T. "The Elaboration Likelihood Model of Persuasion." In L. Berkowitz (ed.), *Advances in Experimental Social Psychology.* Vol. 19. San Diego, Calif.: Academic Press, 1986.

Pignone, M. P., and others. "Counseling to Promote a Healthy Diet In Adults: A Summary of the Evidence for the U.S. Preventive Services Task Force." *American Journal of Preventive Medicine,* 2003, *24,* 75–92.

Prentice-Dunn, S., and Rogers, R. W. "Protection Motivation Theory and Preventive Health: Beyond the Health Belief Model." *Health Education Research,* 1986, *1,* 153–161.

Quinlan, K. B., and McCaul, K. D. "Matched and Mismatched Interventions With Young Adult Smokers: Testing a Stage Theory." *Health Psychology,* 2000, *19,* 165–171.

Riemsma, R. P., and others. "Systematic Review of the Effectiveness of Stage Based Interventions to Promote Smoking Cessation." *BMJ,* 2003, *326,* 1175–1177.

Rimer, B. K., and Glassman, B. "Is There a Use for Tailored Print Communications in Cancer Risk Communication?" *Monographs of the National Cancer Institute,* 1999, *25,* 140–148.

Rosenstock, I. "Historical Origins of the Health Belief Model." *Health Education Monographs,* 1974, *2,* 328–335.

Rosenstock, I. M., Strecher, V. J., and Becker, M. H. "Social Learning Theory and the Health Belief Model." *Health Education Quarterly,* 1988, *15,* 175–183.

Rothman, A. J. "Toward a Theory-Based Analysis of Behavioral Maintenance." *Health Psychology,* 2000, *19,* 64–69.

Rothman, A. J., and Salovey, P. "Shaping Perceptions to Motivate Healthy Behavior: The Role of Message Framing." *Psychology Bulletin,* 1997, *121,* 3–19.

Rudd, J., and Glanz, K. "How Individuals Use Information for Health Action: Consumer Information Processing." In K. Glanz, F. M. Lewis, and B. K. Rimer (eds.), *Health Behavior and Health Education: Theory, Research, and Practice.* San Francisco, Jossey-Bass, 1990.

Sallis, J. F. "Progress in Behavioral Research on Physical Activity." *Annals of Behavioral Medicine,* 2001, *23,* 77–78.

Salovey, P., Rothman, A. J., Detweiler, J. B., and Steward, W. T. "Emotional States and Physical Health." *American Psychologist,* 2000, *55,* 110–121.

Shah, J. Y. "Automatic for the People: How Representations of Significant Others Implicitly Affect Goal Pursuit." *Journal of Personality and Social Psychology,* 2003, *84,* 661–681.

Sheeran, P., Conner, M., and Norman, P. "Can the Theory of Planned Behavior Explain Patterns of Health Behavior Change?" *Health Psychology,* 2001, *20,* 12–19.

Sheeran, P., Trafimow, D., Finlay, K. A., and Norman, P. "Evidence That the Type of Person Affects the Strength of the Perceived Behavioural Control-Intention Relationship." *British Journal of Social Psychology,* 2002, *41*(Pt 2), 253–270.

Smedley, B. D., and Syme, S. L. (eds.) *Promoting Health: Intervention Strategies from Social and Behavioral Sciences.* Washington, D.C.: National Academy Press, 2000.

Stoddard, A. M., and others. "Underusers of Mammogram Screening: Stage of Adoption in Five Subpopulations." *Preventive Medicine* 1998, *27,* 478–487.

Stone, E. G., and others. "Interventions That Increase Use of Adult Immunization and Cancer Screening Services: A Meta-Analysis." *Annals of Internal Medicine,* 2002, *136,* 641–651.

Strecher, V. J., and Rosenstock, I. M. "The Health Belief Model." In K. Glanz, F. M. Lewis, and B. K. Rimer (eds.), *Health Behavior and Health Education: Theory, Research, and Practice.* (2nd ed.) San Francisco: Jossey-Bass, 1996.

Sussman, S., and Wills, T. A. "Rationale for Program Development Needs." In S. Sussman and T. A. Wills (eds.), *Handbook of Program Development for Health Behavior Research and Practice.* Thousand Oaks, Calif.: Sage, 2000.

Sutton, S. "Back to the Drawing Board? A Review of Applications of the Transtheoretical Model to Substance Use." *Addiction,* 2001, *96,* 175–186.

Turkle, S. *Life on the Screen.* New York: Simon & Schuster, 1995.

van Sluijs, E., van Poppel, M., and van Mechelen, W. "Stage-Based Lifestyle Interventions in Primary Care: Are They Effective?" *American Journal of Preventive Medicine,* 2004, *26,* 330–343.

Webb, T. L., and Sheeran, P. "Does Changing Behavioral Intentions Engender Behavior Change? A Meta-Analysis of the Experimental Evidence." *Psychological Bulletin,* 2006, *132,* 249–268.

Weinstein, N. D. "Testing Four Competing Theories of Health-Protective Behavior." *Health Psychology,* 1993, *12,* 324–333.

Weinstein, N. D. "Misleading Tests of Health Behavior Theories." *Annals of Behavioral Medicine,* 2007, *33,* 1–10.

Weinstein, N. D., and Rothman, A. J. "Revitalizing Research on Health Behavior Theories." *Health Education Research,* 2005, *20*(3), 294–297.

Weinstein, N. D., Rothman, A. J., and Sutton, S. R. "Stage Theories of Health Behavior: Conceptual and Methodological Issues." *Health Psychology,* 1998, *17,* 290–299.

West, R. "Time for a Change: Putting the Transtheoretical (Stages of Change) Model to Rest." *Addiction,* 2005, *100,* 1036–1039.

Wilson, T. D., and Gilbert, D. T. "Affective Forecasting: Knowing What to Want." *Current Directions in Psychological Science,* 2005, *14,* 131–134.

Witte, K., and Allen, M. "A Meta-Analysis of Fear Appeals: Implications for Effective Public Health Campaigns." *Health Education and Behavior,* 2000, *27,* 591–615.

PART

3

MODELS OF INTERPERSONAL HEALTH BEHAVIOR

K. Viswanath

Human behaviors are a product of multiple influences. One significant source of influence is the web of interactions people have with others within their social circles. This "web of influence" of members of social circles on health behaviors is the focus of the chapters in Part Three, which covers one major theory and three models to explain how interpersonal interactions may influence individual cognitions, beliefs, and behaviors. Models are valuable, as no single theory may be able to provide a complete explanation for all health behaviors in all contexts.

Chapter Eight reviews the Social Cognitive Theory (SCT), which addresses the tension between two deterministic frameworks that have characterized the explanations of human behaviors: individuals versus the environment. SCT overcomes this dilemma by arguing that both individuals and their environments interact and influence each other—reciprocal determinism—resulting in individual and social change. One of the many virtues of SCT is that it offers a number of constructs that have been used extensively in health education and other theories and models. These include modeling or observational learning and self-efficacy, among others. As the chapter points out, it is often the case that selected constructs from SCT have been applied widely, rather than the complete theory.

Chapter Nine describes conceptualizations of how social networks and social support influence health behavior—a subject of considerable interest to both researchers and practitioners of health education. Recent attention garnered by the idea of social capital has only heightened the interest in social networks. Chapter Nine reviews the different pathways through which social networks influence health and well-being: providing intimacy and companionship, resources to cope with illness, new information, and mobilization of resources to buffer oneself from stress. Social networks may play both a positive and negative role in health—a point worth remembering when considering their role in health behaviors.

In a related vein, Chapter Ten covers work on stress and coping in health behavior. The authors note that stress may contribute negatively to health behavior but in some cases may also provide meaning and purpose to individuals who use positive coping strategies. Chapter Ten reviews the Transactional Model of Stress and Coping and draws interesting parallels between constructs in this model and similar constructs used in other theories.

Interpersonal communication, it is widely agreed, is an important source of influence in health behavior change and maintenance. Chapter Eleven focuses on communication between patients and providers but is a departure from conventional discussion on clinician-patient communications. Instead of reviewing myriad theories of patient-provider communication, Chapter Eleven offers a model of "patient-centered communication," focusing on the key functions of communication that influence health outcomes. The model discussed in Chapter Eleven reviews several pathways that link communication between clinicians and patients to health outcomes—a useful approach that organizes the vast body of work in this area.

Chapter Twelve reviews the work in Part Three, identifying major commonalties and differences among the chapters and discussing the implications for future research and application of interpersonal influences to health behaviors.

CHAPTER

8

HOW INDIVIDUALS, ENVIRONMENTS, AND HEALTH BEHAVIORS INTERACT

Social Cognitive Theory

Alfred L. McAlister

Cheryl L. Perry

Guy S. Parcel

KEY POINTS

This chapter will

■ Define and describe important concepts and principles from Social Cognitive Theory (SCT).

The authors are grateful to Professor Albert Bandura for critical and detailed comments on the first draft, Katherine Sterba for insightful editorial help, Brenda Spence for indispensable technical assistance, and the editors of this volume for their contributions to the final draft. Preparation of this chapter was partly supported by the Michael & Susan Dell Center for Advancement of Healthy Living.

- Describe the fundamental emphasis of SCT on the interaction between individuals and their environments and human capacities for learning and adaptation.
- Demonstrate how this theory has been effectively applied for personal and social change to prevent and manage chronic and infectious diseases, and provide useful insight into other problems such as violence and disaster preparedness.
- Illustrate the measurement and application of key SCT concepts and principles in case studies on smoking cessation and condom use promotion.

Building on previous theorization and research by Miller and Dollard (1941) and Rotter (1954), Social Cognitive Theory (SCT) was first known as *social learning theory,* as it was based on the operation of established principles of learning within the human social context (Bandura, 1977). It was renamed Social Cognitive Theory when concepts from cognitive psychology were integrated to accommodate the growing understanding of human information processing capacities and biases that influence learning from experience, observation, and symbolic communication (Bandura, 1986). With further development, SCT has embraced concepts from sociology and political science to advance the understanding of functioning and adaptive capacities of groups and societies (Bandura, 1997). The theory also has integrated and developed concepts from humanistic psychology by analyzing the processes that underlie self-determination, altruism, and moral behavior (Bandura, 1999).

SCT emphasizes *reciprocal determinism* in the interaction between people and their environments. Most behavioral and social theories focus on individual, social, and environmental factors that determine individual or group behavior (for example, barriers, rewards and punishments, and social norms portrayed in mass communication). SCT posits that human behavior is the product of the dynamic interplay of personal, behavioral, and environmental influences. Although it recognizes how environments shape behavior, this theory focuses on people's potential abilities to alter and construct environments to suit purposes they devise for themselves. In addition to a person's individual capacity to interact with their environment, SCT emphasizes the human capacity for collective action. This enables individuals to work together in organizations and social systems to achieve environmental changes that benefit the entire group. According to Bandura (1997), planned protection and promotion of public health can be viewed as illustrations of this kind of reciprocal determinism, as societies seek to control the environmental and social factors that influence health behaviors and health outcomes.

SCT is applied and discussed in the prodigious body of research and commentary from Albert Bandura of Stanford University. Many classic and recent publications are available at www.des.emory.edu/mfp/Bandura.

CONCEPTS OF SCT

Table 8.1 defines and illustrates the key concepts of SCT. These can be grouped into five categories: (1) psychological determinants of behavior, (2) observational learning, (3) environmental determinants of behavior, (4) self-regulation, and (5) moral disengagement.

TABLE 8.1. **Social Cognitive Theory Concepts.**

Concept	Definition	Illustration
Reciprocal determinism	Environmental factors influence individuals and groups, but individuals and groups can also influence their environments and regulate their own behavior	Planned protection and promotion of public health by changing environmental factors that influence health and behavior
Outcome expectations	Beliefs about the likelihood and value of the consequences of behavioral choices	Changing expectations about the pleasure associated with condoms (McAlister and others, 2000)
Self-efficacy	Beliefs about personal ability to perform behaviors that bring desired outcomes	Improving women's beliefs about their ability to convince partners to use condoms (McAlister and others, 2000)
Collective efficacy	Beliefs about the ability of a group to perform concerted actions that bring desired outcomes	Organization of parents' groups to organize safe parties and advocate other environmental changes to reduce underage alcohol use (Perry and others, 2002)
Observational learning	Learning to perform new behaviors by exposure to interpersonal or media displays of them, particularly through peer modeling	Behavioral journalism promoting condom use (McAlister, Johnson, and others, 2000) and entertainment-education featuring women empowered with literacy skills (Singhal and Rogers, 1999)
Incentive motivation	The use and misuse of rewards and punishments to modify behavior	Laws prosecuting teen smokers may have unwanted effects (Loukas and others, 2006), but taxes can deter the onset of tobacco use (Hopkins and others, 2001).
Facilitation	Providing tools, resources, or environmental changes that make new behaviors easier to perform	Distribution of condoms at no cost (McAlister and others, 2000) and business assistance to help women escape prostitution (Sherman and others, 2006)
Self-regulation	Controlling oneself through self-monitoring, goal-setting, feedback, self reward, self- instruction, and enlistment of social support	Computerized self-management training for asthma patients (Lorig and others, 2001) and telephone counseling for smoking cessation (Rabius and others, 2004)
Moral disengagement	Ways of thinking about harmful behaviors and the people who are harmed that make infliction of suffering acceptable by disengaging self-regulatory moral standards	Dehumanization and diffusion of responsibility influence aggression and corporate transgressions that harm public health (Bandura and others, 1996, 2000)

Psychological Determinants of Behavior in SCT

A number of individual-level psychological determinants have been identified in SCT. One main determinant is *outcome expectations,* defined as "beliefs about the likelihood of various outcomes that might result from the behaviors that a person might choose to perform, and the perceived value of those outcomes." The basic idea— people act to maximize benefits and minimize costs—is fundamental to both animal and human learning theory. SCT builds on this idea by showing that human values and expectations are subjective, that is, people's actions are not based solely on objective reality but on their perceptions of it. SCT also places great importance on how the capacity for foresight makes it possible for people to visualize and work toward distant goals while discounting immediate costs and ignoring the short-term benefits of alternative actions.

SCT and several other health behavior models and theories give special consideration to *social outcome expectations.* These correspond to the concept of social norms in the Theory of Reasoned Action (TRA) and Theory of Planned Behavior (TPB; see Chapter Four), which are defined as expectations about how different people will evaluate our behavior and our willingness to be guided by their evaluation. The concept of *self-evaluative outcome expectation* is important to SCT. It functions like a social outcome, but individuals produce it for themselves. Thus, behavior can be governed partly by people's anticipation of how they will feel about themselves if they do or do not perform a certain behavior. According to SCT, expectations about self-evaluative outcomes can be more powerful than expectations about social and material outcomes for some individuals. The postulation of this category of outcome expectation helps to explain how individuals can resist physical gratifications and social pressures or make unrecognized sacrifices to meet their own standards of approvable conduct.

Self-efficacy belief (Bandura, 1997) is the concept for which SCT is most widely known and which has been integrated into other models and theories (see, for example, Chapter Three). It consists of a person's beliefs about her capacity to influence the quality of functioning and the events that affect her life. Numerous studies have shown that the performance of many behaviors is determined both by outcome expectations and self-efficacy beliefs, with the latter becoming more important for behaviors of progressive complexity or difficulty (Bandura, 1997). Several review papers have presented and discussed methods for measuring self-efficacy in health behavior research (Maibach and Murphy, 1995; Moritz, Feltz, Fahrbach, and Mack, 2000; Contento, Randell, and Basch, 2002). Because many of the things that people seek are achievable only by working together with others, Bandura has extended the concept of perceived efficacy to *collective efficacy,* demonstrating its effects on how people work in organizations and on their political participation (Bandura, 1997; Fernández-Ballesteros and others, 2002).

Observational Learning

The exceptional human capacity for *observational learning,* especially via mass communications, is central to SCT. According to Bandura, four processes govern observational learning (Bandura, 1986, 2002): (1) attention, (2) retention, (3) production, and (4) motivation. Different factors play a role in different processes. For example, access to family, peer, and media models determines what behaviors a person is able to observe, while the perceived functional value of the outcomes expected from the modeled behavior determines what they choose to attend to closely. Cognitive retention of an observed behavior depends on intellectual capacities such as reading ability. Production, that is, the performance of the modeled behavior, depends on physical and communication skills and on self-efficacy for performing, or learning to perform, the observed behavior. Motivation is determined by outcome expectations about the costs and benefits of the observed behavior.

Many studies have shown that models are imitated most frequently when observers perceive the models as similar to themselves, making peer modeling a well-recognized method for influencing behavior (Schunk, 1987). Children are more likely to imitate other children who are their same age or older (Brody and Stoneman, 1981). To help people gain self-efficacy for complex or difficult new behaviors, SCT stresses the usefulness of "coping" models, which confront and successfully struggle with the same challenges and barriers to change that the observers face. Bandura (2006) illustrates this with comments from young women in India who report that they were influenced by a radio serial drama titled *Taru,* in which a mother enrolls her daughters in school despite strong discouragement and many challenges: "When Taru can fight harsh circumstances, why can't we? Before Taru there was darkness, now there is light." This form of peer modeling has been often used in *entertainment education* for social change programs in the United States and internationally (Singhal and Rogers, 1999; Wilkin and others, 2007). Peer modeling, with real stories about community members achieving behavioral change—*behavioral journalism* (McAlister, 1995; McAlister and Fernández, 2002)—is illustrated later in this chapter. For promoting observational learning of health behaviors, storytelling in the form of a narrative may be more effective than the presentation of directly didactic or persuasive messages (Hinyard and Kreuter, 2007).

Environmental Determinants of Behavior

Like ecological models (see Chapter Twenty), SCT includes concepts to describe the powerful influences of environment on behavior. SCT has a reciprocally deterministic viewpoint and hypothesizes that no amount of observational learning will lead to behavior change unless the observers' environments support the new behaviors (Bandura, 2002). One basic form of environmental change to modify behavior is *incentive motivation,* through the provision of rewards or punishments for desired or undesired behaviors. Bandura (1969, 1986) has written extensively on the mechanisms through which public policies do or do not influence behavior, emphasizing the unintended effects that arise with the use of punishment. These unintended effects are illustrated in the enforcement of punitive laws forbidding minors' possession of tobacco in Texas, which appear to be intermittently and selectively enforced with a bias against minority youth (Gottlieb and others, 2004). They are seen as unfair and counterproductive by apprehended violators and their parents (Loukas, Spaulding, and Gottlieb, 2006).

Increasing the prices of smoking through taxation of tobacco products is a less punitive form of incentive motivation; it has been found to be an effective policy to deter teen smoking (Hopkins and others, 2001). It provides the certain and immediate reward of more money to spend on other things for young people who choose not to purchase tobacco. Alternatively, providing financial incentives for participating in smoking cessation and for validated quitting recently has been found to significantly improve quit rates among smokers at a medical center (Volpp and others, 2006).

A second basic approach to influencing behavior through environmental change is *facilitation,* which is the provision of new structures or resources that enable behaviors or make them easier to perform (Bandura, 1998). Motivation seeks to manipulate behavior through external control, whereas facilitation is empowering. SCT joins a number of other theories and models of health behavior in stressing the importance of recognizing barriers to health-promoting behavior change and identifying ways in which those barriers can be removed or overcome. There are many examples of how behavior can be influenced by facilitation, as described in other chapters in this book. A case study later in this chapter describes how education about condom use for HIV protection was combined with the distribution of free condoms, which made them more readily available to those who were at the greatest risk of sexually transmitted disease. Illustrating another form of empowering facilitation that alters behavior, Sherman and colleagues (2006) found that the provision of tools, resources, and training in jewelry making and marketing can enhance the impact of an HIV-risk-reduction program for sex workers by diverting them into a less risky enterprise.

Self-Regulation

SCT emphasizes the human capacity to endure short-term negative outcomes in anticipation of important long-term positive outcomes, that is, to discount the immediate costs of behaviors that lead to a more distant goal. This is achieved through *self-regulation* (Karoly, 1993). According to SCT, self-control does not depend on a person's "will power" but instead on his acquisition of concrete skills for managing himself. The basic idea is that we can influence our own behavior in many of the same ways we would influence another person, that is, through rewards and facilitating environmental changes that we plan and organize for ourselves. Bandura (1997) identifies six ways in which self-regulation is achieved: (1) *self-monitoring* is a person's systematic observation of her own behavior; (2) *goal-setting* is the identification of incremental and long-term changes that can be obtained; (3) *feedback* is information about the quality of performance and how it might be improved; (4) *self-reward* is a person's provision of tangible or intangible rewards for himself; (5) *self-instruction* occurs when people talk to themselves before and during the performance of a complex behavior, and (6) *enlistment of social support* is achieved when a person finds people who encourage her efforts to exert self-control. Instruction in self-regulation techniques is a widely used application of SCT, as described later in this chapter. Further, these strategies are both similar to and overlapping with approaches to change behavior by increasing self-efficacy (see later section and Table 8.2).

Moral Disengagement

SCT describes how people can learn moral standards for self-regulation, which can lead them to avoid violence and cruelty to others. They can violate those standards through what Bandura (1999) labels as mechanisms of *moral disengagement.* These include *euphemistic labeling,* which sanitizes violent acts by using words that make them less offensive; *dehumanization and attribution of blame* to victims by perceiving them as racially or ethnically different and at fault for the punishment they will receive; the *diffusion and displacement of responsibility* by attributing decisions to a group or to authority figures, and *perceived moral justification* for harmful actions by construing them as beneficial and necessary. Quantitative studies of adolescent aggression have explicitly demonstrated how these mechanisms operate and how they determine the likelihood that a young person will commit violent acts (Bandura, Barbaranelli, Caprara, and Pastorelli, 1996; Pelton, Gound, Forehand, and Brody, 2004). Qualitative analyses of statements by participants support the role of these mechanisms in understanding many historical cases of large-scale killings of innocent people (Bandura, 1999). In a study that examined how perceptions of moral justification can influence behavior, McAlister (2006) found that international and regional differences in homicide rates are strongly related to differences in beliefs about the right to kill for protection and revenge.

War has profound implications for public health, and factors that influence support for war may be understood through the use of these concepts from SCT. Structural modeling analyses of a national survey in the United States in 2001 found that increases in public support for the use of military force against Iraq after 9/11 was linked to an increase in measured levels of moral disengagement, that is, an increased proportion of respondents endorsed dehumanizing statements about foreign enemies and believed that pre-emptive use of military force was justified (McAlister, Bandura, and Owen, 2006). In another area of importance to public health, the concepts of moral disengagement have also been employed in qualitative analyses of corporate transgressions that endanger consumers or the public (Bandura, 1999). Tobacco merchandising was made to seem acceptable to those who promote and market tobacco products through displacement and diffusion of responsibility and by justifications based on beliefs about personal freedoms (Bandura, Caprara, and Zsolnai, 2000).

APPLICATIONS TO HEALTH PROMOTION

SCT provides a comprehensive and well-supported conceptual framework for understanding the factors that influence human behavior and the processes through which learning occurs, offering insight into a wide variety of health-related issues. But its greater significance has come from the application of SCT to the design of interventions to meet important practical challenges in medicine and public health (for example, Clark and Zimmerman, 1990; Kok and others, 1996; Elder, Ayala, and Harris, 1999). Some of these applications are described in the next section, with details in two illustrative case studies that follow.

Changing Behavior by Increasing Self-Efficacy

The development of the earliest applications of SCT was preceded by a rejection of the prevailing theories and concepts being applied to psychotherapy, particularly the idea that individual differences in behavior resulted from personality "traits" (Bandura, 2004b). Although it was controversial when introduced, the conceptualization of psychotherapy as a learning process rapidly gained support. Bandura's first comprehensive textbook—*Principles of Behavior Modification*—provided a detailed analysis of a large body of evidence showing that human behavior could be modified and personally regulated, based on knowledge derived from empirical studies of how humans learn from and adapt to their environment (Bandura, 1969). Behavior is a product of an individual's learning history, present perceptions of the environment, and intellectual and physical capacities. Thus, behavior can be changed through new learning experiences, guidance in the adjustment of perceptions, and support for the development of capacities.

In the 1960s, many researchers began to apply behavioral and social learning concepts to the development of more effective cognitive and cognitive-behavioral therapies to help people change or manage unwanted behaviors (for example, Beck, 1995; Meichenbaum, 1977). In Bandura's (1998, 2004a) approach to inducing self-regulatory personal change, challenging behaviors are reduced to a series of small and easily mastered steps, with the therapist providing tools and resources to help the client accomplish them. A central principle in his model of behavior therapy is that the therapist's guidance is necessary at first but that it can be gradually replaced by self-direction as clients learn to master each step in their progress toward the desired behavior. This proved to be highly effective in controlled studies of people with severe snake phobia, as approximately three in four were able to learn to control their fears well enough to handle a snake in a relatively short time (Bandura, Jeffery, and Wright, 1974). Further research showed that increasing self-efficacy was a common mechanism through which different types of treatment achieved changes in behavior (Bandura and Adams, 1977).

SCT identifies four major ways in which self-efficacy can be developed (Bandura, 2004a), as described in Table 8.2: (1) mastery experience, (2) social modeling, (3) improving physical and emotional states, and (4) verbal persuasion.

In a number of recently published examples, interventions have targeted changes in self-efficacy, often along with other cognitive mediating variables. Several such studies have focused on increasing health-promoting physical activity. One study of community-dwelling healthy older adults showed that increases in self-efficacy for exercise were associated with adherence to an exercise intervention at seven- to twelve-month follow-up assessments (Brassington and others, 2002). In another study, self-efficacy improved for completers of an exercise prescription scheme while it deteriorated for dropouts (Jones, Harris, Waller, and Coggins, 2005).

Community-Level Prevention of Chronic Disease and Alcohol Abuse

SCT influenced the development of pioneering community-level projects to prevent heart disease in California (Farquhar and others, 1990) and a well-known, long-term project in Finland to reduce cardiovascular and other chronic disease (Puska,

TABLE 8.2. **Methods for Increasing Self-Efficacy.**

Mastery experience	Enabling the person to succeed in attainable but increasingly challenging performances of desired behaviors. The experience of performance mastery is the strongest influence on self-efficacy belief.
Social modeling	Showing the person that others like themselves can do it. This should include detailed demonstrations of the small steps taken in the attainment of a complex objective.
Improving physical and emotional states	Making sure people are well-rested and relaxed before attempting a new behavior. This can include efforts to reduce stress and depression while building positive emotions—as when "fear" is re-labeled as "excitement."
Verbal persuasion	Telling the person that he or she can do it. Strong encouragement can boost confidence enough to induce the first efforts toward behavior change.

Source: Adapted from Bandura (1997).

2002). The "North Karelia Project" conducted mass media campaigns featuring peer modeling in a "reality television" format: people in North Karelia were followed in news and public affairs programming as they learned to quit smoking, lose or maintain weight, and control hypertension (Puska and others, 1987). Interpersonal communication networks were organized to provide direct modeling and social reinforcement for new behaviors and advocacy of environmental changes such as smoke-free environments and higher cigarette taxes (McAlister and others, 1982). The project also organized important facilitative changes, such as aggressive outreach for hypertension detection and control and loans for farmers converting from dairy to berry production (Kuusipalo, Mikkola, Moisio, and Puska, 1985). Over twenty-five years, these activities led to changes in behavior that translated into a 70 percent reduction in cardiovascular disease, 65 percent reduction in lung cancer, and a six- to seven-year longer life expectancy for women and men, respectively (Puska, 2002).

Long-term effects on chronic disease risk factors were found as a result of some components of the Minnesota Heart Health Program, aimed at youth. Interventions that used peer modeling and facilitative environmental change were carried out for four years at the school and community levels. Two years after the conclusion of the intervention, 12th-grade students in the intervention areas in Minnesota and North Dakota were significantly less likely to smoke and more likely to eat heart-healthy foods and engage in physical activity than students in the control area (Perry, Kelder, and Klepp, 1994). Applications of SCT in peer modeling and building community networks for peer reinforcement, combined with improvements in access to services, have been used to promote cancer screening among Spanish-speaking women (Ramirez and others,

1999). To reduce disparities in the burden of tobacco use, tobacco settlement funds were used to support a regional campaign in Southeast Texas that was explicitly based on SCT. Peer modeling in mass media was designed to modify specific outcome expectations about the stress-reducing effects of tobacco use and its social desirability. School-based programs increased adolescents' self-efficacy for coping with pressures to smoke and provided access to an interactive Web-based program (Shegog and others, 2005). Environmental and policy changes, such as decreased youth access to tobacco products, were implemented concurrently (Meshack and others, 2004). A four-year follow-up found a sharp decrease in cigarette smoking in the Southeast Texas pilot project region where the campaign was conducted (McAlister, Huang, and Ramirez, 2006).

SCT has also been applied in community-level programs to prevent drunk driving and other harms related to alcohol use (for example, Worden and others, 1989; Bandura, 1969). Concepts from the theory were applied to the reduction of underage alcohol abuse in Project Northland—a community-level randomized trial involving twenty-eight communities and twenty-four school districts in Minnesota (Perry and others, 2000). In this project, a major emphasis was placed on creating barriers to drinking for teens and on reducing access to alcohol. Local community teams were organized, using direct action community organizing methods, to assess their communities and then take collective action to reduce access, based on a menu of evidence-based options. These included training of staff in bars and liquor stores and creating safe houses for social events where no alcohol was available (Perry and others, 2000). At the end of the 12th grade, environmental changes to reduce retail access to alcohol were assessed by having young-looking twenty-one-year-old females attempt to purchase beer in all the off-sale outlets in the twenty-eight communities. There was a significant reduction in successful "buys" in the intervention versus control communities. The trajectory of alcohol use and binge drinking also was significantly lower among youth in the intervention communities (Perry and others, 2002), suggesting the long-term impact of this approach.

CASE STUDIES

American Cancer Society Telephone Counseling for Smoking Cessation

Beginning in Texas in June 2000, the American Cancer Society (ACS) offered a telephone counseling service to help smokers quit by providing guidance in self-regulation. The service was subsequently expanded to other states and organizations. More than 250,000 smokers have received assistance. The program is delivered by paraprofessional counselors who receive approximately 140 hours of training and are guided by computer screens that include scripts based on decision trees in the counseling protocol. The decision trees include elements addressing the six self-regulatory processes in SCT: self-monitoring, goal setting, feedback, self-reward, self-instruction, and enlistment of social support (McAlister and others, 2004).

Self-Monitoring. Effective self-monitoring—the systematic observation of one's own behavior—includes observing and recording both the behavior itself and the context and cues or events accompanying the behavior. For a smoker trying to quit, preliminary self-monitoring in advance of quitting can identify the most important cues for smoking. In the ACS's telephone counseling service, this was done by having clients keep simple records of their smoking and the context and cues that were present when they smoked, before making a quit attempt. This enabled clients to identify and begin to develop coping skills that would be needed when they quit, as when a smoker begins to learn anxiety management skills as a result of identifying a link between anxiety and intense cravings for tobacco.

Goal Setting. This is planned behavior in which intentions are formulated in terms of both long-term (distal) and short-term (proximal) goals that will bring people closer to the changes they desire. Gradual steps are needed to achieve the successes that build self-efficacy. In the telephone counseling program, the initial objective for a smoker trying to quit is a single day of not smoking. When that is achieved, a new goal of three days of abstinence is set, with increasing intervals between succeeding sessions, depending on the client's progress.

Feedback. Feedback consists of information about the quantity and quality of the behavior being learned, as provided by others and gleaned from the person's own observations. Informative feedback enables smokers who are struggling with the challenges of cessation to adjust their strategies and efforts and to identify problems that need to be solved. In the telephone counseling program, this occurred when a smoker trying to quit learned that relapses are caused by stress and learned to use relaxation techniques in anticipation of future stressors. To maintain self-efficacy, feedback on an unsuccessful performance should be corrective and framed in a positive way. Thus, a quitter who relapses during the counseling experience is told she made a "good try" and encouraged to learn and benefit from the experience in her next effort to quit.

Self-Reward. At the earliest steps in the self-management process, short-term and frequent rewards that people give themselves may be more effective than rewards that may occur in the distant future. In the ACS counseling program, clients are encouraged to set aside part of their savings from not buying cigarettes for weekly pleasures, while saving the rest for a more expensive gratification in a month or more. The most immediate form of self-reward is the feeling of satisfaction from making progress, and telephone counseling clients are encouraged to actively congratulate themselves for every step they take.

Self-Instruction. When people "talk to themselves" in much the same way an instructor might guide them through a new experience, self-instruction occurs. Effective self-instruction involves speaking to oneself about each subtask in a complex series of tasks. In the ACS counseling program, clients are guided through multiple rehearsals of a combination of deep breathing and self-instruction to help them cope with stress and reduce cravings for tobacco. Self-instructions are also formulated and rehearsed for other situations that might cause relapse, such as social occasions where cigarettes or alcohol are offered.

Enlistment of Social Support. Social support has multiple functions that support the behavior change process. These include verbal persuasion to increase self-efficacy, provision of feedback, and direct cues to action. In the ACS counseling protocol, clients are asked to explicitly identify sources of support and to use them during the counseling process. The counselors are also important sources of short-term social support, and their training focuses on ways to increase clients' self-efficacy, particularly through provision of positive feedback for each small step toward quitting smoking.

Effectiveness and Cost-Effectiveness. In a randomized clinical trial, the ACS telephone counseling service was shown to approximately double a smoker's odds of quitting for one year when those who received telephone counseling were compared to those who received self-help booklets in the mail (McAlister and others, 2004). Counseling was provided at a cost of approximately $100 per client and $1,000 for each successful case of cessation attributable to the service. The service was particularly effective among young adults ages eighteen to twenty-five, presumably due to their shorter duration of smoking and lower levels of addiction (Rabius and others, 2004).

The AIDS Community Demonstration Projects

The AIDS Community Demonstration Projects were funded by the U.S. Centers for Disease Control and Prevention (CDC) to help local health departments in five cities increase condom use among diverse groups believed to be at risk of HIV infection. The target groups included residents of census tracts with high rates of sexually transmitted diseases in Dallas, out-of-treatment injection drug users in Denver and Long Beach, sexual partners of injection drug users in New York City and Long Beach, men who have sex with men but do not disclose that behavior or identify themselves as gay in Seattle, and people who trade sex for money in Long Beach and Seattle. In developing these projects, CDC leaders enlisted scientific guidance in the use of SCT—explicitly seeking to follow the model provided by the North Karelia Project in Finland (Centers for Disease Control and Prevention, 1999; McAlister, Johnson, and others, 2000).

The first phase involved extensive exploratory assessments to determine how to reach the various study groups. Next, qualitative data were gathered in discussions of why and how people use condoms. Based on the findings from this research, quantitative measures were developed to evaluate the programs. Data were collected before and during the implementation of community activities in standardized, twenty-minute street interviews of randomly selected members of the identified research populations. Financial incentives were offered to people who answered anonymous questions about sexual behaviors and condom use. More than 7,000 interviews were completed in nine waves of surveying, conducted every three to six months over a three-year period. Parallel surveys were conducted in experimental and comparison communities for a quasi-experimental evaluation of the projects' effects. The interviews assessed outcome expectations, self-efficacy beliefs (described next), exposure to messages from the project and other sources, the frequency and duration of condom use with main and non-main partners, and whether respondents were carrying a condom when they were interviewed.

Measurement of Outcome Expectations and Self-Efficacy Beliefs. Outcome expectations were measured with the classic semantic differential method (Osgood, 1967) for rating attitudes. Respondents were asked whether condom use was good or bad, wise or foolish, and pleasant or unpleasant. Then they were asked to rate that belief by indicating, for example, whether condom use was extremely unpleasant, very unpleasant, or somewhat unpleasant. Based on their answers, the respondents were given numerical scores for their beliefs, ranging from –3 (extremely unpleasant) to +3 (extremely pleasant). These beliefs about pleasure showed the highest correlation with reported condom use behavior, with most judging condoms to be unpleasant and with greater condom use occurring more often among those who rated them as very unpleasant instead of extremely unpleasant. Self-efficacy was measured by asking respondents how certain they were that they could use a condom if they wanted to. This was measured separately for main partners and other sexual partners, as self-efficacy for condom use was found to be higher for the latter. Additional self-efficacy measures asked respondents to rate their ability to use condoms with each partner type in specific situations, for example, when intoxicated. Interviews also assessed exposure to messages from the project and other sources, the frequency and duration of condom use with main and non-main partners, and whether respondents were carrying a condom when they were interviewed.

Communication and Environmental Change. The activities carried out by local health departments in the experimental communities included three elements: (1) modeling condom use via behavioral journalism in print communications, (2) prompting and reinforcing condom use through peer volunteers, and (3) facilitating use by making free condoms widely available—a controversial policy innovation in some sites. These three elements were brought together through the organization of community networks for distributing condoms, accompanied by various forms of tabloid newsletter displays containing eroticized stories about peer models from the intended audiences learning to use condoms consistently with specific partner types. About 150–200 volunteers participated in organized community networks in the five cities. Seventy peer network participants in Dallas and Long Beach reported more than 3,500 population contacts per month (about 50 contacts each), in which they distributed the printed peer modeling messages and condoms. In some sites, peer volunteers and outreach workers also worked with the target populations to help them advocate for other facilitating environmental changes, such as changes in police practices and the use of condoms as evidence in the prosecution of sex workers.

Program Effects on Cognitions and Behavior. The proportion of respondents carrying condoms increased significantly in the communities where experimental activities were organized, in association with rising levels of reported exposure to the projects (see Figure 8.1). Overall, there was a significant project effect on consistent condom use with non-main partners but *not on condom use with main partners*. Although it required two years of action to produce this effect, the proportion reporting consistent condom use with non-main partners increased from less than one-quarter to more than one-third of the interview respondents in the experimental populations,

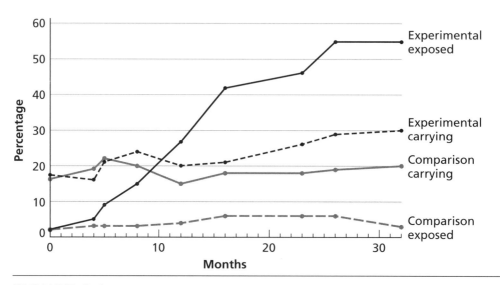

FIGURE 8.1. AIDS Community Demonstration Projects: Exposure and Behavior Change in Carrying Condoms.

while remaining stable in the comparison communities (Centers for Disease Control and Prevention, 1999).

Within the experimental communities, the level of exposure to project messages and materials was strongly related to outcome and self-efficacy expectations. Those reporting more than ten exposures had significantly more positive outcome expectations and self-efficacy beliefs for condom use than those with low exposure levels (McAlister, Johnson, and others, 2000). The project was the most frequently cited source of messages about condom use in the experimental communities, and those reporting exposure to it were as likely to use condoms as those who reported communication with sexual partners about condom use. But, while nearly four in ten respondents reported exposure to the project, fewer than one in ten reported partner communication. Together, these outcome and process evaluation data confirm that the experimental activities effectively accelerated the diffusion of condom use and that the effects were achieved through the theoretical processes for which they were designed.

NEW APPLICATIONS

Potentially important new applications of SCT to interventions for individual and public health are being developed as new technologies and new health threats emerge. Here we describe selected examples of computer and Internet-based applications, as well as strategies for combating intolerance, increasing public health preparedness, and promoting environmentally friendly practices.

New technologies are well suited for the application of SCT, particularly in the development of cognitive and behavioral skills through interactive computer-assisted guidance. For example, computerized assistance in self-directed learning has been shown to be effective in chronic disease management programs for asthma (Lorig and others, 2001). Internet communication can serve both as a source of modeling and of social support and reinforcement in chat rooms and other venues for virtual interaction. Shegog and colleagues (2005) describe an interactive Web-based learning program designed to deter adolescent smoking by testing and reducing susceptibility to tobacco use. The program provides streaming video with tailored peer modeling to refute risky beliefs, for example, that smoking helps people relax. Social skills for avoiding tobacco use are increased by leading visitors through interactive role-plays in which they learn ways to refuse cigarettes with coaching and "virtual" social reinforcement provided by a cartoon character. This Web-based program was evaluated in a single-group pretest-posttest study design in sixth-grade classes of nine middle schools, and was found to significantly influence users' intentions not to smoke, self-efficacy expectations, and personal and social outcome expectations with respect to tobacco use (Shegog and others, 2005).

Following are three more applications.

Combating Intolerance Through Planned Peer Modeling Communications. Efforts to combat intolerance may have many important public health implications, as prejudice may be among the factors that contribute directly and indirectly to disparities in health (Hamburg and Hamburg, 2004). SCT is readily applicable to this topic. McAlister and colleagues (2000) showed how school newsletters featuring behavioral journalism with peer models telling real stories about positive cross-group interactions and reductions in prejudicial thinking could decrease aggression in a multi-ethnic urban school. Other studies have shown that incorporating peer modeling in this kind of narrative, storytelling format can promote tolerance toward immigrants and refugees in Finland (Liebkind and McAlister, 1999) and reduce prejudicial attitudes and intentions toward disabled people in the United Kingdom (Cameron and Rutland, 2006).

Increasing Preparedness for Infectious Diseases and Disasters. SCT can be applied to increasing preparedness to meet emerging awareness of threats from pandemic infectious disease and disasters, as called for by Freimuth, Linnan, and Potter (2000). Applications of the concept of self-efficacy to understanding how people cope with hurricanes were described by Benight and Bandura (2004). Paton (2003) has presented a comprehensive analysis of diverse forms of disaster preparedness based on SCT. McIvor and Paton (2007) recently published research showing how outcome expectations and self-efficacy influence preparatory behaviors.

Promoting Environmentally Responsible Behaviors. Efforts to reduce energy use and promote other environmentally "friendly" behaviors may help ameliorate the public health impact of global warming and environmental degradation. Self-efficacy for restraint in energy use among young people appears to be highly influenced by situational and family factors (Devine-Wright, Devine-Wright, and Fleming, 2004). Berndtsson and Palm (1999) described a campaign to decrease the use of private automobiles in Sweden that was directly based on the North Karelia Project in Finland, combining price changes with peer modeling and "grassroots" outreach to prompt behavior change.

LIMITATIONS IN RESEARCH ON NEW SCT APPLICATIONS

These newly emerging areas of application for SCT have been small in scale, and evaluations have been lacking or incomplete. Much of the research is descriptive or qualitative, particularly with respect to the concept of moral disengagement. Preliminary efforts to use this concept in Internet-based efforts to reduce support for war have been reported (Howard and others, 2007). In the future, it is likely that both old and new concepts from SCT will be used in programs to meet a variety of new and increasing threats to public health. The evaluation of these program and strategies will increase the body of knowledge about whether and how SCT-informed strategies can be mobilized to address new challenges.

SCT is very broad and ambitious, in that it seeks to provide explanations for virtually all human phenomena (Bandura, 1986). However, because it is so broad, it has not been tested comprehensively in the same way that some other health behavior theories have been tested, as described in other chapters in this book. SCT's best-known concept, *self-efficacy,* has been repeatedly validated (see, for example, Moritz, Feltz, Fahrbach, and Mack, 2000). It is found to be associated with behaviors so often that assessments of determinants of behavior may be considered incomplete if self-efficacy is not included. Still, this is not a confirmation of the entire theory. Social cognitive constructs of moral disengagement have been validated in statistical model testing in a few recent studies, but this too is only a part of SCT. Some experimental studies have tested specific concepts from SCT or used them as the basis for experimental interventions. For example, it has been found that the provision of facilitating tools and resources can increase the impact of skills training to reduce unsafe sexual behaviors (Sherman and others, 2006). However, most intervention research on SCT and health behavior has involved the evaluation of multicomponent strategies with many elements and a single or small number of end-points being compared to single interventions or a no-treatment control group (for example, Perry and others, 2002).

To test the theory more fully, different concepts and principles in SCT need to be measured, realized, and manipulated in systematic experiments replicated over diverse behaviors and populations. This could reveal that some of these concepts and principles are more or less useful or feasible for particular behaviors or types of behavior change. For example, future research may show that, to change behaviors related to obesity, incentive motivation and facilitative environmental change are more important than education aimed at influencing individuals' outcome expectations and self-efficacy beliefs. However, environmental changes of the magnitude required to alter nutrition behaviors may not be easy to achieve. Findings from the North Karelia Project in Finland suggest that an extensive campaign of consumer education and advocacy, combined with assistance for food production and marketing innovations, produced a significant long-term impact on nutrition behaviors (Puska, 2002).

To improve the degree to which concepts from SCT and other conceptual models are tested in large-scale evaluations of multicomponent interventions, future research should focus more closely on the measurement and analysis of the theoretical concepts that are presumably influenced by a successful theory-based intervention. For example, in the AIDS Community Demonstration Projects, the program effects on condom carrying and reported condom use were directly linked to program exposure via the effects of that exposure on perceived self-efficacy and on the specific outcome expectations that were hypothesized to influence condom use (McAlister, Johnson, and others, 2000). When any theory or combination of theories is applied to the design of an intervention and evaluated, the investigators should measure all of the concepts used and show the intermediate steps through which they are linked both to behavior change and to effective implementation of the intervention activities. By analyzing mediation processes between programmatic inputs and behavior change outputs, researchers can obtain evidence about the validity of the concepts they are using. This can help advance the understanding of how theoretically based strategies do or do not have positive effects.

SCT provides a very broad and frequently cited source of concepts and principles of behavior change. But health behavior research and action may be enhanced by blending concepts and methods from different theories and models, emphasizing those that focus most closely on the specific health behaviors that are being studied. For example, the Health Belief Model (HBM; see Chapter Three) provides more detail than does SCT with respect to the categorization and measurement of outcome expectations that influence use of preventive services; it was expanded two decades ago to include measurement of self-efficacy as a behavioral determinant. Investigators seeking explanations of why people do or do not obtain vaccinations or cancer screening services may find measurement methods based on that model well suited to their task. For research on physical activity, ecological models may be particularly useful (see Chapter Twenty), as many of the applications of these models have been specific to physical activity. For research on smoking cessation and other addictive behaviors, The Transtheoretical Model (TTM; see Chapter Five) may be an especially helpful source of measurement methods for assessing determinants of behavior change, as it developed from research on those topics. When research moves beyond prediction to evaluate planned actions to change health behaviors, work that is informed by other theories and conceptual models may also be enhanced by incorporating SCT concepts and principles, such as peer modeling in observational learning, self-regulation, incentive motivation, and enabling environmental facilitation.

SUMMARY

SCT seeks to provide a comprehensive understanding of both why and how people change individual health behaviors and the social and physical environments that influence them. SCT is a strong foundation for action-oriented research and practice, using a broad range of approaches to modify diverse behaviors. This chapter defines and describes important concepts and principles from SCT and illustrates their measurement and realization in case studies of theory application.

REFERENCES

Bandura, A. *Principles of Behavior Modification.* New York: Holt, Rinehart & Winston, 1969.

Bandura, A. *Social Learning Theory.* Englewood Cliffs, N.J.: Prentice Hall, 1977.

Bandura, A. *Social Foundations of Thought and Action: A Social Cognitive Theory.* Englewood Cliffs, N.J.: Prentice Hall, 1986.

Bandura, A. *Self-Efficacy: The Exercise of Control.* New York: W. H. Freeman, 1997.

Bandura, A. "Health Promotion from the Perspective of Social Cognitive Theory." *Psychology and Health,* 1998, *13,* 623–649.

Bandura, A. "Moral Disengagement in the Perpetration of Inhumanities." *Personality and Social Psychology Review,* 1999, *3*(3), 193–209.

Bandura, A. "Social Cognitive Theory of Mass Communications." In J. Bryant and D. Zillman (eds.), *Media Effects: Advances in Theory and Research.* (2nd ed.) Hillsdale, N.J.: Erlbaum, 2002.

Bandura, A. "Health Promotion by Social Cognitive Means." *Health Education & Behavior,* 2004a, *31,* 143–164.

Bandura, A. "Swimming Against the Mainstream: The Early Years from Chilly Tributary to Transformative Mainstream." *Behaviour Research and Therapy,* 2004b, *42,* 613–630.

Bandura, A. "On Integrating Social Cognitive and Social Diffusion Theories." In A. Singhal and J. Dearing (eds.), *Communication of Innovations: A Journey with Ev Rogers.* Beverley Hills, Calif.: Sage, 2006.

Bandura, A., and Adams, N. E. "An Analysis of Self-Efficacy Theory of Behavior Change." *Cognitive Therapy and Research,* 1977, *1,* 125–139.

Bandura, A., Barbaranelli, C., Caprara, G. V., and Pastorelli, C. "Mechanisms of Moral Disengagement in the Exercise of Moral Agency." *Journal of Personality and Social Psychology,* 1996, *71,* 364–374.

Bandura, A., Caprara, G. V., and Zsolnai, L. "Corporate Transgressions through Moral Disengagement." *Journal of Human Values,* 2000, *6,* 57–63.

Bandura, A., Jeffery, R. W., and Wright, C. L. "Efficacy of Participant Modeling as a Function of Response Induction Aids." *Journal of Abnormal Psychology,* 1974, *83,* 56–64.

Beck, J. S. *Cognitive Therapy: Basics and Beyond.* New York: Guilford, 1995.

Benight, C. C., and Bandura, A. "Social Cognitive Theory of Posttraumatic Recovery: The Role of Perceived Self-Efficacy." *Behaviour Research and Therapy,* 2004, *42,* 1129–1148.

Berndtsson, A., and Palm, L. "Higher Fuel Taxes or Friendly Persuasion: How to Influence the Environmental Thinking and Behaviour of Car Drivers." Paper presented at Urban Transport Systems, Lund, Sweden, June 1999.

Brassington, G. S., and others. "Intervention-Related Cognitive Versus Social Mediators of Exercise Adherence in the Elderly." *American Journal of Preventive Medicine,* 2002, *23*(2 Suppl), 80–86.

Brody, G. H., and Stoneman, Z. "Selective Imitation of Same-Age, Older and Younger Peer Models." *Child Development,* 1981, *52*(2), 717–720.

Cameron, L., and Rutland, A. "Extended Contact through Story Reading in School: Reducing Children's Prejudice toward the Disabled." *Journal of Social Issues,* 2006, *62*(3), 469–488.

Centers for Disease Control and Prevention (AIDS Community Demonstration Projects Research Group). "Community-Level HIV Intervention in Five Cities: Final Outcome Data from the CDC AIDS Community Demonstration Projects." *American Journal of Public Health,* 1999, *89*(3), 336–345.

Clark, N. M., and Zimmerman, B. J. "A Social Cognitive View of Self-Regulated Learning about Health." *Health Education Research,* 1990, *5*(3), 371–379.

Contento, I. R., Randell, J. S., and Basch, C. E. "Review and Analysis of Evaluation Measures Used in Nutrition Education Research." *Journal of Nutrition Education and Behavior,* 2002, *34*(1), 2–25.

Devine-Wright, P., Devine-Wright, H., and Fleming, P. "Situational Influences upon Children's Beliefs about Global Warming and Energy." *Environmental Education Research,* 2004, *10*(4), 493–506.

Elder, J. P., Ayala, G. X., and Harris, S. "Theories and Intervention Approaches to Health-Behavior Change in Primary Care." *American Journal of Preventive Medicine,* 1999, *17*(4), 275–284.

Farquhar, J. W., and others. "Effects of Communitywide Education on Cardiovascular Disease Risk Factors: The Stanford Five-City Project." *Journal of the American Medical Association,* 1990, *264*(3), 359–365.

Fernández-Ballesteros, R., and others. "Determinants and Structural Relation of Personal Efficacy to Collective Efficacy." *Applied Psychology: An International Review,* 2002, *51,* 107–125.

Freimuth, V., Linnan, H. W., and Potter, P. "Communicating the Threat of Emerging Infections to the Public." *Emerging Infectious Disease,* 2000, *6*(4), 337–347.

Gottlieb, N. H., and others. "Minors' Tobacco Possession Law Violations and Intentions to Smoke: Implications for Tobacco Control." *Tobacco Control,* 2004, *13,* 237–243.

Hamburg, D., and Hamburg, B. *Learning to Live Together: Preventing Hatred and Violence in Child and Adolescent Development.* London: Oxford University Press, 2004.

Hinyard, L. J., and Kreuter, M. W. "Using Narrative Communication as a Tool for Health Behavior Change: A Conceptual, Theoretical, and Empirical Overview." *Health Education and Behavior,* 2007, *34* (5), 777–792.

Hopkins, D. P., and others, for the Task Force on Community Preventive Services. "Reviews of Evidence Regarding Interventions to Reduce Tobacco Use and Exposure to Environmental Tobacco Smoke." *American Journal of Preventive Medicine,* 2001, *20*(2S), 16–66.

Howard, B. H., and others. "www.PeaceTest.org: Development, Implementation and Evaluation of a Web-Based War-Prevention Program in a Time of War." *Journal of Peace Research,* 2007, *44*(4), 559–571.

Jones, F., Harris, P., Waller, H., and Coggins, A. "Adherence to an Exercise Prescription Scheme: The Role of Expectations, Self-Efficacy, Stage of Change and Psychological Well-Being." *British Journal of Health Psychology,* 2005, *10,* 359–378.

Karoly, P. "Mechanisms of Self-Regulation." *Annual Review of Psychology,* 1993, *44,* 23–52.

Kok, G., and others. "Social Psychology and Health Education." *European Review of Social Psychology,* 1996, *7,* 241–282.

Kuusipalo, J., Mikkola, M., Moisio, S., and Puska, P. "The East Finland Berry and Vegetable Project: A Health-Related Structural Intervention Programme." *Health Promotion International,* 1985, *1*(3), 385–391.

Liebkind, K., and McAlister, A. L. "Extended Contact through Peer Modeling to Promote Tolerance in Finland." *European Journal of Social Psychology,* 1999, *29*(5–6), 765–780.

Lorig, K. R., and others. "Chronic Disease Self-Management Programs: Two-Year Health Status and Health Care Utilization Outcomes." *Medical Care,* 2001, *39,* 1217–1223.

Loukas, A., Spaulding, C., and Gottlieb, N. "Examining the Perspectives of Texas Minors Cited for Possession of Tobacco." *Health Promotion Practice,* 2006, *7*(2), 197–205.

Maibach, E., and Murphy, D. A. "Self-Efficacy in Health Promotion Research and Practice: Conceptualization and Measurement." *Health Education Research,* 1995, *10,* 37–50.

McAlister, A. L. "Behavioral Journalism: Beyond the Marketing Model for Health Communication." *American Journal of Health Promotion,* 1995, *9,* 417–420.

McAlister, A. L. "Acceptance of Killing and Homicide Rates in Nineteen Nations." *European Journal of Public Health,* 2006, *16*(3), 260–266.

McAlister, A. L., Huang, P., and Ramirez, A. G. "Settlement-Funded Tobacco Control in Texas: 2000–2004 Pilot Project Effects on Cigarette Smoking." *Public Health Reporter,* 2006, *121*(3), 235–238.

McAlister, A. L., and others. "Theory and Action for Health Promotion Illustrations from the North Karelia Project." *American Journal of Public Health,* 1982, *72*(1), 43–50.

McAlister, A. L., Johnson, W., and others. "Behavioral Journalism for HIV Prevention: Community Newsletters Influence Risk-Related Attitudes and Behavior." *Journalism and Mass Communication Quarterly,* 2000, *77*(1), 143–159.

McAlister, A. L., Bandura, A., and Owen, S. V. "Mechanisms of Moral Disengagement in Support of Military Force: The Impact of September 11." *Journal of Social and Clinical Psychology,* 2006, *25*(2), 141–165.

McAlister, A. L., and Fernández, M. "Behavioral Journalism Accelerates Diffusion of Health Innovations." In R. C. Hornik (ed.), *Public Health Communication: Evidence for Behavior Change.* Hillsdale, N.J.: Erlbaum, 2002.

McAlister, A. L., and others. "Promoting Tolerance and Moral Engagement through Peer Modeling." *Cultural Diversity and Ethnic Minority Psychology,* 2000, *6*(4), 363–373.

McAlister, A. L., and others. "Telephone Assistance for Smoking Cessation: One Year Cost Effectiveness Estimations." *Tobacco Control,* 2004, *13*(1), 85–86.

McIvor, D., and Paton, D. "Preparing for Natural Hazards: Normative and Attitudinal Influences." *Disaster Prevention and Management,* 2007, *16*(1), 79–88.

Meichenbaum, D. *Cognitive-Behavior Modification: An Integrative Approach.* New York: Plenum, 1977.

Meshack, A. F., and others. "Texas Tobacco Prevention Pilot Initiative: Processes and Effects." *Health Education Research,* 2004, *19*(6), 657–668.

Miller, N. E., and Dollard, J. *Social Learning and Imitation.* New Haven, Conn.: Yale University Press, 1941.

Moritz, S. E., Feltz, D. L., Fahrbach, K. R., and Mack, D. E. "The Relation of Self-Efficacy Measures to Sport Performance: A Meta-Analytic Review." *Research Quarterly on Exercise and Sport,* 2000, *71*(3), 280–294.

Osgood, C. E. *The Measurement of Meaning.* Urbana, Ill: University of Illinois Press, 1967.

Paton, D. "Disaster Preparedness: A Social-Cognitive Perspective." *Disaster Prevention and Management: An International Journal,* 2003, *12*(3), 210–216.

Pelton, J., Gound, M., Forehand, R., and Brody, G. "The Moral Disengagement Scale: Extension with an American Minority Sample." *Journal of Psychopathology and Behavioral Assessment,* 2004, *26*(1), 31–39.

Perry, C. L., Kelder, S. H., and Klepp, K. I. "Communitywide Cardiovascular Disease Prevention with Young People: Long-Term Outcomes of the Class of 1989 Study." *European Journal of Public Health,* 1994, *4*(3), 188–194.

Perry, C. L., and others. "Project Northland High School Interventions: Community Action to Reduce Adolescent Alcohol Use." *Health Education and Behavior,* 2000, *27*(1), 29–49.

Perry, C. L., and others. "Project Northland: Long-Term Outcomes of Community Action to Reduce Adolescent Alcohol Use." *Health Education Research,* 2002, *16*(5), 101–116.

Puska, P. "Successful Prevention of Noncommunicable Disease: Twenty-Five Year Experience with the North Karelia Project." *Public Health Medicine,* 2002, *4*(1), 5–7.

Puska, P., and others. "A Television Format for National Health Promotion: Finland's 'Keys to Health.'" *Public Health Reporter,* 1987, *102*(3), 263–269.

Rabius, V., and others. "Telephone Counseling Increases Cessation Rates Among Young Adult Smokers." *Health Psychology,* 2004, *23*(5), 539–541.

Ramirez, A. G., and others. "Advancing the Role of Participatory Communication in the Diffusion of Cancer Screening among Hispanics." *Journal of Health Communication,* 1999, *4*(1), 31–36.

Rotter, J. B. *Social Learning and Clinical Psychology.* Englewood Cliffs, N.J.: Prentice Hall, 1954.

Schunk, D. H. "Peer Models and Children's Behavioral Change." *Review of Educational Research,* 1987, *57*(2), 149–174.

Shegog, R., and others. "Use of Interactive Health Communication to Affect Smoking Intentions in Middle School Students: A Pilot Test of the 'Headbutt' Risk Assessment Program." *American Journal of Health Promotion,* 2005, *19*(5), 334–338.

Sherman, S. G., and others. "The Evaluation of the JEWEL Project: An Innovative Economic Enhancement and HIV Prevention Intervention Study Targeting Drug Using Women Involved in Prostitution." *AIDS Care,* 2006, *18*(1), 1–11.

Singhal, A., and Rogers, E. A. *Entertainment-Education: A Communication Strategy for Social Change.* Hillsdale, N.J.: Erlbaum, 1999.

Volpp, K. G., and others. "A Randomized Controlled Trial of Financial Incentives for Smoking Cessation." *Cancer, Epidemiology, Biomarkers and Prevention,* 2006, *15*(1), 12–18.

Wilkin, H. A., and others. "Does Entertainment-Education Work with Latinos in the United States? Identification and the Effects of a Telenovela Breast Cancer Storyline." *Journal of Health Communication,* 2007, *12*(5), 455–469.

Worden, J. K., and others. "Preventing Alcohol-Impaired Driving through Community Self-Regulation Training." *American Journal of Public Health,* 1989, *79*(3), 287–290.

CHAPTER

SOCIAL NETWORKS AND SOCIAL SUPPORT

Catherine A. Heaney
Barbara A. Israel

KEY POINTS

This chapter will

- Define functions and characteristics of social networks.
- Provide a conceptual framework for understanding the relationship between social networks and health.
- Briefly review the empirical support for this relationship.
- List and describe types of social network interventions.
- Present two examples of social network interventions for promoting health.

The powerful influence that social relationships have on health has garnered great interest among both researchers and practitioners. An understanding of the impact of social relationships on health status, health behaviors, and health decision making can contribute to the design of effective interventions for promoting health. Although no one theory adequately explicates the link between social relationships and health, various conceptual models and theories have guided research in this area.

DEFINITIONS AND TERMINOLOGY

Several key terms have been used in studies of the health-enhancing components of social relationships (Berkman, Glass, Brissette, and Seeman, 2000). The term *social integration* has been used to refer to the existence of social ties. The term *social network* refers to the web of social relationships that surround individuals. The provision of *social support* is one of the important functions of social relationships. Thus, the term *social network* refers to linkages between people that may or may not provide social support and that may serve functions other than providing support. More recently, the term *social capital* has been used to describe certain resources and norms that arise from social networks (Ferlander, 2007).

The structure of social networks can be described in terms of dyadic characteristics (that is, characteristics of specific relationships between the focal individual and other people in the network) and in terms of characteristics of the network as a whole (Israel, 1982; House, Umberson, and Landis, 1988). Examples of dyadic characteristics include the extent to which resources and support are both given and received in a relationship (reciprocity), the extent to which a relationship is characterized by emotional closeness (intensity or strength), the extent to which a relationship is embedded in a formal organizational or institutional structure (formality), and the extent to which a relationship serves a variety of functions (complexity). Examples of characteristics that describe a whole network include the extent to which network members are similar in terms of demographic characteristics such as age, race, and socioeconomic status (homogeneity); the extent to which network members live in close proximity to the focal person (geographic dispersion), and the extent to which network members know and interact with each other (density).

Social networks give rise to various social functions: social influence, social control, social undermining, social comparison, companionship, and social support. This chapter focuses on social networks and the provision of social support. The term *social support* has been defined and measured in numerous ways. According to seminal work by House (1981), social support is the functional content of relationships that can be categorized into four broad types of supportive behaviors or acts:

1. *Emotional support* involves the provision of empathy, love, trust, and caring.
2. *Instrumental support* involves the provision of tangible aid and services that directly assist a person in need.
3. *Informational support* is the provision of advice, suggestions, and information that a person can use to address problems.
4. *Appraisal support* involves the provision of information that is useful for self-evaluation purposes—in other words, constructive feedback and affirmation.

Although these four types of support can be differentiated conceptually, relationships that provide one type often also provide other types, thus making it difficult to study them empirically as separate constructs. (For a comprehensive review of measurement and methodological issues, see Barrera, 2000; Cohen, Underwood, and Gottlieb, 2000.) Table 9.1 summarizes the key concepts and their definitions.

Social support can be distinguished from other functions of social relationships (Burg and Seeman, 1994). Social support is always intended (by the provider of the support) to be helpful, thus distinguishing it from intentional negative interactions (for example, social undermining behaviors such as angry criticism and hassling).

TABLE 9.1. **Characteristics and Functions of Social Networks.**

Concepts	Definitions
Structural characteristics of social networks:	
Reciprocity	Extent to which resources and support are both given and received in a relationship
Intensity or strength	Extent to which social relationships offer emotional closeness
Complexity	Extent to which social relationships serve many functions
Formality	Extent to which social relationships exist in the context of organizational or institutional roles
Density	Extent to which network members know and interact with each other
Homogeneity	Extent to which network members are demographically similar
Geographic dispersion	Extent to which network members live in close proximity to focal person
Directionality	Extent to which members of the dyad share equal power and influence
Functions of social networks:	
Social capital	Resources characterized by norms of reciprocity and social trust
Social influence	Process by which thoughts and actions are changed by actions of others
Social undermining	Process by which others express negative affect or criticism or hinder one's attainment of goals
Companionship	Sharing leisure or other activities with network members
Social support	Aid and assistance exchanged through social relationships and interpersonal transactions
Types of social support:	
Emotional support	Expressions of empathy, love, trust, and caring
Instrumental support	Tangible aid and services
Informational support	Advice, suggestions, and information
Appraisal support	Information that is useful for self-evaluation

Whether or not the intended support is perceived or experienced as helpful by the receiver is an empirical question, and indeed, negative perceptions and consequences of well-intended interpersonal exchanges have been identified (for example, Wortman and Lehman, 1985). In addition, social support is consciously provided, which sets it apart from the social influence exerted through simple observation of the behavior of others (Bandura, 1986) or from receiver-initiated social comparison processes (Wood, 1996). Finally, although the provision of social support, particularly informational support, can attempt to influence the thoughts and behaviors of the receiver, such informational support is provided in an interpersonal context of caring, trust, and respect for each person's right to make his or her own choices. This quality distinguishes social support from some other types of social influence that derive from the ability to provide or withhold desired resources or approval.

Although many investigations of the effects of social relationships on health have narrowly focused on the provision of social support, a broader social network approach has several advantages. First, a social network approach can incorporate functions or characteristics of social relationships other than social support (Israel, 1982; Berkman and Glass, 2000). For example, there is increasing evidence that negative interpersonal interactions, such as those characterized by mistrust, hassles, criticism, and domination, are more strongly related to such factors as negative mood (Fleishman and others, 2000), depression (Cranford, 2004), risky health behaviors such as substance abuse (Oetzel, Duran, Jiang, and Lucero, 2007), and susceptibility to infectious disease (Cohen and others, 1997) than is a lack of social support. Second, whereas a social support approach usually focuses on one relationship at a time, a social network approach allows for the study of how changes in one social relationship affect other relationships. Third, a social network approach facilitates the investigation of how structural network characteristics influence the quantity and quality of social support that are exchanged (McLeroy, Gottlieb, and Heaney, 2001). This information can be important for the development of effective support-enhancing interventions.

BACKGROUND OF THE CONCEPTS

Barnes's (1954) pioneering work in a Norwegian village first presented the concept of a social network to describe patterns of social relationships that were not easily explained by more traditional social units such as extended families or work groups. Much of the early work on social networks was exploratory and descriptive. The findings from these studies provided a knowledge base that helped identify network characteristics. In general, it was found that close-knit networks exchange more affective and instrumental support, and also exert more social influence on members to conform to network norms. Homogenous networks, networks with more reciprocal linkages, and networks with closer geographical proximity were also more effective in providing affective and instrumental support (see Israel, 1982; Berkman and Glass, 2000 for reviews).

The study of social support owes much to the work of social epidemiologist John Cassel (1976). Drawing from numerous animal and human studies, Cassel posited that social support served as a key psychosocial "protective" factor that reduced individuals' vulnerability to the deleterious effects of stress on health. He also specified that psychosocial factors such as social support were likely to play a nonspecific role in the etiology of disease. Thus, social support may influence the incidence and prevalence of a wide array of health outcomes.

From the previous discussion, it is clear that the terms *social network* and *social support* do not connote theories per se. Rather, they are concepts that describe the structure, processes, and functions of social relationships. Various sociological and social psychological theories (such as exchange theory, attachment theory, and symbolic interactionism) have been used to explain the basic interpersonal processes that underlie the association between social relationships and health (Berkman, Glass, Brissette, and Seeman, 2000).

RELATIONSHIP OF SOCIAL NETWORKS AND SOCIAL SUPPORT TO HEALTH

The mechanisms through which social networks and social support may have positive effects on physical, mental, and social health are summarized in Figure 9.1. The model depicts social networks and social support as the starting point or initiator of a causal flow toward health outcomes. In actuality, many of the relationships in Figure 9.1 entail reciprocal influence; for example, health status will influence the extent to which one is able to maintain and mobilize a social network.

In Figure 9.1, Pathway 1 represents a hypothesized direct effect of social networks and social support on health. By meeting basic human needs for companionship, intimacy, a sense of belonging, and reassurance of one's worth as a person, supportive ties may enhance well-being and health, regardless of stress levels (Berkman and Glass, 2000). Pathways 2 and 4 represent a hypothesized effect of social networks and social support on individual coping resources and community resources, respectively. For example, social networks and social support can enhance an individual's ability to access new contacts and information and to identify and solve problems. If the support provided helps to reduce uncertainty and unpredictability or helps to produce desired outcomes, then a sense of personal control over specific situations and life domains will be enhanced. In addition, the theory of symbolic interactionism suggests that human behavior is based on the meaning that people assign to events. This meaning is derived, in large part, from their social interactions (Israel, 1982; Berkman, Glass, Brissette, and Seeman, 2000). Thus, people's social network linkages may help them reinterpret events or problems in a more positive and constructive light (Thoits, 1995).

The potential effects of social networks and social support on organizational and community competence are less well studied. However, strengthening social networks and enhancing the exchange of social support may increase a community's ability to garner its resources and solve problems. Several community-level interventions have shown how intentional network building and the strengthening of social support within communities are associated with enhanced community capacity and control (Minkler,

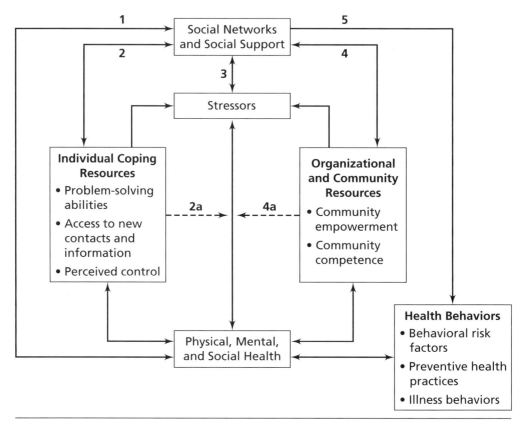

FIGURE 9.1. Conceptual Model for the Relationship of Social Networks and Social Support to Health.

2001; Eng and Parker, 1994). Indeed, these are strategies for building social capital—investing in social relationships so that generalized social trust and norms of reciprocity are strengthened within the community (Ferlander, 2007).

Resources at both the individual and community levels may have direct health-enhancing effects and may also diminish the negative effects on health due to exposure to stressors. When people experience stressors, having enhanced individual or community resources increases the likelihood that stressors will be handled or coped with in a way that reduces both short-term and long-term adverse health consequences. This effect is called a "buffering effect" and is reflected in Pathways 2a and 4a. Research involving people going through major life transitions (such as loss of a job or birth of a child) has shown how social networks and social support influence the coping process and buffer the effects of the stressor on health (see, for example, Hodnett, Gates, Hofmeyr, and Sakala, 2007).

Pathway 3 suggests that social networks and social support may influence the frequency and duration of exposure to stressors. For example, a supportive supervisor may ensure that an employee is not given more work to do than can be completed in the available time. Similarly, having a social network that provides information about new jobs may reduce the likelihood that a person will suffer from long-term unemployment. Reduced exposure to stressors is then, in turn, associated with enhanced mental and physical health.

Pathway 5 reflects the potential effects of social networks and social support on health behaviors. Through the interpersonal exchanges within a social network, individuals are influenced and supported in such health behaviors as adherence to medical regimens (DiMatteo, 2004), help-seeking behavior (McKinlay, 1980; Starrett and others, 1990), smoking cessation (Palmer, Baucom, and McBride, 2000), and weight loss (Wing and Jeffery, 1999). Through influences on preventive health behavior, illness behavior, and sick-role behavior, Pathway 5 makes explicit that social networks and social support may affect the incidence of and recovery from disease.

EMPIRICAL EVIDENCE ON THE INFLUENCE OF SOCIAL RELATIONSHIPS

Numerous reviews of the empirical studies address the influence of social relationships on health (see, for example, Barrera, 2000; Berkman and Glass, 2000; Uchino, 2004). Although there are some inconsistencies in this body of research, few today would disagree with House's summary statement made two decades ago: "Although the results of individual studies are usually open to alternative interpretations, the patterns of results across the full range of studies strongly suggests that what are variously termed social relationships, social networks, and social support have important causal effects on health, exposure to stress, and the relationship between stress and health" (House, 1987).

Prospective epidemiological studies, most often using measures of social integration, consistently find a relationship between a lack of social relationships and all-cause mortality (Berkman and Glass, 2000). More recently, a number of studies documented that intimate ties and the emotional support provided by them increase survival rates among people with severe cardiovascular disease (Berkman and Glass, 2000). Evidence for buffering effects is less conclusive, but studies do suggest that social support mobilized to help a person cope with a stressor reduces the negative effects of the stressor on health (Cohen and Wills, 1985; Thoits, 1995). Although the direct effects and the buffering effects of social networks and social support were initially investigated as either-or relationships, evidence suggests that social support and social networks have both types of effects, and that the predominance of one effect over the other depends on the target population, the situation being studied, and the ways in which the social relationship concept is measured (Cohen and Wills, 1985; House, Umberson, and Landis, 1988; Krause, 1995; Thoits, 1995).

The effect of social relationships on all-cause mortality supports the hypothesis, first put forth by Cassel (1976), that the effect of social relationships on health is not specific to any one disease process. This nonspecific role may explain why studies of the effect of social relationships on specific morbidities have not been conclusive

(House, Umberson, and Landis, 1988; Berkman and Glass, 2000). As our understanding of the influence of social support on the cardiovascular, neuroendocrine, and immune systems deepens (Uchino, 2006), we may be able to make better sense of the pattern of results. Although evidence for a link between social networks and social support and the incidence of particular diseases is inconsistent (Vogt and others, 1992), a positive role for affective support in the processes of coping with and recovering from serious illness has been consistently documented (Spiegel and Diamond, 2001; Wang, Mittleman, and Orth-Gomer, 2005).

The association between social relationships and health does not follow a linear dose-response curve. Rather, very low levels of social integration (that is, having no strong social ties) are most deleterious, with higher levels being less advantageous once a threshold level has been reached (House, 2001). Having at least one strong intimate relationship is an important predictor of good health (Michael, Colditz, Coakley, and Kawachi, 1999). For example, in a study of African American elderly women, severe social isolation (that is, living alone and not having had contact with family or friends during the last two weeks) was associated with a three-fold increase in mortality during a five-year follow-up period (LaVeist, Sellers, Brown, and Nickerson, 1997).

The influence of social network characteristics on social support, health behavior, and health status has been less thoroughly examined than has the relationship between social support and health (Berkman and Glass, 2000). However, the results of earlier reviews of the literature suggest that the social network's reciprocity and intensity were somewhat consistently linked to positive mental health (Israel, 1982; House, Umberson, and Landis, 1988). In addition, networks that were characterized by few ties, high-intensity relationships, high density, and close geographical proximity maintained social identity and the exchange of affective support. Thus, these networks were most health-enhancing when these social network functions were needed. However, during times of transition and change, networks that are larger, more diffuse, and composed of less intense ties may be more adaptive because they are better at facilitating social outreach and exchanging new information (Granovetter, 1983). Furthermore, more recent studies provide evidence that the size and density of social networks that endorse risk-taking norms are associated with higher levels of risk-taking behaviors, such as injection drug use (Berkman and Glass, 2000).

Demographically defined subgroups maintain qualitatively different social networks and experience health benefits from those networks (House, Umberson, and Landis, 1988). Shumaker and Hill (1991) reviewed gender differences in the link between social support and physical health. They suggested that prospective epidemiological studies investigating the effect of social relationships on mortality found a weaker health-protective effect for women than for men. In addition, women of a particular age group (usually over fifty years of age) experienced a positive association between high levels of social support and mortality. Noting that women tend to cast a "wider net of concern" (that is, maintain more strong ties), are more likely to be both the providers and recipients of social support, and are more responsive to the life events of others than are men, the authors suggest that further study is needed to explore the impact of these differences on the health-protective potential of women's social networks.

TRANSLATING THEORY AND RESEARCH INTO PRACTICE

Social epidemiological studies have clearly documented the beneficial effects on health of supportive social networks. However, these observational studies cannot tell us whether we can promote good health by strengthening social networks and increasing the availability of social support. Intervention research is needed to identify the most potent causal agents and critical time periods for social network enhancement. Health education and health behavior researchers who develop and implement social network enhancement interventions face several decision points. House (1981) summarized these decision points in a single question: In order to effectively enhance the health-protective functions of social networks, *who* should provide *what* to whom (and *when*)? The issues of *who, what,* and *when* are discussed next.

Who

Social support can be provided by many types of people, both in one's informal network (for example, family, friends, coworkers, supervisors) and in more formal helping networks (for example, health care professionals, human service workers). Different network members are likely to provide differing amounts and types of support (McLeroy, Gottlieb, and Heaney, 2001). In addition, the effectiveness of the support provided may depend on the source of the support (Agneessens, Waege, and Lievens, 2006). For example, long-term assistance is most often provided by family members; neighbors and friends are more likely to provide short-term aid (McLeroy, Gottlieb, and Heaney, 2001). In medical care settings, patients often need emotional support from family and friends and informational support from health care professionals (Blanchard and others, 1995).

   Thoits offered a more comprehensive approach to defining an effective source of support: the effective provision of support is likely to stem from people who are socially similar to the support recipients and who have experienced similar stressors or situations (Thoits, 1995). These characteristics enhance the "empathic understanding" of the support provider, making it more likely that the support proffered is in concert with the needs and values of the recipient. In addition, the person who desires the support is more likely to overcome the stigma attached to needing help and to seek or mobilize support when the social network member is perceived to be empathic and understanding. Empathic understanding is particularly relevant to the exchange of emotional support but also applies to instrumental and informational support.

   Long-standing, intimate social network ties have unique capabilities to provide social support (Gottlieb and Wagner, 1991; Feeney and Collins, 2003). However, there can be a down side to depending on these types of relationships for support, particularly informational support. Gottlieb and Wagner (1991) noted that people in close relationships are often distressed by the same stressor and that the nature and quality of the support provided is affected by the distress levels of the helper. Also, because the support providers are very interested in the well-being of the support recipients, when support attempts are not well received or do not result in positive changes in the receiver, the helpers can react negatively (Feeney and Collins, 2003).

This is most likely to occur when information or advice is provided. Intimate ties may be best used for emotional support, but other relationships may be better suited for informational support (Gottlieb, 2000).

Considerable debate has focused on whether professional helpers are effective sources of social support. Health education interventions may attempt to enhance the social support available to participants by linking them with professional helpers. Professional helpers often have access to information and resources that are not otherwise available in the social network. However, professional helpers are rarely available to provide social support over long periods of time. Additionally, professional, lay relationships are not typically reciprocal and may involve large power differentials or lack the "empathic understanding" described earlier. Health educators have attempted to overcome these limitations of professional helpers by recruiting members of the community and training them in the knowledge and skills needed to address the target health issue (for example, screening mammography or asthma self-management). These lay health advisers or community health workers can then provide the needed informational support while maintaining their "empathic understanding," gained through life experiences similar to those of recipients (Friedman and others, 2006). In other interventions, professional and informal helpers are integrated into a problem-defined support system created to address specific health issues, such as recovery from stroke (Glass and others, 2000).

What

The *perceptions* of support recipients, rather than the *objective* behaviors involved in interactions, are most strongly linked to recipients' health and well-being (Wethington and Kessler, 1986). Although the perceptions of support recipients are certainly correlated with objective behaviors, this correlation is modest, and it is necessary to identify factors that may influence whether behaviors are perceived as supportive (Haber, Cohen, Lucas, and Baltes, 2007). These factors include the recipient's previous experiences of support with the helper and the social context of the relationship (for example, are the two people in competition for resources? Does one have the power to reward or punish the other?). Other factors are role expectations and individual preferences for types and amounts of social support.

Given the multiple factors that affect how social interactions are perceived, a priori assumptions about which specific behaviors increase perceived social support may be ill-advised. Ways in which social network members can be more supportive can be best identified through involvement of the intended intervention participants. Discussion among the interested parties could include previous successful support efforts and support efforts that have gone awry; such discussion could also generate a set of desired social behaviors and skills specific to the population and problem being addressed. For example, a program designed to enhance coworker and supervisor support used a group format in which employees gleaned suggestions on ways to modify their behavior from the stories of other employees' effective, supportive social interactions (Heaney, 1991). Similar strategies have been used in smoking cessation interventions that attempted to enhance the support for cessation provided by significant others (Palmer, Baucom, and McBride, 2000).

When

Research has suggested that the types of social networks and social support that effectively enhance well-being and health differ according to the age or developmental stage of the support recipient (Kahn and Antonucci, 1980). In addition, people who are experiencing a major life transition or stressor benefit from different types of support during the various stages of coping with the stressor (Thoits, 1995). For example, someone whose spouse has just died may benefit from a closely knit, dense social network that provides strong affective support to the bereaved. However, as the widowed individual makes life modifications to adapt to the loss, more diffuse networks that offer access to new social ties and diverse informational support may be most helpful.

SOCIAL NETWORK AND SOCIAL SUPPORT INTERVENTIONS

Several typologies of social network and social support interventions have been suggested (Israel, 1982; McLeroy, Gottlieb, and Heaney, 2001; Gottlieb, 2000). Table 9.2 presents four categories of interventions: (1) enhancing existing social network linkages, (2) developing new social network linkages, (3) enhancing networks through the use of indigenous natural helpers, and (4) enhancing networks at the community level through participatory problem-solving processes. A fifth category is composed of interventions that use a combination of these types of interventions. Interventions in these five categories are briefly described next, highlighting the challenges and potential benefits of each type. The quantity and quality of the research investigating the effectiveness of social network interventions differs across the types of intervention. Further research is needed to assess the efficacy of the various interventions and the conditions under which each of the types of interventions is most likely to be effective.

Enhancing Existing Network Ties

Existing network ties often offer much untapped potential. Interventions aimed at enhancing existing ties attempt to change the attitudes and behaviors of the support recipient, the support provider, or both. The transactional nature of social exchanges suggests that the last may be most effective, and some research is consistent with this suggestion (Heaney, 1991).

Interventions to enhance existing relationships often include activities to build skills for effective support mobilization, provision, and receipt. They may focus on enhancing the quality of social ties in order to address specific health issues or to provide support across many different situations. For example, cardiac patients were counseled on how to strengthen their social networks, in order to enhance their ability to cope with their illness (ENRICHD Investigators, 2001; see further description

TABLE 9.2. **Typology of Social Network Interventions.**

Intervention Type	Examples of Intervention Activities	Selected References
Enhancing existing network linkages	Training of network members in skills for providing support	Heaney, 1991
	Training of focal individual in mobilizing and maintaining social networks	Sandler and others, 1992
		Wing and Jeffery, 1999
		Palmer, Baucom, and McBride, 2000
	Systems approach (for example, marital counseling or family therapy)	
Developing new social network linkages	Creating linkages to mentors	Helgeson and Gottlieb, 2000
	Developing buddy systems	Chesler and Chesney, 1995
	Facilitating self-help groups	Rhodes, 2002
Enhancing networks through the use of indigenous natural helpers and community health workers (CHWs)	Identification of natural helpers or CHWs	Eng and Hatch, 1991
	Analysis of natural helpers' existing social networks	Kegler and Malcoe, 2004
		Earp and others, 1997
		McQuiston and Flaskerud, 2003
	Training in health topics and community problem-solving strategies	Krieger, Takaro, Song, and Weaver, 2005
Enhancing networks through community capacity building and problem solving	Identification of overlapping networks within the community	Minkler, 2001
	Examination of social network characteristics of members of the selected need or target area	Boutilier, Cleverly, and Labonte, 2000
	Facilitation of ongoing community problem identification and problem solving	

Source: Adapted from Israel, 1982.

later in this chapter.) Partners or significant others were incorporated into smoking cessation programs (Palmer, Baucom, and McBride, 2000) and weight loss programs (Wing and Jeffery, 1999) to provide support for behavior change.

Some of the challenges with this type of intervention include identifying existing network members who are committed to providing support and have the resources to sustain the commitment; identifying the changes in attitudes and behaviors that will result in increased perceived support on the part of the support recipient; and intervening in ways that are consistent with established norms and styles of interaction.

Developing New Social Network Linkages

Interventions designed to develop new social network linkages are most useful when the existing network is small, overburdened, or unable to provide effective support. Sometimes new ties are introduced to alleviate chronic social isolation, such as that experienced by the elderly (Heller and others, 1991). Most often new ties are introduced in response to a major life transition or specific stressor. In these cases, the existing network may lack the requisite experiential or specialized knowledge about the specific stressor.

Some interventions introduce "mentors" or "advisers"—people who have already coped with the situation being experienced by the focal individual (Eckenrode and Hamilton, 2000; Rhodes, 2002). Other interventions introduce "buddies" who are experiencing the stressor or life transition at the same time as the focal person. For example, in some smoking cessation programs and weight control programs, participants are encouraged to "buddy up" with another participant to provide support and encouragement to each other (Palmer, Baucom, and McBride, 2000).

Self-help or mutual aid groups provide a new *set* of network ties. Usually, people come together in self-help groups because they are facing a common stressor or because they want to bring about similar changes, either at the individual level (for example, individual weight loss) or at a community level (for example, increased access to health care in one's community). In self-help or mutual aid groups, the roles of support provider and support recipient are mutually shared among the members. Thus, the ties often entail high levels of reciprocity. Such groups can be particularly effective for participants who cannot mobilize social support from their other social relationships. Although a full description of self-help groups is beyond the scope of this chapter, several good reviews and descriptions exist (see Chesler and Chesney, 1995, and Helgeson and Gottlieb, 2000). Recently, Internet-based support groups have gained in popularity. People with common interests join a virtual community to share experiences and exchange support. Although there is little evidence of their effectiveness to date (Eysenbach and others, 2004), they are likely to be a continuing trend in how people seek information and support for specific life transitions and health problems. Research is needed to identify important components of Internet support groups, and for whom and under what circumstances they can have health-promoting effects.

Use of Indigenous Natural Helpers and Community Health Workers

Natural helpers are members of social networks to whom other network members naturally turn for advice, support, and other types of aid (Israel, 1985). They are respected and trusted network members who are responsive to the needs of others. In addition to providing support directly to network members, natural helpers can link social network members to each other and to resources outside the network. Community health workers (CHWs) are members of the community being served, who are recruited to provide frontline health services and outreach. CHWs are often employed by the health care system to provide a linkage between the community members and formal health services (Love, Gardner, and Legion, 1997).

One of the first tasks in natural helper interventions is to identify the people who currently fill these helping roles. Although various strategies have been used to do this (Eng and Young, 1992), commonly people in the community are asked for the names of people who demonstrate the characteristics of natural helpers. The participation of community members in the identification process is critical. People whose names are repeatedly mentioned can be contacted and recruited. Once the natural helpers are recruited, the health professional can provide the needed information on specific health topics, health and human service resources available in the community, and community problem-solving strategies, and can engage in a consultative relationship with the natural helpers.

Natural helper interventions have been conducted in a number of different communities, including urban neighborhoods, rural counties, Native American communities, migrant farmworker streams, and church congregations (Kegler and Malcoe, 2004; McQuiston and Flaskerud, 2003; Eng and Hatch, 1991). CHWs have also been employed in many different settings (Love, Gardner, and Legion, 1997; Schulz and others, 2002; Krieger and others, 2002).

Enhancing Networks Through Community Capacity Building and Problem Solving

Interventions that involve community members in identifying and resolving community problems may indirectly strengthen the social networks that exist in the community. Such interventions (see, for example, Boutilier, Cleverly, and Labonte, 2000; Rothman, Erlich, and Tropman, 2001) use community organizing techniques with the goals of (1) enhancing the capacity of a community to resolve its problems, (2) increasing the community's role in making decisions that have important implications for community life, and (3) resolving specific problems. Through participating in collective problem-solving processes, community members forge new network ties and strengthen existing ones. For example, in the Tenderloin Senior Outreach Project, elderly residents in the Tenderloin district of San Francisco formed groups and coalitions to address safety and health concerns. Through participation in these groups, the residents became less socially isolated and began to turn to each other for information, advice, and support (Minkler, 2001). See Chapter Thirteen for an extended analysis of community organizing and capacity development.

Although community problem-solving interventions indirectly affect social networks, social network strategies could be incorporated into both the assessment and implementation stages of these interventions (Israel, 1985). The community assessment could determine how people gain information, resources, and support, as well as identify potential problem areas. Examining the extent to which people's networks overlap may aid in the diffusion of new information throughout the community.

Combining Strategies

Some programs have combined the intervention strategies described earlier to maximize the impact of the program. For example, a program that enhances existing network ties and also forges new ties can benefit from well-established social relationships and the infusion of new social resources. In the Family Bereavement Program (Sandler and others, 1992), members of families that had experienced a loss attended workshops, during which they explored ways family members could provide support to each other. During the workshops, the participants also engaged in supportive interactions with other bereaved families. After participating in the workshops, each family was matched with a family adviser, who then provided ongoing emotional and informational support, shoring up overburdened family sources of support.

Combining natural helper interventions with community problem solving is another potentially effective strategy (Eng and Hatch, 1991; Schulz and others, 2002). Although natural helpers can address the needs of the individual network members, the community-level strategy can address some of the broader social, legal, and economic problems facing the community. This results in a more comprehensive ecological approach to enhancing the health of the community. Lay health advisers may be able to enhance the effectiveness of community-level problem solving by integrating community residents more fully into the life of the community and, more specifically, into cooperative problem-solving efforts. Future research is needed to evaluate the efficacy of combining these social network strategies.

HEALTH EDUCATION AND HEALTH BEHAVIOR APPLICATIONS

The two interventions described next illustrate how social network and social support concepts have been applied to practice. The first intervention uses cognitive behavioral therapy to increase social support. The second describes a social network intervention using CHWs.

Enhancing Recovery in Coronary Heart Disease Patients Study (ENRICHD)

Observational studies have consistently demonstrated that patients with coronary heart disease (CHD) who do not have adequate social support are at higher risk for subsequent cardiac mortality and morbidity than are CHD patients who have supportive social networks (Lett and others, 2005). Given that CHD is the leading cause of death in the United States, the potential health benefits associated with enhancing social support for CHD patients are substantial.

The Enhancing Recovery in Coronary Heart Disease Patients (ENRICHD) study was a multicenter, randomized trial conducted to assess the effectiveness of increasing social support among CHD patients. In order to participate in the study, patients must have had a recent myocardial infarction (heart attack) and screened positive for depression or low social support. The intervention was based on the principles of cognitive behavioral therapy. For the patients with low social support, a professional therapist conducted a detailed assessment of the patient's social network, social skills, and problem-solving skills. Counseling sessions then addressed the specific needs identified (ENRICHD Investigators, 2001).

The intervention focused on changing the cognitions and behaviors of the patients in order to enhance their perceived social support. The intent was not for the therapists to become long-term support providers but for them to guide the patients in efforts to enhance their own social networks. Most often, patients were encouraged to strengthen existing relationships rather than seek new social ties. In addition to the individual sessions, some patients (less than a third) participated in group sessions with five to eight other patients. These groups provided opportunities for the patients to exchange social support among themselves, offering both informational and emotional support. Participation in both individual and group sessions continued for six months or until the patient reported being engaged in a supportive social relationship and had achieved a threshold score on a measure of perceived social support (ENRICHD Investigators, 2001).

Of the 2,481 patients who were randomized to the control (that is, usual care) or intervention groups, 39 percent were depressed, 26 percent had low perceived social support, and 34 percent met both criteria. At the six-month follow-up, among those who had been low in social support at baseline, the intervention participants experienced a significantly greater increase in social support than did the usual-care-group participants. This effect was attenuated over time, but some benefit remained up to three years after baseline. Unfortunately, at no point in the four-year follow-up period did the intervention group experience fewer recurrent nonfatal myocardial infarctions nor cardiac deaths than the usual care group (ENRICHD Investigators, 2003).

However, post hoc analyses indicated that participants who were not married and did not have a significant other benefited from the intervention more than did those with partners. Furthermore, participants without a partner but who had moderate levels of social support (as opposed to very low levels) available to them at baseline benefited the most (Burg and others, 2005). The investigators suggest that the therapist may have served as a surrogate partner for those without a partner, whereas a couples therapy approach might have been more effective in enhancing an existing partner relationship. In addition, for those without a partner and with low baseline support levels, additional opportunities to develop new supportive ties (for example, in a support group) may be necessary to achieve and maintain higher levels of support (Burg and others, 2005). Thus, conducting an assessment of the participants' social networks first and then matching them with an appropriate mode of intervention might have resulted in larger and more durable increases in social support. The ENRICHD investigators admit that the magnitude or the duration of the increase achieved in the trial may simply not have been sufficient to protect against subsequent morbidity and mortality.

Also, patients were enrolled in the study while still hospitalized due to their myocardial infarction. Although negative health-related life events can be viewed as windows of opportunity for health behavior change, the time immediately subsequent to a myocardial infarction might be a particularly difficult time to depend solely on the patient to bring about long-lasting changes in his or her own social network. Including other social network members in the intervention and developing a shared responsibility for increasing the exchange of support might have been more effective.

The Seattle–King County Healthy Homes Project

Asthma is the most common chronic disease of childhood, disproportionately affecting low-income children and children of color (American Lung Association, 2006). Indoor air quality is a major contributor to the development and exacerbation of asthma (Institute of Medicine, 2000). The SKCHHP (Seattle–King County Healthy Homes Project) had the goal of improving the asthma-related health status of low-income children by reducing exposure to allergens and irritants in their homes. The project was developed under the auspices of Seattle Partners for Healthy Communities, with its commitment to principles of community-researcher collaboration (Krieger and others, 2002).

CHWs were recruited from the communities being served by the project. All six CHWs hired by the project lived within the targeted areas and were either personally affected by asthma or had a close family member with asthma. CHWs, because they are members of the community, have an "insider perspective"—an understanding of the culture and workings of the community (Love, Gardner, and Legion, 1997). Thus, the CHWs are perceived to have more empathic understanding (Thoits, 1995) for the community participants and to be credible sources of information and advice. Often, CHWs are hired to work in underserved, low-income areas where they provide a culturally appropriate linkage between the community and the medical system or other service providers (Love, Gardner, and Legion, 1997).

The SKCHHP CHWs completed a forty-hour training that focused on knowledge and skills relevant to assessing and changing the home environment to reduce exposure to asthma triggers. Once trained, the CHWs made home visits to families who had enrolled in the project. Rather than conducting the assessments and carrying out the change strategies *for* the families, the CHWs provided the knowledge, resources, and support necessary to empower the families to take action for themselves. The CHWs worked with each of the families to develop a Home Action Plan, based on the results of the home environment assessment, and then assisted families in carrying out the plans. CHWs visited the homes of participants five to nine times over the course of a year, with each visit averaging forty-five to fifty minutes (Krieger and others, 2002).

The CHWs were expected to use a caring and empathic approach with each family. They provided instrumental, informational, and emotional support. They educated the families about the various asthma triggers in the homes and how best to reduce them, assisted with some of the cleaning and repair tasks called for by the Home Action Plan, and identified community resources that could help meet the needs of the families, whether asthma-related or not. Perhaps most important, the CHWs were attentive to the concerns of each family, providing individualized advice, assistance, and encouragement. In general, participants were impressed with the efforts of the CHWs, with 84 percent of them rating their CHWs as excellent or very good (Krieger and others, 2002).

The effectiveness of the project was evaluated through a randomized trial with a one-year follow-up period. Households (n = 274) were randomly assigned to either a high-intensity intervention (the program as described earlier) or a low-intensity intervention (one home visit by a CHW to assess the home environment, create an action plan, and provide limited education and resources). After one year, the children of families in the high-intensity group had a larger decrease in the number of days with activity limited by asthma and in the number of times urgent health services were used than did the children in the low-intensity group. In addition, the children's caregivers in the high-intensity group reported more improvement in quality of life than did those in the low-intensity group. Behaviors intended to reduce asthma triggers in the home also increased more among the families in the high-intensity group. Some limited data suggested that these gains in health outcomes and behaviors were sustained for at least another six months after the first follow-up (Krieger, Takaro, Song, and Weaver, 2005).

FUTURE DIRECTIONS FOR RESEARCH AND PRACTICE

Both of the interventions described here illustrate the importance of tailoring social network interventions to the needs and resources of participants. No generic social network intervention is likely to be effective for everyone. Thus, establishing participatory assessment processes, during which individuals and communities describe the strengths and weaknesses of their social networks, will help structure programs to be optimally effective.

Social network interventions are most likely to be effective if developed and implemented within an ecological framework that considers multiple levels of influence (McLeroy, Gottlieb, and Heaney, 2001). For example, interventions that enhance individuals' motivation and skills for performing healthy behaviors while also enhancing the health-promoting qualities of social networks have great potential. In addition, given our growing understanding of the extent to which broad social forces (for example, crime rates and income disparities) influence the structure and function of social networks (Berkman, Glass, Brissette, and Seeman, 2000), interventions that attempt to enhance social networks within the context of community-based problem-solving efforts hold promise. Thus, an important direction for future research is to develop and evaluate social network interventions that include strategies across multiple units of practice (for example, individual, family, and community).

It is important to evaluate both intervention processes and outcomes (Israel and others, 1995). Effective social network interventions will be advanced through (1) carefully describing the intervention activities, (2) monitoring the effects of these activities on the amount and quality of social support both delivered and received, and (3) assessing changes in knowledge, health behaviors, community capacity, or health status. Rigorous and comprehensive evaluation studies will improve our ability to consistently translate the health-protective effects of social networks and social support into effective interventions.

SUMMARY

Social networks influence health and well-being in various ways, including by facilitating the exchange of social support. Consistent empirical evidence suggests that people who maintain strong social relationships are healthier and live longer. However, our understanding of how to enhance social networks and increase the exchange of social support among network members is just beginning. Evaluation of carefully designed and meticulously theory-informed social network interventions will help advance our ability to answer the question posed earlier: In order to effectively enhance the health-protective functions of social networks, *who* should provide *what* to *whom* (and *when*)?

REFERENCES

Agneessens, F., Waege, H., and Lievens, J. "Diversity in Social Support by Role Relations: A Typology." *Social Networks,* 2006, *28,* 427–441.

American Lung Association. "Trends in Asthma Mortality and Morbidity." [http://www.lungusa.org/atf/cf/{7A8D42C2-FCCA-4604–8ADE-7F5D5E762256}/ASTHMA06FINAL.PDF]. July 2006.

Bandura, A. *Social Foundations of Thought and Action.* Englewood Cliffs, N.J.: Prentice Hall, 1986.

Barnes, J. A. "Class and Committees in a Norwegian Island Parish." *Human Relations,* 1954, *7,* 39–58.

Barrera, M. "Social Support Research in Community Psychology." In J. Rappaport and E. Seidman (eds.), *Handbook of Community Psychology.* New York: Kluwer Academic/Plenum, 2000.

Berkman, L. F., and Glass, T. "Social Integration, Social Networks, Social Support, and Health." In L. F. Berkman and I. Kawachi (eds.), *Social Epidemiology.* New York: Oxford University Press, 2000.

Berkman, L. F., Glass, T., Brissette, I., and Seeman, T. E. "From Social Integration to Health: Durkheim in the New Millennium." *Social Science and Medicine,* 2000, *51,* 843–857.

Blanchard, C. G., and others. "The Role of Social Support in Adaptation to Cancer and to Survival." *Journal of Psychosocial Oncology,* 1995, *13,* 75–95.

Boutilier, M., Cleverly, S., and Labonte, R. "Community as a Setting for Health Promotion." In B. D. Poland, L. W. Green, and I. Rootman (eds.), *Settings for Health Promotion: Linking Theory and Practice.* Thousand Oaks, Calif.: Sage, 2000.

Burg, M. M., and Seeman, T. E. "Families and Health: The Negative Side of Social Ties." *Annals of Behavioral Medicine,* 1994, *16,* 109–115.

Burg, M. M., and others. "Low Perceived Social Support and Post-Myocardial Infarction Prognosis in the Enhancing Recovery in Coronary Heart Disease Clinical Trial: The Effects of Treatment." *Psychosomatic Medicine,* 2005, *67,* 879–888.

Cassel, J. "The Contribution of the Social Environment to Host Resistance." *American Journal of Epidemiology,* 1976, *104,* 107–123.

Chesler, M. A., and Chesney, B. K. *Cancer and Self-Help: Bridging the Troubled Waters of Childhood Illness.* Madison: University of Wisconsin Press, 1995.

Cohen, S., Underwood, L. G., and Gottlieb, B. H. (eds.). *Social Support Measurement and Intervention.* New York: Oxford University Press, 2000.

Cohen, S., and Wills, T. "Stress, Social Support, and the Buffering Hypothesis." *Psychological Bulletin,* 1985, *98,* 310–357.

Cohen, S., and others. "Social Ties and Susceptibility to the Common Cold." *Journal of the American Medical Association,* 1997, *277,* 1940–1944.

Cranford, J. A. "Stress-Buffering or Stress-Exacerbation? Social Support and Social Undermining as Moderators of the Relationship Between Perceived Stress and Depressive Symptoms Among Married People." *Personal Relationships,* 2004, *11,* 23–40.

DiMatteo, M. "Social Support and Patient Adherence to Medical Treatment: A Meta-Analysis." *Health Psychology,* 2004, *23,* 207–218.

Earp, J. L., and others. "Lay Health Advisors: A Strategy for Getting the Word Out About Breast Cancer." *Health Education and Behavior,* 1997, *24,* 432–451.

Eckenrode, J., and Hamilton, S. "One-to-One Support Interventions: Home Visitation and Mentoring." In S. Cohen, L. G. Underwood, and B. H. Gottlieb (eds.), *Social Support Measurement and Intervention.* New York: Oxford University Press, 2000.

Eng, E., and Hatch, J. W. "Networking Between Agencies and Black Churches: The Lay Health Advisor Model." *Prevention in Human Services,* 1991, *10,* 123–146.

Eng, E., and Parker, E. "Measuring Community Competence in the Mississippi Delta: The Interface between Program Evaluation and Empowerment." *Health Education Quarterly,* 1994, *21,* 199–220.

Eng, E., and Young, R. "Lay Health Advisors as Community Change Agents." *Family and Community Health,* 1992, *15,* 24–40.

ENRICHD Investigators. "Enhancing Recovery in Coronary Heart Disease (ENRICHD) Study Intervention: Rationale and Design." *Psychosomatic Medicine,* 2001, *63,* 747–755.

ENRICHD Investigators. "Effects of Treating Depression and Low Perceived Social Support on Clinical Events After Myocardial Infarction." *Journal of the American Medical Association,* 2003, *289,* 3106–3116.

Eysenbach, G., and others. "Health Related Virtual Communities and Electronic Support Groups: Systematic Review of the Effects of Online Peer to Peer Interactions." *BMJ,* 2004, *328,* 1166.

Feeney, B., and Collins, N. "Motivations for Caregiving in Adult Intimate Relationships: Influences on Caregiving Behaviors and Relationship Functioning." *Personality and Social Psychology Bulletin,* 2003, *29,* 950–968.

Ferlander, S. "The Importance of Different Forms of Social Capital for Health". *Acta Sociologica,* 2007, *50,* 115–128.

Fleishman, J. A., and others. "Coping, Conflictual Social Interactions, Social Support, and Mood Among HIV-Infected Persons." *American Journal of Community Psychology,* 2000, *28*(4), 421–430.

Friedman, A. R., and others. "Allies Community Health Workers: Bridging the Gap." *Health Promotion Practice,* 2006, *7*(2 Suppl), 96S–107S.

Glass, T. A., and others. "Psychosocial Intervention in Stroke: Families in Recovery From Stroke Trial (FIRST)." *American Journal of Orthopsychiatry,* 2000, *70,* 169–181.

Gottlieb, B. H. "Selecting and Planning Support Interventions." In S. Cohen, L. G. Underwood, and B. H. Gottlieb (eds.), *Social Support Measurement and Intervention.* New York: Oxford University Press, 2000.

Gottlieb, B. H., and Wagner, F. "Stress and Support Processes in Close Relationships." In J. Eckenrode (ed.), *The Social Context of Coping.* New York: Plenum Press, 1991.

Granovetter, M. "The Strength of Weak Ties." *Sociological Theory,* 1983, *1,* 201–233.

Haber, M. G., Cohen J. L., Lucas, T., and Baltes, B. B. "The Relationship Between Self-Reported Received and Perceived Social Support: A Meta-Analytic Review." *American Journal of Community Psychology,* 2007, *39,* 133–144.

Heaney, C. A. "Enhancing Social Support at the Workplace: Assessing the Effects of the Caregiver Support Program." *Health Education Quarterly,* 1991, *18,* 477–494.

Helgeson, V. S., and Gottlieb, B. H. "Support Groups." In S. Cohen, L. G. Underwood, and B. H. Gottlieb (eds.), *Social Support Measurement and Intervention.* New York: Oxford University Press, 2000.

Heller, K., and others. "Peer Support Telephone Dyads for Elderly Women: Was This the Wrong Intervention?" *American Journal of Community Psychology,* 1991, *19,* 53–74.

Hodnett, E., Gates, S., Hofmeyr, G., and Sakala, C. "Continuous Support for Women During Childbirth." *Cochrane Database Systematic Reviews,* 2007, *3,* CD003766.

House, J. S. *Work Stress and Social Support.* Reading, Mass.: Addison-Wesley, 1981.

House, J. S. "Social Support and Social Structure." *Sociological Forum,* 1987, *2,* 135–146.

House, J. S. "Social Isolation Kills—But How and Why?" *Psychosomatic Medicine,* 2001, *63,* 273–274.

House, J. S., Umberson, D., and Landis, K. R. "Structures and Processes of Social Support." *Annual Review of Sociology,* 1988, *14,* 293–318.

Institute of Medicine. *Clearing the Air: Asthma and Indoor Air Exposures.* Washington, D.C.: National Academy Press, 2000.

Israel, B. A. "Social Networks and Health Status: Linking Theory, Research, and Practice." *Patient Counseling and Health Education,* 1982, *4,* 65–79.

Israel, B. A. "Social Networks and Social Support: Implications for Natural Helper and Community Level Interventions." *Health Education Quarterly,* 1985, *12,* 65–80.

Israel, B. A., and others. "Evaluation of Health Education Programs: Current Assessment and Future Directions." *Health Education Quarterly,* 1995, *22,* 364–389.

Kahn, R. L., and Antonucci, T. C. "Convoys Over the Life Course: Attachments, Roles and Social Support." In P. B. Baltes and O. Brim (eds.), *Life Span Development and Behavior.* Volume 3. New York: Academic Press, 1980.

Kegler, M., and Malcoe, L. H. "Results from a Lay Health Advisor Intervention to Prevent Lead Poisoning Among Rural Native American Children." *American Journal of Public Health,* 2004, *94,* 1730–1735.

Krause, N. "Assessing Stress-Buffering Effects: A Cautionary Note." *Psychology and Aging,* 1995, *10,* 518–526.

Krieger, J. W., Takaro, T. K., Song, L., and Weaver, M. "The Seattle-King County Healthy Homes Project: A Randomized, Controlled Trial of a Community Health Worker Intervention to Decrease Exposure to Indoor Asthma Triggers." *American Journal of Public Health,* 2005, *95,* 652–659.

Krieger, J., and others. "The Seattle-King County Healthy Homes Project: Implementation of a Comprehensive Approach to Improving Indoor Environmental Quality for Low Income Children with Asthma." *Environmental Health Perspectives,* 2002, *110,* 311–322.

LaVeist, T. A., Sellers, R. M., Brown, K. A., and Nickerson, K. J. "Extreme Social Isolation, Use of Community-Based Senior Support Services, and Mortality Among African American Women." *American Journal of Community Psychology,* 1997, *25,* 721–732.

Lett, H. S., and others. "Social Support and Coronary Heart Disease: Epidemiologic Evidence and Implications for Treatment." *Psychosomatic Medicine,* 2005, *67,* 869–878.

Love, M. B., Gardner, K., and Legion, V. "Community Health Workers: Who They Are and What They Do." *Health Education and Behavior,* 1997, *24,* 510–522.

McKinlay, J. B. "Social Network Influences on Morbid Episodes and the Career of Help Seeking." In L. Eisenberg and A. Kleinman (eds.), *The Relevance of Social Science for Medicine.* Dordrecht,, The Netherlands: D. Reidel Publishing, 1980.

McLeroy, K. R., Gottlieb, N. H., and Heaney, C. A. "Social Health." In M. P. O'Donnell and J. S. Harris (eds.), *Health Promotion in the Workplace.* (3rd ed.) Albany, New York: Delmar, 2001.

McQuiston, C., and Flaskerud, J. "If They Don't Ask About Condoms, I Just Tell Them: A Descriptive Case Study of Latino Lay Health Advisors' Helping Activities." *Health Education and Behavior,* 2003, *30,* 79–96.

Michael, Y. L., Colditz, G. A., Coakley, E., and Kawachi, I. "Health Behaviors, Social Networks, and Healthy Aging: Cross-Sectional Evidence from the Nurses' Health Study." *Quality of Life Research,* 1999, 8, 711–722.

Minkler, M. "Community Organizing Among the Elderly Poor in San Francisco's Tenderloin District." In J. Rothman, J. L. Erlich, and J. E. Tropman (eds.), *Strategies of Community Intervention.* Itasca, Ill.: Peacock Publishers, 2001.

Oetzel, J., Duran, B., Jiang, Y., and Lucero, J. "Social Support and Social Undermining as Correlates for Alcohol, Drug, and Mental Disorders in American Indian Women Presenting for Primary Care at an Indian Health Service Hospital." *Journal of Health Communication,* 2007, *12,* 187–206.

Palmer, C. A., Baucom, D. H., and McBride, C. M. "Couple Approaches to Smoking Cessation." In K. B. Schmaling and T. G. Sher (eds.), *The Psychology of Couples and Illness: Theory, Research, and Practice.* Washington, D.C.: American Psychological Association, 2000.

Rhodes, J. E. *Stand by Me: The Risks and Rewards of Mentoring Today's Youth.* Cambridge, Mass.: Harvard University Press, 2002.

Rothman, J., Erlich, J. L., and Tropman, J. E. *Strategies of Community Intervention.* Itasca, Ill.: Peacock, 2001.

Sandler, I. N., and others. "Linking Empirically Based Theory and Evaluation: The Family Bereavement Program." *American Journal of Community Psychology,* 1992, *20,* 491–521.

Schulz, A. J., and others. "Addressing Social Determinants of Health through Community-Based Participatory Research: The East Side Village Health Worker Partnership." *Health Education and Behavior,* 2002, *29,* 326–341.

Shumaker, S. A., and Hill, D. R. "Gender Differences in Social Support and Physical Health." *Health Psychology,* 1991, *10,* 102–111.

Spiegel, D., and Diamond, S. "Psychosocial Interventions in Cancer, Group Therapy Techniques." In A. Baum and B. L. Andersen (eds.), *Psychosocial Interventions for Cancer.* Washington, D.C.: American Psychological Association, 2001.

Starrett, R. A., and others. "The Role of Environmental Awareness and Support Networks in Hispanic Elderly Persons' Use of Formal Social Services." *Journal of Community Psychology,* 1990, *18,* 218–227.

Thoits, P. A. "Stress, Coping, and Social Support Processes: Where Are We? What Next?" *Journal of Health and Social Behavior,* 1995, *Spec. No.,* 53–79.

Uchino, B. *Social Support and Physical Health: Understanding the Health Consequences of Relationships.* New Haven, Conn.: Yale University Press, 2004.

Uchino, B. "Social Support and Health: A Review of Physiological Processes Potentially Underlying Links to Disease Outcomes." *Journal of Behavioral Medicine,* 2006, *29,* 377–387.

Vogt, T. M., and others. "Social Networks as Predictors of Ischemic Heart Disease, Cancer, Stroke, Hypertension—Incidence, Survival, and Mortality." *Journal of Clinical Epidemiology,* 1992, *45,* 659–666.

Wang, H.-X., Mittleman, M., and Orth-Gomer, K. "Influence of Social Support on Progression of Coronary Artery Disease in Women." *Social Science and Medicine,* 2005, *60,* 599–607.

Wethington, E., and Kessler, R. C. "Perceived Support, Received Support, and Adjustment to Stressful Life Events." *Journal of Health and Social Behavior,* 1986, *27,* 78–89.

Wing, R. R., and Jeffery, R. W. "Benefits of Recruiting Participants with Friends and Increasing Social Support for Weight Loss and Maintenance." *Journal of Consulting and Clinical Psychology,* 1999, *67,* 132–138.

Wood, J. V. "What Is Social Comparison and How Should We Study It?" *Personality and Social Psychology Bulletin,* 1996, *22*(5), 520–537.

Wortman, C. B., and Lehman, D. R. "Reactions to Victims of Life Crises: Support Attempts that Fail." In I. G. Sarason and B. R. Sarason (eds.), *Social Support: Theory, Research, and Applications.* Dordrecht, The Netherlands: Martinus Nijhoff, 1985.

CHAPTER

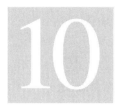

STRESS, COPING, AND HEALTH BEHAVIOR

Karen Glanz
Marc D. Schwartz

KEY POINTS

This chapter will

- Review major theories, research, and applications related to stress, coping, and health.
- Summarize historical concepts of health, stress, and coping.
- Describe an influential theoretical framework—the Transactional Model of Stress and Coping—and key variables, definitions, and research approaches to studying this framework.
- Discuss theoretical extensions of the Transactional Model, including information-seeking styles, social support, optimism, and psychoneuroimmunology.
- Illustrate applications of the Transactional Model to understanding the use of coping strategies and the design and evaluation of health behavior interventions.

Understanding stress and coping is essential to health education, health promotion, and disease prevention. *Stressors* are demands made by the internal or external environment that upset balance or homeostasis, thus affecting physical and psychological well-being and requiring action to restore balance or equilibrium (Lazarus and Cohen, 1977). Stress can contribute to illness through its direct physiological effects or indirect effects via maladaptive health behaviors (for example, smoking, poor eating habits). Stress does not affect all people equally; some people live through terribly threatening experiences, yet manage to cope well and do not get ill. Further, many people experience growth and find positive lessons from stressful experiences, as studies of cancer survivors demonstrate (see, for example, Carver and Antoni, 2004). The ways in which individuals who are ill or at risk for illness have for coping can be important influences on their psychological and physical health outcomes. Support from friends, family, and health care providers in the face of stress can also have profound effects on psychological and physical outcomes.

The illness experience, medical treatment, a diagnosis of illness, and fear of developing an illness all can provoke stressful reactions. How individuals experience and cope with stress affects whether and how they seek medical care and social support, and how well they adhere to health professionals' advice. Reactions to stressors can promote or inhibit healthful practices, and influence motivation to practice habits that promote health. Issues related to stress and coping have taken on expanded public health relevance in recent years, in the face of emerging issues such as preparedness for natural disasters and human-made acts of terrorism, as well as in the growing numbers of survivors of once-fatal diseases, such as cancer.

A better understanding of theory and the empirical literature on stress and coping is essential to developing effective strategies and programs for individuals to improve coping and enhance psychological and physical well-being. The purpose of this chapter is to review major theories, research, and applications related to stress, coping, and health.

HISTORICAL CONCEPTS OF HEALTH, STRESS, AND COPING

Conceptualizations of health, stress, and coping are derived from numerous branches of research, with the earliest work conducted by scientists in the fields of biology and psychophysiology (for example, Cannon, 1932). Diverse health and behavioral science disciplines, including epidemiology, personality psychology, cognitive and social psychology, and medicine, have contributed to understanding stress and coping.

Early work on stress focused on physiological reactions to stressful stimuli. Cannon (1932) is credited with first describing the "fight-or-flight" reaction to stress. Hans Selye, the father of modern stress research, extended Cannon's studies with clinical observations and laboratory research. He hypothesized that all living organisms exhibited nonspecific changes in response to stressors, labeled as a three-stage General Adaptation Syndrome (GAS). This syndrome consists of an alarm reaction, resistance, and exhaustion (Selye, 1956). Each stage evokes both physiological and behavioral responses. Without curative measures, physical and/or psychological deterioration occurs.

Another major stream of stress research in the 1960s and 1970s focused on identifying and quantifying potential stressors, or *stressful life events*. Holmes and Rahe (1967) developed the Social Readjustment Rating Scale (SRRS), a tool to measure stressful life events. Studies showed that people with high scores on the SRRS had more illness episodes than those with low scores. This scale stimulated a substantial body of research (Dohrenwend and Dohrenwend, 1981), despite numerous methodological limitations.

Beginning in the 1960s and 1970s, stress was considered to be a transactional phenomenon dependent on the meaning of the stimulus to perceivers (Lazarus, 1966;

Antonovsky, 1979). The central concept is that a given event or situation is perceived in different ways by different people. Moreover, these perceptions, rather than the objective stressors, are the main determinants of effects on behaviors and on health status. Some researchers in the field of occupational stress and health used this concept as a foundation for a model that viewed occupational stress as resulting from the interactions between individual workers' characteristics and the work environment, or the "person-environment fit" (House, 1974). These lines of theory led to an examination of possible buffering, or moderating factors, and, in particular, to a focus on the role of social support (Cohen and Wills, 1985).

Parallel research in biology and epidemiology shows that some personality dispositions and psychological states (for example, fatalism, hostility, and emotional suppression) are linked to disease endpoints (Scheier and Bridges, 1995). Chronic stressors and responses to them affect the sympathetic nervous system and endocrine functions, thus influencing the occurrence and progression of health problems, including cancer, infectious diseases, and HIV/AIDS (Glaser and Kiecolt-Glaser, 2005). Research in stress and coping has often been challenged by the view that both psychological and biological factors account for some effects on health status and health behavior.

Clearly, there are numerous and important areas of research and theory on stress and health. In this chapter, we emphasize cognitive-behavioral theory and research because of the direct relevance to public health, health education, and health behavior change.

THE TRANSACTIONAL MODEL OF STRESS AND COPING: OVERVIEW, KEY CONSTRUCTS, AND EMPIRICAL SUPPORT

The Transactional Model of Stress and Coping is a framework for evaluating processes of coping with stressful events. Stressful experiences are construed as person–environment *transactions,* in which the impact of an external stressor, or demand, is mediated by the person's appraisal of the stressor and the psychological, social, and cultural resources at his or her disposal (Lazarus and Cohen, 1977; Cohen, 1984). When faced with a stressor, a person evaluates potential threats or harms (*primary appraisal),* as well as his or her ability to alter the situation and manage negative emotional reactions (*secondary appraisal*). Actual *coping efforts,* aimed at problem management and emotional regulation, give rise to *outcomes* of the coping process (for example, psychological well-being, functional status, and adherence).

Recent extensions of coping theory suggest that positive psychological states should also be taken into account. Thus, during a stressful period, numerous affect-inducing events occur that may allow for a co-occurrence of negative and positive affect during the same period of time (Folkman and Moskowitz, 2000). For example, positive affect may facilitate processing of self-relevant information, serve as a buffer against adverse physiological consequences of stress, and protect against clinical depression (Moskowitz, Folkman, Collette, and Vittinghoff, l996). Accordingly, Folkman proposed that a cognitive theory of stress and coping should accommodate positive psychological states (Folkman and Moskowitz, 2000). The extension of this theory to positive psychological states is discussed in more detail later in this chapter.

Table 10.1 summarizes key concepts, definitions, and applications of the Transactional Model of Stress and Coping. Figure 10.1 (see page 216) illustrates interrelationships among these concepts. As shown in the figure, positive psychological states may be the result of meaning-based coping processes, and they can also lead back to appraisal and coping. For more extensive discussions of theoretical underpinnings of the model, readers should refer to the work of Lazarus, Folkman, and Moskowitz (Lazarus and Folkman, 1984; Folkman and Moskowitz, 2000).

TABLE 10.1. Transactional Model of Stress and Coping.

Concept	Definition	Application
Primary appraisal	Evaluation of the significance of a stressor or threatening event	Perceptions of an event as threatening can cause distress. If an event is perceived as positive, benign, or irrelevant, little negative threat is felt.
Secondary appraisal	Evaluation of the controllability of the stressor and a person's coping resources	Perception of one's ability to change the situation, manage one's emotional reaction, and/or cope effectively can lead to successful coping and adaptation.
Coping efforts	Actual strategies used to mediate primary and secondary appraisals	
Problem management	Strategies directed at changing a stressful situation	Active coping, problem solving, and information seeking may be used.
Emotional regulation	Strategies aimed at changing the way one thinks or feels about a stressful situation	Venting feelings, avoidance, denial, and seeking social support may be used.
Meaning-based coping	Coping processes that induce positive emotion, which in turn sustains the coping process by allowing reenactment of problem- or emotion-focused coping	Positive reappraisal, revised goals, spiritual beliefs, positive events.
Outcomes of coping (adaptation)	Emotional well-being, functional status, health behaviors	Coping strategies may result in short- and long-term positive or negative adaptation.

TABLE 10.1. **Transactional Model of Stress and Coping, Cont'd.**

Concept	Definition	Application
Dispositional coping styles	Generalized ways of behaving that can affect a person's emotional or functional reaction to a stressor; relatively stable across time and situations	
Information seeking	Attentional styles that are vigilant (monitoring) versus those that involve avoidance (blunting)	Monitoring may increase distress and arousal; it may also increase active coping. Blunting may mute excessive worry but may reduce adherence.
Optimism	Tendency to have generalized positive expectancies for outcomes	Optimists may experience fewer symptoms and/or faster recovery from illness.

Primary Appraisal

Primary appraisal is a person's judgment about the significance of an event as stressful, positive, controllable, challenging, benign, or irrelevant. Health problems are usually evaluated initially as threatening or as negative stressors. Two basic primary appraisals are perceptions of *susceptibility* to the threat and perceptions of *severity* of the threat. According to the Transactional Model of Stress and Coping, appraisals of personal risk and threat severity prompt efforts to cope with the stressor. For example, a woman who perceives herself at risk for breast cancer may be motivated to obtain mammograms (problem-focused coping) and may seek social support to cope with her concerns about the threat (emotion-focused coping). However, heightened perceptions of risk can also generate distress. Among women with a family history of ovarian cancer, those who perceive themselves as highly susceptible are more prone to experience aversive, intrusive thoughts and psychological distress (Schwartz and others, 1995). Appraisals of high severity and susceptibility can also prompt escape-avoidance behaviors (Lazarus and Folkman, 1984). This can have the paradoxical effect of reducing adherence to health-promoting practices, such as adherence to recommended breast cancer screening guidelines (Lerman and others, 1993).

Primary appraisals also act to minimize the significance of threats, particularly when the threat is ambiguous or uncertain. This "appraisal bias" was demonstrated in a series of well-designed studies by Croyle and colleagues (Ditto and Croyle, 1995). Employing a test for a fictitious enzyme disorder, they showed that those who were informed of abnormal test results rated the disorder as less serious and the test itself as less valid than did those who received "normal" test results. Such "minimizing" appraisals also have been shown to reduce distress associated with real health threats.

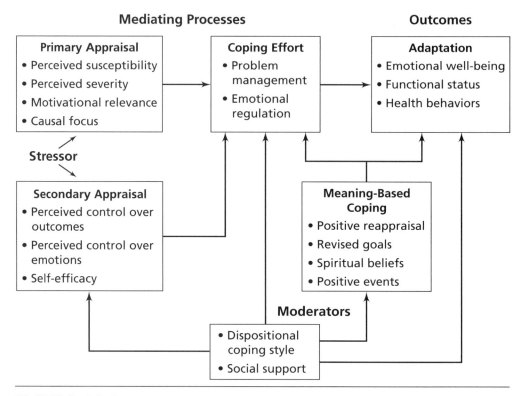

FIGURE 10.1. Transactional Model of Stress and Coping.

For example, beliefs of invulnerability among breast cancer patients and HIV-positive men were associated with reduced distress, enhanced perceived control and active coping, and better overall adjustment (Taylor and others, 1992). However, other studies suggest that minimizing appraisals may also diminish motivation to adopt recommended preventive health behaviors such as dietary restrictions and smoking cessation (Chapman, Wong, and Smith, 1993).

Other primary appraisals involve the *motivational relevance* and *causal focus* of the stressor. When a stressor is appraised as having a major impact on a person's goals or concerns (high motivational relevance), that person is likely to experience anxiety and situation-specific distress (Smith and Lazarus, 1993). This may be especially true when the relevance is to one's own physical health or well-being. Perceiving oneself as responsible for the stressor (self-causal focus) may be more likely to generate guilt and depression, rather than anxiety (Smith, Haynes, Lazarus, and Pope, 1993). However, the most important aspect of causal appraisals of illness may be whether or nor they are generated at all.

Secondary Appraisal

Secondary appraisal is an assessment of a person's coping resources and options (Cohen, 1984). In contrast to primary appraisals that focus on features of the stressful situation, secondary appraisals address what one can do about the situation. Key examples of secondary appraisals are *perceived ability to change the situation* (for example, perceived control over the threat), *perceived ability to manage one's emotional reactions* to the threat (for example, perceived control over feelings), and *expectations about the effectiveness of one's coping resources* (for example, coping self-efficacy).

Positive associations between perceptions of control over illness and psychological adjustment have been observed across a wide variety of diseases. These include cancer (Norton and others, 2005), heart disease (Moser and others, 2007), and HIV/AIDS (Taylor and others, 1992). Moreover, perceived control over illness may improve physical well-being by increasing the likelihood that a person will adopt recommended health behaviors. For example, perceived control over health outcomes is related positively to safe sexual behaviors (Taylor and others, 1992; Kok, Hospers, Harterink, and de Zwart, 2007). In situations that cannot be altered (such as severe or fatal disease), high levels of perceived control may increase distress and dysfunction (Affleck, Tennen, Pfeiffer, and Fifield, 1987). Beliefs about personal control are likely to be adaptive only to the extent that they "fit" with reality.

Beliefs about one's ability to perform the behaviors necessary to exert control (that is, self-efficacy) play a central role in performance of a variety of health behaviors. For example, self-efficacy beliefs predict success with smoking cessation attempts, as well as maintenance of exercise and diet regimens (Bandura, 1997). Self-efficacy—a central construct of Social Cognitive Theory (SCT; see Chapter Eight)—is specific to a given behavior, not a global personality trait. For example, a sedentary nonsmoker may have high self-efficacy for avoiding tobacco use but low self-efficacy for exercising regularly.

Coping Efforts

According to the Transactional Model, emotional and functional effects of primary and secondary appraisals are mediated by actual *coping strategies* (Lazarus and Folkman, 1984). Original formulations of the model conceptualized coping efforts along two dimensions: (1) problem management and (2) emotional regulation. Also referred to as problem-focused coping, problem-management strategies are directed at changing the stressful situation. Examples of problem-focused coping include active coping, problem solving, and information seeking. By contrast, emotion-focused coping efforts are directed at changing the way one thinks or feels about a stressful situation. These strategies include seeking social support and venting feelings, as well as avoidance, and denial. The model predicts that problem-focused coping strategies will be most adaptive for stressors that are changeable, whereas emotion-focused strategies are most adaptive when the stressor is unchangeable or when this strategy is used in conjunction with problem-focused coping strategies.

Empirical studies of coping have focused on the extent to which an individual engages versus disengages with the stressor (Carver and others, 1993). When a stressor is perceived as highly threatening and uncontrollable, a person may be more likely to use disengaging coping strategies (Taylor and others, 1992). Examples of disengaging coping strategies include distancing, cognitive avoidance (that is, trying not to think about a stressor), behavioral avoidance (for example, not going for a follow-up test due to fear that an abnormal screening result means a cancer diagnosis), distraction, and denial. Each of these strategies shifts attention away from the stressor. This attentional shift may allow individuals to minimize their initial distress by avoiding thoughts and feelings about the stressor (Suls and Fletcher, 1985). Ultimately, however, avoidance or denial may lead to intrusive thoughts that can generate increased distress over time (Carver and others, 1993; Schwartz and others, 1995) and keep people from developing healthier coping strategies. For that reason, avoidance and denial are often considered maladaptive. By contrast, when a stressor is appraised as controllable and a person has favorable beliefs about self-efficacy, he or she is more likely to use engaging coping strategies. Examples of engaging coping strategies include active coping, planning problem solving, information seeking, and making use of social support.

Other common coping responses to health threats use *meaning-based coping,* which can induce positive emotion. These include positive reinterpretation, acceptance, and use of religion and spirituality (Carver and others, 1993). These processes involve interpretation of a stressful situation in a personally meaningful way.

There are interesting parallels between the coping strategies in the Transactional Model and the change processes in the Transtheoretical Model, also known as the Stages of Change Model (see Chapter Five). For example, self-reevaluation is a change process that can facilitate progression from the contemplation stage of behavior change to the preparation stage. Similar to emotion-focused coping strategies such as reappraisal, self-reevaluation involves assessing and, in some cases, altering how one feels about a problem. Likewise, change processes such as stimulus control and counter-conditioning (or substitution of alternatives for problem behaviors) could be considered problem-focused coping strategies.

Several theoretically driven scales have been developed to assess coping efforts. Typically, respondents are asked to describe a stressful situation they have experienced and to answer questions about how they would evaluate and respond to the situation. The most widely used subscales address problem-focused coping and emotion-focused coping (Stone, Greenberg, Kennedy-Moore, and Newman, 1991). Examples of available tools include the Ways of Coping Inventory (WOC) (Folkman and Lazarus, 1988), the Multidimensional Coping Inventory (Endler and Parker, 1990), and the Coping Orientations to Problems Experienced (COPE) scale (Carver, Scheier, and Weintraub, 1989). The COPE questionnaire uses twelve subscales to measure types of coping strategies, including active coping, suppression of competing activities, planning, restraint, social support, positive reframing, religion, acceptance, denial, disengagement, use of humor, and self-distraction (Carver and others, 1993). Scales to measure daily use of coping strategies may provide more precise assessments of coping transactions (Stone, Kennedy-Moore, and Neale, 1995). The Cancer Behavior Inventory (CBI) (Merluzzi and others, 2001)—a new measure of self-efficacy for coping with cancer—provides a refined tool to assess secondary appraisal. The CBI includes eight subscales: maintenance of activity and independence, seeking and understanding medical information, stress management, coping with treatment-related side effects, accepting cancer/maintaining positive attitude, affective regulation, and seeking support.

The Transactional Model has generated an extensive body of literature on coping strategies, adjustment to illness, and health behavior (Stanton, Revenson, and Tennen, 2007). In general, these studies provide evidence for the psychological benefits of active coping strategies and acceptance/reappraisal over avoidant or disengaging strategies (for example, Carver and others, 1993; Taylor and others, 1992). More recent studies have reinforced the significant association between use of avoidant coping (for example, avoiding others, hiding feelings, and refusing to think about the illness) and higher levels of psychological distress (Baider and others, 1997), poorer quality of life (Trask and others, 2001), and risky health behaviors.

By contrast, benefits of more "healthy" or adaptive coping strategies are increasingly evident in the literature. For example, breast cancer patients scoring lowest in avoidant coping were more likely to be actively involved in treatment decision making (Hack and Degner, 1999). In addition, emotionally expressive coping predicted both psychological and physical adjustment to breast cancer (Stanton and others, 2000). Use of spirituality and seeking social support may reduce the chances that a person will engage in risky behaviors, such as unprotected sexual intercourse (Folkman, Chesney, Pollack, and Phillips, 1992). Use of spirituality has also been associated with growth and the capacity to derive positive meaning from being an ovarian cancer survivor (Wenzel and others, 2002). These are examples from a growing body of literature that describes the physical and mental health benefits of active coping efforts, including both problem-focused and emotion-focused efforts.

Most research on coping strategies evaluates efforts to cope with a particular situation, distinct from generalized coping styles (Stone and Porter, 1995). However, as discussed next, the effects of specific coping strategies on emotional and functional outcomes of a health threat and the accompanying stress may depend on a person's dispositional coping style and perceptions of support in the environment.

Coping Outcomes

Coping outcomes represent a person's adaptation to a stressor, following from appraisal of the situation (primary appraisal) and resources (secondary appraisal) and influenced by coping efforts. Because a problem or stressor may change over time, outcomes may occur in differing timeframes. Three main categories of outcomes are emotional well-being, functional status (or health status, disease progression, and so forth), and health behaviors. These outcomes may also interact with one another. For example, clinically meaningful links have been made between endocrine function and cancer. In particular, the hormone cortisol, which is highly involved in the stress response, has been found to be associated with a variety of health outcomes, including breast cancer. Recent studies have demonstrated an association between loss of daily variation in cortisol and shorter survival time from breast cancer (Stephton, Sapolsky, Kraemer, and Spiegel, 2000). A link between social support and cortisol in breast cancer has been confirmed in a clinical trial demonstrating that group support for breast cancer patients reduced mean cortisol levels (Cruess and others, 2000). These recent studies provide support for the premise that reactions to stress may affect health status through physiological processes of the endocrine, immune, and nervous systems (Glaser and Kiecolt-Glaser, 2005). However, caution should be used when interpreting relationships between psychological factors and disease progression. Tross and colleagues (1996) examined contributions of potential psychological predictors to length of disease-free and overall survival over a fifteen-year period. This study, conducted within a randomized clinical trial, found no significant predictive effect of distress levels on disease outcomes.

Health behaviors, such as seeking care, communicating with health providers, and adhering to treatment recommendations, may be influenced by physical limitations (functional status) and emotional reactions (worry, depression, denial). Similarly, desirable health behaviors may be influenced by meaning-based processes, such as positive reappraisal, which may decrease worry and enhance positive affect.

THEORETICAL EXTENSIONS

Coping Styles

In contrast to situation-specific coping efforts, coping styles are conceptualized as stable dispositional characteristics that reflect generalized tendencies to interpret and respond to stress in particular ways (Lazarus, 1993). Thus, coping efforts can be considered "mediators" of the effects of stress and appraisals on emotional and functional outcomes—in other words, the mechanism by which these effects are exerted. By contrast, coping styles are enduring traits that are believed to drive appraisal and coping efforts (Lazarus, 1993). Individual differences in coping styles can be considered "moderators" of the impact of stress on coping processes and outcomes. That is, the specific effect of a stressful event or a specific coping behavior on adjustment may depend, in part, on the person's coping style. Coping styles can also have direct effects on the emotional and physical outcomes of stressful events.

Information Seeking. Uncertainty can hinder the coping process by making it difficult to appraise the degree of threat associated with a stressor and to choose a coping response (Lazarus and Folkman, 1984). Because uncertainty is ever-present in the health care setting (Eton, Lepore, and Helgeson, 2005; Mishel and others, 2005), information seeking is a frequently used coping response (Case, Andrews, Johnson, and Allard, 2005). Although there is substantial evidence that information seeking can lead to reduced distress and adaptive health behaviors (van Zuuren and others, 2006), there is also evidence that individuals differ in the extent to which they seek information in the face of a health threat. Those who typically seek information are called "monitors," and those who avoid information are called "blunters." Compared to blunters, monitors seek and attend to stressor-related information (Koo, Krass, and Asiani, 2006; Rees and Bath, 2000). Several studies have shown that the vigilant style of monitors contributes to heightened perceived risk, worry, and distress about health threats (Schwartz and others, 1995; Andrykowski and others, 2002). These studies suggest that a monitoring coping style may be associated with more threatening primary appraisals of health threats. Effects of monitoring on physical outcomes of stressful events also have been demonstrated. For example, monitors exhibit more physical distress and arousal during invasive medical procedures than blunters (Miller and Mangan, 1983).

However, in some situations, monitoring may be more adaptive than blunting. When stressors are short term and monitors' needs for information are satisfied (for example, by preparation for stressful medical procedures), active coping is enhanced and emotional and physical distress is minimized (Miller and Mangan, 1983; van Zuuren and others, 2006). Further, monitors may be more inclined to seek health-related information that could have significant medical benefits (Lerman, Daly, Masny, and Balshem, 1994; Koo, Krass, and Asiani, 2006) and may also play a more active role in medical decision making (Ong and others, 1999) and be less likely to experience regret following difficult medical decisions (Sheehan, Sherman, Lam, and Boyages, 2007).

Research has also shown that monitors and blunters may benefit differentially from information, depending on how it is presented. In a study to enhance cervical dysplasia screening follow-up, recommendations were either loss-framed (emphasizing costs), gain-framed (emphasizing benefits), or neutrally framed (no emphasis). Monitors reported more distress when the message was presented in a loss frame, because the sense of risk was heightened (Miller and others, 1999). In a more recent study of mammography messages, monitors were more likely to obtain mammograms when provided with detailed reassuring messages and less likely to obtain mammograms when presented with more concise, simple messages. Conversely, blunters were more motivated by the less detailed message (Williams-Piehota and others, 2005).

Optimism. Perhaps the most widely studied coping style is dispositional optimism—the tendency to have positive rather than negative generalized expectancies for outcomes. These expectancies are relatively stable over time and across situations (Scheier and Carver, 1992). Direct benefits of optimism on psychological adjustment and quality of life have been demonstrated in prospective studies of a variety of illnesses, including cancer patients (Kung and others, 2006; Carver and others, 1993) and HIV-positive men (Taylor and others, 1992).

Studies examining the association between optimism and disease outcomes have been more mixed. A recent prospective study found no association between optimism and lung cancer survival (Schofield and others, 2004). In contrast, previous studies have reported associations between optimism and survival from head and neck cancer (Allison, Guichard, Fung, and Gilain, 2003), reduced cardiovascular mortality (Giltay and others, 2004, 2006), and slower HIV progression (Ironson and others, 2005).

Studies exploring effects of optimism on coping responses are relevant to understanding the Transactional Model. For example, Carver and colleagues (1993) found that active coping, planning, and problem solving mediated the beneficial effects of optimism on psychological well-being among early-stage breast cancer patients. Further, optimism was related inversely to avoidance—a coping strategy that generated distress in this sample. Among gay men at risk for AIDS, dispositional optimism was associated with perceived lower risk of AIDS (primary appraisal), higher perceived control over AIDS (secondary appraisal), more active coping strategies, less distress, and more risk-reducing health behaviors (Taylor and others, 1992). Thus, dispositional optimism appears to exert effects on each of the key processes of the Transactional Model. These effects, in turn, influence how optimists and pessimists respond emotionally and physically to health threats and illness.

Social Support

Social support has been conceptualized in a variety of ways. Some definitions focus on the quantitative and tangible dimensions (for example, number of friendships), while others focus on nontangible aspects such as feelings of interconnectedness, or qualitative aspects involving subjective appraisals of adequacy of support networks (Heitzmann and Kaplan, 1988). Substantial evidence shows the direct effects of social support on well-being and health outcomes (for example, Kroenke and others, 2006). However, evidence also exists for "stress-buffering" effects of social support (for example, Cohen and Wills, 1985; Christian and Stoney, 2006). The stress-buffering hypothesis predicts that social support will have stronger positive effects on adjustment and physical well-being when a stressor becomes more intense or persistent.

By influencing key processes posited in the Transactional Model, social support can influence how people adapt to stressful events. For example, availability of confidants could affect a person's perceptions of personal risk or the severity of illness (primary appraisal). These interactions could also bolster beliefs about one's ability to cope with situations and manage difficult emotions (secondary appraisal) (Cohen and McKay, 1984). Social support can also serve as a mechanism for downward comparison—that is, to compare oneself to someone who is worse off (Cohen and Wills, 1985). Resultant increases in self-esteem and self-efficacy could increase the likelihood of active coping rather than avoidance (Holahan and Moos, 1986). A supportive environment also can protect against stress by providing opportunities to explore different coping options and to evaluate their effectiveness (Holahan and Moos, 1986).

Just as a supportive environment is related to positive psychosocial and health outcomes, a nonsupportive environment can adversely affect one's ability to cope with a health threat. When key social supports actively discourage the disclosure of feelings about a stressor, avoidant coping and adverse psychosocial outcomes can increase. For example, Cordova and colleagues (2001) reported that breast cancer survivors who reported feeling socially constrained had higher levels of depression and poorer quality of life. Similar findings have been observed among prostate cancer survivors (Zakowski and others, 2004).

Social support also influences health behaviors and outcomes (Myers and others, 2007). Low social support predicts more rapid progression of HIV (Leserman, 2000), mortality among individuals with heart disease (Williams and others, 1992; Brummett and others, 2005), and mortality following myocardial infarction (Frasure-Smith and others, 2000). Recent data from the Nurses' Health Study demonstrated a prospective association between social isolation and both breast cancer and all-cause mortality (Kroenke and others, 2006). Although the association between social support and health is fairly robust, some findings are also inconsistent (Thong and others, 2007).

Despite consistent associations between social support and health outcomes in observational studies, the results of intervention studies are less clear-cut. If coping strategies facilitate adjustment to a cancer diagnosis, psychosocial support should be a potent factor in mediating emotional distress and improving health outcomes. Preliminary evidence to support this came from two studies that reported that support group interventions for cancer patients improved emotional adjustment and influenced survival (Fawzy and others, 1993; Spiegel, Bloom, Kraemer, and Gottheil, 1989). However, more recent studies have failed to replicate these findings in cancer patients (Spiegel and others, 2007) and other populations. For example, a randomized controlled trial of an intervention designed to improve social support, reduce depression, and reduce mortality among myocardial infarction patients failed to decrease mortality, despite successfully enhancing social support and reducing depression (Berkman and others, 2003). Although there is ample evidence to demonstrate a link between low social support and unhealthy behaviors, such as smoking and sedentary lifestyles (Brummett and others, 2005), it remains to be determined whether these behaviors and positive health outcomes can be improved via social support interventions.

Positive Psychology

"Positive" psychology examines how people develop and sustain characteristics, such as hope, wisdom, future mindedness, courage, spirituality, and perseverance in the face of significant stress (Seligman and Csikszentmihalyi, 2000). Early research in this area focused on characterizing people who remained relatively healthy while undergoing stressful life experiences. Antonovsky (1979) and Kobasa (1979) suggested that people who exhibited healthful adaptation to internal and environmental stressors had strong resistance resources and a sense of meaningfulness in their lives. Antonovsky (1979) described a "sense of coherence," which involves a strong sense of confidence that the world is predictable and that things will work out well. Similarly, Kobasa identified a constellation of features she called "hardiness," marked by a strong sense of meaningfulness and commitment to self, a vigorous attitude toward life, and an internal locus of control (Kobasa, 1979). This work was a forerunner of more recent research on purpose and dispositional optimism, which can be considered aspects of positive psychology. The consideration of positive outcomes is important to future progress in coping theory and research (Folkman and Moskowitz, 2000).

Several studies have found positive associations between a sense of purpose in life and life satisfaction, positive mood states, and happiness (Gustavsson-Lilius, Julkunen, Keskivaara, and Hietanen, 2007; Ryff and Keyes, 1995; Ryff, Lee, Essex, and Schmutte, 1994). This research also suggests that purpose in life is negatively associated with depression. In general, these studies suggest that people who endorse a strong purpose in life are likely to experience better emotional well-being. Also, as noted earlier in the section on coping styles, dispositional optimism appears to exert effects on each of the key processes of the Transactional Model.

Although much of positive psychology has focused on dispositional characteristics such as optimism, hardiness, purpose in life, and sense of coherence, increasing attention is being paid to situational characteristics such as benefit finding. *Benefit finding* refers to the identification of positive life changes that have resulted from major stressors (Helgeson, Reynolds, and Tomich, 2006). Several studies have shown that benefit finding is significantly associated with the use of positive reappraisal and other forms of active coping (Lechner and others, 2006; Kinsinger and others, 2006). Benefit finding has been associated with positive adjustment to a variety of health stressors such as rheumatoid arthritis (Danoff-Burg and Revenson, 2005), cardiovascular disease (Affleck, Tennen, Pfeiffer, and Fifield, 1987), and HIV (McGregor and others, 2004). Among cancer patients, evidence is more mixed (Lechner and others, 2006). Although many studies have reported associations between benefit finding and well-being/quality of life (for example, Carver and Antoni, 2004), some studies reported no association (for example, Sears, Stanton, and Danoff-Burg, 2003) or suggested that there might be an association between benefit finding and increased distress/poorer quality of life (Tomich and Helgeson, 2004). Recent longitudinal studies have suggested that these inconsistencies may be attributable to a curvilinear relationship between benefit finding and adjustment (Lechner and others, 2006) or to a distinction between initial benefit finding and longitudinal changes in benefit finding (Schwarzer and others, 2006).

Stress, Coping, and Psychoneuroimmunology

The physiological manifestations of stress have long been recognized. Acute stress is characterized by the "fight or flight" response and involves activation of the hypothalmic-pituitary-adrenal (HPA) axis and/or the sympathetic nervous system (SNS) (Glaser and Kiecolt-Glaser, 2005). While acute stress may lead to enhanced or impaired immune function (Moynihan, 2003), chronic stress clearly has an adverse impact on immune function (Moynihan, 2003). Although the mechanisms in humans are not entirely clear, it is believed that ongoing exposure to elevated levels of catecholamines (for example, epinephrine and norepeinephrine), cortisol, and other stress hormones likely contribute to the immune dysregulation associated with chronic stress (Glaser and Kiecolt-Glaser, 2005; Antoni, 2003).

Numerous studies have demonstrated that chronic stress impairs immune function. Stressed individuals have poorer immune responses to viral vaccination, greater reactivation of latent herpes viruses, suppressed lymphocyte production, and greater susceptibility to viral infection (Kiecolt-Glaser and others, 1987; Cohen, Tyrrell, and Smith, 1991).

Given these associations, the Transactional Model predicts that appraisals and coping should be related to immune function and health. Although not entirely consistent, there is evidence to support these hypotheses. For example, at least two studies among breast cancer patients and bereaved individuals found that coping by finding meaning was associated with reduced cortisol levels (Cruess and others, 2000) and increased natural killer cell activity (Bower, Kemeny, Taylor, and Fahey, 2003). Further, intervention studies in which individuals are taught strategies for adaptive coping have demonstrated benefits on a variety of neuroendocrine and immune parameters among healthy, stressed individuals (for example, Gaab, Sonderegger, Scherrer, and Ehlert, 2006) and women with breast cancer (for example, McGregor and others, 2004).

Public Health Perspectives

Stress affects individuals in their relationships to other people and situations, and it can be experienced at the community level as well. The public health relevance of stress and coping is underscored by the idea that health and illness are products of both individual-level risk and protective factors *and* contextual factors (Kawachi and Subramanian, 2006).

The Transactional Model has been applied to public health issues such as the effects of racism on health disparities. Racism has been conceptualized to have both direct and indirect effects on health. Although racism may indirectly influence health via socioeconomic status (SES), it may also directly affect health by serving as an acute and chronic stressor (Williams, 1999). Evidence for the role of racism as a stressor comes from laboratory studies in which perceived racism has been associated with increased cardiovascular reactivity (for example, Clark and Gochett, 2006; Merritt and others, 2006), particularly among African Americans (Lepore and others, 2006). Although lab data are relatively consistent, epidemiological studies of the link between racism and health have yielded mixed results (Brondolo, Rieppi, Kelly, and Gerin, 2003). Several studies examining relationships between perceived racism and hypertension have found positive associations (Cozier and others, 2006; Krieger and Sidney, 1996), but others have reported no association (Davis, Liu, Quarells, and Din-Dzietharn, 2005; Dressler, Bindon, and Neggers, 1998).

Effects of stress due to racism, low SES, and other environmental stressors may be moderated by specific coping styles. One such widely studied coping style is *John Henryism*—a term referring to a strong behavioral predisposition to cope actively with psychosocial and environmental stressors (James, Hartnett, and Kalsbeek, 1983). According to the John Henryism hypothesis, when coupled with severe constraints (low education, low SES, and persistent racism, for example), persistent and highly active coping results in adverse health effects (Dressler, Bindon, and Neggers, 1998). A number of studies have found that individuals rated high on John Henryism and with limited resources are more likely to have hypertension and exhibit higher cardiovascular reactivity (Merritt and others, 2004). However, other studies have failed to find such associations (for example, McKetney and Ragland, 1996). More recent studies have suggested that the association between John Henryism and health may be more complicated than originally thought. For example, among individuals of higher SES, it appears that John Henryism may be associated with reduced perceived stress (Haritatos, Mahalingam, and James, 2007), better self-reported physical health

(Haritatos, Mahalingam, and James, 2007; Bonham, Sellers, and Neighbors, 2004), and lower rates of nicotine dependence (Fernander and others, 2005).

Stress Management Interventions

A variety of techniques to manage stress, improve coping, and reduce deleterious effects of stressors on physical and psychological health have been developed and tested. Techniques such as relaxation training and visual imagery can be conceptualized as coping efforts directed at emotional regulation, which is consistent with the original formulation of the Transactional Model (Lazarus and Folkman, 1984). Relaxation strategies focus on the interplay between biological and psychological responses to stressors (Critchley and others, 2001). Use of relaxation techniques assumes that individuals possess alternative responses to fight-or-flight—responses that counteract the effects of stress. Relaxation training has been shown to decrease chemotherapy side effects (Burish and Jenkins, 1992) and lead to improved mood and quality of life (Walker and others, 1999).

Although not derived directly from the Transactional Model, cognitive-behavioral stress management (CBSM) approaches, which integrate relaxation with coping skills training, are consistent with the approach. Interventions derived from the CBSM approach focus on teaching individuals to identify sources and indicators of stress, and train them to improve coping skills in order to manage the stress. Antoni and colleagues (2006b) showed that interventions based on CBSM led to improved quality of life and reduced distress among breast cancer patients, prostate cancer patients (Penedo and others, 2006), and HIV-positive men (Antoni and others, 2005), and improved quality of life among patients with heart disease (Blumenthal and others, 2005).

Stress management interventions also can affect physiological outcomes. In a study of patients with ischemic heart disease, patients randomized to a sixteen-week CBSM intervention exhibited significant improvements in cardiovascular risk markers compared to patients who received usual care (Blumenthal and others, 2005). In contrast, another study among women with ischemic heart disease found that a similar intervention did not improve cardiovascular risk markers (Claesson and others, 2006).

APPLICATIONS TO SPECIFIC HEALTH BEHAVIOR RESEARCH AREAS

Examples of the application of the Transactional Model of Stress and Coping are given in two applications that follow. The first application describes a study of cancer survivors' use of online support groups informed by stress and coping concepts. The second application describes studies of cognitive-behavioral intervention strategies to improve coping and adaptation among HIV-positive men.

Cancer Survivors' Use of Online Support Groups

For patients with cancer and those at increased risk for cancer, psychological adjustment and adherence to early detection and treatment may be affected by concerns about their prognosis or personal risk. The Transactional Model of Stress and Coping has been used as the theoretical foundation for interventions to promote adjustment after cancer treatment among patients and their families (Northouse, Kershaw, Mood, and Schafenacker, 2005), to understand the role of spirituality in adjustment to cancer (Laubmeier, Zakowski, and Bair, 2004), and to evaluate a risk counseling intervention for relatives of colorectal cancer patients (Glanz, Steffen, and Taglialatela, 2007).

Cancer survivors increasingly are turning to online communities, often referred to as Electronic Support Groups (ESGs), but relatively little is known about how cancer survivors and their caregivers use these growing resources. The Health eCommunities Study is a multimethod project designed to assess, among other things, why people join online cancer support groups and the types of messages they send to request or offer support (Rimer and others, 2005; Meier and others, 2007). The conceptual framework for the Health eCommunities Study was based on Lazarus and Folkman's theory (1984), with a particular focus on exploring problem-focused and emotion-focused coping strategies.

A Web-based survey of 293 new subscribers to online cancer mailing lists showed that the most common purposes for joining were to obtain information on how to deal with cancer (62 per cent strongly agree), for support (42 per cent strongly agree), and to help others (37 per cent strongly agree) (Rimer and others, 2005). An analysis of themes from a sample of 2,755 messages revealed that emotional support was provided in the form of emotional coping strategies, empathy, encouragement, prayers, and esteem support. An unexpected finding was that survivors were more likely to offer than to request support, thus potentially using online connections to promote their own coping resources as well as those of others (Meier and others, 2007).

Methods and findings of the Health eCommunities Study illustrate important challenges of studying virtual communities, as well as new approaches for understanding and increasing the way patients and caregivers manage the stress of illness. The use of an integrated conceptual framework of stress and coping to organize the research questions in this study bridges the gap between individual clinical concerns and public health challenges with broad reach. It also illustrates how new communication technologies are being used by patients to cope with illness and manage stress.

Cognitive Behavioral Stress Management for HIV-Positive Men

Individuals who are diagnosed with HIV face a variety of challenges that can result in chronic stress (Antoni, 2003). These stressors can include financial hardships, social stigma, multiple bereavements, and stress associated with following complex medication regimens (Antoni and others, 2000). Such stressors have the potential to overwhelm the coping resources of affected individuals, leading to poor adjustment (Carrico and others, 2005a). In turn, poor psychosocial adjustment can result in an adverse impact on the already compromised immune system of this population and ultimately contribute to more rapid disease progression (Antoni, 2003). Thus, interventions designed to help HIV-positive individuals manage the stressors associated with their disease have the potential to improve psychological adjustment and beneficially affect immune function and disease state.

The Transactional Model of Stress and Coping served as a guiding framework for the development of a Cognitive Behavioral Stress Management (CBSM) intervention, delivered and evaluated by Antoni and colleagues in a series of studies. CBSM has been evaluated in randomized trials in breast and prostate cancer patients, and HIV-infected men. This application describes the methods and results of a long-term study evaluating CBSM among early-symptomatic, HIV-positive homosexual and bisexual men. The CBSM intervention was designed to promote adjustment to HIV-associated stressors and subsequently to have an impact on immune function and potentially on HIV progression (Antoni, 2003). CBSM was delivered in a group format, typically over ten weekly 135-minute sessions; the content of the CBSM intervention has been described in detail in several reports (Carrico and others, 2005b).

CBSM addresses several key elements of the Transactional Model. The goal of the initial sessions is to help participants understand the link between cognitive appraisals and their physiological and emotional responses to stress. Thus, initial sessions focus on (1) identifying stressors, (2) recognizing the stress response, and (3) understanding the role of cognitive appraisals. The next few sessions teach techniques for identifying cognitive distortions in the appraisal process and fostering more realistic and adaptive appraisals. Once participants understand how to recognize and modify cognitive distortions, thus reducing their sense that nothing can be done to deal with their overwhelming stressors, subsequent sessions provide detailed instruction about how to generate and execute coping strategies. The final sessions focus on assertiveness training and accessing social support. Across all of the sessions, participants receive detailed training in the use of relaxation as a coping strategy. Thus, the CBSM intervention touches on the three key elements of the Transactional Model—primary appraisal, secondary appraisal, and coping. The intervention also includes several extensions of the model—relaxation training, social support, and positive psychology.

Participants were seventy-three HIV-positive men randomized in a 2:1 ratio to CBSM and a wait-list control condition. The groups did not differ at baseline on any sociodemographic, disease-related, psychological, or immune variables. Consistent with the Transactional Model, the CBSM intervention led to significant reductions in perceptions of stress and distress over the ten-week intervention (Antoni and others, 2000). A subsequent analysis examined the one-year impact of the CBSM on a subset of participants from this study. CBSM participants exhibited reduced depression relative to control participants. Further, consistent with the Transactional Model, these sustained reductions in depression were mediated by increases in adaptive coping during the intervention period (Carrico and others, 2005b).

The investigators also evaluated the impact of the CBSM intervention on a variety of immunological and hormonal outcomes. Compared to control participants, those assigned to the CBSM arm exhibited reduced levels of the stress hormones norepinephrine and urinary cortisol (Antoni and others, 2000), increases in T-cytotoxic/suppressor cells (Antoni and others, 2000), and increased production of naïve T-cells—a marker of immune system reconstitution. This effect was found in both the short and long term, and was partially mediated by reduced depression in the CBSM group (Antoni and others, 2002, 2005).

These data are consistent with other studies conducted by Antoni and colleagues in a variety of populations. CBSM led to improved quality of life and reductions in distress among breast cancer patients (Antoni and others, 2006a) and prostate cancer patients (Penedo and others, 2006). Other investigators using similar interventions have also reported beneficial effects in heart disease patient populations (for example, Blumenthal and others, 2005). Finally, more recent research by Antoni and colleagues evaluated the impact of CBSM, in combination with medication-adherence training among HIV-positive men. The most recent study showed that CBSM, in combination with medication-adherence training, led to reduced depression and decreased HIV-viral load (Antoni and others, 2006b). Taken together, these studies strongly support the benefit of CBSM across a variety of psychosocial and physiological outcomes.

RESEARCH GAPS AND FUTURE DIRECTIONS

In 2000, Lazarus observed that the field of research on stress and coping is maturing and that the research is being applied increasingly in clinical practice (2000). Researchers are using longitudinal and prospective designs and randomized controlled trials of interventions to improve coping (Stanton, Revenson, and Tennen, 2007). The use of day-to-day and real-time measures (Stone, Shiffman, Atienza, and Nebeling, 2007) are advancements that complement more general measures over long periods. There is growing interest in the role of positive emotions in coping, including ideas such as love and hope, that warrant further examination (Seligman and Csikszentmihalyi, 2000; Folkman and Moskowitz, 2000). Although it was not covered in this chapter, research on coping during childhood and adolescence that examines how coping is developed is an active emphasis of some health-related stress research (Skinner and Zimmer-Gembeck, 2007). The recognition that people can react with resilience to stress is a powerful driver of new research.

There are both opportunities and needs to apply theory on stress and coping to public health issues such as terrorism, disasters, and other mass traumatic events (Matthieu and Ivanoff, 2006; Kawachi and Subramanian, 2006). Although most recent research on these issues appears to lack a theoretical basis, some major studies have been interpreted as consistent with the Transactional Model of Stress and Coping (Schuster and others, 2001).

Although it is difficult to offer simple generalizations about the adaptability of specific coping processes or the efficacy of interventions, the extensive research conducted in this area has several implications for the practice of health promotion and health education. First, because individuals' emotional and health behavior responses to health threats are influenced to a large degree by their subjective interpretations, these appraisals should be assessed. For example, to improve understanding of determinants of cancer patients' lifestyle practices following treatment, one should assess primary appraisals (such as perceptions of risk of recurrence), secondary appraisals (for example, self-efficacy in adopting health behavior recommendations), and specific coping strategies (problem-focused coping, emotion-focused coping, and meaning-based coping). These assessments could provide useful information about appraisals that facilitate or hinder such practices. This information would be useful for designing motivational messages and coping skills training techniques to be incorporated into standardized interventions.

A second implication of research on stress and coping relates to dispositional coping styles. As described in this chapter, coping strategies are likely to be beneficial to the extent that they fit with the features of the stressful situation and with the individual's own needs for information, control, and level of optimism versus pessimism. Incorporation of coping styles assessments into health promotion and psycho-educational interventions will facilitate the tailoring of these strategies to individual needs. Research on stress, coping, and health behavior suggests that interventions tailored to individual appraisals and coping behaviors are likely to be most effective in terms of enhancing coping, reducing stress, and improving health behavior and physical well-being.

SUMMARY

The theory and research presented in this chapter illustrate the complexities of stress and coping and their effects on psychological well-being, health behavior, and health. This work suggests that the outcomes of the stress and coping process are determined by the interplay of situational factors, individual appraisals of the situation, and coping strategies. No particular pattern of relationships among these factors has been related consistently to positive outcomes of the coping process across all behaviors and health concerns. Rather, effects of the stress and coping processes depend on context (for example, controllability of the stressor), timing (short- versus long-term adaptation), and individual characteristics (for example, information processing styles and meaning-based coping processes).

The core concepts of the Transactional Model of Stress and Coping—primary appraisal, secondary appraisal, coping efforts, meaning-based coping, and outcomes of coping—and theoretical extensions related to dispositional coping styles comprise a useful framework for understanding and analyzing perceptions of and reactions to stress. They also warrant attention in applications that respond to emerging and contemporary public health issues, including natural disasters (for example, hurricanes, tsunamis) and disasters due to human actions or technology failure (for example, terrorism, plane crashes).

REFERENCES

Affleck, G., Tennen, H., Pfeiffer, C., and Fifield, H. "Appraisals of Control and Predictability in Adapting to a Chronic Stress." *Journal of Personality & Social Psychology,* 1987, *53,* 273–279.

Allison, P. J., Guichard, C., Fung, K., and Gilain, L. "Dispositional Optimism Predicts Survival Status 1 Year After Diagnosis in Head and Neck Cancer Patients." *Journal of Clinical Oncology,* 2003, *21,* 543–548.

Andrykowski, M. A., and others. "Psychological Impact of Benign Breast Biopsy: A Longitudinal, Comparative Study." *Health Psychology,* 2002, *21*(5), 485–494.

Antoni, M. H. "Stress Management and Psychoneuroimmunology in HIV Infection." *CNS Spectrums,* 2003, *8,* 40–51.

Antoni, M. H., and others. "Cognitive-Behavioral Stress Management Intervention Effects on Anxiety, 24-Hour Urinary Norepinephrine Output, and T-Cytotoxic/Suppressor Cells Over Time Among Symptomatic HIV-Infected Gay Men." *Journal of Consulting & Clinical Psychology,* 2000, *68,* 31–45.

Antoni, M. H., and others. "Stress Management and Immune System Reconstitution in Symptomatic HIV-Infected Gay Men Over Time: Effects on Transitional Naive T Cells (CD4(+)CD45RA(+)CD29(+))." *The American Journal of Psychiatry,* 2002, *159,* 143–145.

Antoni, M. H., and others. "Increases in a Marker of Immune System Reconstitution are Predated by Decreases in 24-Hour Urinary Cortisol Output and Depressed Mood During a 10-Week Stress Management Intervention in Symptomatic HIV-Infected Men." *Journal of Psychosomatic Research,* 2005, *58,* 3–13.

Antoni, M. H., and others. "Reduction of Cancer-Specific Thought Intrusions and Anxiety Symptoms with a Stress Management Intervention Among Women Undergoing Treatment for Breast Cancer." *The American Journal of Psychiatry,* 2006a, *163,* 1791–1797.

Antoni, M. H., and others. "Randomized Clinical Trial of Cognitive Behavioral Stress Management on Human Immunodeficiency Virus Viral Load in Gay Men Treated with Highly Active Antiretroviral Therapy." *Psychosomatic Medicine,* 2006b, *68,* 143–151.

Antonovsky, A. *Health, Stress, and Coping.* San Francisco: Jossey-Bass, 1979.

Baider, L., and others. "The Role of Psychological Variables in a Group of Melanoma Patients: An Israeli Sample." *Psychosomatics,* 1997, *38,* 45–53.

Bandura, A. *Self-Efficacy: The Exercise of Control.* New York: W. H. Freeman, 1997.

Berkman, L. F., and others. "Effects of Treating Depression and Low Perceived Social Support on Clinical Events After Myocardial Infarction: The Enhancing Recovery in Coronary Heart Disease Patients (ENRICHD) Randomized Trial." *Journal of the American Medical Association,* 2003, *289,* 3106–3116.

Blumenthal, J. A., and others. "Effects of Exercise and Stress Management Training on Markers of Cardiovascular Risk in Patients With Ischemic Heart Disease: A Randomized Controlled Trial." *Journal of the American Medical Association,* 2005, *293,* 1626–1634.

Bonham, V. L., Sellers, S. L., and Neighbors, H. W. "John Henryism and Self-Reported Physical Health Among High-Socioeconomic Status African American Men." *American Journal of Public Health,* 2004, *94,* 737–738.

Bower, J. E., Kemeny, M. E., Taylor, S. E., and Fahey, J. L. "Finding Positive Meaning and its Association with Natural Killer Cell Cytotoxicity Among Participants in a Bereavement-Related Disclosure Intervention." *Annals of Behavioral Medicine,* 2003, *25,* 146–155.

Brondolo, E., Rieppi, R., Kelly, K. P., and Gerin, W. "Perceived Racism and Blood Pressure: A Review of the Literature and Conceptual and Methodological Critique." *Annals of Behavioral Medicine,* 2003, *25,* 55–65.

Brummett, B. H., and others. "Perceived Social Support as a Predictor of Mortality in Coronary Patients: Effects of Smoking, Sedentary Behavior, and Depressive Symptoms." *Psychosomatic Medicine,* 2005, *67,* 40–45.

Burish, T. G., and Jenkins, R. S. "Effectiveness of Biofeedback and Relaxation Training in Reducing the Side Effects of Cancer Chemotherapy." *Health Psychology,* 1992, *11,* 17–23.

Cannon, W. B. *The Wisdom of the Body.* New York: W. W. Norton, 1932.

Carrico, A. W., and others. "Cognitive-Behavioural Stress Management with HIV-Positive Homosexual Men: Mechanisms of Sustained Reductions in Depressive Symptoms." *Chronic Illness,* 2005a, *1,* 207–215.

Carrico, A. W., and others. "Cognitive Behavioral Stress Management Effects on Mood, Social Support, and a Marker of Antiviral Immunity are Maintained up to 1 Year in HIV-Infected Gay Men." *International Journal of Behavioral Medicine,* 2005b, *12,* 218–226.

Carver, C. S., and Antoni, M. H. "Finding Benefit in Breast Cancer During the Year After Diagnosis Predicts Better Adjustment 5 to 8 Years After Diagnosis." *Health Psychology,* 2004, *23,* 595–598.

Carver, C. S., and others. "How Coping Mediates the Effect of Optimism on Distress: A Study of Women with Early Stage Breast Cancer." *Journal of Personality and Social Psychology,* 1993, *65*(2), 375–390.

Carver, C. S., Scheier, M. F., and Weintraub, J. K. "Assessing Coping Strategies: A Theoretically Based Approach." *Journal of Personality and Social Psychology,* 1989, *56,* 267–283.

Case, D. O., Andrews, J. E., Johnson, J. D., and Allard, S. L. "Avoiding Versus Seeking: The Relationship of Information Seeking to Avoidance, Blunting, Coping, Dissonance, and Related Concepts." *Journal of the Medical Library Association,* 2005, *93,* 353–362.

Chapman, S., Wong, W. L., and Smith, W. "Self-Exempting Beliefs About Smoking and Health: Differences Between Smokers and Ex-Smokers." *American Journal of Public Health,* 1993, *83,* 215–219.

Christian, L. M., and Stoney, C. M. "Social Support Versus Social Evaluation: Unique Effects on Vascular and Myocardial Response Patterns." *Psychosomatic Medicine,* 2006, *68,* 914–921.

Claesson, M., and others. "Cognitive-Behavioural Stress Management Does Not Improve Biological Cardio-vascular Risk Indicators in Women With Ischaemic Heart Disease: A Randomized-Controlled Trial." *Journal of Internal Medicine,* 2006, *260,* 320–331.

Clark, R., and Gochett, P. "Interactive Effects of Perceived Racism and Coping Responses Predict a School-Based Assessment of Blood Pressure in Black Youth." *Annals of Behavioral Medicine,* 2006, *32,* 1–9.

Cohen, F. "Coping." In J. D. Matarazzo, S. M. Weiss, J. A. Herd, N. E. Miller, and S. M. Weiss (eds.), *Behavioral Health: A Handbook of Health Enhancement and Disease Prevention.* New York: Wiley, 1984.

Cohen, S., and McKay, G. "Social Support, Stress and the Buffering Hypothesis: A Theoretical Analysis." In A. Baum, J. E. Singer, and S. E. Taylor (eds.), *Handbook of Psychology and Health* (Vol. 4). Hillsdale, N.J.: Erlbaum, 1984.

Cohen, S., Tyrrell, D. A., and Smith, A. P. "Psychological Stress and Susceptibility to the Common Cold." *The New England Journal of Medicine,* 1991, *325,* 606–612.

Cohen, S., and Wills, T. A. "Stress, Social Support, and the Buffering Hypothesis." *Psychological Bulletin,* 1985, *98*(2), 310–357.

Cordova, M. J., Cunningham, L. L., Carlson, C. R., and Andrykowski, M. A. "Posttraumatic Growth Following Breast Cancer: A Controlled Comparison Study." *Health Psychology,* 2001, *20,* 176–185.

Cozier, Y., and others. "Racial Discrimination and the Incidence of Hypertension in US Black Women." *Annals of Epidemiology,* 2006, *16,* 681–687.

Critchley, H. D., and others. "Brain Activity During Biofeedback Relaxation: A Functional Neuroimaging Investigation." *Brain,* 2001, *124*(5), 1003–1012.

Cruess, D. G., and others. "Cognitive-Behavioral Stress Management Reduces Serum Cortisol by Enhancing Benefit Finding Among Women Being Treated for Early Stage Breast Cancer." *Psychosomatic Medicine,* 2000, *62,* 304–308.

Danoff-Burg, S., and Revenson, T. A. "Benefit-Finding Among Patients With Rheumatoid Arthritis: Positive Effects on Interpersonal Relationships." *Journal of Behavioral Medicine,* 2005, *28,* 91–103.

Davis, S. K., Liu, Y., Quarells, R. C., and Din-Dzietharn, R. "Stress-Related Racial Discrimination and Hypertension Likelihood in a Population-Based Sample of African Americans: The Metro Atlanta Heart Disease Study." *Ethnicity & Disease,* 2005, *15,* 585–593.

Ditto, P. H., and Croyle, R. T. "Understanding the Impact of Risk Factor Test Results: Insights From a Basic Research Program." In R. T. Croyle (ed.), *Psychosocial Effects of Screening for Disease Prevention and Detection.* New York: Oxford University Press, 1995.

Dohrenwend, B. S., and Dohrenwend, B. P. *Stressful Life Events and Their Contexts.* New York: Prodist, 1981.

Dressler, W. W., Bindon, J. R., and Neggers, Y. H. "John Henryism, Gender, and Arterial Blood Pressure in an African American Community." *Psychosomatic Medicine,* 1998, *60,* 620–624.

Endler, N., and Parker, J. "Multidimensional Assessment of Coping: A Critical Evaluation." *Journal of Personality and Social Psychology,* 1990, *58,* 844–854.

Eton, D. T., Lepore, S. J., and Helgeson, V. S. "Psychological Distress in Spouses of Men Treated for Early-Stage Prostate Carcinoma." *Cancer,* 2005, *103,* 2412–2418.

Fawzy, F. I., and others. "Malignant Melanoma: Effects of an Early Structured Psychiatric Intervention, Coping, and Affective State on Recurrence and Survival 6 Years Later." *Archives of General Psychiatry,* 1993, *50,* 681–689.

Fernander, A. F., and others. "Exploring the Association of John Henry Active Coping and Education on Smoking Behavior and Nicotine Dependence among Blacks in the USA." *Social Science & Medicine,* 2005, *60,* 491–500.

Folkman, S., Chesney, M. A., Pollack, L., and Phillips, C. "Stress, Coping, and High-Risk Sexual Behavior." *Health Psychology,* 1992, *11,* 218–222.

Folkman, S., and Lazarus, R. S. *The Ways of Coping Questionnaire.* Palo Alto, Calif.: Consulting Psychologists Press, 1988.

Folkman, S., and Moskowitz, J. "Positive Affect and the Other Side of Coping." *American Psychologist,* 2000, *55,* 647–654.

Frasure-Smith, N., and others. "Social Support, Depression, and Mortality During The First Year After Myocardial Infarction." *Circulation,* 2000, *101,* 1919–1924.

Gaab, J., Sonderegger, L., Scherrer, S., and Ehlert U. "Psychoneuroendocrine Effects of Cognitive-Behavioral Stress Management in a Naturalistic Setting—A Randomized Controlled Trial." *Psychoneuroendocrinology,* 2006, *31,* 428–438.

Giltay, E. J., and others. "Dispositional Optimism and All-Cause and Cardiovascular Mortality in a Prospective Cohort of Elderly Dutch Men and Women." *Archives of General Psychiatry,* 2004, *61,* 1126–1135.

Giltay, E. J., and others. "Dispositional Optimism and the Risk of Cardiovascular Death: The Zutphen Elderly Study." *Archives of Internal Medicine,* 2006, *166,* 431–436.

Glanz, K., Steffen, A. D., and Taglialatela, L. A. "Effects of Colon Cancer Risk Counseling for First-Degree Relatives." *Cancer, Epidemiology, Biomarkers and Prevention,* 2007, *16,* 1485–1491.

Glaser, R., and Kiecolt-Glaser, J. K. "Stress-Induced Immune Dysfunction: Implications for Health." *Nature Reviews. Immunology,* 2005, *5,* 243–251.

Gustavsson-Lilius, M., Julkunen, J., Keskivaara, P., and Hietanen, P. "Sense of Coherence and Distress in Cancer Patients and Their Partners." *Psycho-Oncology,* 2007, *16*(12), 1100–1110.

Hack, T. F., and Degner, L. F. "Coping with Breast Cancer: A Cluster Analytic Approach." *Breast Cancer Research and Treatment,* 1999, *54*(3), 185–194.

Haritatos, J., Mahalingam, R., and James, S. A. "John Henryism, Self-Reported Physical Health Indicators, and the Mediating Role of Perceived Stress Among High Socio-Economic Status Asian Immigrants." *Social Science & Medicine,* 2007, *64,* 1192–1203.

Heitzmann, C. A., and Kaplan, R. M. "Assessment of Methods for Measuring Social Support." *Health Psychology,* 1988, *7,* 75–109.

Helgeson, V. S., Reynolds, K. A., and Tomich, P. L. "A Meta-Analytic Review of Benefit Finding and Growth." *Journal of Consulting and Clinical Psychology,* 2006, *74,* 797–816.

Holahan, C. J., and Moos, R. H. "Personality, Coping, and Family Resources in Stress Resistance: A Longitudinal Analysis." *Journal of Personality and Social Psychology,* 1986, *51,* 389–395.

Holmes, T. H., and Rahe, R. H. "The Social Readjustment Rating Scale." *Journal of Psychosomatic Research,* 1967, *11,* 213–218.

House, J. S. "Occupational Stress and Coronary Heart Disease: A Review and Theoretical Integration." *Journal of Health and Social Behavior,* 1974, *15,* 12–27.

Ironson, G., and others. "Dispositional Optimism and the Mechanisms by which it Predicts Slower Disease Progression in HIV: Proactive Behavior, Avoidant Coping, and Depression." *International Journal of Behavioral Medicine,* 2005, *12,* 86–97.

James, S., Hartnett, S. A., and Kalsbeek, W. D. "John Henryism and Blood Pressure Among Black Men." *Journal of Behavioral Medicine,* 1983, *6,* 259–278.

Kawachi, I., and Subramanian, S. V. "Measuring and Modeling the Social and Geographic Context of Trauma: A Multilevel Modeling Approach." *Journal of Traumatic Stress,* 2006, *19,* 195–203.

Kiecolt-Glaser, J. K., and others. "Chronic Stress and Immunity in Family Caregivers of Alzheimer's Disease Victims." *Psychosomatic Medicine,* 1987, *49,* 523–535.

Kinsinger, D. P., and others. "Psychosocial and Sociodemographic Correlates of Benefit-Finding in Men Treated for Localized Prostate Cancer." *Psychooncology,* 2006, *15,* 954–961.

Kobasa, S. C. "Stressful Life Events, Personality, and Health: An Inquiry into Hardiness." *Journal of Personality and Social Psychology,* 1979, *37,* 1–11.

Kok, G., Hospers, H. J., Harterink, P., and de Zwart, O. "Social-Cognitive Determinants of HIV Risk-Taking Intentions Among Men Who Date Men Through the Internet." *AIDS Care,* 2007, *19*(3), 410–417.

Koo, M., Krass, I., and Asiani, P. "Enhancing Patient Education about Medicines: Factors Influencing Reading and Seeking of Written Medicine Information." *Health Expectations,* 2006, *9,* 174–187.

Krieger, N., and Sidney, S. "Racial Discrimination and Blood Pressure: The CARDIA Study of Young Black and White Adults." *American Journal of Public Health,* 1996, *86,* 1370–1378.

Kroenke, C. H., and others. "Social Networks, Social Support, and Survival After Breast Cancer Diagnosis." *Journal of Clinical Oncology,* 2006, *24,* 1105–1111.

Kung, S., and others. "Association of Optimism-Pessimism with Quality of Life in Patients with Head and Neck and Thyroid Cancers." *Mayo Clinic Proceedings,* 2006, *81,* 1545–1552.

Laubmeier, K. K., Zakowski, S. G., and Bair, J. P. "The Role of Spirituality in the Psychological Adjustment to Cancer: A Test of the Transactional Model of Stress and Coping." *International Journal of Behavioral Medicine,* 2004, *11,* 48–55.

Lazarus, R. S. *Psychological Stress and the Coping Process.* New York: McGraw-Hill, 1966.

Lazarus, R. S. "Toward Better Research on Stress and Coping." *American Psychologist,* 2000, *55,* 665–673.

Lazarus, R. S. "Coping Theory and Research: Past, Present, and Future." *Psychosomatic Medicine,* 1993, *55,* 234–247.

Lazarus, R. S., and Cohen, J. B. "Environmental Stress." In I. Altman and J. F. Wohlwill (eds.), *Human Behavior and Environment*. Vol. 2. New York: Plenum, 1977.

Lazarus, R. S., and Folkman, S. *Stress, Appraisal, and Coping*. New York: Springer, 1984.

Lechner, S. C., and others. "Curvilinear Associations Between Benefit Finding and Psychosocial Adjustment to Breast Cancer." *Journal of Clinical and Consulting Psychiatry*, 2006, *74*, 828–840.

Lepore, S. J., and others. "Effects of Social Stressors on Cardiovascular Reactivity in Black and White Women." *Annals of Behavioral Medicine*, 2006, *31*, 120–127.

Lerman, C., Daly, M., Masny, A., and Balshem, A. "Attitudes about Genetic Testing for Breast-Ovarian Cancer Susceptibility." *Journal of Clinical Oncology*, 1994, *12*, 843–850.

Lerman, C., and others. "Mammography Adherence and Psychological Distress among Women at Risk for Breast Cancer." *Journal of the National Cancer Institute*, 1993, *85*, 1074–1080.

Leserman, J. "The Effects of Depression, Stressful Life Events, Social Support, and Coping on the Progression of HIV Infection." *Current Psychiatry Reports*, 2000, *2*, 495–502.

Matthieu, M. M., and Ivanoff, A. "Using Stress, Appraisal, and Coping Theories in Clinical Practice: Assessments of Coping Strategies after Disasters." *Brief Treatment and Crisis Intervention*, 2006, *6*, 337–348.

McGregor, B. A., and others. "Cognitive-Behavioral Stress Management Increases Benefit Finding and Immune Function Among Women with Early-Stage Breast Cancer." *Journal of Psychosomatic Research*, 2004, *56*, 1–8.

McKetney, E. C., and Ragland, D. R. "John Henryism, Education, and Blood Pressure in Young Adults. The CARDIA Study. Coronary Artery Risk Development in Young Adults Study." *American Journal of Epidemiology*, 1996, *143*, 787–791.

Meier, A., and others. "How Cancer Survivors Provide Support on Cancer-Related Internet Mailing Lists." *Journal of Medical Internet Research*, 2007, *9*(2), e12.

Merritt, M. M., and others. "Low Educational Attainment, John Henryism, and Cardiovascular Reactivity to and Recovery from Personally Relevant Stress." *Psychosomatic Medicine*, 2004, *66*, 49–55.

Merritt, M. M., and others. "Perceived Racism and Cardiovascular Reactivity and Recovery to Personally Relevant Stress." *Health Psychology*, 2006, *25*, 364–369.

Merluzzi, T., and others. "Self-Efficacy for Coping with Cancer: Revision of the Cancer Behavior Inventory (Version 2.0)." *Psycho-Oncology*, 2001, *10*(3), 206–217.

Miller, S. M., and others. "Monitoring Styles in Women at Risk for Cervical Cancer: Implications for the Framing of Health-Relevant Messages." *Annals of Behavioral Medicine*, 1999, *21*, 27–34.

Miller, S. M., and Mangan, C. E. "The Interacting Effects of Information and Coping Style in Adapting to Gynecological Stress: Should the Doctor Tell All?" *Journal of Personality and Social Psychology*, 1983, *45*, 223–236.

Mishel, M. H., and others. "Benefits from an Uncertainty Management Intervention for African-American and Caucasian Older Long-Term Breast Cancer Survivors." *Psycho-Oncology*, 2005, *14*, 962–978.

Moser, D. K., and others. "Impact of Anxiety and Perceived Control on In-Hospital Complications after Acute Myocardial Infarction." *Psychosomatic Medicine*, 2007, *69*(1), 10–16.

Moskowitz, J. T., Folkman, S., Collette, L., and Vittinghoff, E. "Coping and Mood During AIDS-Related Caregiving and Bereavement." *Annals of Behavioral Medicine*, 1996, *18*, 49–57.

Moynihan, J. A. "Mechanisms of Stress-Induced Modulation of Immunity." *Brain, Behavior, and Immunity*, 2003, *17*(Suppl 1), S11–S16.

Myers, R. E., and others. "A Randomized Controlled Trial of the Impact of Targeted and Tailored Interventions on Colorectal Cancer Screening." *Cancer*, 2007, *110*, 2083–2091.

Northouse, L., Kershaw, T., Mood, D., and Schafenacker, A. "Effects of a Family Intervention on the Quality of Life of Women with Recurrent Breast Cancer and Their Family Caregivers." *Psycho-Oncology*, 2005, *14*, 478–491.

Norton, T. R., and others. "Ovarian Cancer Patients' Psychological Distress: The Role of Physical Impairment, Perceived Unsupportive Family and Friend Behaviors, Perceived Control, and Self-Esteem." *Health Psychology*, 2005, *24*(2), 143–152.

Ong, L. M., and others. "Cancer Patients' Coping Styles and Doctor-Patient Communication." *Psycho-Oncology*, 1999, *8*, 155–166.

Penedo, F. J., and others. "A Randomized Clinical Trial of Group-Based Cognitive-Behavioral Stress Management in Localized Prostate Cancer: Development Of Stress Management Skills Improves Quality Of Life And Benefit Finding." *Annals of Behavioral Medicine*, 2006, *31*, 261–270.

Rees, C. E., and Bath, P. A. "The Psychometric Properties of the Miller Behavioral Style Scale with Adult Daughters of Women with Early Stage Breast Cancer: A Literature Review and Empirical Study." *Journal of Advanced Nursing*, 2000, *32*, 366–374.

Rimer, B. K., and others. "How New Subscribers Use Cancer-Related Online Mailing Lists." *Journal of Medical Internet Research,* 2005, *7*(3), e32.

Ryff, C. D., and Keyes, C. L. "The Structure of Psychological Well-Being Revisited." *Journal of Personality and Social Psychology,* 1995, *69,* 719–727.

Ryff, C. D., Lee, Y. H., Essex, M. J., and Schmutte, P. S. "My Children and Me: Midlife Evaluations of Grown Children and Self." *Psychology and Aging,* 1994, *9,* l95–205.

Scheier, M. F., and Bridges, M. W. "Person Variables and Health: Personality and Predispositions and Acute Psychological States as Shared Determinants for Disease." *Psychosomatic Medicine,* 1995, *57,* 255–268.

Scheier, M. F., and Carver, C. S. "Effects of Optimism on Psychological and Physical Well-Being: Theoretical Overview and Empirical Update." *Cognitive Therapy and Research,* 1992, *16,* 201–228.

Schofield, P., and others. "Optimism and Survival in Lung Carcinoma Patients." *Cancer,* 2004, *100,* 1276–1282.

Schuster, M. A., and others. "A National Survey of Stress Reactions after the September 11, 2001, Terrorist Attacks." *The New England Journal of Medicine,* 2001, *345,* 1507–1512.

Schwartz, M., and others. "Coping Disposition, Perceived Risk, and Psychological Distress Among Women at Increased Risk for Ovarian Cancer." *Health Psychology,* 1995, *14,* 232–235.

Schwarzer, R., and others. "Changes in Finding Benefit After Cancer Surgery and the Prediction of Well-Being One Year Later." *Social Science & Medicine,* 2006, *63,* 1614–1624.

Sears, S. R., Stanton, A. L., and Danoff-Burg, S. "The Yellow Brick Road and the Emerald City: Benefit Finding, Positive Reappraisal Coping and Posttraumatic Growth in Women with Early-Stage Breast Cancer." *Health Psychology,* 2003, *22,* 487–497.

Seligman, M., and Csikszentmihalyi, M. "Positive Psychology: An Introduction." *American Psychologist,* 2000, *55*(1), 5–14.

Selye, H. *The Stress of Life.* New York: McGraw-Hill, 1956.

Sheehan, J., Sherman, K. A., Lam, T., and Boyages, J. "Association of Information Satisfaction, Psychological Distress and Monitoring Coping Style with Post-Decision Regret Following Breast Reconstruction." *Psycho-Oncology,* 2007, *16*(4), 342–351.

Skinner, E. A., and Zimmer-Gembeck, M. J. "The Development of Coping." *Annual Review of Psychology,* 2007, *58,* 119–144.

Smith, C. A., Haynes, K. N., Lazarus, R. S., and Pope, L. K. "In Search of the 'Hot' Cognitions: Attributions, Appraisals, and Their Relation to Emotion." *Journal of Personality and Social Psychology,* 1993, *65,* 916–929.

Smith, C. A., and Lazarus, R. S. "Appraisal Components, Core Relational Themes, and the Emotions." *Cognition and Emotion,* 1993, *7,* 233–269.

Spiegel, D., Bloom, J., Kraemer, H., and Gottheil, E. "Effect of Psychosocial Treatment on Survival of Patients with Metastatic Breast Cancer." *Lancet,* 1989, *2*(8668), 888–891.

Spiegel, D., and others. "Effects of Supportive-Expressive Group Therapy on Survival of Patients with Metastatic Breast Cancer: A Randomized Prospective Trial." *Cancer,* 2007, *110*(5), 1130–1138.

Stanton, A. L., and others. "Emotionally Expressive Coping Predicts Psychological and Physical Adjustment to Breast Cancer." *Journal of Consulting and Clinical Psychology,* 2000, *68*(5), 875–882.

Stanton, A. L., Revenson, T. A., and Tennen, H. "Health Psychology: Psychological Adjustment to Chronic Disease." *Annual Review of Psychology,* 2007, *58,* 565–592.

Stephton, S. E., Sapolsky, R. M., Kraemer, H. C., and Spiegel, D. "Diurnal Cortisol Rhythm as a Predictor of Breast Cancer Survival." *Journal of the National Cancer Institute,* 2000, *92,* 994–1000.

Stone, A., Greenberg, M., Kennedy-Moore, E., and Newman, M. "Self Report, Situation-Specific Coping Questionnaires: What Are They Measuring?" *Journal of Personality and Social Psychology,* 1991, *61,* 648–658.

Stone, A., Kennedy-Moore, E., and Neale, J. "Coping with Daily Problems." *Health Psychology,* 1995, *14,* 341–349.

Stone, A. A., and Porter, L. S. "Psychological Coping: Its Importance for Treating Medical Problems." *Mind/Body Medicine,* 1995, *1,* 46–54.

Stone, A., Shiffman, S., Atienza, A., and Nebeling, L. (eds.). *The Science of Real-Time Data Capture: Self-Reports in Health Research.* New York: Oxford University Press, 2007.

Suls, J., and Fletcher, B. "The Relative Efficacy of Avoidant and Nonavoidance Coping Strategies: A Meta-Analysis." *Health Psychology,* 1985, *4,* 249–288.

Taylor, S. E., and others. "Optimism, Coping, Psychological Distress, and High-Risk Sexual Behavior Among Men at Risk for Acquired Immunodeficiency Syndrome (AIDS)." *Journal of Personality and Social Psychology,* 1992, *63,* 460–473.

Thong, M. S., and others. "Social Support Predicts Survival in Dialysis Patients." *Nephrology, Dialysis, Transplantation,* 2007, *22,* 845–850.

Tomich, P. L., and Helgeson, V. S. "Is Finding Something Good in the Bad Always Good? Benefit Finding Among Women with Breast Cancer." *Health Psychology,* 2004, *23,* 16–23.

Trask, P. C., and others. "Psychosocial Characteristics of Individuals with Non-Stage IV Melanoma." *Journal of Clinical Oncology,* 2001, *19*(11), 2844–2850.

Tross, S., and others. "Psychological Symptoms and Disease-Free and Overall Survival in Women With Stage II Breast Cancer: Cancer and Leukemia Group B." *Journal of the National Cancer Institute,* 1996, *88*(10), 629–631.

van Zuuren, F. J., and others. "The Effect of an Information Brochure on Patients Undergoing Gastrointestinal Endoscopy: A Randomized Controlled Study." *Patient Education and Counseling,* 2006, *64*(1–3), 173–182.

Walker, L. G., and others. "Psychological, Clinical and Pathological Effects of Relaxation Training and Guided Imagery During Primary Chemotherapy." *British Journal of Cancer,* 1999, *80,* 262–268.

Wenzel, L. B., and others. "Resilience, Reflection, and Residual Stress in Ovarian Cancer Survivorship." *Psycho-Oncology,* 2002, *11,* 142–153.

Williams, D. R. "Race, Socioeconomic Status, and Health: The Added Effects of Racism and Discrimination." *Annals of the New York Academy of Sciences,* 1999, *896,* 173–188.

Williams, R. B., and others. "Prognostic Importance of Social and Economic Resources Among Medically Treated Patients with Angiographically Documented Coronary Artery Disease." *Journal of the American Medical Association,* 1992, *267,* 520–524.

Williams-Piehota, P., and others. "Matching Health Messages to Monitor-Blunter Coping Styles to Motivate Screening Mammography." *Health Psychology,* 2005, *24,* 58–67.

Zakowski, S. G., and others. "Written Emotional Disclosure Buffers the Effects of Social Constraints on Distress Among Cancer Patients." *Health Psychology,* 2004, *23,* 555–556.

CHAPTER

KEY INTERPERSONAL FUNCTIONS AND HEALTH OUTCOMES

Lessons from Theory and Research on Clinician-Patient Communication

Richard L. Street Jr.
Ronald M. Epstein

KEY POINTS

This chapter will

- Discuss the major pathways between clinician-patient communications and their outcomes on health.
- Define key functions of clinician-patient communications.

■ Describe key factors that may moderate the health outcomes as a result of patient-provider communications.

■ Provide an example that applies the key concepts to clinical practice guidelines for smoking cessation counseling.

■ Discuss directions for future research.

Interpersonal communication is one of the key sources of social influence, a process critical to change in health behavior. Interpersonal communication may take place in informal relationships, such as families and friends, or in more formal relationships, such as physicians and patients. There are several advantages to delineating how interpersonal communications may influence health behavior. The resulting understanding can lead to the design of effective interventions to change health behaviors and improve patient-provider communications. It also helps to distinguish interpersonal influence from related areas, such as social support and social networks (see Chapter Nine). This chapter describes theory and research on clinician-patient communication as a specific type of interpersonal influence. There is a rich literature in this area of study, and much of it can be related to influence and communication in other types of interactions related to health behavior (for example, with friends, family, coworkers).

One of the most interesting yet least understood aspects of medical care is the way clinicians and patients communicate with one another. Good communication is often associated with improved physical health, more effective chronic disease management, and better health-related quality of life long after the encounter (Ong, de Haes, Hoos, and Lammes, 1995; Arora, 2003). This suggests that "good" communication can lead to better health. However, over forty years of research on clinician (mostly physician)-patient communication has resulted in few significant advances toward formulating theoretical models to address questions such as what the key elements of effective communication are and how and in what ways clinician-patient communication affects health outcomes and health behaviors.

As there are virtually thousands of published papers on this topic, we have organized this chapter around key *functions* of clinician-patient communication and how they may lead to better health outcomes through a selective review of the literature. A functional approach is advantageous for two main reasons. First, it taps into the "work" that communication does, as it is aimed toward accomplishing certain tasks (for example, reach a diagnosis, make treatment decisions). Second, a functional approach provides a useful framework for organizing a review of the literature and the various theoretical and conceptual approaches that have been applied to clinician-patient communication. We will start with a discussion of the pathways through which communication may lead to better health outcomes, before discussing the six key functions of clinician-patient communication and the moderators of this relationship. The focus will be on physician-patient communication because this has been the topic of the vast majority of previous research. However, this analysis should be applicable to other types of clinicians, including nurses, allied health professionals, and health educators.

COMMUNICATION BETWEEN HEALTH CARE PROVIDERS AND PATIENTS: HISTORICAL PERSPECTIVE

Health care provider-patient interactions have been studied for over fifty years by medical sociologists and health services researchers (Parsons, 1951; Roter and Hall, 1992). During provider-patient interactions, the level of patient involvement may vary on a continuum from totally passive (Parsons, 1951) to extremely active (Roter and Hall, 1992; Haug and Lavin, 1983). The different types of provider-patient encounters are best illustrated by Roter and Hall's (1992) typology of provider-patient relationships. The level of control that the provider and patient possess determines which of the four typologies is operating.

Descriptive models of patient-provider communication—a subject of interest for several decades—categorized communication into several types, based on the degree of control exercised between the patient and the provider (Parsons, 1951; Lewis, DeVellis, and Sleath, 2002; Roter and Hall, 1992). Roter and Hall (1992) identify at least four different types of interactions, based on the degree of control between the provider and the patient. The relationship is considered *paternalistic* when the provider has greater control over the interaction and is characterized by a low degree of involvement by the patient (Roter and Hall, 1992). *Mutuality* is characterized by balance in control between the provider and the patient, and the interactions and decision making are more likely to be participatory (Roter and Hall, 1992; Sleath, 1996). A *default* interaction is when neither party has control and could result in patient dissatisfaction and nonparticipation (Roter and Hall, 1992). Finally, *consumerism* is when patients exercise greater control in the interactions relative to physicians (Haug and Lavin, 1983). A patient is likely to have a greater say, and the health care provider is likely to be more sensitive to the goals and needs of the patients in such situations (Kaplan and others, 1996; Stewart, 2001). This chapter goes beyond descriptive models to organize the voluminous literature into critical pathways that link clinician-patient communications with health outcomes and to key functions of clinician-patient communication.

PATHWAYS BETWEEN CLINICIAN-PATIENT COMMUNICATION AND HEALTH OUTCOMES

Before describing the key functions of clinician-patient communication, we preface this analysis with general observations about theory in the study of communication in medical encounters and its relationship to health outcomes. Even though a number of studies offered descriptive models of relationship factors affecting communication processes and health outcomes, the explanatory mechanisms for why elements of clinician-patient interactions are associated with health outcomes are not as well understood. In part, this is because any number of cognitive, affective, behavioral, cultural, organizational, and even economic factors could moderate or mediate relationships between communication and subsequent improvement in health. Consider two very different examples.

First, clinician-patient communication could help the patient understand how to follow a complex medication regimen. By taking the medication appropriately, chemical agents can treat the disease and improve the patient's health. But if these agents are ineffective, the patient's understanding of the treatment regimen would be for naught. Second, clinician-patient communication could affect motivational and cognitive processes underlying health-related behaviors (for example, smoking, diet, exercise). These processes might enhance the patient's decision-making and problem-solving skill for adopting a healthier lifestyle that, in turn, could lead to better health. But if the patient's social environment does not support these behavior changes, the patient may experience insurmountable barriers, in spite of the quality of the clinician-patient encounter. In short, any number of theoretical processes may be involved, from the communicative dynamics of the consultation itself to the actualization of health outcomes in the days, weeks, and months after the encounter.

Figure 11.1 offers a starting point for identifying possible theoretical mechanisms that might account for ways in which clinician-patient communication affects health outcomes. Clinician-patient communication can affect health directly or can affect it indirectly through the mediating effects of proximal outcomes (such as greater mutual understanding, trust, patient satisfaction, and patient involvement in decision making) and intermediate outcomes (such as changes in patient health behaviors, self-care skills, adherence to treatment, and better medical decisions). For example, a

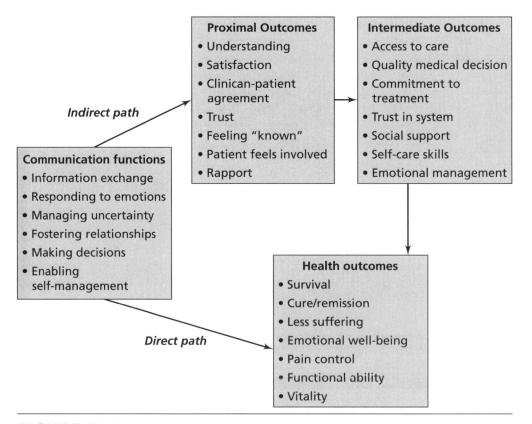

FIGURE 11.1. Direct and Indirect Pathways from Communication to Health Outcomes.

physician can alleviate emotional distress directly by telling a patient that a diagnostic test result is normal. Or a physician who is reassuring and offers clear, understandable explanations may help a hospitalized patient to experience lower anxiety, better sleep, and improved appetite immediately after the clinical encounter (Montazeri, Gillis, and McEwen, 1998; Ong, Visser, Lammes, and de Haes, 2000).

In most situations, however, a more complex series of mechanisms links communication to health outcomes (Arora, 2003). Physician-patient communication that is characterized by effective information exchange and positive affect can lead to greater patient trust (a proximal outcome) and a greater willingness to follow through with commitment to treatment (an intermediate outcome), which in turn may affect survival. Or patient participation in consultations could help the physician to understand the patient's values and preferences and discover possible misperceptions the patient might have about treatment effects. The doctor can then communicate clinical information in a way the patient understands (a proximal outcome) and, together with the patient, arrive at a higher-quality decision that best matches the patient's circumstances (intermediate outcome) and leads to improved health.

Whether direct or indirect, communication may improve health through various causal mechanisms or pathways. These might include improved patient knowledge and clinician-patient agreement on diagnosis and treatment, improved therapeutic alliances for coordinating patient care and involving the patient in care, helping the patient manage negative emotions more effectively, building stronger family/social support, higher-quality medical decisions (for example, informed, clinically sound, concordant with patient values, and mutually endorsed), and enhanced patient agency (self-efficacy, empowerment, and enablement) (Epstein and Street, 2007). If a researcher hypothesizes that one of these pathways operates to mediate the relationship between communication and health, then he or she can identify the relevant theoretical mechanisms that account for this influence.

Table 11.1 presents examples of theoretical and conceptual models that are pertinent to specific functions of clinician-patient communication. The following sections illustrate how the models are related to these key functions.

TABLE 11.1. **Representative Models of Patient-Centered Communication Functions.**

Communication Function	Theoretical/Conceptual Models	Key Theme
Fostering healing relationships	Paternalism (Parsons, 1951)	Advocates paternalistic physician-patient relationships with professional distance
	Consumerism (Reeder, 1972)	Advocates consumerist (patient as consumer) approach to physician-patient relationship

TABLE 11.1. Representative Models of Patient-Centered Communication Functions, Cont'd.

Communication Function	Theoretical/Conceptual Models	Key Theme
Fostering healing relationships *(continued)*	Three models of physician-patient relationships (Szasz and Hollender, 1956)	Activity/passivity model—the physician makes the decisions
		Guidance/cooperation model—the physician provides instructions, the patient carries them out
		Mutual participation model—the physician assists patients in helping themselves; the patient participates in decision making
	Four types of physician-patient relationships (Roter and Hall, 1992)	Paternalism—high physician control, low patient control
		Mutuality—high physician and patient control
		Default—low physician and patient control
		Consumerism—low physician control, high patient control
	Model of relational topoi (Burgoon, Buller, Hale, and deTurck, 1984)	Identifies twelve dimensions of relational communication: dominance-submission, intimacy, affection-hostility, involvement, inclusion-exclusion, trust, depth, emotional arousal, composure, similarity, formality, and task-social orientation
Information exchange	Cognitive Model (Ley, 1988)	Hypothesizes (1) patient understanding of medical information enhances memory, (2) memory and understanding increase patient satisfaction, and (3) satisfaction increases compliance

TABLE 11.1. **Representative Models of Patient-Centered Communication Functions, Cont'd.**

Communication Function	Theoretical/Conceptual Models	Key Theme
Responding to emotions	Burgoon, Buller, Hale, and deTurck's (1984) model of relational topoi	Identifies four dimensions of relational communication that focus on emotional communication: intimacy, affection-hostility, emotional arousal, and composure
	Model of empathic understanding (Squier, 1990)	Posits that empathic understanding is a function of perspective-taking skill and emotional reactivity and that better understanding of a patient's health problems will be achieved through self-disclosure, open communication, and better labeling of feelings and sensations
Managing uncertainty	Mishel's uncertainty theory (Mishel, 1999)	Posits that uncertainty is experienced when aspects of the illness, treatment, and recovery are perceived as inconsistent, random, complex, and unpredictable
	Problematic integration theory (Babrow, 2001)	Posits that discrepancies between the likelihood of certain events and the value of those events create four kinds of cognitive states that are problematic: divergence (difference between what is desired and what is likely), ambiguity (uncertainty about the likelihood of an event), ambivalence (uncertainty about the value of an event), and impossibility (an event will not happen)
	Uncertainty management theory (Brashers, 2001)	Posits that the management of uncertainty involves multiple options ranging from efforts to reduce uncertainty (for example, to alleviate anxiety) to efforts to maintain or create uncertainty (for example, to have hope)

TABLE 11.1. **Representative Models of Patient-Centered Communication Functions, Cont'd.**

Communication Function	Theoretical/Conceptual Models	Key Theme
Making decisions	A model of decision making (Charles and others, 1999)	Posits three types of medical decision making—paternalistic, shared, and informed—and that each unfolds in three phases—information exchange, deliberation, and the decision
	A linguistic model of patient participation in care (Street, 2001)	Posits that patient participation in consultations, including in decision making, is a function of predisposing factors (for example, motivation, beliefs about patient involvement), enabling factors (for example, knowledge, communication skill), and provider behavior (for example, partnership building)
	Integrative model of shared decision making (Makoul and Clayman, 2006)	Identifies 9 degrees of "sharedness" in medical decision making: doctor alone, doctor led and patient acknowledgment, doctor led and patient agreement, doctor led and patient views/opinions, shared equally, patient led and doctor's views/opinions, patient led and doctor agreement, patient led and doctor acknowledgment, patient alone
Enabling patient self-management	Self-determination theory (Ryan and Deci, 2000)	Human behavior is driven to meet three basic needs—competence, autonomy, and relatedness
	Transtheoretical Model (Prochaska and Velicer, 1997)	Posits that behavior change is on a continuum: precontemplation, contemplation, preparation, action, maintenance, termination

TABLE 11.1. **Representative Models of Patient-Centered Communication Functions, Cont'd.**

Communication Function	Theoretical/Conceptual Models	Key Theme
Enabling patient self-management *(continued)*	Integrative model of health behavior (Fishbein and Cappella, 2006)	Health behavior is a function of attitudes, social norms, and self-efficacy, which emanate from behavioral, normative, and control beliefs
	Patient agency model (O'Hair and others, 2003)	Identifies three steps to patient agency (control of health—cope with uncertainty), empowerment (having a "voice" in clinical encounters), and agency (self-efficacy, control, and behavioral actualization)

KEY FUNCTIONS OF CLINICIAN-PATIENT COMMUNICATION

Most studies of physician-patient communication focus on patients' perceptions of their own and the physician's behavior (Smith and others, 2006) or a coder's ratings of the physician's and patient's communicative profiles or styles (for example, frequency of physician information giving, number of questions patients asked, proportion of communication that is patient-centered) (Kaplan, Greenfield, and Ware, 1989; Street and others, 2005). To link these behaviors to outcomes, one must consider the key functions of physician-patient communication that could affect outcomes. These functions include fostering the physician-patient relationship, exchanging and managing information, validating and responding to emotions, managing uncertainty, making decisions, and enabling patient self-management. Table 11.2 provides examples of measures used to assess communication related to these functions and whether they are patient or physician perceptions derived from surveys or whether they are coded by observers of the interactions between patients and physicians (either live or from audio or video recordings). These measures are the foundation of research on clinician-patient communication, and some of them are based in measurement techniques that have been used in broader studies of interpersonal influence and communication.

TABLE 11.2. **Representative Measures and Coding Systems of Patient-Centered Communication Functions.**

Communication Function	Measure	Key Dimensions
Fostering healing relationships	Provider-Patient Orientation Scale (Krupat, Yeager, and Putnam, 2000)	Self-report measures of "caring" (affiliation) and "sharing" (control) preferences in the provider-patient relationship (self-report)
	Patient Reactions Assessment (PRA) (Galassi, Schanberg, and Ware, 1992)	PRA subscale, "affective communication" measures patient perception of physician's respect and concern for the patient (self-report)
	Patient perceptions of physician communication measure (PPC) (Street, Gordon, and Haidet, 2007)	PPC subscale, "interpersonal sensitivity," measures patient's perceptions of doctor affect toward the patient (self or observer rating)
		PPC subscale, "partnership-building," measures patient perceptions of physician interest in the patient's perspective (self or observer rating)
	Roter Interaction Analysis System (RIAS) (Roter and Larson, 2002)	Socio-emotional categories of RIAS identify fifteen types of relationship-related utterances (for example, laughs, disagrees, shows interest) (observer coding)
	Active Patient Participation Coding System (APPC) (Street and Millay, 2001)	Physician facilitation categories of APPC, including partnership-building (utterances that solicit patient views and perspective) and supportive communication (utterances that reassure, praise, comfort, and so on) (observer coding)
	Measure of patient-centered communication (MPCC) (Brown, Stewart, and Ryan, 2001)	Assesses physician's responsiveness to patient's concerns (observer coding)

TABLE 11.2. **Representative Measures and Coding Systems of Patient-Centered Communication Functions, Cont'd.**

Communication Function	Measure	Key Dimensions
Information exchange	Information Preference Scale (Blanchard, Labrecque, Ruckdeschel, and Blanchard, 1988)	Measures patients' preferences type and amount of information from physicians
	Information Styles Questionnaire (Cassileth Zupkis, Sutton-Smith, and March, 1980)	Measures patients' preferences for amount of information from physicians
	Willingness to discuss psychosocial and physical aspects of health (Street, Cauthen, Buchwald, and Wiprud, 1995)	Measures patients' willingness to discuss physical and psychosocial aspects of health
	Preferences for discussing health-related quality of life (Detmar and others, 2000)	Measures patients' and physicians' preferences for discussing health-related quality of life issues
	Preferences for discussing prognostic information (Hagerty and others, 2004)	Patient preference regarding • Specific prognostic information • When to discuss prognosis and who should initiate the discussion • Prognostic information, timing, and manner of presentation
	Patient Reactions Assessment (PRA) (Galassi, Schanberg, and Ware, 1992)	PRA subscale, "information," measures patient's perception of physicians' information-giving
	Patient perceptions of physician communication measure (PPC) (Street, Gordon, and Haidet, 1997)	PPC subscale, "information-giving," measures patient's perceptions of doctor's information-giving (self-report and observer rating)
	Perceived Involvement in Care Scale (Lerman and others, 1990)	Patient involvement subscale measures patient's perception of his or her involvement in the interaction (self-report)

TABLE 11.2. **Representative Measures and Coding Systems of Patient-Centered Communication Functions, Cont'd.**

Communication Function	Measure	Key Dimensions
Information exchange *(continued)*	Krantz Health Opinion Survey (Krantz, Baum, and Wideman, 1980)	Active participation subscale taps into patient preferences for information seeking during consultations (self-report)
	Roter Interaction Analysis System (RIAS) (Roter and Larson, 2002)	Task categories of RIAS identify information seeking and information-giving utterances across five categories: medical condition, therapeutic regimen, psychosocial information, lifestyle information, and other (observer coded)
	Physician-Patient Verbal Coding Scheme (Gordon, Street, Sharf, and Souchek, 2006)	Measures physician information giving across seven categories: health status/condition, treatment, rationale for treatment, prognosis, risks, instructions, and other (observer coded)
Making decisions	Informed decision-making coding (Braddock and others, 1999)	Measures degree to which physician recommendations satisfy informed decision making (observer coded)
	Control Preferences Scale (Degner, Sloan, and Venkatesh, 1997)	Uses a card sort technique to measure patients' preferences for control in medical decision making (self-report)
	Rochester Participatory Decision-Making Scale (RPAD) (Shields and others, 2005b)	Measures patient-physician collaborative decision making (observer coded)
Responding to emotions	RIAS Global affect scales (Roter and Larson, 2002)	Measures physician and patient affect in medical encounters (observer-coded)
	Physician empathy scale (Hojat and others, 2002)	Measure of physician empathy (self-report)

TABLE 11.2. **Representative Measures and Coding Systems of Patient-Centered Communication Functions, Cont'd.**

Communication Function	Measure	Key Dimensions
Responding to emotions *(continued)*	Empathic Communication Coding System (ECCS) (Bylund and Makoul, 2002)	Measures patient-created empathic opportunities and physician responses to those opportunities (observer coding)
Managing uncertainty	Mishel Uncertainty in Illness Scale (Mishel, 1999)	Measures two dimensions of uncertainty in illness (self-report)
Enabling patient self-management	Health Care Climate Questionnaire (Williams and others, 2005)	Measures degree to which physicians support patient autonomy in self-care (self-report)
	The 5-As model (Glasgow, Emont, and Miller, 2006)	Can be used to measure four steps to physician facilitation of patient health behavior change: ask, advise, assess, assist, and arrange follow-up (observer coding)
	Ory and others, 2006 Russel and Roter, 1993 Tai-Seale and others, 2007	Example of studies that used observers to code for whether lifestyle issues were discussed in medical consultations

Fostering Healing Physician-Patient Relationships

Interpersonal relationships, including the physician-patient relationship, can be characterized along two primary dimensions: how the participants distribute control in the relationship and their affective orientation to one another (for example, liking, affiliation, friendliness). Early models of the physician-patient relationship focused prescriptively on the importance of medical expertise to legitimize physician control in the relationship, especially to help sick patients in an affective neutral way or with benevolence (Parsons, 1951). The last thirty years have seen a shift away from advocating a paternalistic physician-patient relationship toward approaches that recognize that patients may also be consumers (Reeder, 1972) or partners in care (Holman and Lorig, 2000).

Physicians and patients generally desire a relationship that is characterized by mutual trust, engagement, respect, and agreement on one another's roles in the relationship (Fuertes and others, 2007). For patients, trust is greater when the physician is perceived as informative, respectful, emotionally supportive, and genuinely interested in the patient's views (Gordon and others, 2006). Showing respect and engagement are accomplished verbally, by expressing interest in another's views and circumstances, and nonverbally, through eye contact and facial expressions of attentiveness (Epstein and others, 2005a; Roter, Frankel, Hall, and Sluyter, 2006). Studies of factors affecting physicians' perceptions of their relationships with patients are rare, although some research shows that physicians have less favorable impressions of some patients (for example, minority [van Ryn and Burke, 2000], unkempt [Harris, Rich, and Crowson, 1985]), which in turn may lead to less involved, positive, and informative communication with these patients (Street, Gordon, and Haidet, 2007).

Although trust and respect, arguably, are desirable in all physician-patient relationships, there is often considerable variability in physician and patient preferences for their respective roles in the relationship. For example, patients and physicians may have differing views of the patient's level of involvement in decision making and the appropriateness of discussing psychosocial topics in the consultation (Krupat and others, 2000; Street, Cauthen, Buchwald, and Wiprud, 1995). When physician and patient expectations for the relationship are concordant, patients are more likely to evaluate the physician more favorably, be satisfied with care, and intend to adhere to treatment (Krupat and others, 2000; Krupat and others, 2001). However, physicians are often not aware of the patient's expectations (Bruera, Willey, Palmer, and Rosales, 2002). The discordance can be subtle, and effective alignment of physician and patient expectations depends on both parties openly discussing their preferences and the reasons underlying them so that they can establish mutually agreeable norms for the relationship (Epstein, 2006).

A strong physician-patient relationship is particularly important for patients because of the fear and worry associated with threats to health and well-being (McWilliam, Brown, and Stewart, 2000). Indicators of a strong therapeutic alliance between physician and patient include mutual trust and a patient's feeling respected and supported emotionally. These alliances are considered therapeutic because the quality of the physician-patient (and family) relationships can affect health outcomes in two respects. First, a strong relationship can directly promote emotional well-being through the patient's sense of feeling known, cared for, and understood (Salkeld, Solomon, Short, and Butow, 2004; Henman and others, 2002). Second, a strong physician-patient relationship can indirectly improve health through continuity of care, patient satisfaction, and commitment to treatment plans (Fuertes and others, 2007; Cabana and Jee, 2004).

Exchanging and Managing Information

Information exchange is the most widely studied function of physician-patient communication. Historically, research in this area has embraced a deficit perspective on physician-patient information exchange. For example, researchers have focused on patients' lack of health literacy (Davis and others, 2002), dissatisfaction with the amount of information they receive from clinicians (Arora, 2003; Champman and

Rush, 2003), their failure to remember information (Ley, 1988), and on physicians' lack of understanding of the patient's perspective (Teutsch, 2003; Rothschild, 1998; Simon and Kodish, 2005). A more recent alternative is a process model of information exchange that focuses on the reciprocal efforts of both clinicians and patients to manage information and achieve, even negotiate, a shared understanding of the medical and personal issues underlying the patient's health condition. Information exchange is more successful when patients participate actively to garner more and clearer information from physicians (Cegala, Post, and McClure, 2001; Street, 1991), when physicians use partnering and supportive communication to elicit the patient's beliefs and understandings (Street and others, 2005; Zandbelt and others, 2007), and when physicians can explain risk and clinical evidence in ways patients understand (Hagerty and others, 2005).

Moreover, information exchange is as much "managed" as it is "exchanged." Although most patients want to know all about their disease and treatment options (Fallowfield, Saul, and Gilligan, 2001), many may become overwhelmed by the volume of information provided by clinicians, the mass media, and the Internet (Hoffman, 2005). The informing process is complicated by the emotional salience of some types of information (Fallowfield and Jenkins, 2004), discrepancies between physician and patient understandings of disease and treatment (Williams and Wood, 1986), the challenges of communicating risk information (Epstein, Alper, and Quill, 2004), and literacy and communication skills needed for more active patient participation (Street, 2001). When successful, management of information can increase satisfaction (Davidson and Mills, 2005), facilitate participation in the consultation (Charles, Gafni, and Whelan, 1999), increase the patient's ability to cope with illness (Hagerty and others, 2005), and help the patient make informed decisions about treatment (Braddock and others, 1999).

The relationship of clinician-patient information exchange to outcomes involves more than simply the recall of information. It depends on clinician and patient achieving a shared understanding of the clinical evidence, the patient's health beliefs, and the patient's values and preferences. However, achieving a shared understanding can be difficult because physicians and patients often understand illness through different lenses. Patients' health beliefs are dynamic and complex, often based on more on "common sense" than on clinical evidence (Kleinman, 1980). This explains why patients might tend only to take medications for hypertension when they feel "tense" (Blumhagen, 1982) or why patients who believe that surgery spreads cancer (Gansler and others, 2005) might choose radiation or noninvasive treatments. When physicians and patients understand one another's respective illness representations, they are in better position to reconcile differences in viewpoints and come to some agreement on the patient's condition and options for treatment. When this occurs, patients can participate in decision making to the degree they wish, make informed decisions (Woolf and others, 2005), gain a sense of control, and place greater trust in the physician and health care system (Gordon and others, 2006), each of which can contribute to better health directly by lowering anxiety or indirectly by improving the quality of decision making and the patient's commitment to treatment.

Validating and Managing Emotions

An important, but rarely studied, function of communication is validating and managing the emotional aspects of the physician-patient encounter. Patients who are diagnosed with serious disease or worry that they might have a life-threatening condition often experience a range of negative emotions, including fear, sadness, anxiety, frustration, and anger. If sustained, these emotional states lower health-related quality of life and may even cause physiological harm (Luecken and Compas, 2002). However, physicians typically are not very effective at uncovering patients' fears and concerns (Beach, Easter, Good, and Pigeron, 2005), partly because few patients express their emotions explicitly (Butow and others, 2002) and partly because physicians do not recognize or are not comfortable discussing patients' emotional distress (Lang, Floyd, and Beine, 2000).

Physicians can help patients manage their emotions in several ways. Clear and understandable communication of disease-specific information can help patients better understand their health status and achieve a greater sense of control, more hopefulness, and better management of uncertainty (Schofield and others, 2003). Validating patients' emotional experiences and encouraging patients to express emotions also can help reduce patient anxiety and depression (Iwamitsu and others, 2003; Zachariae and others, 2003). Communication that enhances the patient's self-confidence, sense of worth, and hope may confer the meaning, motivation, and energy needed to pursue work or leisure activities, and allow the patient to enjoy better quality of life, despite the disease. In short, physician-patient communication can promote emotional well-being directly by alleviating distress and enhancing positive feelings and indirectly by facilitating the patient's ability to cope with post-consultation stress, uncertainty, and setbacks which, in turn, may lead to improvements in patients' physical symptoms (Rosenberg and others, 2002).

Managing Uncertainty

Uncertainty in illness occurs when a person perceives aspects of the illness, treatment, and recovery as inconsistent, random, complex, and unpredictable (Mishel, 1999). Managing uncertainty is distinct from other communicative functions because providing information, offering emotional support, and making decisions do not necessarily mean a reduction of uncertainty. Uncertainty may be due to a lack of information (for example, "Do I have diabetes?"), too much information (for example, "There are so many options for treatment"), or information that can be interpreted in multiple ways (for example, "Is no change in tumor marker status a positive sign?") (Babrow, 2001). In addition, although a patient's experience of uncertainty can lead to emotional distress, a loss of sense of control, and lower quality of life (Clayton, Mishel, and Belyea, 2006), uncertainty also may have self-protective value for some patients and families by allowing for hope (Brashers and others, 1999). Thus, uncertainty is best viewed as something managed rather than something simply reduced.

Making Decisions

Effective decision making is one of the most important and complicated aspects of physician-patient communication. Although decisions emerging from a consultation can have profound effects on health outcomes, little is known about what constitutes a quality medical decision. At the very least, a good medical decision is one that the physician and patient mutually agree on, where all parties are satisfied with their level of involvement in the process, the decision aligns with the patient's values and the best available clinical evidence, and the decision is feasible to implement (Epstein and Street, 2007). Only recently have researchers tried to incorporate some of these criteria in developing measures of decision quality (Sepucha and others, 2007). Also, patients vary greatly in their desire to be involved in medical decision making (Bruera and others, 2001), and physicians often do not know patients' preferences for involvement (Bruera, Willey, Palmer, and Rosales, 2002). Further, patient preferences for involvement may change during the course of a consultation or from one visit to the next (Butow and others, 1997). Physician understanding and accommodation of patients' preferences for involvement is important because patients who believe their actual level of involvement in the consultation is congruent with their preferred level are more satisfied with care and with the decision (Lantz and others, 2005).

It is difficult to understand the nature and impact of patients' preferences for involvement because existing research often fails to distinguish patient preferences to be involved in the decision-making process from who assumes responsibility for the decision. Charles and colleagues' (Charles, Gafni, and Whelan, 1999) model of medical decision making offers a useful starting point for addressing these issues because it distinguishes active patient participation in the discussion from control in making the decision. The model identifies three types of decision making—paternalistic (physician makes decision), shared (physician and patient decide together), and informed (patient decides after considering physician input)—each of which proceeds through three stages: exchanging information, deliberating, and deciding treatment. Many patients want to be actively involved in exchanging information about treatment possibilities and in deliberating on the pros, cons, and value of different treatment options. Yet these same patients may prefer not to assume responsibility for the decision. Thus, a shared decision is not inherently a positive outcome of the decision-making process, although active patient participation in information exchange and deliberation is important because it helps physician and patient achieve a shared understanding of the patient's condition and the best options for treatment.

Communication associated with medical decision making is often problematic in ways that can lower decision quality and adversely affect health. First, patients do not always achieve their preferred level of involvement in decision making (Bruera, Willey, Palmer, and Rosales, 2002; Davidson, Brundage, and Feldman-Stewart, 1999). When this happens, patients' values and preferences may not be discussed, and patients may not have an opportunity to clarify conflicting goals and needs. Moreover, when patients are not adequately involved in the decision-making process, physicians may not discover patients' beliefs about health and treatment, which may be inconsistent with scientific evidence. One example would be a patient who chooses less effective herbal treatments instead of chemotherapy because of the belief that herbs are "natural" (Peele, Siminoff, Xu, and Ravdin, 2005). When patients are part of the decision-making process by actively participating in the encounter, regardless of who assumes responsibility for the decision, they often have less post-decision regret and anxiety and experience better health after the consultation (Kaplan, Greenfield, and Ware, 1989; Ward and others, 2003).

Further, the clinical evidence supporting particular treatment options may be complicated and even inconsistent. For example, different experts may give conflicting recommendations, forcing patients to choose among different sources of authority. Research also may produce contradictory findings, such as whether some level of alcohol consumption has health benefits (Meyerhoff and others, 2005). Difficulties also arise when trying to understand risk in the context of decision making. Physicians typically approach risk analytically by focusing on epidemiological evidence, but patients may perceive risk experientially, that is, based on personal experience and associated meanings (Hunt, Castaneda, and de Voogd, 2006). When physicians and patients cannot achieve a shared understanding of the risks and benefits associated with different treatment possibilities, a lower-quality decision may occur, the patient's choice for treatment may not be fully informed, and the patient's commitment to treatment may be lower (Gattellari, Voigt, Butow, and Tattersall, 2002).

Enabling Patient Self-Management

Helping patients to manage their own health is another important, though understudied, function of physician-patient communication. This aspect of communication is aimed at enabling patients to self-manage important aspects of their illnesses, such as finding health-related information, coping with treatment effects, seeking appropriate care, and effectively navigating the health care system (Howie and others, 1999; O'Hair and others, 2003). Enabling patient self-management is more than information exchange because it also comprises recommendations, instructions, and advocacy. Physicians can help patients help themselves by providing navigational help, supporting patient autonomy, and providing guidance and advice on better self-care.

Patients with long-term and chronic diseases such as cancer and diabetes must navigate a complex health care system to obtain care. Examples of providing navigational help include helping patients to get follow-up testing, giving directions to specialists' offices, arranging for support groups or social work referrals, and coordinating care among specialists (Dohan and Schrag, 2005). Supporting patient autonomy involves communicating in a way that bolsters the patient's sense of self-efficacy and motivates the patient to take control of her health. Autonomy-supportive behaviors include exploring patients' ambivalence about taking action, providing alternative options to achieve the same goal, and giving patients time to consider choices rather than forcing a premature decision. This approach has been applied with success to smoking cessation, weight loss, adherence, and exercise (Williams and others, 1998; Williams and others, 2005). Providing patients with guidance and advice can also help patients to help themselves. Physicians can do this by giving instructions and recommendations that are patient-focused, that is, clear, using nontechnical language, including repetition, summarization, categorization, and asking patients to repeat complex recommendations so that it is clear that they understand and can remember the advice (Ellis, Hopkin, Leitch, and Crofton, 1979; King, 1992).

Physician-patient communication can improve health by empowering patients to be active, capable agents in managing their health. O'Hair describes a three-stage process through which communication can enhance the patient's capacity for agency (O'Hair and others, 2003). In the first stage, patients confront and try to cope with the uncertainty imposed by their health condition. The second stage involves empowerment, including having a voice in the clinical environment. Empowering behaviors include actively seeking information, participating in decisions, and openly expressing concerns and feelings (Street and Millay, 2001). The third stage, agency, is characterized by self-efficacy in managing one's health, a sense of control, the ability and volition to follow through with appropriate treatment recommendations, and the ability to solve problems and cope with health-related complications (see also Chapter Eight). Although theories of interpersonal communication can help explain processes related to empowerment, other health behavior theories help to account for processes related to agency (see Chapter Four and Eight).

The value of enhanced patient agency has been demonstrated in several studies. Cancer patients' sense of control over their disease has been linked to emotional well-being and coping during survivorship (Street and Voigt, 1997). In diabetes, more effective self-management has led to better metabolic control and improved functioning (Lorig, Ritter, and Jacquez, 2005).

MODERATORS OF COMMUNICATION-OUTCOME RELATIONSHIPS

Thus far, we have discussed key functions of clinician-patient communication that can affect health either directly or indirectly through both proximal and intermediate outcomes (see Figure 11.1). These relationships may also be moderated by any number of factors. A moderator is a qualitative or quantitative variable that affects the direction or strength of the relationship between an independent variable and a dependent variable (Baron and Kenny, 1986). Figure 11.2 provides examples of potential moderators along two continua, one related to the degree to which the factor is intrinsic or extrinsic to physicians, patients, and their relationship, and the other related to the degree to which the factor is mutable. Intrinsic moderators are characteristics of individuals and of the clinician-patient relationship that either directly or implicitly tap into affective and cognitive processes (for example, emotional state, health literacy, knowledge about the illness, goals, self-efficacy). Extrinsic moderators include characteristics of disease, the family and social environment, cultural values and beliefs, the health care system, and economic factors. The stable-mutable dimension reflects the degree to which the moderator is susceptible to change. Understanding which factors are changeable is critically important because modifiable factors can be targeted for interventions to increase the chances that communication will accomplish desired outcomes.

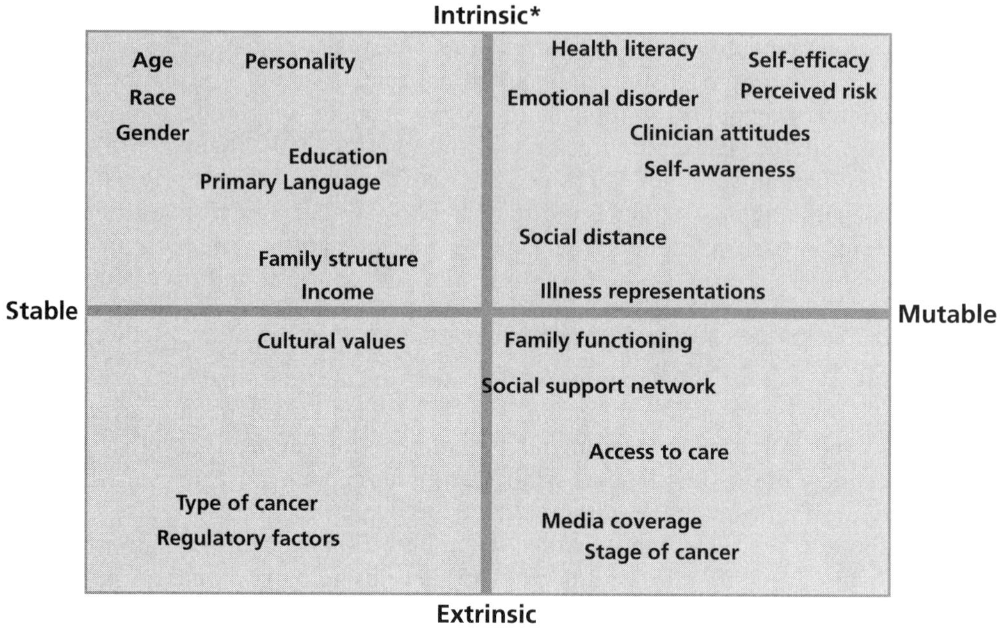

Intrinsic*

Age   Personality

Race

Gender

Education
Primary Language

Family structure

Income

Stable

Cultural values

Type of cancer

Regulatory factors

Health literacy   Self-efficacy

Emotional disorder   Perceived risk

Clinician attitudes

Self-awareness

Social distance

Illness representations

Mutable

Family functioning

Social support network

Access to care

Media coverage

Stage of cancer

Extrinsic

*Intrinsic to clinicians, patients, and their relationships.

FIGURE 11.2. Examples of Potential Moderators of Clinician-Patient Health Outcomes.

Next we discuss four intrinsic moderators that can influence the relationships between communication and health outcomes, yet are modifiable: (1) health literacy, (2) social distance, (3) clinician attitudes toward patients, and (4) patient preferences for clinician and patient roles in care. In addition, context is discussed as an important source of extrinsic moderators.

Health Literacy

Health literacy is a person's capacity to obtain, process, and communicate information about health (Baker, 2006). Health literacy is a modifiable factor and an important moderator of relationships between communication and outcomes, because it affects patients' ability to understand clinical and health-related information. Low health literacy may restrict the patient's ability to be an active participant in medical consultations because of limited familiarity with health-related terms (Davis and others, 2002; Street, 2001) and because of embarrassment due to this limited understanding (Baker and others, 1996). Hence, several of the pathways linking communication to improved outcomes, such as improved patient knowledge and shared understanding, better medical decisions, and enhanced patient agency, may not be achieved for low-literacy patients.

The communication challenges facing people with low health literacy may account for some disparities related to race (Sentell and Halpin, 2006), access to care (Sudore and others, 2006), and poorer health outcomes among people with chronic diseases such as diabetes (Schillinger and others, 2003; Sarkar, Fisher, and Schillinger, 2006). Health care organizations can help address literacy-related barriers by providing patients with culturally appropriate health education that helps them to understand their health issues, encourages patient participation in discussing concerns and beliefs, and provides suggestions for how to talk with their physicians (Cegala, Post, and McClure, 2001; Street, 2003a).

Social Distance

In the context of this chapter, *social distance* refers to the number and importance of dissimilarities between physicians and patients. Social distance may be a perception or may be based on objective indicators, and the two may or may not correlate. Differences in demographic characteristics such as race, gender, or age may not translate automatically into perceived social distance because people may be similar or dissimilar on multiple dimensions, each of which has varying degrees of perceptual salience. For example, a middle-aged, black female patient with children may feel that she has much more in common with a white male physician with children of the same age than with a younger, single black female physician.

Social distance can moderate the relationship between communication and outcomes for several reasons. Clinician-patient differences in beliefs about health, use of language, and health-related values create the risk of misunderstanding or bias. This can lead to situations in which patients' needs are not understood and false assumptions are made about their needs and capabilities (Balsa and McGuire, 2001, 2003). Also, social distance can make it more difficult to establish strong physician-patient relationships. Patients appreciate clinicians who can understand and empathize with their life circumstances (Saha, Komaromy, Koepsell, and Bindman, 1999; Henman and others, 2002). Physician communication intended to enhance the relationship, such as expressions of empathy and shared understanding, may not be as effective in building the therapeutic alliance if the patient does not perceive the communication as sincere or believes the doctor is not capable of empathic understanding.

Finally, although objective aspects of social distance may be difficult to change, perceived social distance is mutable. By showing attentiveness, avoiding interruption, asking about the patient's beliefs and values, and giving clinical information in a way the patient understands, the physician communicates commitment, respect, and an interest in the patient as a person. In turn, when patients share their beliefs, values, and preferences, they are sharing information that provides opportunities for the doctor to understand them better and for both parties to discover common ground. The power of effective communication in decreasing perceived social distance is suggested in studies showing that patient trust increases during the consultation when clinicians are perceived as more informative, caring, and interested in the patient's views (Gordon and others, 2006).

Physician Attitudes Toward Patients

Differences in race, gender, and class between patients and physicians may have sub-conscious or implicit influences on physicians' attitudes, perceptions, and communi-cations with patients (Burgess, van Ryn, Crowley-Matoka, and Malat, 2006). These perceptions can influence the physician's communication, such as following up on the concerns of some patients but not others, the detail with which doctors provide explanations about disease and treatment, and the degree to which they offer encour-agement and support (Horgan, Stein, and Roter, 2002). Under these circumstances, there is a greater burden on patients to communicate effectively. For example, one study found that physicians recommended more intensive cancer diagnostic proce-dures for white patients, regardless of their communication behavior, but recom-mended the same procedures for black women only for those who were more assertive in asking about them (Krupat and others, 1999). The belief that clinicians have more negative attitudes toward certain types of patients may explain why more black pa-tients and poor patients report that a positive self-presentation is important in getting good medical care than do white patients and those of higher SES (Malat, van Ryn, and Purcell, 2006). However, this can lead to a situation in which patients who are already socially disadvantaged and are less inclined to assert themselves bear a greater burden for achieving effective communication than do their more socially privileged counterparts (Street and others, 2005; Wiltshire, Cronin, Sarto, and Brown, 2006). Ultimately, physicians' negative perceptions of patients can disrupt pathways linking communication to better health because they limit the degree to which physician and patient can achieve shared understanding, make informed decisions, build thera-peutic alliances, and adequately deal with the patient's emotions and concerns.

Patient Preferences for Physician and Patient Roles

Patients have expectations for their own roles and the physician's role in health care, especially with regard to what issues are discussed and who has control over deci-sion making. Patient preferences may be an important moderator of communica-tion-outcome relationships in several respects. First, a substantial number of patients fail to achieve their desired level of participation in the decision-making process (Deg-ner and others, 1997), which can lower satisfaction with care, increase post-deci-sion regret, and increase patient anxiety. Thus, a physician's well-intentioned but mismatched communication, such as partnership building with a patient who prefers clinician control of decisions or assuming decisional control for a patient who wants to be involved in decision making, may lower the quality of the decision, interfere with the patient's ability to manage emotions, and lower the patient's motivation or confidence in following a treatment plan.

Patients also vary in their expectations for physician and patient roles, and this has often been found to be associated with demographic characteristics. Older and less educated patients are more likely to prefer paternalistic decision-making mod-els, whereas younger and more educated patients desire more active and collabora-tive roles (Degner and others, 1997; Cassileth, Zupkis, Sutton-Smith, and March,

1980). Some evidence indicates that women prefer explicit emotional support from physicians, whereas men primarily want information rather than to discuss their feelings (Clarke, Booth, Velikova, and Hewison, 2006; Kiss and Meryn, 2001).

Patients' preferences for physician and patient roles in the encounter may change from visit to visit, or even over the course of a consultation. For example, a patient who is sicker or more distressed may prefer to relinquish decisional control to a health care provider (Butow and others, 1997; Degner and others, 1997). Some research indicates that patients' perceived roles in the consultation, not their preferred roles, were stronger predictors of evaluations of care. Patients who reported a shared role with their physicians were more satisfied and evaluated their physicians' communication more favorably than did patients who felt that their actual role matched their previously stated role preference. However, a match between preferred and perceived roles was associated with less post-consultation anxiety (Gattellari, Butow, and Tattersall, 2001).

In summary, patient preferences for their own and the clinician's communication vary and can moderate the effectiveness of different functions of communication to achieve better outcomes. Because clinicians are not very good judges of patient preferences and because patients and clinicians often do not perceive the decision-making process in the same way, clinicians should directly assess patient preferences prior to or early in the consultation. This will help determine how to manage communication over time and help to better align clinician and patient perspectives.

Context as an Important Source of Extrinsic Moderators

The discussion of moderators has emphasized intrinsic moderators because they can have powerful effects on communication processes and health outcomes and because they can be the targets of interventions aimed at improving physician-patient communication. However, extrinsic moderators are also powerful influences on communication-health outcome relationships (see Figure 11.2). It is important to take into account contextual elements of an interaction, because they are the primary source of extrinsic moderators of communication-outcome relationships.

Clinician-patient interactions, like other forms of communication, are "situated"— that is, they take place within multiple layers of context, including organizational, political, geographic, and media (Street, 2003b). These contextual elements can affect both how physicians and patients communicate with one another and whether the outcomes of the consultation can lead to improved health. Although any number of contextual elements may influence health care, three particularly important aspects of context are (1) the family and social environment, (2) the media environment, and (3) the health care system.

The patient's social environment, consisting of extended family, friends, and coworkers, can affect clinician-patient communication and outcomes in several ways. Family and friends can either reinforce or undermine the decisions reached by physicians and patients and thus affect adherence and health outcomes. Even the best medical decision, in terms of physician-patient agreement and the clinical evidence, may be for naught if family and friends fail to support it. Also, the physicians' emotional support of the patient and navigational and self-care help can be enhanced when social networks are supportive and provide tangible help, such as providing transportation to medical appointments and assisting in the patient's self-care (Albrecht and Goldsmith, 2003). Family members' presence in clinical encounters can either facilitate the interaction or interfere with the communication, thus affecting the degree to which key functions of communication are achieved (Greene, Majerovitz, Adelman, and Rizzo, 1994; Ishikawa, Roter, Yamazaki, and Takayama, 2005; Shields and others, 2005a).

The media environment also affects patient-clinician communication processes and outcomes in several ways. Media coverage of a health issue can influence patients' beliefs and expectations, especially when the media reach a large audience. This was demonstrated dramatically in an Italian study (Passalacqua and others, 2004) of a widespread media campaign promoting Di Bella therapy—an unproven cancer treatment that significantly raised expectations and hope among cancer patients. Later, the treatment was publicly shown to be ineffective. Drug companies use mass media for direct-to-consumer advertising in the hopes that patients will ask clinicians for their products, and this ploy is often effective (Kravitz and others, 2005). Finally, the media environment, the Internet in particular, offers extensive resources for health-related information and social support. Patients may benefit from this information by understanding their conditions and treatment expectations better and participating more effectively in medical interactions (Hesse and others, 2005; Street, 2003c). However, some of this information may be scientifically suspect, and patients may be overwhelmed with the amount of information available.

Both the physical and procedural features of the health care facility can affect clinician-patient communication and outcomes. Facilities offering an effective "team" approach provide care that is coordinated and characterized by good communication among multidisciplinary team members. They also may offer informational and social support resources to clinicians and patients in person, through shared electronic patient records, and via the Internet (Boyle, Robinson, Heinrich, and Dunn, 2004). In contrast, loosely integrated care may require that patients use medical services at multiple facilities. Even simple organizational practices, such as longer scheduled visits, can have a significant effect on clinician-patient communication to the extent that they constrain or encourage patient involvement in decision making. Longer visits are characterized by greater patient participation, and patients control proportionally more of the conversation (Dugdale, Epstein, and Pantilat, 1999; Street and Gordon, 2006). Physical aspects of the health care facility, such as ambient noise, privacy, and décor, can affect how comfortable patients are in seeking care and discussing their concerns with physicians (Lindberg, Lewis-Spruill, and Crownover, 2006). It is helpful to be aware of how organizational practices affect the quality of communication in medical encounters, especially since poorer communication may lead to poorer outcomes, unnecessary tests, more readmissions, and higher costs (Epstein and others, 2005b; Little and others, 2001).

CLINICIAN-PATIENT COMMUNICATION: APPLICATION IN HEALTH EDUCATION AND HEALTH BEHAVIOR

This section describes an application that illustrates outcomes of effective clinician-patient communication, within the "functions of clinician-patient communication" approach discussed in this chapter. The example relates to evidence for the influence of provider directives in patient smoking cessation attempts. Elsewhere in this book, readers will find discussions of barriers in the social environment that may constrain health-promoting behaviors (see Part Four and Chapter Eight). Considering those social and contextual barriers and taking other predictors of behavior into account, clinician recommendations explain much of the variation in a number of outcomes for people who have access to a regular source of care. The positive influence of the clinician recommendations highlighted in this section can be partially described by the high levels of trust placed in health care providers. Data from the National Cancer Institute's Health Information National Trends Survey (HINTS) reveal that despite newly available communication channels, physicians remain the most highly trusted source of health information (Hesse and others, 2005).

Treatment of Tobacco Use and Dependence

The U.S. Public Health Service's clinical practice guidelines for smoking cessation, *Treating Tobacco Use and Dependence,* outline a process known as the "5 As" of provider-to-patient communication: *Ask, Advise, Assess, Assist, and Arrange* (Fiore, 2000). These five clinician-patient communication directives dovetail with the functions of communication described in this chapter. The directives may work directly or indirectly to achieve attempts in smoking cessation among patients, as Figure 11.1 suggests. A provider's movement through each of the 5 As fulfills each of the stated functions of clinician-patient communication, thereby enhancing the likelihood that patients exposed to the interaction will make a quit attempt. Several studies have documented the importance of clinician involvement in smoking cessation, and others have lauded the guidelines as an essential starting point for clinician-patient communication about quitting smoking.

The 5 As were not explicitly constructed from tests of the various theories (for example, paternalism, self-determination) that underlie the given functions of clinician-patient communication discussed in this chapter. However, they were based on empirical evidence, much of which comes from theoretically grounded research. This set of recommended actions describes how various clinician cues may work to influence smoking cessation outcomes, by performing each of the functions of communication. For example, *Ask* fulfills the functions of information exchange and fostering relationships; *Advise* fulfills the function of information exchange; *Assess* fulfills the functions of responding to emotions and managing uncertainty; *Assist* fulfills the functions of making decisions and enabling self-management, and *Arrange* fulfills the function of enabling self-management.

Communication style is highly dependent on the individual clinician, but any approach can be used to implement the recommendation that clinicians discuss smoking cessation with patients. To this end, the clinical practice guidelines provide strength-of-evidence ratings for several types of provider-patient exchanges (for example, brief interactions, counseling, pharmacotherapy recommendations), to assist clinicians with choosing appropriate and effective strategies for helping patients to quit smoking.

DIRECTIONS FOR FUTURE RESEARCH

The conceptual framework offered in this chapter has important implications for future research on physician-patient communication. As mentioned at the outset, researchers should be guided by or develop theoretical models linking the communication process to health outcomes. We have identified key communication functions, as well as potential pathways to improved health. To test the importance of these functions along particular pathways, researchers will need to develop measures that tap into these key processes. Longitudinal studies will be needed to track outcomes, following the interactions and events that occur along the pathways than can affect communication-outcome relationships. Studies of patients' experiences over time may best be completed using designs of physicians nested within patients, the opposite of the traditional "patient-nested-within-clinician" design used in most physician-patient communication studies. Longitudinal studies are rare, likely due to their expense and complexity, but are greatly needed.

Although this chapter identifies six key communication functions, psychometrically sound measures of all six functions are lacking. Often, existing measures use similar nomenclature to measure distinct behaviors or use different nomenclature for similar behaviors (Stewart, 2001). Measures based on audio- or videotaped coding schemes of the actual interaction often do not correlate strongly with measures based on patient perceptions of the same encounter collected via surveys (Street, 1992). To successfully monitor and improve the delivery and impact of communication in clinical practice, measures of the key functions must capture, over time, in a reliable and valid manner, the interactions of patients and their families with members of the health care delivery team. Ideally, communication measures should be theory-based and empirically validated, reflect what is important to patients and families, account for all relevant participants in the interaction, and achieve a balance between general and function-specific aspects of communication (Stewart, 2001).

Given the complex set of factors affecting physician-patient communication processes, the pathways through which communication achieves desired outcomes, and the moderators of these relationships, researchers will need to use multilevel modeling in their analytical techniques in order to determine the unique influences of various factors on communication and outcomes (Street, 1991; Street, Gordon, and Haidet, 2007). Failure to account for multiple influences on communication may result in misleading findings. In one study, physicians appeared to give more information to white patients than black patients. However, when communication variables were entered into the equation, physician information giving was no longer related to race per se but rather to the degree to which patients were active participants (Gordon, Street, Sharf, and Souchek, 2006). In short, black patients received less information because they were less actively involved in eliciting information from physicians. In another study, the finding that black patients had lower post-visit trust in physicians than whites became nonsignificant after an indicator of the patients' perceptions of the physicians' communication was entered into the model (Gordon and others, 2006). Black patients viewed their doctors as less informative and supportive during the interaction, which accounted for their lower trust ratings.

SUMMARY

Models of clinician-patient communication should be simple enough to be understandable and guide empirical research yet complex enough to approximate clinical reality. We have proposed a model of pathways linking clinician-patient communication to health outcomes and identified six communication functions that are key to promoting improve health outcomes: establishing and maintaining the physician-patient relationship, exchanging and managing information, validating and responding to emotions, managing uncertainty, making decisions, and enabling patient self-management. The pathways through which effective communication leads to better health outcomes include, but are not limited to, improved patient knowledge and shared understanding, improved access to care, improved therapeutic alliances among health professionals and patients/family, improved management of negative emotions, stronger family/social support, improved quality of medical decisions, and improved patient agency.

Studies of moderators of the relationship between communication and proximal, intermediate, and health and societal outcomes suggest that relationship factors need to be studied in greater depth. Furthermore, underlying and modifiable moderating factors may affect communication-outcomes relationships, such as the patient's health literacy, social distance, physicians' attitudes toward patients, and physician and patient preferences for their roles in the interaction, as well as a number of extrinsic moderators embedded in the context of medical encounters. Future research should use more theoretically, methodologically, and ecologically sound research designs in order to better understand the linkages between good physician-patient communication and improved health.

REFERENCES

Albrecht, T. L., and Goldsmith, D. "Social Support, Social Networks, and Health." In T. Thompson, A. Dorsey, K. Miller, and R. Parrott (eds.), *The Handbook of Health Communication.* Mahwah, N.J.: Erlbaum, 2003.

Arora, N. K. "Interacting with Cancer Patients: The Significance of Physicians' Communication Behavior." *Social Science & Medicine,* 2003, *57,* 791–806.

Babrow, A. "Uncertainty, Value, Communication, and Problematic Integration." *Journal of Communication,* 2001, *51*(3), 553–573.

Baker, D. W. "The Meaning and the Measure of Health Literacy." *Journal of General Internal Medicine,* 2006, *21,* 878–883.

Baker, D. W., and others. "The Health Care Experience of Patients with Low Literacy." *Archives of Family Medicine,* 1996, *5,* 329–334.

Balsa, A. I., and McGuire, T. G. "Statistical Discrimination in Health Care. *Journal of Health Economics,* 2001, *20,* 881–907.

Balsa, A. I., and McGuire, T. G. "Prejudice, Clinical Uncertainty and Stereotyping as Sources of Health Disparities." *Journal of Health Economics,* 2003, *22,* 89–116.

Baron, R. M., and Kenny, D. A. "The Moderator-Mediator Variable Distinction in Social Psychological Research: Conceptual, Strategic, and Statistical Considerations." *Journal of Personality and Social Psychology,* 1986, *51,* 1173–1182.

Beach, W. A., Easter, D. W., Good, J. S., and Pigeron, E. "Disclosing and Responding to Cancer 'Fears' During Oncology Interviews. *Social Science & Medicine,* 2005, *60,* 893–910.

Blanchard, C. G., Labrecque, M. S., Ruckdeschel, J. C., and Blanchard, E. B. "Information and Decision-Making Preferences of Hospitalized Adult Cancer Patients." *Social Science & Medicine,* 1988, *27,* 1139–1145.

Blumhagen, D. "The Meaning of Hypertension." In N. Chrisman and T. Maretzki (eds.), *Clinically Applied Anthropology.* Dordrecht, Holland: Reidel, 1982.

Boyle, F. M., Robinson, E., Heinrich, P., and Dunn, S. M. "Cancer: Communicating in the Team Game." *ANZ Journal of Surgery,* 2004, *74,* 477–481.

Braddock, C. H., and others. "Informed Decision Making in Outpatient Practice: Time to Get Back to Basics." *Journal of the American Medical Association,* 1999, *282,* 2313–2320.

Brashers, D. E., and others. "'In an Important Way, I Did Die': Uncertainty and Revival in Persons Living with HIV or AIDS." *AIDS Care,* 1999, *11,* 201–219.

Brashers, D. E. "HIV and Uncertainty: Managing Treat Decision Making." *Focus,* 2001, *16*(9), 5–6.

Brown, J. B., Stewart, M. A., and Ryan, B. L. *Assessing Communication Between Patients and Physicians: The Measure of Patient-Centered Communication (MPCC).* Working Paper Series, Paper # 95–2. (2nd ed.) London, Ontario, Canada: Thames Valley Family Practice Research Unit and Centre for Studies in Family Medicine, 2001.

Bruera, E., Willey, J. S., Palmer, J. L., and Rosales, M. "Treatment Decisions for Breast Carcinoma: Patient Preferences and Physician Perceptions." *Cancer,* 2002, *94,* 2076–2080.

Bruera, E., and others. "Patient Preferences Versus Physician Perceptions of Treatment Decisions in Cancer Care." *Journal of Clinical Oncology,* 2001, *19*(11), 2883–2885.

Burgess, D. J., van Ryn, M., Crowley-Matoka, M., and Malat, J. "Understanding the Provider Contribution to Race/Ethnicity Disparities in Pain Treatment: Insights from Dual Process Models of Stereotyping." *Pain Medicine,* 2006, *7,* 119–134.

Burgoon, J. K., Buller, D. B., Hale, J. L., and deTurck, M. A. "Relational Messages Associated with Nonverbal Behaviors." *Human Communication Research,* 1984, *10*(3), 351–378.

Butow, P. N., and others. "The Dynamics of Change: Cancer Patients' Preferences for Information, Involvement and Support." *Annals of Oncology,* 1997, *8,* 857–863.

Butow, P. N., and others. "Oncologists' Reactions to Cancer Patients' Verbal Cues." *Psychooncology,* 2002, *11,* 47–58.

Bylund, C. L., and Makoul, G. "Empathic Communication and Gender in the Physician-Patient Encounter." *Patient Education and Counseling,* 2002, *48,* 207–216.

Cabana, M. D., and Jee, S. H. "Does Continuity of Care Improve Patient Outcomes?" *Journal of Family Practice,* 2004, *53,* 974–980.

Cassileth, B. R., Zupkis, R. V., Sutton-Smith, K., and March, V. "Information and Participation Preferences Among Cancer Patients." *Annals of Internal Medicine,* 1980, *92,* 832–836.

Cegala, D. J., Post, D. M., and McClure, L. "The Effects of Patient Communication Skills Training on the Discourse of Older Patients During a Primary Care Interview." *Journal of the American Geriatrics Society,* 2001, *49,* 1505–1511.

Champman, K., and Rush, K. "Patient and Family Satisfaction with Cancer-Related Information: A Review of the Literature." *Canadian Oncology Nursing Journal,* 2003, *13,* 107–116.

Charles, C., Gafni, A., and Whelan, T. "Decision-Making in the Physician-Patient Encounter: Revisiting the Shared Treatment Decision-Making Model." *Social Science & Medicine,* 1999, *49*(5), 651–661.

Clarke, S. A., Booth, L., Velikova, G., and Hewison, J. "Social Support: Gender Differences in Cancer Patients in the United Kingdom." *Cancer Nursing,* 2006, *29,* 66–72.

Clayton, M. F., Mishel, M. H., and Belyea, M. "Testing a Model of Symptoms, Communication, Uncertainty, and Well-Being, in Older Breast Cancer Survivors." *Research in Nursing & Health,* 2006, *29*(1), 18–39.

Davidson, J. R., Brundage, M. D., and Feldman-Stewart, D. "Lung Cancer Treatment Decisions: Patients' Desires for Participation and Information." *Psychooncology,* 1999, *8,* 511–520.

Davidson, R., and Mills, M. E. "Cancer Patients' Satisfaction with Communication, Information and Quality of Care in a UK Region." *European Journal of Cancer Care,* 2005, *14,* 83–90.

Davis, T. C., and others. "Health Literacy and Cancer Communication." *CA: A Cancer Journal for Clinicians,* 2002, *52,* 134–149.

Degner, L. F., Sloan, J. A., and Venkatesh P. "The Control Preferences Scale." *Canadian Journal of Nursing Research,* 1997, *29,* 21–43.

Degner, L. F., and others. "Information Needs and Decisional Preferences in Women with Breast Cancer." *Journal of the American Medical Association,* 1997, *277,* 1485–1492.

Detmar, S. B., and others. "How Are You Feeling? Who Wants To Know? Patients' and Oncologists' Preferences For Discussing Health-Related Quality-Of-Life Issues." *Journal of Clinical Oncology,* 2000, *18,* 3295–3301.

Dohan, D., and Schrag, D. "Using Navigators to Improve Care of Underserved Patients: Current Practices and Approaches." *Cancer,* 2005, *104,* 848–855.

Dugdale, D. C., Epstein, R., and Pantilat, S. Z. "Time and the Patient-Physician Relationship." *Journal of General Internal Medicine,* 1999, *14*(Suppl 1), S34–S40.

Ellis, D. A., Hopkin, J. M., Leitch, A. G., and Crofton, J. "'Doctors' Orders': Controlled Trial of Supplementary, Written Information for Patients." *British Medical Journal,* 1979, *1,* 456.

Epstein, R. M. "Making Communication Research Matter: What Do Patients Notice, What Do Patients Want, and What Do Patients Need?" *Patient Education and Counseling,* 2006, *60,* 272–278.

Epstein, R. M., Alper, B. S., and Quill, T. E. "Communicating Evidence for Participatory Decision Making." *Journal of the American Medical Association,* 2004, *291,* 2359–2366.

Epstein, R. M., and Street, R. L., Jr. *Patient-Centered Communication in Cancer Care: Promoting Healing and Reducing Suffering.* Bethesda, Md.: National Cancer Institute, 2007.

Epstein, R. M., and others. "Measuring Patient-Centered Communication in Patient-Physician Consultations: Theoretical and Practical Issues. *Social Science & Medicine,* 2005a, *61,* 1516–1528.

Epstein, R. M., and others. "Patient-Centered Communication and Diagnostic Testing." *Annals of Family Medicine,* 2005b, *3,* 415–421.

Fallowfield, L., and Jenkins, V. "Communicating Sad, Bad, and Difficult News in Medicine." *Lancet,* 2004, *363,* 312–319.

Fallowfield, L., Saul, J., and Gilligan, B. "Teaching Senior Nurses How to Teach Communication Skills in Oncology." *Cancer Nursing,* 2001, *24*(3), 185–191.

Fiore, M. C., and others. *Treating Tobacco Use and Dependence.* Clinical Practice Guideline. Rockville, Md.: U.S. Department of Health and Human Services. Public Health Service, 2000.

Fishbein, M., and Cappella, J. N. "The Role of Theory in Developing Effective Health Communications." *Journal of Communication,* 2006, *56,* S1–S17

Fuertes, J. N., and others. "The Physician-Patient Working Alliance." *Patient Education and Counseling,* 2007, *66,* 29–36.

Galassi, J. P, Schanberg, R., and Ware, W. B. "The Patient Reactions Assessment: A Brief Measure Of The Quality Of The Patient-Provider Relationship." *Psychological Assessment,* 1992, *4,* 346–351.

Gansler, T., and others. "Sociodemographic Determinants of Cancer Treatment Health Literacy." *Cancer,* 2005, *104,* 653–660.

Gattellari, M., Butow, P. N., and Tattersall, M. H. "Sharing Decisions in Cancer Care." *Social Science & Medicine,* 2001, *52*(12), 1865–1878.

Gattellari, M., Voigt, K. J., Butow, P. N., and Tattersall, M. H. "When the Treatment Goal is Not Cure: Are Cancer Patients Equipped to Make Informed Decisions?" *Journal of Clinical Oncology,* 2002, *20,* 503–513.

Glasgow, R. E., Emont, S., and Miller, D. C. "Assessing Delivery of the Five 'As' for Patient-Centered Counseling." *Health Promotion International,* 2006, *21,* 245–255.

Gordon, H. S., Street, R. L., Jr., Sharf, B. F., and Souchek, J. "Racial Differences in Doctors' Information-Giving and Patients' Participation." *Cancer,* 2006, *107,* 1313–1320.

Gordon, H. S., and others. "Racial Differences in Trust and Lung Cancer Patients' Perceptions of Physician Communication." *Journal of Clinical Oncology,* 2006, *24,* 904–909.

Greene, M. G., Majerovitz, S. D., Adelman, R. D., and Rizzo, C. "The Effects of the Presence of a Third Person on the Physician-Older Patient Medical Interview." *Journal of the American Geriatrics Society,* 1994, *42,* 413–419.

Hagerty, R. G., and others. "Cancer Patient Preferences for Communication of Prognosis in the Metastatic Setting." *Journal of Clinical Oncology,* 2004, *22,* 1721–1730.

Hagerty, R. G., and others. "Communicating with Realism and Hope: Incurable Cancer Patients' Views on the Disclosure of Prognosis." *Journal of Clinical Oncology,* 2005, *23,* 1278–1288.

Harris, I. B., Rich, E. C., and Crowson, T. W. "Attitudes of Internal Medicine Residents and Staff Physicians Toward Various Patient Characteristics." *Journal of Medical Education,* 1985, *60,* 192–195.

Haug, M. R., and Lavin, B. *Consumerism in Medicine: Challenging Physician Authority.* Thousand Oaks, Calif.: Sage, 1983.

Henman, M. J., and others. "Lay Constructions of Decision-Making in Cancer." *Psychooncology,* 2002, *11,* 295–306.

Hesse, B. W., and others. "Trust and Sources of Health Information: The Impact of the Internet and its Implications for Health Care Providers: Findings from the First Health Information National Trends Survey." *Archives of Internal Medicine,* 2005, *165,* 2618–2624.

Hojat, M., and others. "Physician Empathy: Definition, Components, Measurement, and Relationship to Gender and Specialty." *The American Journal of Psychiatry,* 2002, *159,* 1563–1569.

Hoffman, J. "Awash in Information, Patients Face a Lonely, Uncertain Road." *New York Times,* 2005.

Holman, H., and Lorig, K. "Patients as Partners in Managing Chronic Disease: Partnership is a Prerequisite for Effective and Efficient Health Care." *BMJ,* 2000, *320,* 526–527.

Horgan, T. G., Stein, T. S., and Roter, D. L. "Liking in the Physician-Patient Relationship." *Patient Education and Counseling,* 2002, *48,* 69–77.

Howie, J. G., and others. "Quality at General Practice Consultations: Cross Sectional Survey." *British Medical Journal,* 1999, *319,* 738–743.

Hunt, L. M., Castaneda H., and de Voogd, K. B. "Do Notions of Risk Inform Patient Choice? Lessons from a Study of Prenatal Genetic Counseling." *Medical Anthropology,* 2006, *25,* 193–219.

Ishikawa, H., Roter, D. L., Yamazaki, Y., and Takayama, T. "Physician-Elderly Patient-Companion Communication and Roles of Companions in Japanese Geriatric Encounters." *Social Science & Medicine,* 2005, *60,* 2307–2320.

Iwamitsu, Y., and others. "Differences in Emotional Distress Between Breast Tumor Patients with Emotional Inhibition and Those with Emotional Expression." *Psychiatry and Clinical Neurosciences,* 2003, *57,* 289–294.

Kaplan, S., and others. "Characteristics of Physicians with Participatory Decision-Making Styles." *Annals of Internal Medicine,* 1996, *124*(5), 497–504.

Kaplan, S. H., Greenfield, S., and Ware, J. E., Jr. "Assessing the Effects of Physician-Patient Interactions on the Outcomes of Chronic Disease." *Medical Care,* 1989, *27,* S110–S127.

King, A. "Comparison of Self-Questioning, Summarizing, and Notetaking-Review as Strategies for Learning from Lectures." *American Educational Research Journal,* 1992, *29,* 303–323.

Kiss A., Meryn S. "Effect of Sex and Gender on Psychosocial Aspects of Prostate and Breast Cancer." *British Medical Journal,* 2001, *323,* 1055–1058.

Kleinman, A. *Patients and Healers in the Context of Culture.* Berkeley, Calif.: University of California Press, 1980.

Krantz, D. S., Baum, A., and Wideman, M. "Assessment of Preferences for Self-Treatment and Information in Health Care." *Journal of Personality and Social Psychology,* 1980, *39,* 977–990.

Kravitz, R. L., and others. "Influence of Patients' Requests for Direct-to-Consumer Advertised Antidepressants: A Randomized Controlled Trial." *Journal of the American Medical Association,* 2005, *293,* 1995–2002.

Krupat, E., Yeager, C. M., and Putnam, S. "Patient Role Orientations, Doctor-Patient Fit, and Visit Satisfaction." *Psychology and Health,* 2000, *15,* 707–719.

Krupat, E., and others. "Patient Assertiveness and Physician Decision-Making Among Older Breast Cancer Patients." *Social Science & Medicine,* 1999, *49,* 449–457.

Krupat, E., and others. "The Practice Orientations of Physicians and Patients: The Effect of Doctor-Patient Congruence on Satisfaction." *Patient Education and Counseling,* 2000, *39,* 49–59.

Krupat, E., and others. "When Physicians and Patients Think Alike: Patient-Centered Beliefs and Their Impact on Satisfaction and Trust." *Journal of Family Practice,* 2001, *50,* 1057–1062.

Lang, F., Floyd, M. R., and Beine, K. L. "Clues to Patients' Explanations and Concerns About Their Illnesses: A Call for Active Listening." *Archives of Family Medicine,* 2000, *9,* 222–227.

Lantz, P. M., and others. "Satisfaction with Surgery Outcomes and the Decision Process in a Population-Based Sample of Women with Breast Cancer." *Health Services Research,* 2005, *40*(3), 745–767.

Lerman, C. E., and others. "Patients' Perceived Involvement in Care Scale: Relationship to Attitudes About Illness and Medical Care." *Journal of General Internal Medicine,* 1990, *5,* 29–33.

Lewis, M. A., DeVellis, B. M., and Sleath, B. "Social Influence and Interpersonal Communication in Health Behavior." In K. Glanz, F. M. Lewis, and B. K. Rimer (eds.), *Health Behavior and Health Education: Theory, Research, and Practice.* (3rd ed.) San Francisco: Jossey-Bass, 2002.

Ley, P. *Communicating with Patients: Improving Communication, Satisfaction, and Compliance.* London: Croom Helm, 1988.

Lindberg, C., Lewis-Spruill, C., and Crownover, R. "Barriers to Sexual and Reproductive Health Care: Urban Male Adolescents Speak Out." *Issues in Comprehensive Pediatric Nursing,* 2006, *29,* 73–88.

Little, P., and others. "Observational Study of Effect of Patient Centeredness and Positive Approach on Outcomes of General Practice Consultations." *British Medical Journal,* 2001, *323,* 908–911.

Lorig, K. R., Ritter, P. L., and Jacquez, A. "Outcomes of Border Health Spanish/English Chronic Disease Self-Management Programs." *Diabetes Educator,* 2005, *31,* 401–409.

Luecken, L. J., and Compas, B. E. "Stress, Coping, and Immune Function in Breast Cancer." *Annals of Behavioral Medicine,* 2002, *24,* 336–344.

Makoul, G., and Clayman, M. L. "An Integrative Model of Shared Decision Making in Medical Encounters." *Patient Education and Counseling,* 2006, *60*(3), 301–312.

Malat, J. R., van Ryn, M., and Purcell, D. "Race, Socioeconomic Status, and the Perceived Importance of Positive Self-Presentation in Health Care." *Social Science & Medicine,* 2006, *62,* 2479–2488.

McWilliam, C. L., Brown, J. B., and Stewart, M. "Breast Cancer Patients' Experiences of Patient-Doctor Communication: A Working Relationship." *Patient Education and Counseling,* 2000, *39,* 191–204.

Meyerhoff, D. J., and others. "Health Risks of Chronic Moderate and Heavy Alcohol Consumption: How Much Is Too Much?" *Alcoholism, Clinical and Experimental Research,* 2005, *29,* 1334–1340.

Mishel, M. H. "Uncertainty in Chronic Illness." *Annual Review of Nursing Research,* 1999, *17,* 269–294.

Montazeri, A., Gillis, C. R., and McEwen, J. "Quality of Life in Patients With Lung Cancer: A Review of Literature from 1970 to 1995." *Chest,* 1998, *113*(2), 467–481.

O'Hair, D., and others. "Cancer Survivorship and Agency Model: Implications for Patient Choice, Decision Making, and Influence." *Health Communication,* 2003, *15,* 193–202.

Ong, L. M., de Haes, J. C., Hoos, A. M., and Lammes, F. B. "Doctor-Patient Communication: A Review of the Literature." *Social Science & Medicine,* 1995, *40,* 903–918.

Ong, L. M., Visser, M. R., Lammes, F. B., and de Haes, J. C. "Doctor-Patient Communication and Cancer Patients' Quality of Life and Satisfaction." *Patient Education and Counseling,* 2000, *41,* 145–156.

Ory, M. G., and others. "Prevalence and Correlates of Doctor-Geriatric Patient Lifestyle Discussions: Analysis of ADEPT Videotapes." *Preventive Medicine,* 2006, *43,* 494–497.

Parsons, T. *The Social System.* Glencoe, Ill.: Free Press, 1951.

Passalacqua, R., and others. "Effects of Media Information on Cancer Patients' Opinions, Feelings, Decision-Making Process and Physician-Patient Communication." *Cancer,* 2004, *100,* 1077–1084.

Peele, P. B., Siminoff, L. A., Xu, Y., and Ravdin, P. M. "Decreased Use of Adjuvant Breast Cancer Therapy in a Randomized Controlled Trial of a Decision Aid with Individualized Risk Information." *Medical Decision Making,* 2005, *25,* 301–307.

Prochaska, J. O., and Velicer, W. F. "The Transtheoretical Model of Health Behavior Change." *American Journal of Health Promotion,* 1997, *12*(1), 38–48.

Reeder, L. G. "The Patient-Client as a Consumer: Some Observations on the Changing Professional-Client Relationship." *Journal of Health and Social Behavior,* 1972, *13,* 406–412.

Rosenberg, H. J., and others. "Expressive Disclosure and Health Outcomes in a Prostate Cancer Population." *International Journal of Psychiatry in Medicine,* 2002, *32,* 37–53.

Roter, D. L., Frankel, R. M., Hall, J. A., and Sluyter, D. "The Expression of Emotion Through Nonverbal Behavior in Medical Visits: Mechanisms and Outcomes." *Journal of General Internal Medicine,* 2006, *21*(Suppl 1), S28–S34.

Roter, D. L., and Hall, J. A. *Doctors Talking to Patients/Patients Talking to Doctors: Improving Communication in Medical Visits.* Westport, Conn.: Auburn House, 1992.

Roter, D. L., and Larson, S. "The Roter Interaction Analysis System (RIAS): Utility and Flexibility for Analysis of Medical Interactions." *Patient Education and Counseling,* 2002, *46,* 243–251.

Rothschild, S. K. "Cross-Cultural Issues in Primary Care Medicine." *Disease-a-Month: DM,* 1998, *44,* 293–319.

Russell, N. K., and Roter, D. L. "Health Promotion Counseling of Chronic-Disease Patients During Primary Care Visits." *American Journal of Public Health,* 1993, *83,* 979–982.

Ryan, R. M., and Deci, E. L. "Self-Determination Theory and the Facilitation of Intrinsic Motivation, Social Development, and Well-Being." *American Psychologist,* 2000, *55*(1), 68–78.

Saha, S., Komaromy, M., Koepsell, T. D., and Bindman, A. B. "Patient-Physician Racial Concordance and the Perceived Quality and Use of Health Care." *Archives of Internal Medicine,* 1999, *159,* 997–1004.

Salkeld, G., Solomon, M., Short, L., and Butow, P. N. "A Matter of Trust—Patient's Views on Decision-Making in Colorectal Cancer." *Health Expectations,* 2004, *7,* 104–114.

Sarkar, U., Fisher, L., and Schillinger, D. "Is Self-Efficacy Associated with Diabetes Self-Management Across Race/Ethnicity and Health Literacy?" *Diabetes Care,* 2006, *29,* 823–829.

Schillinger, D., and others. "Closing the Loop: Physician Communication with Diabetic Patients Who Have Low Health Literacy." *Archives of Internal Medicine,* 2003, *163,* 83–90.

Schofield, P. E., and others. "Psychological Responses of Patients Receiving a Diagnosis of Cancer." *Annals of Oncology,* 2003, *14,* 48–56.

Sentell, T. L., and Halpin, H. A. "Importance of Adult Literacy in Understanding Health Disparities." *Journal of General Internal Medicine,* 2006, *21,* 86–866.

Sepucha, K., and others. "An Approach to Measuring the Quality of Breast Cancer Decisions." *Patient Education and Counseling,* 2007, *65,* 261–269.

Shields, C. G., and others. "Influence of Accompanied Encounters on Patient-Centeredness with Older Patients." *Journal of the American Board of Family Practice,* 2005a, *18,* 344–354.

Shields, C. G., and others. "Rochester Participatory Decision-Making Scale (RPAD): Reliability and Validity." *Annals of Family Medicine,* 2005b, *3,* 436–442.

Simon, C. M., and Kodish, E. D. "Step into my Zapatos, Doc: Understanding and Reducing Communication Disparities in The Multicultural Informed Consent Setting." *Perspectives in Biology and Medicine,* 2005, *48,* S123–S138.

Sleath, B. "Pharmacist-Patient Interactions: Paternalism, Participatory, or Default?" *Patient Education and Counseling,* 1996, *28,* 253–263.

Smith, M. Y., and others. "Patient-Physician Communication in the Context Of Persistent Pain: Validation of a Modified Version of the patients' Perceived Involvement in Care Scale." *Journal of Pain and Symptom Management,* 2006, *32*(1), 71–81.

Squier, R. S. "A Model of Empathic Understanding and Adherence to Treatment Regimens in Practitioner-Patient Relationships." *Social Science & Medicine,* 1990, *30*(3), 325–329.

Stewart, M. "Towards a Global Definition of Patient Centred Care: The Patient Should Be the Judge of Patient Centred Care." *British Medical Journal,* 2001, *322,* 444–445.

Street, R. L. "Information-Giving in Medical Consultations: The Influence of Patients' Communicative Styles and Personal Characteristics." *Social Science & Medicine,* 1991, *32*(5), 541–548.

Street, R. L. "Analyzing Communication in Medical Consultations. Do Behavioral Measures Correspond to Patients' Perceptions?" *Medical Care,* 1992, *30,* 976–988.

Street, R. L. "Active Patients as Powerful Communicators." In W. P. Robinson, and H. Giles (eds.), *The New Handbook of Language and Social Psychology.* New York: Wiley, 2001.

Street, R. L. "Interpersonal Communication Skills in Health Care Contexts." In J. O. Greene and B. R. Burleson (eds.), *Handbook of Communication and Social Interaction Skills.* Mahwah, N.J.: Erlbaum, 2003a.

Street, R. L. "Communication in Medical Encounters: An Ecological Perspective." In T. Thompson, A. Dorsey, K. Miller, and R. Parrott (eds.), *The Handbook of Health Communication.* Mahwah, N.J.: Erlbaum, 2003b.

Street, R. L. "Mediated Consumer-Provider Communication in Cancer Care: The Empowering Potential of New Technologies." *Patient Education and Counseling,* 2003c, *50,* 99–104.

Street, R. L., Cauthen, D., Buchwald, E., and Wiprud, R. "Patients' Predispositions to Discuss Health Issues Affecting Quality of Life." *Family Medicine,* 1995, *27,* 663–670.

Street, R. L., and Gordon, H. S. "The Clinical Context and Patient Participation in Post-Diagnostic Consultations." *Patient Education and Counseling,* 2006, *64*(1–3), 217–224.

Street, R. L., Gordon, H., and Haidet, P. "Physicians' Communication and Perceptions of Patients: Is It How They Look, How They Talk, Or Is It Just The Doctor?" *Social Science & Medicine,* 2007, *65*(3), 586–598.

Street, R. L., and Millay, B. "Analyzing Patient Participation in Medical Encounters." *Health Communication,* 2001, *13*(1), 61–73.

Street, R. L., and Voigt, B. "Patient Participation in Deciding Breast Cancer Treatment and Subsequent Quality of Life." *Medical Decision Making,* 1997, *17*(3), 298–306.

Street, R. L., and others. "Patient Participation in Medical Consultations: Why Some Patients are More Involved Than Others." *Medical Care,* 2005, *43,* 960–969.

Sudore, R. L., and others. "Limited Literacy in Older People and Disparities in Health and Healthcare Access." *Journal of the American Geriatrics Society,* 2006, *54,* 770–776.

Szasz, T. S., and Hollender, M. H. "A Contribution to the Philosophy of Medicine: The Basic Models of the Doctor-Patient Relationship." *Archives of Internal Medicine,* 1956, *97,* 585–592.

Tai-Seale, M., and others. "Two-Minute Mental Health Care for Elderly Patients: Inside Primary Care Visits." *Journal of the American Geriatrics Society,* 2007, *55,* 1903–1911.

Teutsch, C. "Doctor-Patient Communication." *Medical Clinics of North America,* 2003, *87*(5), 1115–1145.

van Ryn, M., and Burke, J. "The Effect of Patient Race and Socio-Economic Status on Physicians' Perceptions of Patients." *Social Science & Medicine,* 2000, *50,* 813–828.

Ward, M. M., and others. "Participatory Patient-Physician Communication and Morbidity in Patients with Systemic Lupus Erythematosus." *Arthritis and Rheumatism,* 2003, *49,* 810–818.

Williams, G. C., and others. "Autonomous Regulation and Long-Term Medication Adherence in Adult Outpatients." *Health Psychology,* 1998, *17,* 269–276.

Williams, G. C., and others. "Variation in Perceived Competence, Glycemic Control, and Patient Satisfaction: Relationship to Autonomy Support from Physicians." *Patient Education and Counseling,* 2005, *57,* 39–45.

Williams, G. H., and Wood, P. H. "Common-Sense Beliefs About Illness: A Mediating Role for the Doctor." *Lancet,* 1986, *2,* 1435–1437.

Wiltshire, J., Cronin, K., Sarto, G. E., and Brown, R. "Self-Advocacy During the Medical Encounter: Use of Health Information and Racial/Ethnic Differences." *Medical Care,* 2006, *44,* 100–109.

Woolf, S. H., and others. "Promoting Informed Choice: Transforming Health Care to Dispense Knowledge for Decision Making." *Annals of Internal Medicine,* 2005, *143,* 293–300.

Zachariae, R., and others. "Association of Perceived Physician Communication Style with Patient Satisfaction, Distress, Cancer-Related Self-Efficacy, and Perceived Control Over the Disease." *British Journal of Cancer,* 2003, *88,* 658–665.

Zandbelt, L. C., and others. "Patient Participation in the Medical Specialist Encounter: Does Physicians' Patient-Centered Communication Matter?" *Patient Education and Counseling,* 2007, *65,* 396–406.

CHAPTER

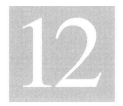

PERSPECTIVES ON MODELS OF INTERPERSONAL HEALTH BEHAVIOR

K. Viswanath

KEY POINTS

This chapter will

- Identify defining characteristics of theories involving interpersonal interactions.
- Highlight important features of the theories discussed in Part Three of the book: Social Cognitive Theory, social networks and social support, stress and coping, and interpersonal communication between clinicians and patients.
- Discuss the cross-level linkages between individual-based health behavior theories and more macro-level theories.
- Draw attention to ways in which health disparities may be affected by behaviors at the interpersonal level.

Two simple questions are implied in the quest for better theories of health education and health behavior and are part of the rationale for studying these theories. First, what set of factors influences health-related behaviors among individuals? Second, what are the determinants that could lead to changes in behaviors that maintain good health? Behind these seemingly simple questions lies a complex and linked set of factors that drive human behaviors when it comes to health. The complexity stems from the fact that health behavior is a product of influences at multiple levels—individual, interpersonal, organizational, and societal—and temporal constraints such as life cycle, age, or time (Smedley and Syme, 2000). Theories and hypotheses abound at each level. For example, some theories focus on individual cognitions and affect and how they explain health behaviors (Chapters Four to Seven). Others focus on larger social forces external to the human agency and how they may interact with intra-individual factors to affect health behaviors (Chapters Thirteen to Seventeen). A third group—the focus of this chapter—are theories that focus on external forces in more proximal geographical and psychological spheres, the realms of interpersonal interactions (Chapters Eight to Eleven). Often, attempts to change health behaviors require an understanding of these multiple influences.

SOME DEFINING CHARACTERISTICS OF INTERPERSONAL INTERACTIONS

Theories in this section focus on the mid-level, interpersonal interactions among people both as individuals and social actors, and how these interactions may influence health behaviors. Individuals' cognitions, beliefs, emotions, and feelings are products of their informal "web of relationships"—a phenomenon Simmel commented on more than eight decades ago (1955/1922). Members of the family, friends, and coworkers—actors in such informal interactions—are significant sources of social support, information, and social capital (Chapters Nine and Eleven). Some interactions serve as models for health behaviors, good or bad (Chapter Eight). Interactions may also occur in formal relationships, such as between patients and providers (Chapter Eleven) or between community health workers, such as *promotoras* and their clients. Although formal interactions provide support and information, they may be different to the extent that they are based on asymmetrical power relationships in which one party is an expert and the other is a layperson.

The nature of relationships among formal actors, particularly between providers and patients, has been changing from paternalistic models to more participatory models of communication and interactions leading to increased focus on shared and informed decision making (Kaplan and others, 1996; Rimer and others, 2004). Some have attributed this shift from the so-called "paternalistic model" to a "consumerist" model to controversies in medicine, greater availability of health information—abetted by the communication and informatics revolutions and social movements that promote patient and consumer interests (Rimer and others, 2004). Indeed, a large amount of health-related information is easily available on the World Wide Web, though the Web itself is not accessible to everyone (Viswanath, 2006). Chapter Eight reviews some of the effects of the shift from paternalistic to consumer models on patient outcomes and areas of future research.

Another defining characteristic of the work in these chapters is that they focus on models and theories. Some types of human behaviors are too complex for one theory to provide a complete explanation. A model is a description of a complex phenomenon based on a set of assumptions, which are drawn from multiple theories to explain the relationship between variables in the model (Earp and Ennett, 1991). Models have some advantages. They rationalize several different factors that influence a behavior and attempt to tell a coherent story. They bring order and posit how interactions between and among different variables may occur and under what conditions. Causal pathways and relationships in the pathways allow interventionists to identify potential levers for intervention to influence the targeted health behavior. Despite these uses, the disadvantage is that some models are not easily amenable to testing in an integrated manner. One might test individual factors and the posited relationship among them, but not the complete model.

THEORIES AND MODELS AT THE INTERPERSONAL LEVEL

The chapters in Part Three review some of the major theories and models that inform our understanding of interpersonal-level influence on health behaviors. We briefly highlight here some features and issues with the theories discussed in those chapters.

Social Cognitive Theory

Social Cognitive Theory (SCT), formalized by Albert Bandura, addresses the classic tension between human agency and the social structure by offering the construct of *reciprocal determinism*, which suggests that human agency and the environment interact and influence each other, leading to individual and social change. As McAlister, Perry, and Parcel argue in Chapter Eight, while conceding that the environment is powerfully influential on human behavior, SCT privileges human agency by proposing that individuals have the capacity to change or even build the environment. By emphasizing the *dynamism in the interactions* between the individual and the environment, SCT moved away from the deterministic approach of focusing exclusively on one level or the other, which limited the explanatory power of the variables. In explaining individual and social change, Bandura introduced a series of concepts such as *observational learning* or *modeling, self-regulation, moral disengagement*, and *self-efficacy,* which have provided a fertile vein to be mined by students of health behavior theories and practice.

The various constructs and the relationships among them are detailed in the chapter, but it is worth noting that some constructs rather than the entire model have found broad appeal among health behavior researchers. Two are worth drawing attention to: self-efficacy and observational learning or modeling.

Self-efficacy and its counterpart at the group level—collective efficacy—have proved to be widely used constructs by health behavior theorists and practitioners. Self-efficacy is the individual's belief in his capacity to perform a given behavior when faced with a variety of challenges. Collective efficacy is a shared belief of a group, aggregated from beliefs of the individual members, that it is capable of action to achieve collective goals. A cursory search of Medline revealed more than eight thousand citations for *self-efficacy!* The idea that self-efficacy beliefs influence the feelings, choices of humans, and their motivations has been widely used to study a variety of behaviors from increasing physical activity among children (Kelder and others, 2005) to smoking cessation among adults (Gotay, 2005) and improved disease management for arthritis (Theis, Helmick, and Hootman, 2007), among others.

Self-efficacy has been applied to so many specific domains of health behavior that it has been adopted for use in other theories, such as the Health Belief Model (HBM; Chapter Three), the Theory of Planned Behavior (TPB) and Integrated Behavioral Model (IBM; Chapter Four). A major appeal of self-efficacy in health behavior stems from the fact that it is a modifiable factor that can be intervened on because sources of self-efficacy include personal experiences, persuasion, and vicarious experiences learned from observing others, or modeling.

Observational learning (or modeling) is another construct that has been adopted widely. It is rooted in human capacity to learn from observing the behaviors of others and enacting those behaviors (or avoiding them in case of expected negative outcomes). Learning may be from direct experience or personal observation or may be vicarious through various media, including mass media and interpersonal channels. People use others as models in developing their knowledge and modeling their behaviors, particularly when the referents are similar to them. Modeling and observational learning have been applied in understanding pro-social change, such as entertainment education to promote condom use (Keller and Brown, 2002), as well as negative outcomes, such aggressive behavior after watching violent TV programs (Huesmann, 2007; also see Chapter Eight).

Despite the intuitive sense that vicarious learning through media has a powerful influence on knowledge, beliefs, and behaviors, particularly in the context of so-called "entertainment-education" (or edutainment), it is difficult to test this assumption empirically using SCT without isolating other factors that influence social change and the mechanisms that contribute to it. Other theories have incorporated modeling to offer a more elaborate explanation of why and how narratives may lead to real-world behavior change. Using "transportation theory," they argue that exposure to narratives, whether as short public service announcements or longer dramas or serials, transports viewers to the fictional world, making the experience more enjoyable (Green and Brock, 2000). Transportation may encourage the consumer of messages to identify with characters, reduce counterarguments, and provide vivid exemplars for the real world (Green, 2006; Zillmann, 2002), thus leading to behavior change. The audience may even believe that the fictional world reflects reality (Gerbner and others, 2002). Although the theory of narratives does not substitute for SCT's hypothesis about observational learning, it offers greater elaboration of how observation may work and delineates mechanisms that lead to behavior change. Overall, the power and appeal of SCT lies less in its goal to provide a complete explanation of human behavior (though that seems to be Bandura's intention) and more in offering powerful constructs such as self-efficacy, modeling, and a few others that are widely used in theory and practice.

Social Networks, Social Support, and Health Behavior

Long before the idea of social capital and social networks entered the arena of health research, social theorists, such as Durkheim (1964/1933) and Simmel (1955/1922), grappled with the ways in which the web of social relationships (social networks) influences human cognitions and behavior and acts as glue to hold the society together. They proposed that social relationships, characterized by both the nature and degree of interactions, may offer social support, perform social control, and manage social conflict.

Social relationships and how they affect health have received considerable attention over the past three decades (Berkman and Glass, 2000; Berkman and Kawachi, 2000; Berkman, 1984). Chapter Nine offers a review of the defining features of social networks and their functions in providing social support. Heaney and Israel present a model that shows at least four distinct pathways between social networks and social support, and physical, mental, and social health. One is a direct pathway where social ties provide intimacy and companionship and promote health and well-being. Social networks may also provide resources to cope with illness, contacts, new information, and access to community resources, which in turn affect health. Resource mobilization through networks performs a "buffering" function, enabling individuals to cope with stressors. Last, social networks may influence health behaviors, such as exercising with friends, which in turn may influence health (Voorhees and others, 2005).

In addition to proposing a model with pathways that connect social networks and social support, Heaney and Israel present some useful generalizations. One—the effect of social networks and social support on health—is diffused and not specific to any one disease process. Two, the number of ties matter, up to a point. The complete absence of any network (social isolation) is harmful, while at some point more ties do not bring a corresponding benefit. Three, while characteristics of networks matter, the relationships among social networks, social support, and health are not simple. In general, intense and strong ties may be helpful at times, such as during life transitions, yet weaker ties are better at offering new information and new contacts, captured famously by Granovetter (1973) as the "strength of weak ties." Ties to social organizations may be a powerful source of health information (Viswanath, 2005). Four, types of support, such as emotional or instrumental, may vary by the relationship between the focal person and the person offering the support. Heaney and Israel clearly show that not all members of social networks are equally effective in offering social support. Five, interventions have attempted to enhance existing networks, develop new networks, identify natural helpers, and build community capacity to solve problems, or combine these strategies.

Some additional issues are worth noting about social networks and health. Heaney and Israel suggest that no claims can be made that the causal pathways are unidirectional. In fact, it is possible that ill health may limit one's social networks and fray social relationships. The causal influences of social networks and social support on health require more careful elucidation under different conditions and for different groups of people. For example, it remains to be seen if social support is influenced by social class and social determinants such as race, ethnicity, or neighborhood context and how these factors affect interventions to promote health.

Although Chapter Nine proffered the positive functions of social networks and social ties, a review of work on the influence of social networks on health behaviors suggests that effects are both positive and negative. For example, friends within networks may serve as models for adopting risk behaviors such as smoking or substance abuse (Valente, Unger, and Johnson, 2005) or may share risk factors such as obesity (Christakis and Fowler, 2007).

Introduction of new communication technologies, such as the Internet, has made the study of social networks all the rage. A lot of attention is being paid to such social network sites as MySpace™ and Facebook™ and their influence on members' beliefs and behaviors. The presence of online support groups has multiplied, extending the proffering of social support to communities without geographical proximity (Rimer and others, 2005).

Communication is central to social networks, both in initiating and in maintaining such networks, and is an important antecedent to social capital (Viswanath, 2007). The mechanisms connecting social capital and health behavior are complex and require further research (Kawachi, Subramanian, and Kim, 2007). The relationships among social network, social support, and health remains a fruitful area for future research.

Stress, Coping, and Health Behavior

At the outset, readers may wonder how stress and coping fit into this section on interpersonal influences. As Glanz and Schwartz (Chapter Ten) point out, interpersonal interactions and communications play a crucial role in helping people cope with stress by providing social support, potentially mitigating the impact of stress or providing ways to cope with it. As the authors suggest, stress may have a negative physiological effect on health or contribute indirectly to behaviors that are not conducive to good health. For example, smoking may be one way for people to cope with stress (Ackerson, Kawachi, Barbeau, and Subramanian, 2007). Social conditions, such as potential for an influenza pandemic, bioterrorism, and natural catastrophes, have made stress and coping important concerns for health education researchers and practitioners. For example, an assessment of mental illness and suicidal ideation among victims of Hurricane Katrina found high levels of hurricane-related post-traumatic stress disorder and other mental illnesses (Kessler and others, 2008).

An important observation that could be made from the review of literature on stress and coping in Chapter Ten is that constructs used in that literature draw from and are closely connected to constructs in other theories and models discussed elsewhere in this book. Glanz and Schwartz focus on the Transactional Model of Stress and Coping, which proposes that stressful experiences are a product of how a person assesses an external stressor and the psychological, social, and cultural resources she can draw on to manage stress, leading to outcomes such as well-being and functional status, among others. Constructs used in the model are related to theories discussed in other chapters in this book. For example, *primary appraisal*—the perception of an external event as stressful or positive—is composed of two types of appraisals, personal susceptibility and severity, constructs also used in the Health Belief Model (HBM; Chapter Three). Similarly, primary appraisal may result in actions to cope with the stress, either by addressing the problem or seeking support to manage emotions. Acute stress may also overwhelm an individual seeking to avoid taking action, a concern also addressed by those working on theories informing the use of fear appeals (Witte and Allen, 2000).

In a related vein, active coping efforts depend on such factors as perceived ability to change the situation, ability to manage stress, and perceived effectiveness of resources—all related to the construct of self-efficacy, which is central to Social Cognitive Theory (SCT; Chapter Eight). Similarly, there are parallels between coping strategies of the Transactional Model and the change processes in the Transtheoretical Model (TTM; Chapter Five). One coping style is to draw on social support, and discussions in Chapter Ten complement the ideas about social support presented in Chapter Nine. Although there is considerable evidence suggesting that social support is related to health behaviors and health outcomes, there are also inconsistent findings on how social support can be improved by interventions. The applications described in Chapter Nine are helpful exemplars of how social support and social networks may affect coping responses to stress.

One of the more interesting developments in the study of stress and coping comes from research that examined how individual stress and coping may be affected by social structural conditions, including socioeconomic status (SES) and neighborhood conditions. For example, one of the coping styles is information seeking—an effort to reduce or manage uncertainty and reduce distress (Rutten and others, 2005). Active seekers of information have been labeled as "monitors," compared to those who avoid information, called "blunters." Although individual-level explanations for blunting and monitoring have been examined extensively, the structural constraints that may deter people from seeking information and acting on it are less understood. For example, some work suggests that information seekers have higher SES, and active seeking was associated with higher levels of physical activity, higher consumption of fruits and vegetables, and weekly exercise (Ramanadhan and Viswanath, 2006). These data raise the issue of how at least one coping style of stress—information seeking—may mediate outcomes such as physical health and functioning, and how it is influenced by SES.

Community-level violence (for example, witnessing violent incidents in the neighborhood) is associated with anxiety and depressive symptoms among low-SES women, even when they are not directly affected by it (Clark and others, 2007). Similarly, people living in states with higher or intermediate levels of social capital reported better physical and mental health, compared to those living in states with lower social capital (Kim and Kawachi, 2007). There is tentative evidence that perceptions of "organizational justice" may be related to workers' psychosocial well-being (Kawachi, 2006). Recent research shows how discrimination may have both indirect and direct pathways to negative health outcomes, by restricting minorities to low-SES conditions, greater exposure to stressors, internalized racism, and subjective experiences

(Ahmed, Mohammed, and Williams, 2007). These exemplar pieces identify another fruitful area of research, for elucidating both the mechanisms linking structural conditions with individual stress and how interventions may be developed to reduce stress and improve well-being.

Interpersonal Communication and Health

One underlying theme of chapters in Part Three is that interpersonal communication may contribute to individual health by developing and maintaining social networks, providing social support, and helping to manage stress. Interpersonal communication varies, depending on whether it occurs among people in more formal relationships, such as physicians and patients, or in informal cliques, such as with friends and families. Chapter Eleven focuses on one such formal relationship: clinician-patient communications. Research in this area has been pursued for at least five decades, resulting in thousands of studies and papers. It has become even more important because of greater availability of health information in the public environment, informatics and communication revolutions, the consumerist movement in health care, and technological developments that place greater responsibility on patients to make complex health-related decisions (Rimer and others, 2004; Viswanath, 2005).

Street and Epstein (Chapter Eleven) organized work in this area around key functions of clinician-patient communication and how they may be related to health outcomes. To capture the complexity of the relationship between clinician-patient communication and health outcomes, they offer a model of "patient-centered communication," identifying several pathways that link communications to health outcomes and how they are related to critical functions of clinician-patient communications. The pathways suggest that clinician-patient communication could have direct effects on health, or it could have indirect effects through proximal outcomes, like understanding, trust, and satisfaction, or intermediate outcomes like health behaviors, adherence, and decision making.

Key functions they identify include fostering the physician-patient relationship, exchanging and managing information, validating and managing emotions, managing uncertainty, decision making, and enabling patient self-management. They also identify a set of moderator variables such as health literacy, social distance, physician attitudes toward patients, patient preferences for physician and patient roles, and external environment (including context).

Their approach offers some advantages over conventional discussions of physician-patient communication. By taking this approach, they go beyond descriptive models of medical encounters to trying to explain the underlying mechanisms between communications and health outcomes and various theories that could connect them. Also, the communication functions of clinician-patient communication and the pathways linking the communications to health outcomes are general enough that they could be extended to other interpersonal communications and how they may affect health. For example, research can focus on how communication with people in close social networks helps in managing uncertainty and validating emotions, leading to less psychological distress (Brashers, Goldsmith, and Hsieh, 2002).

The approach taken in Chapter Eleven suggests leverage points where health education interventions can be effective in influencing subsequent health outcomes. For example, interventions might focus on training physicians to assess and be sensitive to patients' emotional and informational needs (Brédart, Bouleuc, and Dolbeault, 2005) or on decision making to improve patient satisfaction and well-being. In summary, the value of Street and Epstein's patient-centered communication approach is that it is in line with the recent movements in the field, which place the patients' needs at the center and promote the notion of the more empowered patient.

SUMMARY AND FUTURE DIRECTIONS

The chapters in this section of the book, by focusing on the interpersonal level, offer the critical cross-level linkages between individual-based health behavior theories and the macro-level models discussed in chapters in the next section. One practical advantage for health educators in theorizing at the meso-level is the possibility of developing interventions that are practical but still take the context of interpersonal influences into account. A second advantage is that meso-level theories explain the variety of influences on individuals and how these influences—family members, coworkers, friends, and providers among others—may affect health behaviors.

The theories in Chapters Eight through Eleven offer guidance for promoting health behavior change, as well as the settings and types of interventions that could be developed. For example, interventions could promote physical activity by offering social support through one's social network either at home, in the neighborhood, or with a coworker in the workplace.

Another lesson from these chapters is that they offer guidance on how to organize the large number of theories of health behavior though model building. The assumption is that no single theory captures the web of influences on an individual. Models are one way to develop parsimonious explanations for complex health behaviors. In addition, the theories point to a core group of concepts that appear in different theories and settings, which may help a student or practitioner of health education develop a target for research or application.

Despite the voluminous body of work reviewed here, much work remains to be done. One, it is not clear what role interpersonal communication will play in how we link larger social forces of increasing immigration into the United States, global migration of peoples across national borders, and globalization of economies with individual health. For example, it is conceivable that physicians and patients are increasingly likely to be from different racial, ethnic, and social-class backgrounds, with implications of these changes on physician-patient interactions and health outcomes. Or coworkers from different cultures may have to adjust to each others' working styles, leading to stress and tensions in the workplace and possibly affecting health. Or recent immigrants may suffer from the loss of social networks in their place of origin, with negative health outcomes. Of equal or greater importance, beliefs about interpersonal communication and relationships may vary tremendously across cultures. One can easily think of the gender segregation that still exists in some countries and orthodox cultures and how they affect social ties.

Changes in health care financing are encouraging people other than physicians to play an increasing role in health care and health promotion. These include such roles as *promotoras* (nurse practitioners), who may take on more active roles (see also Chapter Eighteen). Massachusetts recently passed a law allowing the pharmacy chain CVS to open "Minute Clinics" staffed by nurse practitioners to permit consultation and resolution of minor illnesses (Smith, 2008). The impact on health behaviors of interactions with different types of health care practitioners and in varied settings will remain an important area of inquiry.

The informatics and communication revolutions are having a broad and deep impact on interpersonal relationships in all realms, and health is no exception. The booming number of social networking groups and support groups for patients on the Internet and their influence on health behavior is only beginning to be explored (Rimer and others, 2005) and remains an important area for future research.

Last, the growing disparities between different social groups separated by social class, race, and ethnicity may be addressed in important ways by drawing on what happens at the interpersonal level. People who suffer from material disadvantages may also suffer from lack of resources within their social networks to help them cope with stress, manage uncertainty, and obtain information and instrumental and social support to maintain good health (Krieger, 2007; Viswanath, 2006). An urgent moral imperative is to understand how theories at the interpersonal level can offer a useful bridge between the macro and micro levels to ameliorate the conditions of the poor and reduce disparities.

REFERENCES

Ackerson, L. K., Kawachi, I., Barbeau, E. M., and Subramanian, S. V. "Exposure to Domestic Violence Associated with Adult Smoking in India: A Population Based Study." *Tobacco Control*, 2007, *16*(6), 378–383.

Ahmed, A. T., Mohammed, S. A., and Williams, D. R. "Racial Discrimination and Health: Pathways and Evidence." *Indian Journal of Medical Research*, 2007, *126*(4), 318–327.

Berkman, L. F. "Assessing the Physical Health Effects of Social Networks and Social Support." *Annual Review of Public Health*, 1984, *5*, 413–432.

Berkman, L. F., and Glass, T. "Social Integration, Social Networks, Social Support, and Health." In L. F. Berkman and I. Kawachi (eds.), *Social Epidemiology*. New York: Oxford University Press, 2000.

Berkman, L. F., and Kawachi, I. (eds.). *Social Epidemiology*. New York: Oxford University Press, 2000.

Brashers, D. E., Goldsmith, D. J., and Hsieh, E. "Information Seeking and Avoiding in Health Contexts." *Human Communication Research*, 2002, *28*, 258–271.

Brédart, A., Bouleuc, C., and Dolbeault, S. "Doctor-Patient Communication and Satisfaction with Care in Oncology." *Current Opinions in Oncology*, 2005, *17*(4), 351–354.

Christakis, N. A., and Fowler, J. H. "The Spread of Obesity in a Large Social Network Over 32 Years." *New England Journal of Medicine*, 2007, *357*(4), 370–379.

Clark C., and others. "Witnessing Community Violence in Residential Neighborhoods: A Mental Health Hazard for Urban Women." *Journal of Urban Health*, 2007, *85*(1), 22–38.

Durkheim, E. *The Division of Labor in Society*. Translated by G. Simpson. New York: Free Press, 1964. (Originally published 1933.)

Earp, J. A., and Ennett, S. T. "Conceptual Models for Health Education Research and Practice." *Health Education Research*, 1991, *6*(2), 163–171.

Gerbner, G., and others. "Growing Up with Television: Cultivation Processes." In J. Bryant and D. Zillman (eds.), *Media Effects: Advances in Theory and Research*. Mahwah, N.J.: Erlbaum, 2002.

Gotay, C. C. "Behavior and Cancer Prevention." *Journal of Clinical Oncology*, 2005, *23*(2), 301–310.

Granovetter, M. S. "Strength of Weak Ties." *American Journal of Sociology*, 1973, *78*(6), 1360–1380.

Green, M. "Narratives and Cancer Communication." *Journal of Communication,* 2006, *56*(Suppl), S163–S183.

Green, M., and Brock, T. C. "The Role of Transportation in the Persuasiveness of Public Narratives." *Journal of Personality and Social Psychology*, 2000, *79*, 701–721.

Huesmann, L. R. "The Impact of Electronic Media Violence: Scientific Theory And Research." *Journal of Adolescent Health*, 2007, *41*(6 Suppl 1), S6–S13.

Kaplan, S., and others. "Characteristics of Physicians with Participatory Decision-Making Styles." *Annals of Internal Medicine*, 1996, *124*(5), 497–504.

Kawachi, I. "Injustice at Work and Health: Causation or Correlation?" *Occupational and Environmental Medicine*, 2006, *63*(9), 578–579.

Kawachi, I., Subramanian, S. V., and Kim, D. (eds.). *Social Capital and Health*. New York: Springer, 2007.

Kelder, S., and others. "The CATCH Kids Club: A Pilot After-School Study for Improving Elementary Students' Nutrition and Physical Activity." *Public Health Nutrition*, 2005, *8*(2), 133–140.

Keller, S. N., and Brown, J. D. "Media Interventions to Promote Responsible Sexual Behavior." *Journal of Sex Research*, 2002, *39*(1), 67–72.

Kessler, R. C., and others. "Trends in Mental Illness and Suicidality after Hurricane Katrina." *Molecular Psychiatry*, 2008, January 8.

Kim, D., and Kawachi, I. "U.S. State-Level Social Capital and Health-Related Quality of Life: Multilevel Evidence of Main, Mediating, and Modifying Effects." *Annals of Epidemiology*, 2007, *17*(4), 258–269.

Krieger, N. "Why Epidemiologists Cannot Afford to Ignore Poverty." *Epidemiology*, 2007, *18*(6), 658–663.

Ramanadhan, S., and Viswanath, K. "Health and the Information Non-Seekers: A Profile." *Health Communication*, 2006, *20*(2), 131–139.

Rimer, B. K., and others. "Informed Decision Making: What Is Its Role in Cancer Screening?" *Cancer,* 2004, *101*(5 Suppl), 1214–1228.

Rimer, B. K., and others. "How New Subscribers Use Cancer-Related Online Mailing Lists." *Journal of Medical Internet Research*, 2005, *7*(3), e32.

Rutten, L. J., and others. "Information Needs and Sources of Information Among Cancer Patients: A Systematic Review of Research (1980–2003)." *Patient Education and Counseling*, 2005, *57*, 250–261.

Smedley, B. D., and Syme, S. L. *Promoting Health: Intervention Strategies from Social and Behavioral Research*. Washington, D.C.: National Academy Press, 2000.

Simmel, G. *Conflict and the Web of Group Affiliations*. New York: Free Press, 1955. (Originally published 1922.)

Smith, S. "In-Store Healthcare Wins State Approval." *Boston Globe,* January 10, 2008.

Theis, K. A., Helmick, C. G., and Hootman, J. M. "Arthritis Burden and Impact are Greater Among U.S. Women Than Men: Intervention Opportunities." *Journal of Women's Health*, 2007, *16*(4), 441–453.

Valente, T. W., Unger, J., and Johnson, A. C. "Do Popular Students Smoke? The Association Between Popularity and Smoking Among Middle School Students." *Journal of Adolescent Health*, 2005, *37*, 323–329.

Viswanath, K. "The Communications Revolution and Cancer Control." *Nature Reviews Cancer*, 2005, *5*(10), 828–835.

Viswanath, K. "Public Communications and its Role in Reducing and Eliminating Health Disparities." In G. E. Thomson, F. Mitchell, and M. B. Williams (eds.), *Examining the Health Disparities Research Plan of the National Institutes of Health: Unfinished Business*. Washington, D.C.: Institute of Medicine; 2006.

Viswanath, K. "Social Capital and Health Communications." In I. Kawachi, S. V. Subramanian, and D. Kim (eds.), *Social Capital and Health*. New York: Springer, 2007.

Voorhees, C. C., and others. "The Role of Peer Social Network Factors and Physical Activity in Adolescent Girls." *American Journal of Health Behavior*, 2005, *29*(2), 183–190.

Witte, K., and Allen, M. "A Meta-Analysis of Fear Appeals: Implications for Effective Public Health Campaigns." *Health Education and Behavior,* 2000, *27*(5), 591–615.

Zillmann, D. "Exemplification Theory of Media Influence." In J. Bryant and D. Zillmann (eds.), *Media Effects: Advances in Theory and Research*. Mahwah, N.J.: Erlbaum, 2002.

PART

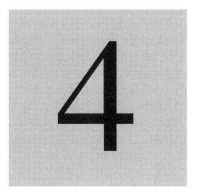

4

COMMUNITY AND GROUP MODELS OF HEALTH BEHAVIOR CHANGE

Karen Glanz

An understanding of the functioning of groups, organizations, large social institutions, and communities is vital to health enhancement. Designing health behavior and environmental change initiatives to serve communities and targeted populations, not just single individuals, is at the heart of a public health orientation. The collective well-being of communities can be fostered by creating structures and policies that support healthy lifestyles and by reducing or eliminating health hazards and constraints in the social and physical environments. Both approaches require an understanding of how social systems operate, how change occurs within and among systems, and how community and organizational changes influence people's behavior and health.

Health behavior today occurs in the context of rapid technological change and important policy debates around the world. Health concerns, such as substance abuse, AIDS prevention and education, smoking prevention and control, prevention and treatment of obesity, bioterrorism, and new health care technologies raise issues that cannot be addressed adequately through individual or small-group interventions alone (Smedley and Syme, 2000). Rather, health professionals need to view and understand health behavior and organizational changes in the context of social institutions and communities. Theories and frameworks in this part of *Health Behavior and Health Education* can help professionals understand the health behavior of large groups, communities, organizations, and coalitions, and can guide organizationwide and communitywide health promotion and education interventions. These social systems are both viable and essential units of practice when widespread and long-term maintenance of behavior change and social change are important goals. In many cases, community and organization-level interventions should be paired with those aimed at individuals.

Community-level models are frameworks for understanding how social systems function and change, and how communities and organizations can be activated. They complement individually oriented behavior change goals with broad aims that include advocacy and policy development. Community-level models suggest strategies and initiatives that are planned and led by organizations and institutions whose missions are to protect and improve health—schools, worksites, health care settings, community groups, and government agencies. Other institutions for which health enhancement is not a central mission, such as the mass media, also play a critical role. These settings and structures—and the mass media—and people's interactions with them are increasingly being shaped by new information technologies, particularly the Internet and Web.

The chapters in this section represent state-of-the-art descriptions of four types of models for behavior change and community development in social systems or large populations. Some chapters address theoretical perspectives on changing the health behavior of populations. Others are concerned primarily with conceptual frameworks for intervention methods that are *based on* theoretical foundations from the social sciences.

In Chapter Thirteen, Minkler, Wallerstein, and Wilson provide a comprehensive overview of principles and methods of community organization and community building for health improvement. They discuss the main theoretical and conceptual bases of community organization, processes and models for community organization, and emerging concepts and methods of community building for health. They also discuss progress and tools for measuring and evaluating community organizing and community building. The authors then describe a case study of community organization—the YES! Program for youth development.

In Chapter Fourteen, Oldenburg presents diffusion of innovations theory, which focuses on how new ideas, products, programs, and social practices spread within a society or from one society (or social system) to another. He then discusses how diffusion theory was applied to increase adoption, maintenance, and sustainability of a skin cancer prevention program at swimming pools and in international dissemination of diabetes prevention strategies found efficacious in the landmark Diabetes Prevention Trial.

In Chapter Fifteen, Butterfoss, Kegler, and Francisco analyze four theories of organizational change: Stage Theory, Organizational Development Theory, Interorganizational Relations Theory, and Community Coalition Action Theory. Each of these theories can be used to create specific intervention strategies directed at levels of a single organization or at coalitions of multiple organizations, thus improving adoption and implementation of health promotion programs and community strategies. Further, strategies based on each of these theories can be used simultaneously to produce optimal effects. Butterfoss and colleagues then illustrate how these theories can be used as a basis for health promotion interventions for heart disease prevention and cancer control in Canada and the United States.

Finnegan and Viswanath introduce the Media Studies Framework for health behavior change in Chapter Sixteen. Their chapter describes communication theories that are especially relevant to public health and health behavior change. Four perspectives on the effects of media are introduced: the Knowledge Gap hypothesis, Agenda Setting, Cultivation Studies, and Risk Communication. They then present two applications of media studies to health: (1) a countermarketing campaign to prevent teen smoking and (2) the reframing of media coverage of the causes of and solutions for childhood obesity.

Part Four concludes with a summary, comparison, and critique of organizational and community interventions in health promotion and education. Chapter Seventeen discusses parallel elements in concept and strategies, as well as converging applications of community and group intervention models of health behavior change.

An understanding of theory, research, and practice in communities, systems, and organizations will be critical to wide improvement of health in the future. This part of *Health Behavior and Health Education* provides a diverse set of frameworks and applications for consideration of both researchers and practitioners.

REFERENCE

Smedley, B. D., and Syme, S. L. (eds.). *Promoting Health: Intervention Strategies from Social and Behavioral Research.* Washington, D.C.: National Academy Press, 2000.

CHAPTER

13

IMPROVING HEALTH THROUGH COMMUNITY ORGANIZATION AND COMMUNITY BUILDING

Meredith Minkler

Nina Wallerstein

Nance Wilson

KEY POINTS

This chapter will

- Provide a historical summary of the field and process of community organization and the emergence of community-building practice.
- Examine the concept of community.
- Present models of community organization and community building.
- Explore key theoretical and conceptual bases of community organization and community building.
- Analyze a case study to demonstrate the relevance of these models in practice.

Community organizing is the process by which community groups are helped to identify common problems or goals, mobilize resources, and develop and implement strategies to reach goals they have set collectively (Minkler and Wallerstein, 2004). The newer and related concept of community building (Blackwell and Colmenar, 2000) may be seen not as a method so much as an orientation to the ways in which people who identify as members of a shared community engage together in the process of community change (Walter, 2004).

Implicit in the definitions of both *community organizing* and *community building* is the concept of empowerment, viewed as an enabling process through which individuals or communities take control over their lives and environments (Rappaport, 1984). A multi-level construct involving "participation, control and critical awareness" (Zimmerman, 2000), empowerment embodies both social change processes and outcomes of transformed conditions (Wallerstein, 2006). Without empowerment, community organizing cannot be said to have taken place.

Community organization is important in health education, partially because it reflects one of the field's most fundamental principles, that of "starting where the people are" (Nyswander, 1956). The health education professional who begins with the community's felt needs is more likely to be successful in the change process and in fostering true community ownership of programs and actions. Community organizing also is important in light of evidence that social involvement and participation can themselves be significant factors in improving perceived control, empowerment, individual coping capacity, health behaviors, and health status (Eng, Briscoe, and Cunningham, 1990; Wandersman and Florin, 2000; Link and Phelan, 2000; Wallerstein, 2006). Finally, the heavy emphasis on community partnerships and community-based health initiatives by government agencies and foundations suggests the need for further refining theory, methods, and measurement techniques. This chapter describes the history of community organization and community-building practice, examines models of community organization and community building, explores key theoretical and conceptual bases, and presents a case study to illustrate these models in practice.

HISTORICAL PERSPECTIVE

The term *community organization* was coined by American social workers in the late 1800s in reference to their efforts to coordinate services for newly arrived immigrants and the poor (Garvin and Cox, 2001). As Garvin and Cox pointed out, although community organization typically is portrayed as having been born of the settlement house movement, several important milestones by rights should be included in any history of community organization practice. Prominent among these are (1) the post-Reconstruction period organizing by African Americans to salvage newly won rights that were rapidly slipping away, (2) the Populist movement, which began as an agrarian revolution and became a multisectoral coalition and a major political force, and (3) the Labor movement of the 1930s and 1940s, which taught the value of forming coalitions around issues, the importance of full-time professional organizers, and the use of conflict as a means of bringing about change (Garvin and Cox, 2001).

Within the field of social work, early approaches to community organization stressed collaboration and the use of consensus and cooperation, as communities were helped to self-identify and to increase their problem-solving ability (Garvin and Cox, 2001; Ross, 1955). By the 1950s, however, a new brand of community organization, which stressed confrontation and conflict strategies for social change, was gaining popularity. Most closely identified with Saul Alinsky (1969, 1972), social action organizing emphasized redressing power imbalances by creating dissatisfaction with the status quo among the disenfranchised, building communitywide identification, and helping members devise winnable goals and nonviolent conflict strategies as a means to bring about change.

Since the 1950s, strategies and tactics of community organization increasingly have been applied to achieve broader social change objectives, through movements that included civil rights, women's rights, gay rights, anti-Vietnam war organizing, and disability rights. The 1980s and 1990s also witnessed new community organization tactics and strategies in areas as diverse as the AIDS crisis and the New Right's organizing to ban abortions. From the mid-1990s to the present, use of computer technology also has greatly increased, with groups across the political spectrum building online communities and identifying and organizing support on a mass scale (Herbert, 2004).

Within the health field, in the mid-1980s the World Health Organization (WHO) adopted a new approach to health promotion that stressed increasing people's control over the determinants of their health, high-level public participation, and intersectoral cooperation (World Health Organization, 1986). Reflecting this new approach, the WHO-initiated Healthy Cities movement emerged and grew to involve thousands of healthy cities and communities worldwide. It aims to create sustainable environments and processes through which governmental and nongovernmental sectors partner to create public policies, achieve high-level participation in community-driven projects, and, ultimately, to reduce inequities and disparities among groups (Norris and Pittman, 2000).

Finally, alongside these developments has been a growing appreciation of the importance of facilitating community *building,* conceptualized as an orientation to community that stresses community assets and shared identity, whether or not task-oriented organizing takes place (Walter, 2004; Chávez, Minkler, Wallerstein, and Spencer, 2007).

The community-building orientation is reflected in efforts such as the National Black Women's Health Project (www.BlackWomensHealth.org)—a twenty-six-year-old organization that stresses empowerment through self-help and consciousness-raising for social change. Through local efforts, such as its annual seven-city Walking for Wellness event, a Leadership Development Institute, policy briefings, and other activities, the organization also melds community building with more traditional community-organizing methods to improve black women's health. Such community-building projects are strength-based, borrowing from feminist organizing an accent on the process of practice (Hyde, 1996) and on the use of dialogue to integrate personal and political experiences (Gutierrez and Lewis, 2004). Although theoretical work, practical applications, and research in the area of community building remain underdeveloped, community-building practice increasingly is becoming an important complement to more traditional notions of community organization.

THE CONCEPT OF COMMUNITY

The concept of community is integral to a discussion of community organization and community building. Although typically thought of in geographical terms, communities may also be based on shared interests or characteristics such as ethnicity, sexual orientation, or occupation (Fellin, 2001). Communities have been defined as (1) *functional spatial units* meeting basic needs for sustenance, (2) *units of patterned social interaction,* and (3) *symbolic units of collective identity* (Hunter, 1975). Eng and Parker (1994) add a fourth definition to community as a social unit where people come together politically to make changes.

Two sets of theories are relevant to understanding the concept of community. The first—the *ecological system perspective*—is particularly useful in the study of autonomous geographical communities, focusing as it does on population characteristics such as size, density, and heterogeneity, the physical environment, the social organization or structure of the community, and the technological forces affecting it (see Chapter Twenty). In contrast, the *social systems perspective* focuses primarily on formal organizations that operate within a given community, exploring the interactions of community subsystems (economic, political, and so on), both horizontally within the community and vertically, as they relate to other, extra-community systems (Fellin, 2001; see Chapter Fifteen). Warren's (1963) classic approach to community clearly fits within the latter perspective, envisioning communities as entities that change their structure and function to accommodate various social, political, and economic developments. Similarly, Alinsky's (1972) view of communities as reflecting the social problems and processes of an urban society provides a good example of a social systems perspective. Finally, as discussed next, the power of the Internet for creating cyber communities across time and distance has added a critical new dimension to our understanding of the meaning and power of community (Herbert, 2004).

The perspective on community that one adopts will influence one's view of the appropriate domains and functions of the community organization process. Community development specialists, such as agricultural extension workers and Peace Corps volunteers, have focused on *geographical communities.* In contrast, proponents of a broader approach, typified by social action organizers (Alinsky, 1972; Rinku Sen, 2003), have encouraged organizing around *issues* such as public housing and unemployment, in recognition of the tremendous impact of those larger socioeconomic issues on local communities. Finally, as Chávez and colleagues (2007), Rivera and Erlich (1995), and Gutierrez and Lewis (2004) have suggested, an appreciation of the unique characteristics of communities of color should be a major consideration. In African American communities, for example, West (1993) argues that market exploitation has led to a shattering of the religious and civic organizations that have historically buffered these communities from hopelessness and nihilism. He calls for community change through re-creating a sense of agency and political resistance based on "subversive memory—the best of one's past without romantic nostalgia" (West, 1993). A view of community that incorporates such a perspective would support building on pre-existing social networks and structures, emphasizing self-determination and empowerment (Gutierrez and Lewis, 2004).

MODELS OF COMMUNITY ORGANIZATION

Although community organization frequently is treated as though it were a singular model of practice, several typologies of community organization have been developed. Different models of community organization and community building illustrate how alternative assumptions about the nature and meaning of community shape how community organization and community building are conceptualized and practiced. The best-known typology is Rothman's (2001) categorization of community organization as consisting of three distinct models of practice: locality development, social planning, and social action. *Locality development* is heavily process-oriented, stressing consensus and cooperation and aimed at building group identity and a sense of community. By contrast, *social planning* is heavily task-oriented, stressing rational-empirical problem solving—usually by an outside expert—as a means of problem solving. Finally, the *social action model* is both task- and process-oriented. It is concerned with increasing the problem-solving ability of the community and with achieving concrete changes to redress imbalances of power and privilege between an oppressed or disadvantaged group and the larger society (Rothman, 2001). Professionals frequently use a blend of two or more of the models.

For close to three decades, Rothman's typology has remained the dominant framework for community organization and, as such, has had a significant impact on practice (Walter, 2004). However, the typology and its underlying assumptions have a number of important limitations. Use of the term *locality development,* for example, may be unnecessarily restrictive, discouraging organizing along nongeographical lines. Second, inclusion of a social planning model that often relies heavily on outside technical experts and may not increase the problem-solving ability of the community appears to contradict one of the most basic criteria of effective organizing. Third, as Walter (2004) argued, the fact that this typology is problem-based and organizer-centered constitutes a philosophical and practical limitation that may be particularly problematic, as organizing increasingly occurs in multicultural contexts. Finally, the approach misses several other critical dimensions, including ideology, longitudinal development, and the fundamentals of social movements (Hyde, 1996).

Partially in reaction to the perceived limitations of the Rothman typology, Hyde (1996), Walter (2004), and others (Gardner, 1991; Labonte, 1994; Wallerstein, Sanchez-Merki, and Dow, 2004) have proposed newer models of collaborative empowerment and community-building practice that provide important alternative approaches. These models can be seen as descendants of the community development model in their emphases on self-help and collaboration, yet they extend beyond community development, which is externally driven and may implicitly accept the status quo. They take their parentage from community-driven development in which community concerns direct the organizing in a process that creates healthy and more equal power relations (Hyde, 1996; Labonte, 1994; see Figure 13.1). Feminist and "women-centered" models (Hyde, 1996) also are reflected in these alternative approaches.

These newer community-building models emphasize community strengths as a diversity of groups and systems that identify and nurture shared values and goals (Walter, 2004). In an unpublished 1992 paper, Arthur Himmelman described a "collaborative empowerment model" that, for example, includes many of the steps stressed in more traditional organizing (for example, clarifying a community's purpose and vision, examining what others have done, and building a community's power base) but puts its heaviest accent on enabling communities to play the lead role so that real empowerment, rather than merely "community betterment," is achieved. McKnight's (1987) notion of "community regeneration" has at its heart enabling people to recognize and contribute their "gifts," which represent the building blocks or assets of a community that enable it to care for its members.

Along similar lines, Walter's (2004) community-building approach is described as "a way of orienting one's self in community" that places community "at the center of practice." In this approach, community building attempts to balance and blend such elements of community as history, identity, and autonomy, with the dimensions of community development, community planning, community action, community consciousness, and "the commons" (which encompasses the relationship between community and its broader environment). As such, the community-building approach significantly contrasts with more traditional notions of community organization practice that are "community based" but not necessarily *of* and *by* the community (Walter, 2004).

The increasing accent on "cultural humility" in community organizing and community-building practice also should be noted. Described by Tervalon and Garcia (1998) as an openness to others' cultures and an ability to listen to our own internal dialogue, this concept is well captured in the work of organizations like the Oakland, California-based Prevention Institute (Chávez, Minkler, Wallerstein, and Spencer, 2007). The Institute approaches health and social problems within a broad cultural context and emphasizes both organizing and strength-based community-building approaches.

The coalition-building model is alternately defined as one of community organization practice and as a strategy used across models. Coalitions are increasingly popular in diverse areas of health, including chronic disease, drugs and alcohol, violence, and the fight against budget cuts (Butterfoss and Kegler, 2002; see Chapter Fifteen).

In sum, several models of community organizing and community building have surfaced in the last decade to complement earlier organizing approaches. Figure 13.1 presents a typology that incorporates both need- and strength-based approaches of new perspectives and older models. Along the needs-based axis, "community development," as primarily a consensus model, is contrasted with Alinsky's "social action" conflict-based model. The newer strength-based models contrast a community-building capacity approach with an empowerment-oriented social action approach. Several concepts span these two approaches, such as community competence, leadership development, and the multiple perspectives on gaining power. Looking at primary strategies, consensus approaches primarily use collaboration strategies, whereas conflict approaches use advocacy strategies and ally building to support advocacy efforts.

As illustrated in Figure 13.1, community organizing and community building are fluid endeavors. Although some organizing efforts primarily have focused in one quadrant, the majority incorporate concepts from multiple quadrants. It is important for organizing efforts to clarify their assumptions and decide on primary strategies based on group history, member skills, willingness to take risks, or comfort level with different approaches.

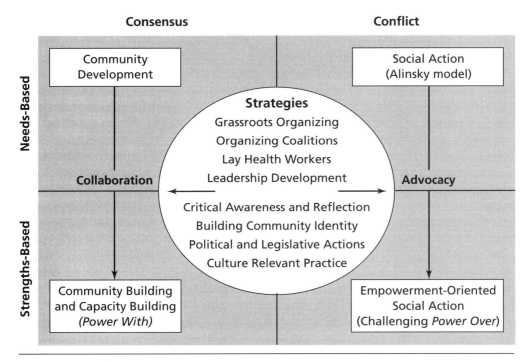

| Consensus | | Conflict |

FIGURE 13.1. Community Organization and Community-Building Typology.

CONCEPTS IN COMMUNITY ORGANIZATION AND COMMUNITY-BUILDING PRACTICE

Although no single unified model of community organization or community build-ing exists, some key concepts are central to the most often used models. Several of these concepts—empowerment, critical consciousness, community capacity, issue selection, and participation and relevance—are discussed next and summarized in Table 13.1.

Empowerment and Critical Consciousness

Although the term *empowerment* has been justifiably criticized as a "catch-all phrase" in social science (Rappaport, 1984), it remains a central tenet of community organi-zation and community-building practice. Within public health, empowerment (or com-munity empowerment) has been variously defined as communities achieving equity (Katz, 1984), communities having the capacity to identify problems and solutions (Cottrell, 1983), participatory self-competence in the political life of the commu-nity (Wandersman and Florin, 2000), and the "expansion of assets and capabilities of people to participate in, negotiate with, influence, control, and hold accountable in-stitutions that affect their lives" (Narayan, 2002).

TABLE 13.1. **Key Concepts in Community Organization and Community Building.**

Concept	Definition	Application
Empowerment	Social action process for people to gain mastery over their lives and the lives of their communities	Community members assume greater power or expand their power from within to create desired changes.
Critical consciousness	A consciousness based on reflection and action in making change	Engage people in dialogue that links root causes and community actions
Community capacity	Community characteristics affecting its ability to identify, mobilize, and address problems	Community members actively participate in identifying and solving their problems and become better able to address future problems collaboratively
Social capital	Relationships between community members including trust, reciprocity, and civic engagement	Community members collectively improve leadership, social networks, and quality of neighborhood life
Issue selection	Identifying winnable and specific targets of change that unify and build community strength	Identify issues through community participation; decide targets as part of larger strategy.
Participation and relevance	Community organizing should "start where the people are" and engage community members as equals	Community members create their own agenda based on felt needs, shared power, and awareness of resources.

In these definitions, empowerment is an action-oriented concept with a focus on removal of barriers and on transforming power relations among communities, institutions, and governmental agencies. It is based on an assumption of community cultural strengths and assets that can be strengthened. The dialogue process of Paulo Freire (1970), with its accent on critical consciousness or action based on critical reflection through dialogue, is central, as is the understanding that empowerment is exercised in multiple domains, from personal through political and collective action (Narayan, 2002; Wallerstein, 2006).

Bearing this in mind, a broader definition is most useful—one that considers empowerment a social action process by which individuals, communities, and organizations gain mastery over their lives in the context of changing their social and political environment to improve equity and quality of life (Rappaport, 1984; Wallerstein, 1992, 2006).

As a theory and methodology, community empowerment is multilayered, representing both processes and outcomes of change for individuals, the organizations of which they are a part, and the community social structure itself. At the level of individuals, "psychological empowerment" includes people's perceived control in their lives, their critical awareness of their social context, and their political efficacy and participation in change (Zimmerman, 2000). For individuals, empowerment challenges the perceived or real "powerlessness" that comes from the health injuries of poverty, chronic stressors, lack of control, and few resources.

Organizational empowerment incorporates both *processes* of organizations (for example, whether they are acting to influence societal change) and *outcomes,* such as their effectiveness in gaining new resources. At the community level, as individuals engage in community organizing efforts, community empowerment outcomes can include an increased sense of community, greater participatory processes and community competence, and outcomes of actual changes in policies, transformed conditions, or increased resources that may reduce inequities. As communities become empowered, key health and social indicators such as rates of alcoholism, divorce, suicide, and other social problems may begin to decline.

Community Capacity and Social Capital

Closely related to the concept of empowerment is the notion of *community capacity,* defined as "the characteristics of communities that affect their ability to identify, mobilize, and address social and public health problems" (Goodman and others, 1999). Community capacity has multiple dimensions: active participation, leadership, rich support networks, skills and resources, critical reflection, sense of community, understanding of history, articulation of values, and access to power (Goodman and others, 1999).

Definitions of *community capacity* have drawn from related concepts, such as "community competence" and "social capital." *Community competence* originally was defined by Cottrell (1983) as "the various component parts of the community being able to collaborate effectively on identifying the problems and needs of the community; to achieve a working consensus on goals and priorities; to agree on ways and means to implement the agreed upon goals; to collaborate effectively in the required actions."

Social capital has more recently captured the imagination of public health. From its origins in political science, *social capital* is defined as the features of social organization that facilitate coordination and cooperation for mutual benefit (Putnam, 1996, 2007). In sociology, it is viewed as a resource stemming from the structure of social relationships that facilitates achievement of specific goals (Coleman, 1988). Within epidemiology, social capital has been predominantly operationalized as a horizontal relationship between neighbors or community members, with variables including trust, reciprocity, and civic engagement such as in voluntary organizations, soccer leagues, parent-teacher organizations, and the like (Kawachi, Kennedy, Lochner, and Prothrow-Stith, 1997; Kim and Kawachi, 2007). More recent research, however, has explored the importance of bridging and linking social capital, connecting people across boundaries and across levels of power or hierarchy (Szreter and Woolcock, 2004). Lack of social capital has been correlated with poor health status, all-cause mortality and other morbidities, and health-related quality of life, and may mediate the relationship between income inequality and health (Kawachi, Kennedy, Lochner, and Prothrow-Stith, 1997; Kim and Kawachi, 2007). New research showing lower social capital in neighborhoods characterized by racial/ethnic heterogeneity (Putnam, 2007) is particularly disturbing in underscoring how far we have to go in developing cross-cultural understanding and trust (Minkler and Wallerstein, 2008).

Social networks—the web of relationships in which people are embedded—and social support—the tangible and intangible resources they give and receive through these networks (Cohen and Syme, 1985)—are important to consider in the context of community capacity building (see Chapter Nine). Social network techniques may be used in identifying natural helpers or leaders within a community, as well as high-risk groups, and may involve network members in undertaking the community assessment and actions necessary to strengthen networks within the community. Leadership development is another key aspect of fostering community capacity and is key to building group capacity and effectiveness. As Gutierrez and Lewis (2004) suggested, an emphasis on leadership development may be especially important in communities of color, where "a unidirectional outreach approach" often treats such communities as "targets of change rather than active participants and collaborators."

Issue Selection, Participation, and Relevance

One of the most important steps in community organization practice involves effective differentiation between problems, or things that are troubling, and issues the community feels strongly about (Miller, 1985). As Alinsky (1972) and Staples (2004) suggest, a good issue must be *winnable,* simple and *specific,* and *unifying* rather than *divisive*; it should also *involve* them in a meaningful way in achieving problem resolution. It should *affect many people* and *build up the community or organization* (giving leadership experience, increased visibility, and so on). Last, it should be *part of a larger plan or strategy.* Thus, participation and relevance—"starting where the people are" (Nyswander, 1956)—is an integral aspect of issue selection.

A variety of methods may be used to help a community group obtain the data needed for issue selection, while ensuring their participation and the relevance of issues ultimately selected (see Chapter Eighteen). Face-to-face data collection processes include focus groups, Nominal Group Process (NGP) (Delbecq, Van de Ven, and

Gustafson, 1975), door-to-door surveys, and interviews, which also can be useful in assessing felt needs and in increasing a sense of participation. These methods are useful for issue selection only to the extent that they enable the discovery of the real issues of concern to the community.

Freire's (1970) dialogical problem-posing method is an approach to issue selection that has proven especially helpful to engage participants in identifying themes that elicit social and emotional involvement and therefore increase motivation to participate. Community organizers in the United States also have adopted strategies from organizational development in creating strategic action plans to prioritize issues by available resources, appropriate timelines, and barriers to reaching goals (French and Bell, 1990; see Chapter Fifteen).

Thoughtfully undertaken, issue selection processes can contribute to community empowerment and serve as a positive force for social change. However, calls have been made increasingly for approaches that emphasize community strengths and assets along with issue selection. Among the useful new approaches to combining issue selection with this more positive emphasis on community strengths and assets is the "photovoice" method (Wang and Burris, 1997). Using this technique, health education professionals provide cameras and skills training to community residents, who then use the cameras to convey their own images of their community, including problems in need of redress and community strengths and assets. Participants then work together to select the pictures that best capture their collective wisdom and use these both to tell their stories and to stimulate change through local organizing and institutional- and policy-level action.

Another major new contributor to community organizing and community building that has emerged in the past decade involves harnessing the power of the Internet for collecting data, selecting issues, planning, and assessing allies and opposition (Herbert, 2004). In addition to providing extensive access to data about public health issues and concerns, the Internet can provide tools for assessing community needs and strengths, and also for later steps in community building and advocacy. For example, Fawcett and colleagues' (2000) "Community Tool Box" (http://ctb.ku.edu) is organized around sixteen core competencies, ranging from assessing community needs and resources to creating and maintaining coalitions, influencing policy development, and evaluating and sustaining the work. The site both supports online organizers and provides links to off-line assistance.

The advent and rapid growth of online organizing has not been without challenges. Poor communities still have too few onramps to the information superhighway, and although promising efforts to close the digital divide are under way, socioeconomic, linguistic, disability-related, generational, and other barriers remain a significant problem. As Herbert (2004) notes, "urging people to take action" over a listserv is not the same as meeting face-to-face and having group discussions, dialogues, and trainings that can lead to longer-term, sustainable change. Despite these limitations, however, the Internet is likely to become a more important resource for community organizing and community building in the years ahead.

MEASUREMENT AND EVALUATION ISSUES

A major limitation of most community organizing and community-building efforts has been failure to address evaluation processes and outcomes adequately. Some of the factors that hinder meaningful evaluation include funding constraints, lack of evaluation skills, and difficulty identifying appropriate outcomes of such work. Also, the continually evolving nature of community organizing initiatives and the fact that these projects often seek change on multiple levels can make traditional evaluation approaches inappropriate or ill-suited to such organizing endeavors. Finally, the focus of many standard evaluation approaches on long-term change in health and social indicators may fail to capture the shorter-term, system-level effects with which community organizing is heavily concerned, such as improvements in organizational collaboration, community involvement, capacity, and healthier public policies or environments.

The lack of formal evaluations of most community organizing efforts, coupled with the failure of many engaged in these projects to write up and publish their results, have made it difficult to amass a literature of "successful" and "unsuccessful" organizing efforts and the hallmarks of each, which are critical parts of building evidence for the field. Although some characteristics of successful community collaborations have been identified, such as shared vision, strong leadership, and a focus on process and not merely task achievement (Connell and others, 1995), much remains to be examined and assessed. Careful evaluation and documentation of both successful and unsuccessful community organizing projects are vitally needed.

Several key resources exist for professionals interested in evaluating community organizing and related efforts. Among them are *New Approaches to Evaluating Community Initiatives* (Connell and others, 1995; Fulbright-Anderson and others, 1998), which explored dilemmas commonly faced in the design, measurement, and interpretation of community initiatives, and articles on the measurement of internal and external effectiveness. A two-part issue of *Health Education Quarterly* titled "Community Empowerment, Participatory Education and Health" remains highly relevant to practitioners today and includes both tools and case studies (Wallerstein and Bernstein, 1994).

Well-established measures of community empowerment, capacity, and social capital that remain highly useful include assessments of sense of community (Chavis and Pretty, 1999), community competence (Eng and Parker, 1994), multi-level perceived control (Israel, Checkoway, Schulz, and Zimmerman, 1994), and social cohesion and social influence. Also useful are measures of trust, reciprocity, social capital, and civic engagement (Kreuter, Lezin, and Koplan, 1997; Kawachi, Kennedy, Lochner, and Prothrow-Stith, 1997), collective efficacy and social norm control (Sampson, Raudenbush, and Earls, 1997), psychological empowerment beliefs of perceived control, critical understanding of one's social environment, and participation in social action (Zimmerman, 1990, 2000). More recent measures for perceived neighborhood control and neighborhood participation (Parker and others, 2001) and measures of community empowerment can be found on the World Bank Web site (http://www.worldbank.org/), as well as in specific literature on youth, women, and interventions with vulnerable populations (Wallerstein, 2006).

Despite advances in measurement for capturing these kinds of changes, however, any tool or set of scales has limits. Self-report measures of individuals cannot completely capture organizational and community-level processes over time. Qualitative approaches are needed to enhance understanding of the context, dynamics of change, and outcomes such as transformed conditions, new policies, participation, and political voice.

The process by which communities develop their own sets of capacity and empowerment indicators is equally important to the development of validated scales. Some community groups have already developed indicators of capacity and sustainability (Norris 1997; The Aspen Institute, 1996; Bauer, 1997). A useful resource for communities wishing to develop their own indicators is the self-reflection workbook developed in New Mexico to evaluate community organizing and community building in the context of creating healthier communities (Wallerstein, Polacsek, and Maltrud, 2002). The workbook focuses on changes in community processes, such as grassroots participation, and changes in short-term, system-level outcomes, such as the development of new programs, as a result of the organizing experience. As noted earlier, it is these middle-level outcomes, rather than long-term changes in self-rated health and other health or social indicators, that are often most important in documenting changes in community capacity and empowerment. A Pan American Health Organization task force created a participatory evaluation handbook for healthy municipalities, which contains both a participatory cycle of gathering evidence and recommendations on multi-level indicators and outcomes (Pan American Health Organization, 2005).

A major contribution to the literature in this area is a key text on empowerment evaluation edited by Fetterman and Wandersman (2005), which defines *empowerment evaluation* as "the use of evaluation concepts, techniques and findings to foster improvement and self determination." Through this process, "the community, in collaboration with the support team, identifies its own health issues, decides how to address them, monitors progress toward its goals and uses the information to adapt and sustain the initiative" (Fawcett and others, 1996).

Fawcett and his colleagues (2001) have helped tailor empowerment evaluation methods more directly to the evaluation of community coalitions for health and related organizing efforts. Their Community Tool Box Web site (http://ctb.ku.edu), discussed earlier, can be used to guide more rigorous and empowering approaches to such evaluation.

The availability of new tools to help with the evaluation of community organizing does not solve the problem of insufficient funding and commitment to carrying out high-quality evaluative research. If the current increase in attention that foundation and government funders are giving to evaluation and measurement issues in community-based initiatives translates into increased funding, this should help spur major advances in the evaluation and documentation of community organizing and community building.

APPLICATION OF COMMUNITY ORGANIZATION AND COMMUNITY BUILDING

The next section of this chapter describes an application of the concepts and methods of community organizing and community building. The Youth Empowerment Strategies (YES!) project in California provides a case study of a multiyear project conducted with youth living in distressed neighborhood environments.

The Youth Empowerment Strategies (YES!) Project

In the United States, alcohol, tobacco and other drug use, fighting, bullying, and other risk behaviors among youth are serious concerns. Although risk behaviors often are seen as matters of individual choice, they are shaped in part by the broader societal context in which they take place. Individually based interventions that offer refusal skills, scare tactics, or health information as the sole component of the intervention often have disappointing results, in part because they do not address the underlying cause—the risk behavior environment.

In contrast to more traditional approaches, the Youth Empowerment Strategies (YES!) project, conducted in West Contra Costa County, California, from 2002–2005, was designed to engage pre-adolescent youth as critical thinkers and problem solvers. In so doing, this three-year after-school empowerment program and research project incorporated many of the principles and practices of community building and community organizing discussed earlier. Funded by a Centers for Disease Control and Prevention (CDC) grant to the Public Health Institute, YES! was built, in part, on the earlier Adolescent Social Action Project in New Mexico (Wallerstein and Sanchez-Merki, 1994; Wallerstein, Sanchez-Merki, and Dow, 2004) and used a strengths-based approach to empowerment. The program trained local high school and college students as cofacilitators to work with youth in after-school settings. At the heart of the YES! intervention were thirty-seven small, four- to twelve-member social action groups at five schools, in which students, led by pairs of trained facilitators, engaged in problem-posing dialogue and other community-building and organizing methods (for example, risk and asset mapping and photovoice) to identify resources and strengths in their environment and then to design and carry out action plans to address their shared concerns.

The approaches used in the YES! program were designed to build a sense of community and create a group context in which cognitive and social skills were taught and practiced in the course of democratic decision making. Participants' skills in collaborative problem solving were, in turn, used to facilitate group-designed and implemented social action projects in the participants' school and neighborhood communities (Wilson and others, 2006a; Wilson and others, 2007). Incorporated in YES!'s empowerment education approach were components of positive youth development, as stated by various interventionists and researchers (for example, Catalano and others, 2004), as fostering the building of competence (skills and resources for developing healthy options, developmentally appropriate skill-building activities), confidence (opportunities for making decisions, positive self-identity), connection (primary or secondary support, bonding with others, relationships with caring adults and peers), character (a sense of responsibility for self and for others), caring (a sense of belonging), and contribution to the community (participation in meaningful community work). To this list, YES! added empowerment education's emphasis on the participatory strategy of having youth identify their community concerns, then plan and engage in social action to change underlying conditions that cause distress and ill health.

Conceptual and Intervention Models

The conceptual model underlying the YES! program posits that individuals living in distressed neighborhood environments have higher levels of exposure to environmental and social distress (Wilson and others, 2007). The increased exposure leads to negative changes in beliefs and attitudes, which may, in turn, result in decreased health-promoting behaviors (Wilson and others, 2005; Sanders-Phillips, 1996; Wallerstein, 1992). As illustrated in Figure 13.2, problems in early adolescence such as fighting and bullying, engaging in other troubling school behaviors, and using alcohol, tobacco, and other drugs are markers for later adverse health outcomes.

The YES! intervention model (Figure 13.3) suggests that participation in YES! groups can have a positive influence on beliefs (for example, future orientation and efficacy at personal and group levels) and teaches a repertoire of behaviors (for example, collaboration skills). These may positively influence proximal outcomes, such as willingness to use conflict resolution skills and group collaborative decision making, in the pursuit of meaningful community participation, ultimately resulting in increased health and wellness outcomes (Wilson and others, 2006a). Although the models are depicted as linear, the components also can be thought of as a continuum and as interactive.

The YES! Program

We next describe how these conceptual and intervention models were operationalized at the program level and how principles and processes of community organizing and community building were central to this work.

Participants. Participants in the YES! program were fifth- and sixth-graders who attended academically underperforming elementary schools. School populations ranged from 90 percent to 98 percent students of color, with 74 percent to 92 percent living in or near poverty and thus qualifying for free or reduced-price lunch, compared to 33 percent overall for the county. Across the three years of the YES! program's operation, 301 boys and girls participated in the project's research component, with 189 also participating in the YES! after-school program and the remainder serving as comparisons at nearby schools in the same neighborhood.

Facilitators. Careful selection and training of local high school, college, and graduate student pairs who cofacilitated the groups was critical to the success of YES!

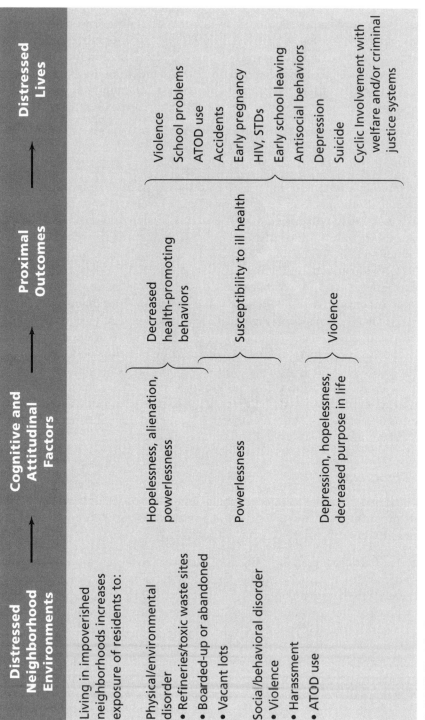

FIGURE 13.2. Conceptual Risk Model.

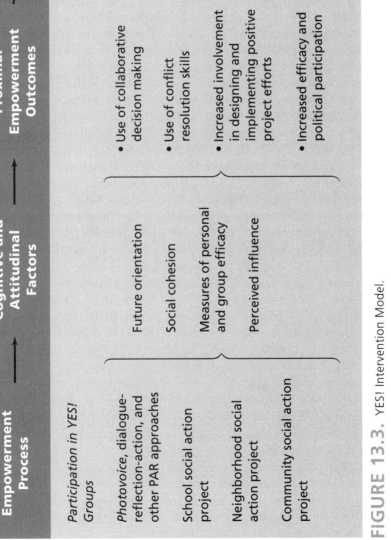

Empowerment Process

Participation in YES! Groups

Photovoice, dialogue-reflection-action, and other PAR approaches

School social action project

Neighborhood social action project

Community social action project

Cognitive and Attitudinal Factors

Future orientation

Social cohesion

Measures of personal and group efficacy

Perceived influence

Proximal Empowerment Outcomes

• Use of collaborative decision making

• Use of conflict resolution skills

• Increased involvement in designing and implementing positive project efforts

• Increased efficacy and political participation

Health and Wellness Outcomes

Increased

• Awareness of risky behaviors

• Health-promoting behaviors

Reduced

ATOD use

Accidents

Antisocial behaviors

Violence

Depression

FIGURE 13.3. YES! Intervention Model.

group social action projects (Wilson and others, 2006b). Across the three years of the program, over seventy-five group cofacilitators completed thirty to sixty hours of training. Cofacilitators also met weekly with YES! staff and met monthly as a group. The cofacilitators were paid for their time and received college or community service credits.

Curriculum. The YES! group cofacilitators completed a curriculum to learn participatory education techniques such as facilitating critical dialogue and community organizing strategies, youth development, group facilitation and management, multicultural understanding, and conducting social action projects with youth. The curriculum included activities in community building and group bonding, photography (sessions and photographic assignments on light, balance, perspective, and so on, and looking at others' photographs to interpret their meaning), photovoice, and community organizing strategies. Organizing strategies included school community mapping, issue selection, democratic decision making about social action project goals and methods, strategies for action planning, recruiting allies for support, and school and community engagement on multiple levels (Wilson and others, 2007).

Photovoice (described earlier) was central to the YES! program's empowerment education approach (Wang and Burris, 1997). After learning and practicing the basics of photography, participants took photographs documenting qualities of their schools, wrote about the images, and placed them on a group-drawn school community map. The photovoice assignment was to take photographs of assets (people, places, or things that made participants feel healthy, happy, or safe at school), as well as photographs of issues of concern at school. Using the acronym SHOWeD, facilitators then asked students to reflect on their own photographs by doing "freewrites," in which they wrote about a picture of their choosing, responding to the questions: What do you **S**ee in this picture? What's really **H**appening? How does this relate to **O**ur lives? **W**hy does it exist? What can we **D**o about it? (Wallerstein and Auerbach, 2004).

After presenting their freewrites to a partner, who asked clarifying questions, and then to the group, participants engaged in facilitated discussion about the effects of the assets and issues at the school. The task for the facilitators was to elicit deeper thinking or critical consciousness (Freire, 1973) and to guide group members in discussing how and why their individual experiences were public concerns and clarifying the underlying root cause of the issues from the participants' perspectives. SHOWeD questions again were used in group discussions of the photographs, with additional "but why?" questions included as part of the Freirian problem-posing dialogical process. Through these discussions, the group explored the social context and the causality of each asset or issue to help frame the purpose and goal of the social action project. Each group ranked the importance of the issues and assets identified and used some of the criteria for issue selection already discussed (for example, Is the issue winnable? Do people care deeply about it? Does it affect a lot of people?) to choose a social action project topic, either by consensus or voting. The group members posted comments about potential project ideas on flip chart pages placed around the room to solicit input from everyone. Responses then were discussed, with each group choosing both the project topic and the specific method or methods for the project it would pursue and presenting the project to school personnel for support and approval (Wilson and others, 2007).

Social Action Projects. The groups came up with four distinct types of social action projects: (1) *awareness campaigns about conditions at school,* for example, poster campaigns concerning potential teacher layoffs, a school vote to have the school district fix a shack on campus that was covered with graffiti and bullet holes (three groups); (2) *school behavior campaigns,* for example, skits on subjects such as why rumors cause fights, good and bad ways to get attention, the importance of talking to adults about what is bothering you (five groups); (3) *clean-up projects,* for example, painting bathrooms to remove graffiti, cleaning up litter on a playground (two groups), and (4) projects to *improve school spirit,* for example, school spirit T-shirts and a yearbook (two groups) (Wilson and others, 2006a). With the exception of one group that was unable to move beyond creating an exhibition of its issue and asset photographs, each of the groups moved from issue selection to developing and carrying out a social action plan (see Table 13.2 for a list of the social action projects; Wilson and others, 2007). Although far more modest in scope than the projects typically associated with community building and organizing by older youth and adults, these outcomes, and the sense of empowerment that came from identifying goals and collectively working to achieve them, were of real consequence to the students involved.

Evaluation of the YES! Program

Methods. Confidential questionnaires were administered by YES! staff to both YES! group participants and to students at comparison schools after obtaining parent/grandparent written informed consent and written student assent. The second-year questionnaire was modified, based on the first-year responses. Questionnaire items were drawn from published scales and included the types of outcomes presented in the models (see Figures 13.2 and 13.3), including variables such as exposure to gangs, community violence, and friends' delinquent behaviors; cognitive and attitudinal factors, including sense of hope, depression, attitudes toward violence, likelihood of violence and delinquency, adapted measures of perceptions of individual, group, and community control (Israel, Checkoway, Schulz, and Zimmerman, 1994), and measures of democratic awareness, belief in community action effectiveness, sense of community, leadership, political participation, and political efficacy (adapted from Wallerstein, 2006). In addition to questionnaires, qualitative data on each group's work and process were collected by YES! staff, and year-end interviews were conducted with individual group members, as well as with school personnel.

Data Analysis and Impact of Participation. Sample size and attrition across the three years of the project precluded rigorous statistical outcome evaluation. Descriptive analyses indicated that the YES! program resulted in a number of positive effects on participating youth. In addition to the direct effects of youth organizing and youth-designed and implemented social action projects, preliminary study results for program

TABLE 13.2. **Examples of YES! Group Social Action Projects.**

Issue or Asset Selected	Social Action Theme	Social Action Project
Fighting	Rumors get started in the bathrooms and cause fights	Presented skit to school on how to react to rumors to avoid fights
Unclean bathrooms	People have to be responsible for their behavior in the bathrooms	Classroom presentations and pledges of commitment; placed framed pledge posters in each classroom
Playground litter	Raise awareness and get students involved in playground cleanup	Organized a "delitterization" pledge in classrooms and a Cleanup Afternoon
Graffiti in the bathrooms	Unchecked graffiti encourages others to do it	Cleaned and painted two bathrooms and posted before and after pictures
Loss of sports and teachers due to school district finances	Raise district awareness about students' concerns regarding personnel cuts	Petition campaign (using posters from photovoice)
Dangerous shed on campus	Get the school district to fix up or tear down "The Scary Place" shed	Organized vote of third- to fifth- graders. Wrote request to school district to fix shed.
Gangs and drugs	Peer pressure to use drugs	Presented skit to school on how gangs push drugs on younger kids and cause violence; created and distributed photonovellas
Creek clean-up	People throwing trash, broken appliances, and other items into creek	Original idea: hold a creek clean-up. Second idea: distribute passes to the dump at street fair Actual project: perform a rap about keeping the creek clean and safe

participants and students from comparison schools indicated that those involved with YES! were significantly more likely to engage with friends who participated in pro-social behaviors (such as participating in clubs in and outside of school) and to participate more in problem solving for school social problems. Participants also were significantly less likely to engage in physically aggressive behaviors and in theft.

Also, pre and post surveys of 195 participants showed that following their participation in the program, these students were significantly more likely to report an intention to register to vote at age eighteen, to report feeling an increased voice in "having a say in what our school does," and to say they had increased understanding of important societal issues.

Finally, exit interviews with a number of the YES! participants showed that many had a strong desire to continue to engage in social action in their school and the broader community, and project staff developed and gave each participant a nicely bound booklet summarizing the participant's efforts and achievements, as well as resources to connect participants with other social action opportunities in their community.

COMMUNITY ORGANIZING AND COMMUNITY BUILDING WITH YOUTH: CHALLENGES AND CONSIDERATIONS

Community building and organizing with preadolescent and adolescent youth face significant limits. First, these youth still depend on older individuals as mentors and as facilitators of the logistics of organizing. Elementary and middle school youth, in particular, need parental permission and transportation to and from meetings and events; situations like changes in a parent's work schedule can interfere with participation in group meetings.

Second, children often have limited ability to initiate real social change, so modest community building and organizing outcomes, or simply community service, should be emphasized. By limiting the boundaries of the community primarily to the school, YES! afforded its participants a familiar arena and ready allies in the school staff.

Third, time may be a significant constraint for the scope of the community organizing projects. Time is needed to allow critical reflection, dialogue, and resultant learning to take place (Freire, 1973). Our experience suggests that with this age group, four months (90 minutes × 16 weeks) would be a good period of time for participants to develop and evaluate a meaningful social action project.

The degree of empowerment that group members experience depends both on the level of effort and the success of that effort, which may be heavily influenced by external factors. Therefore, it is essential for the projects to have multiple markers of success. Several groups did not have the opportunity to assess the impact of their work because, for example, they did not receive a response to letters they sent to the "powers that be" requesting remediation of a problem they had uncovered. Based on this experience, the YES! project built a self-evaluation component into the social action planning process and expanded and modified the curriculum to promote more richly developed social action projects.

An additional consideration in community building and organizing with youth within an empowerment framework work is that, in an after-school context, program activities cannot be exclusively "school-like." Building in time for parties, games, and other non-school-like activity is critical to participant retention and overall program success with youth. It also is consistent with good community organizing and community building with any age group, which reminds us to balance the group's work with social activities, and to celebrate even small successes with parties and refreshments (Minkler and Wallerstein, 2004).

A final challenge in community building and organizing with youth involves the key role of older facilitators, who can both catalyze participant empowerment and decision making and provide structure and guidance to help the group and its social action efforts move forward. Advance training for the facilitators and a detailed curriculum covering the period up to the groups' actual selection of their social action projects proved critical to project success. Facilitators also needed a clear understanding of their role and how to serve as the "headlight," or keeper of the vision, of the program if a group was stuck. Continuous dialogue between facilitators and program staff and frequent opportunities to debrief and discuss how to handle difficult situations also are critical to effective community organizing and community-building work with early adolescents (Wilson and others, 2006a, 2007).

Despite the challenges, the YES! project offers a promising example of a theoretically driven approach to community organizing and community building with youth. It is grounded in principles of empowerment and emphasizes critical thinking and moving into action. The program also revealed that while external constraints, participants' maturity levels, and a host of other factors limit what can realistically be accomplished, this type of program has real potential for involving pre-adolescent youth in identifying, designing, and conducting social action projects to create solutions for things of concern in their world. At least as important, such involvement may plant the seeds for future involvement in community building and organizing, and youth experience early on the excitement of working together to identify problems, dialogue about their causes and possible solutions, and develop action plans to promote change.

THE CHALLENGE OF COMMUNITY ORGANIZATION APPROACHES

Often, health and social service professionals are employed by an agency with specific agendas and categorical funding. The practitioner in this setting may not be able to undertake community organizing in the strictest sense of the word, because an outside group already has identified the specific health problem or problems to be addressed. Yet professionals in these situations can apply many of the core principles and approaches of community organization and community-building practice. They can elicit high-level community participation or involvement and can strive to build leadership skills and increase community competence as an integral part of the overall health education project. Further, even when the overall problem area (for example, heart disease or HIV/AIDS) has been identified initially by an outside group or agency, the health education professional, using community organizing and community-building skills and approaches, can help communities identify, within this broader framework, those specific issues of greatest relevance.

Most important, professionals can challenge themselves to examine their own dynamic of power with their professional colleagues and members of the community, to understand the complexities of working in partnership toward the goals of community ownership of projects undertaken and increased empowerment and community competence (Wallerstein, 1999). In sum, both community organization and newer models of community-building practice have essential messages for health education professionals in a wide variety of settings and hold great relevance in the changing sociopolitical climate of the twenty-first century.

SUMMARY

The continued pivotal role of community organization in health education practice reflects its time-tested efficacy and its fit with the most fundamental principles of effective community health education. Community organization stresses the principles of relevance and participation, or starting where the people are, and the importance of creating environments in which individuals and communities become empowered as they increase their community competence or problem- solving ability.

Newer models of community building stress many of the same principles, within an overall approach that focuses on community growth and change through increased group identification; discovery, nurturing, and mapping of community assets, and creation of "critical consciousness"—all toward the end of building stronger and more caring communities. New communication tools and online strategies have increased the reach of these methods over the last decade. A variety of tools are now available for evaluation of community organizing efforts, though the need continues for innovative designs and measurement approaches.

The YES! project illustrates how principles and methods of community building and community organizing can be adapted for use with youth in an underserved community to increase feelings of empowerment, facilitate the development of critical thinking skills, and promote social justice through social action. Although the outside public health professionals and researchers who initially designed the program had identified some particular outcome areas of interest (for example, alcohol, tobacco and other drug use, and other risky behaviors), they clearly "started where the people are" in inviting student participants to identify their own issues of concern and relevant resources, and to act together to address their collective goals.

REFERENCES

Alinsky, S. D. *Reveille for Radicals.* Chicago, Ill.: University of Chicago Press, 1969.

Alinsky, S. D. *Rules for Radicals.* New York: Random House, 1972.

The Aspen Institute. *Measuring Community Capacity Building: A Workbook-in-Progress for Rural Communities.* The Aspen Institute Rural Economic Policy Program. Aspen, Colo.: Aspen Institute, 1996.

Bauer, G. *Community Health Indicators on the Neighborhood Level: A Prototype for the Fruitvale/San Antonio Area in Oakland.* Oakland Community-Based Public Health Initiative (OCBPHI), 1997.

Blackwell, A. G., and Colmenar, R. "Community Building: From Local Wisdom to Public Policy." *Public Health Reports,* 2000, *113*(2 and 3), 167–173.

Butterfoss, F. D., and Kegler, M. C. "Toward a Comprehensive Understanding of Community Coalitions: Moving from Practice to Theory." In R. DiClemente, L. Crosby, and M. C. Kegler (eds.), *Emerging Theories in Health Promotion Practice and Research.* San Francisco: Jossey-Bass, 2002.

Catalano, R. F., and others. "Positive Youth Development in the United States: Research Findings on Evaluations of Positive Youth Development Programs." *Annals of the American Academy of Political and Social Science,* 2004, *591,* 98–124.

Chávez, V., Minkler, M., Wallerstein, N., and Spencer, M. *Community Organizing for Health and Social Justice.* San Francisco: Jossey-Bass, 2007.

Chavis, D. M., and Pretty, G.M.H. "Sense of Community: Advances in Measurement and Application." *Journal of Community Psychology,* 1999, *27*(6), 635–642.

Cohen, S., and Syme, S. L. (eds.). *Social Support and Health.* Orlando, Fla.: Academic Press, 1985.

Coleman, J. S. "Social Capital in the Creation of Human Capital." *American Journal of Sociology,* 1988, *94,* S95–S121.

Connell, J. P., and others (eds.). *New Approaches to Evaluating Community Initiatives: Concepts, Methods and Contexts.* Washington, D.C.: The Aspen Institute, 1995.

Cottrell, L. S., Jr. "The Competent Community." In R. Warren and L. Lyon (eds.), *New Perspectives on the American Community.* Homewood, Ill.: Dorsey Press, 1983.

Delbecq, A., Van de Ven, A. H., and Gustafson, D. H. *Group Techniques for Program Planning: A Guide to Nominal Group and Delphi Processes.* Glenview, Ill: Scott, Foresman, 1975.

Eng, E., Briscoe, J., and Cunningham, A. "The Effect of Participation in State Projects on Immunization." *Social Science and Medicine,* 1990, *30*(12), 1349–1358.

Eng, E., and Parker, E. "Measuring Community Competence in the Mississippi Delta: The Interface between Program Evaluation and Empowerment." *Health Education Quarterly,* 1994, *21*(2), 199–220.

Fawcett, S. B., and others. "Evaluating Community Initiatives for Health and Development." In I. Rootman, and others (eds.), *Evaluation in Health Promotion Approaches.* Copenhagen: WHO European Series No. 92, 2001.

Fawcett, S. B., and others. "Empowering Community Health Initiatives Through Evaluation." In D. Fetterman, S. Kaftarian, and A. Wandersman (eds.), *Empowerment Evaluation,* Thousand Oaks, Calif.: Sage, 1996.

Fawcett, S. B., and others. "The Community Tool Box: A Web-Based Resource for Building Healthier Communities." *Public Health Reports,* 2000, *115*(2 and 3), 274–278.

Fellin, P. "Understanding American Communities." In J. Rothman, J. Erlich, and J. Tropman (eds.), *Strategies of Community Intervention.* (5th ed.) Itasca, Ill.: Peacock, 2001.

Fetterman, D., and Wandersman, A. (eds.) *Empowerment Evaluation: Principles in Practice.* New York: Guilford Press, 2005.

Freire, P. *Pedagogy of the Oppressed.* New York: Seabury Press, 1970.

Freire, P. *Education for Critical Consciousness.* New York: Seabury Press, 1973.

French, W., and Bell, C. *Organization Development: Behavioral Science Interventions for Organization Improvement.* (2nd ed.) Englewood Cliffs, N.J.: Prentice Hall, 1990.

Fulbright-Anderson, K., Kubisch, A. C., and Connell, J. P. (eds.). *New Approaches to Evaluating Community Initiatives,* Vol. 2: *Theory, Measurement, and Analysis.* Aspen, Colorado: The Aspen Institute, 1998.

Gardner, J. *Building Community.* Washington, D.C.: Independent Sector Leadership Studies Program, 1991.

Garvin, C. D., and Cox, F. M. "A History of Community Organizing Since the Civil War with Special Reference to Oppressed Communities." *Strategies of Community Intervention.* (5th ed.) Itasca, Ill.: Peacock, 2001.

Goodman, R. M., and others. "Identifying and Defining the Dimensions of Community Capacity to Provide a Basis for Measurement." *Health Education and Behavior,* 1999, *25*(3), 258–278.

Gutierrez, L., and Lewis, E. "Education, Participation and Capacity Building in Community Organizing with Women of Color." In M. Minkler (ed.), *Community Organizing and Community Building For Health.* New Brunswick, N.J.: Rutgers, 2004.

Herbert, S. "Harnessing the Power of the Internet for Advocacy and Organizing." In M. Minkler (ed.), *Community Organizing and Community Building For Health.* (2nd ed.) New Brunswick, N.J.: Rutgers, 2004.

Hunter, A. "The Loss of Community: An Empirical Test Through Replication." *American Sociology Review,* 1975, *40*(5), 537–552.

Hyde, C. "A Feminist Response to Rothman's 'The Interweaving of Community Intervention Approaches.'" *Journal of Community Practice,* 1996, *3*(3/4), 127–145.

Israel, B., Checkoway, B., Schulz, A., and Zimmerman, M. "Health Education and Community Empowerment: Conceptualizing and Measuring Perceptions of Individual, Organizational, and Community Control." *Health Education Quarterly,* 1994, *21*(2), 149–170.

Katz, R. "Empowerment and Synergy: Expanding the Community's Healing Resources." *Prevention in Human Services, 1984, 3,* 201–226.

Kawachi, I., Kennedy, B. P., Lochner, K., and Prothrow-Stith, D. "Social Capital, Income Equality, and Mortality." *American Journal of Public Health, 1997, 87,* 1491–1497.

Kim, D., and Kawachi, I. "U.S. State-Level Social Capital and Health-Related Quality of Life: Multilevel Evidence of Main, Mediating, and Modifying Effects." *Annals of Epidemiology, 2007, 17,* 258–269.

Kreuter, M. W., Lezin, N. A., and Koplan, A. N. *Social Capital: Evaluation Implications for Community Health Promotion.* Atlanta: World Health Organization (WHO), 1997.

Labonte, R. "Health Promotion and Empowerment: Reflections on Professional Practice." *Health Education Quarterly,* 1994, *21*(2), 253–268.

Link, B. G., and Phelan, J. C. "Evaluating the Fundamental Cause Explanation for Social Disparities in Health." In C. D. Bird, P. Conrad, and A. M. Fremont (eds.), *Handbook of Medical Sociology.* (5th ed.) Upper Saddle River, N.J.: Prentice Hall, 2000.

McKnight, J. "Regenerating Community." *Social Policy,* Winter 1987, 54–58.

Miller, M. *Turning Problems into Actionable Issues.* San Francisco: Organize Training Center, 1985.

Minkler, M., and Wallerstein, N. "Improving Health Through Community Organization and Community Building." In M. Minkler (ed.), *Community Organizing and Community Building For Health.* (2nd ed.) New Brunswick, N.J.: Rutgers, 2004.

Minkler, M., and Wallerstein, N. "Introduction to Community-Based Participatory Research: New Issues and Emphases." In M. Minkler and N. Wallerstein (eds.), *Community-Based Participatory Research for Health.* San Francisco: Jossey-Bass, 2008.

Narayan, D. *Empowerment and Poverty Reduction: A Sourcebook.* Washington, D.C.: World Bank, 2002.

Norris, T. *The Community Indicators Handbook, Redefining Progress.* Boulder, Colo.: Tyler Norris Associates, 1997.

Norris, T., and Pittman, M. "The Healthy Communities Movement and the Coalition for Healthier Cities and Communities." *Public Health Reports,* 2000, *113,* 118–124.

Nyswander, D. B. "Education for Health: Some Principles and their Application." *Health Education Monographs,* 1956, *14,* 65–70.

Pan American Health Organization. *Participatory Evaluation of Healthy Municipalities: A Practical Resource Kit for Action.* Washington, D.C.: Pan American Health Organization, 2005.

Parker, E. A., and others. "Disentangling Measures Of Individual Perceptions Of Community Social Dynamics: Results of a Community Survey." *Health Education and Behavior,* 2001, *28*(4), 462–486.

Putnam, R. "E Pluribus Unum: Diversity and Community in the Twenty-first Century." The 2006 Johan Skytte Prize Lecture. *Scandinavian Political Studies,* 2007, *30*(2).

Putnam, R. D. "The Strange Disappearance of Civic America." *The American Prospect,* 1996, *24,* 34–48.

Rappaport, J. "Studies in Empowerment: Introduction to the Issue." *Prevention in Human Services,* 1984, *3*(2/3), 1–7.

Rinku Sen, R. *Stir It Up.* San Francisco: Jossey-Bass, 2003.

Rivera, F., and Erlich, J. "An Option Assessment Framework for Organizing in Emerging Minority Communities." In J. Tropman and others (eds.), *Tactics and Techniques of Community Intervention.* (3rd ed.) Itasca, Ill.: Peacock Publishers, 1995.

Ross, M. *Community Organization: Theory and Principles.* New York: Harper and Brothers, 1955.

Rothman, J. "Approaches to Community Intervention." In J. Rothman, J. L. Erlich, and J. E. Tropman (eds.), *Strategies of Community Intervention.* Itasca, Ill: Peacock Publishers, 2001.

Sampson, R. J., Raudenbush, S. W., and Earls, F. "Neighborhoods and Violent Crime: A Multilevel Study of Collective Efficacy." *Science,* 1997, *277,* 918–924.

Sanders-Phillips, K. "The Ecology of Urban Violence: Its Relationship to Health Promotion Behaviors in Low-Income Black and Latino Communities." *American Journal of Health Promotion,* 1996, *10,* 308–317.

Staples, L. "Selecting and Cutting the Issue." In M. Minkler (ed.), *Community Organizing and Community Building for Health.* (2nd ed.) New Brunswick, N.J.: Rutgers University Press, 2004.

Szreter, S., and Woolcock, M. "Health by Association? Social Capital, Social Theory, and the Political Economy of Public Health." *International Journal of Epidemiology,* 2004, *33,* 650–667.

Tervalon, M., and Garcia, J. "Cultural Humility Versus Cultural Competence: A Critical Distinction in Defining Physician Training Outcomes in Multicultural Education." *Journal of Health Care for the Poor and Underserved,* 1998, *9*(2), 117–125.

Wallerstein, N. "Powerlessness, Empowerment, and Health: Implications for Health Promotion Programs." *American Journal of Health Promotion,* 1992, *6,* 197–205.

Wallerstein, N. "Power Between Evaluator and Community: Research Relationships within New Mexico's Healthier Communities." *Social Science and Medicine,* 1999, *49,* 39–53.

Wallerstein, N. "The Effectiveness of Empowerment Strategies to Improve Health." Copenhagen: Health Evidence Network, World Health Organization, 2006. Available at www.euro.who.int/HEN/Syntheses/empowerment/20060119_10.

Wallerstein, N., and Auerbach, E. *Problem-Posing at Work: Popular Educators Guide.* Edmonton, Alberta, Canada: Grass Roots Press, 2004.

Wallerstein, N., and Bernstein, E. (eds.) "Community Empowerment Participatory Education and Health." *Health Education Quarterly,* Summer and Fall 1994, *21*(2 and 3).

Wallerstein, N., Polacsek, M., and Maltrud, K. "Participatory Evaluation Model for Coalitions: A Systems Indicator Approach from New Mexico." *Health Promotion Practice,* 2002, *3*(3), 361–373.

Wallerstein, N., and Sanchez-Merki, V. "Freirian Praxis in Health Education: Research Results from an Adolescent Prevention Program." *Health Education Research,* 1994, *9*(1), 105–118.

Wallerstein, N., Sanchez-Merki, V., and Dow, L. "Freirian Praxis in Health Education and Community Organizing: A Case Study of an Adolescent Prevention Program." In M. Minkler (ed.), *Community Organizing and Community Building for Health.* (2nd ed.) New Brunswick, N.J.: Rutgers University Press, 2004.

Walter, C. "Community Building Practice" In M. Minkler (ed.), *Community Organizing and Community Building for Health.* (2nd ed.) New Brunswick, N.J.: Rutgers University Press, 2004.

Wandersman, A., and Florin, P. "Citizen Participation and Community Organizing." In J. Rappaport and E. Seidman (eds.), *Handbook of Community Psychology.* New York: Plenum, 2000.

Wang, C., and Burris, M. A. "Photovoice: Concept, Methodology and Use for Participatory Assessment." *Health Education and Behavior,* 1997, *24,* 369–387.

Warren, R. *The Community in America.* Chicago, Ill.: Rand McNally, 1963.

West, C. *Race Matters.* Boston: Beacon Press, 1993.

Wilson, N., and others. "Adolescent Alcohol, Tobacco, and Marijuana Use: The Influence of Neighborhood Disorder and Hope." *American Journal of Health Promotion,* 2005, *20*(1), 11–19.

Wilson, N., and others. "Getting to Social Action: The Youth Empowerment Strategies (YES!) Project." *Health Promotion Practice.* First published on July 17, 2006a, as doi:10.1177/1524839906289072.

Wilson, N., and others. "Training Students as Facilitators in the Youth Empowerment Strategies (YES!) Project." Co-published simultaneously in *Journal of Community Practice,* 2006b, 14(1/2), 201–217; and B. N. Checkoway and L. M. Guitiérrez (eds.), *Youth Participation and Community Change.* Binghamton, N.Y.: Haworth Press, 2006b.

Wilson, N., and others. "Engaging Young Adolescents in Social Action through Photovoice: The Youth Empowerment Strategies (YES!) Project." *Journal of Early Adolescence,* 2007, *27*(2), 1–21.

World Health Organization. Ottawa Charter for Health Promotion, 1986.

Zimmerman, M. "Taking Aim on Empowerment Research: On the Distinction Between Individual and Psychological Conceptions." *American Journal of Community Psychology,* 1990, *18,* 169–177.

Zimmerman, M. "Empowerment Theory: Psychological, Organizational and Community Levels of Analysis." In E. S. Julian Rappaport (ed.), *Handbook of Community Psychology.* New York: Kluwer Academic/Plenum Publishers, 2000.

CHAPTER

14

DIFFUSION OF INNOVATIONS

Brian Oldenburg

Karen Glanz

KEY POINTS

This chapter will

- Describe the Diffusion of Innovations model and its key concepts.
- Provide an overview of factors that influence the process of diffusion.
- Describe two applications in detail and use them to illustrate some of the key concepts and features of the model.
- Identify limitations of the model and future directions for improved understanding and application of the model.

The history of innovations teaches us that usually it takes far too long for proven concepts and programs to become part of practice. One of the best illustrations of this principle was the recognition that, although citrus juice was shown effective in preventing scurvy in 1601, the British merchant navy did not introduce citrus juice into sailors' shipboard diets until 1795, nearly two centuries later (Mosteller, 1981).

Diffusion of effective programs and ideas is a significant challenge for public health and health promotion. Practitioners often find that research-based interventions

Thanks to Jan Nicholson, Steve Bunker, and Barbara Rimer for their helpful comments and advice during the preparation of this manuscript. Prasuna Reddy and Pilvikki Absetz also gave invaluable advice and comments on the diabetes prevention case example presented in this chapter.

are difficult to conduct in less controlled community settings and that the research base is not adequate to meet practitioners' needs (Glanz and Oldenburg, 1997; Oldenburg, Sallis, French, and Owen, 1999). Further, public health decision makers are often reluctant to consider "new" interventions when effectiveness has not been demonstrated in their particular locality, setting, or population (Brownson and others, 2007b). Practitioners and policymakers want strategies and interventions they can use to solve problems in their communities. They may not know or be able to search the research or evidence literatures to learn what has worked in other settings. By contrast, in developing efficacious programs, researchers usually are most concerned about internal rather than external validity (Green and Glasgow, 2006). Until recently, there has been little incentive for researchers to consider issues related to wider implementation and diffusion of effective programs. Slowly, this is beginning to change, as government and other agencies emphasize the importance of diffusion, dissemination, and translation. If effective public health programs, products, and practices are not widely and effectively disseminated, they will not achieve their potential impact to improve the public's health. The Diffusion of Innovations model has been used over several decades to understand the steps and processes required to achieve widespread dissemination and diffusion of public health innovations.

Major reports have noted the substantial gap between knowledge and practice in health and medicine, and have drawn attention to the fact that the failure to use available research findings is both costly and harmful to society (for example, Institute of Medicine, 2001). The knowledge-practice gap exists across all fields of medical and public health practice, as well as other fields as diverse as education and agriculture. In public health, even for interventions such as tobacco control, where a compelling evidence base has existed for decades, implementation remains inadequate in most developed countries and even poorer in many developing countries. The challenge of promoting the uptake of innovations that have been shown to be effective is great. As Kerner, Rimer, and Emmons (2005) noted: "Efforts to move effective preventive strategies into widespread use too often have been unsystematic, uncoordinated, and insufficiently capitalized, and little is known about the best strategies to facilitate active dissemination and rapid implementation of evidence-based practices."

In this chapter, we define *diffusion* as the process by which an innovation is communicated through certain channels over time among the members of a social system (Rogers, 2003). We refer to *dissemination* as planned, systematic efforts designed to make a program or innovation more widely available to a target audience or members of a social system.

DEVELOPMENT OF THE FIELD AND RELATED RESEARCH TRADITIONS

In the 2003 edition (the fifth) of his book, *Diffusion of Innovations*, Rogers noted that there were about 5,200 publications on the diffusion of such diverse innovations as agricultural practices, technology, fertility control methods, policy innovations, consumer products, educational curricula, political reforms, and health promotion programs (Rogers, 2003). The majority of authors analyzed diffusion narrowly and according to specific applications (Wejnert, 2002). Three notable exceptions to this trend are the writings of Rogers (1962, 1983, 1995, 2003), Strang and Soule (1998), Wejnert (2002), and Greenhalgh and colleagues (2004, 2005), who have considered diffusion relevant to a broad range of fields of human endeavor and behavior. Because the literature on diffusion is vast, readers should refer to these sources for detailed reviews of research associated with specific concepts and variables.

The development of diffusion studies has emerged from multiple conceptual and research traditions over the last fifty years. Rogers (2003) identified nine major diffusion research traditions, estimating that four of these account for nearly two-thirds of all diffusion publications: rural sociology, marketing and management, communication, and public health. In a recent extensive systematic review, Greenhalgh and others (2004, 2005) identified thirteen research traditions that have contributed to an improved understanding of the diffusion of innovations as applied to health. Some of these overlap with Rogers's most recent overview, with some notable additions. According to Greenhalgh and others, early diffusion research areas include *rural sociology, medical sociology, communication studies*, and *marketing*. Findings from these areas yielded robust empirical findings about how adoption decisions are influenced by the attributes of innovations, characteristics and behaviors of adopters, and the nature and extent of interpersonal and mass media factors. However, the collective work from these fields had many limitations. In particular, this work has had an almost exclusive focus on relatively simple innovations and individual adopters as the unit of analysis; in nonexperimental settings, most programs are more complex and consist of multiple components.

Three recent research areas can be seen as building on the earlier approaches: (1) *development studies*, where the emphasis is on the political, technological, or ideological context of the innovation, (2) *health promotion*, and (3) *evidence-based medicine*. In the last field, it has been recognized recently that the implementation of clinical guidelines depends both on organizational and system changes and on individual clinicians' behaviors.

Five additional research areas prominent in the organization, management, and organizational psychology literatures have become important to diffusion research. As the emphasis has shifted toward understanding the behavior of organizations and broader systems, these research traditions have addressed diffusion of innovations: studies of structural determinants of organizational innovativeness; studies of organizational process, context, and culture; interorganizational studies; knowledge-based approaches to innovation in organizations; narrative organizational studies, and complexity studies (Greenhalgh and others, 2004).

Ideas about the diffusion of innovations also have been popularized by the publication of books such as Malcolm Gladwell's best-seller *The Tipping Point: How Little Things Can Make a Big Difference* (Gladwell, 2000). Gladwell's central argument is that a number of patterns and factors are important in virtually every influential trend, ranging from the spread of communicable diseases to the popularity of a children's television show. Three key factors usually determine whether a particular trend will "tip" into wide-scale popularity. First, the new idea or innovation needs some influential early adopters or champions. Second, the innovation needs to have a quality or attributes that people find compelling. Third, the physical and broader social environment can be enormously influential (Gladwell, 2000). Readers may find

Gladwell's writings useful in relating their work in public health to lay audiences such as business and political leaders.

In relation to health promotion and public health, Orlandi and others (1990) identified the need to address the gap between innovation development and diffusion planning. Systematic reviews in the 1990s revealed both inattention to diffusion and dissemination and mixed findings. Oldenburg and others (1999) conducted a content analysis of 1,210 articles published in twelve public health and health promotion journals in the early 1990s, and classified 89 percent of the published studies as basic research and development (including efficacy trials), 5 percent innovation development studies, and less than 1 percent dissemination and diffusion research. Similarly, in a content analysis of four journals, Sallis, Owen, and Fotheringham (2000) found that less than 20 percent of articles addressed the translation of research into practice. A recent systematic review of thirty-one dissemination studies in cancer control concluded that there was no strong evidence to recommend any single dissemination strategy as effective or to improve the uptake of cancer control interventions (Ellis and others, 2005). There simply was too little research to reach conclusions.

The landscape is changing, and the evidence base for diffusion in public health and health promotion has begun to expand more rapidly in recent years. The interdisciplinary evidence review of 495 sources conducted by Greenhalgh and colleagues (2004, 2005) provides important research synthesis for those working in health behavior and health education. Several relevant special issues or sections of journals have been published in relation to the dissemination of physical activity, cancer control, AIDS education and prevention programs, and relevant concepts and methods (Buller, 2006; Kerner, Rimer, and Emmons, 2005; *American Journal of Public Health*, 2006; "Moving Science into Practice," 2006; Ratzan, 2004). These publications reflect an increasingly diverse range of research on diffusion that expands on earlier research and extends to areas such as physical activity, sexual practices, drug use, mental health, and reproductive health.

In recent health behavior and health education research, applications of diffusion models are noteworthy in their focus on *active* dissemination. This is in stark contrast to the well-established diffusion research emphasis on survey research to explain how innovations spread (Rogers, 2003). In the physical activity field, the SPARK (Sports, Play, and Active Recreation for Kids) and CATCH (Coordinated Approach to Child Health) programs for school-based physical education have been widely disseminated, and use some of the core constructs of the Diffusion of Innovations model to describe the dissemination efforts (Owen, Glanz, Sallis, and Kelder, 2006). In the cancer control field, the Pool Cool sun-safety program for aquatic settings is an example of a health behavior change program that has progressed from an efficacy trial to program dissemination and a diffusion trial (Glanz, Steffen, Elliott, and O'Riordan, 2005). Body and Soul—a nutrition intervention to increase fruit and vegetable intake and conducted through African American churches—was widely disseminated through a partnership of the American Cancer Society, the Centers for Disease Control and Prevention (CDC), and the National Cancer Institute, and was rigorously evaluated (Campbell and others, 2007; Resnicow and others, 2004). In HIV/AIDS, the Diffusion of Innovations model has been used extensively in the development, implementation, and wide diffusion of programs in both developed and developing countries (Bertrand, 2004).

KEY CONCEPTS

We describe key concepts of Diffusion of Innovations in two categories: (1) foundational concepts and stages of diffusion (Table 14.1) and (2) characteristics of innovations that determine diffusion (Table 14.2). Diffusion and dissemination are distinct concepts, as described at the beginning of this chapter; diffusion is the process by

TABLE 14.1. **Key Concepts and Stages of Diffusion.**

Concept	Definition*
Diffusion	The overall spread of an innovation, the process by which an innovation is communicated through certain channels over time among the members of a social system.
Dissemination	The planned, systematic efforts designed to make a program or innovation more widely available. Diffusion is the direct or indirect outcome of those efforts.
Innovation	An idea, practice, or object that is perceived as new by an individual or other unit of adoption.
Communication Channels	Means by which messages are spread, including mass media, interpersonal channels, and electronic communications.
Social System	Set of interrelated units that are engaged in joint problem solving to accomplish a common goal. Social systems have structure, including norms and leadership.
Innovation Development	All the decisions and activities (and their impacts) that occur from the early stage of an idea to its development and production.
Adoption	Uptake of the program or innovation by the target audience.
Implementation	The active, planned efforts to implement an innovation within a defined setting.
Maintenance	The ongoing use of an innovation over time.
Sustainability	The degree to which an innovation or program of change is continued after initial resources are expended.
Institutionalization	Incorporation of the program into the routines of an organization or broader policy and legislation.

*Definitions adapted from Rogers, 2003, and Oldenburg and Parcel, 2002.

which an innovation is communicated through certain channels over time among members of a social system (Rogers, 2003), whereas dissemination involves planned, systematic efforts to maximize the reach and adoption of new programs, strategies, or policies. Diffusion is also the outcome of dissemination efforts.

Although diffusion of most innovations involves both passive and active features, the spread of an innovation can be conceptualized on a continuum. *Passive* diffusion (in which the spread is unplanned, informal, and largely mediated horizontally by peers and social networks) lies at one end of the continuum and *active* dissemination (in which the spread is much more planned, formal, centralized and likely to occur through vertical hierarchies) is at the other end. There are three general pathways by which health behavior programs or innovations can be actively disseminated. These include (1) "direct to practice" distribution of materials and tools, (2) enactment and implementation of policies, legislation, or regulations, and (3) a systematic, sustained, and long-term approach that uses multiple strategies and methods, including ongoing evaluation over time (Owen, Glanz, Sallis, and Kelder, 2006).

In addition to providing succinct definitions of other basic concepts, including *innovation, communication channels*, and *social system*, we describe the various stages in the multistep diffusion process. The first stage is *innovation development*, followed by *dissemination, adoption, implementation, maintenance, sustainability*, and *institutionalization* (Orlandi, Landers, Weston, and Haley, 1990; Oldenburg and Parcel, 2002). During the innovation development phase, social marketing often has been used to design, target, refine, and implement health promotion innovations or "products" (see Chapter Nineteen). Innovation development is included in several familiar models of intervention development and testing for health promotion, such as Intervention Mapping (Bartholomew, Parcel, Kok, and Gottlieb, 2006). The dissemination process requires planning to persuade target groups to adopt an innovation, but it is critical that the intervention has been developed with the target population in mind and is appropriate to the intended settings.

During the adoption phase, several issues require attention: the needs of target adopters, their current attitudes and values, how they will respond to the innovation, what factors will increase likelihood of adoption, how potential adopters can be influenced to change their behaviors, and barriers to adoption of an innovation and how they can be overcome. The decision to adopt is influenced by three types of knowledge: (1) *awareness knowledge* that the innovation exists, (2) *procedural knowledge* about how to use the innovation, and (3) *principles knowledge* or understanding about how the innovation works (Rogers, 2003). The decision to adopt is not based solely on knowledge and inevitably also requires attitude change. Often a partial trial of the innovation leads to a choice to adopt or reject the innovation (Cain and Mittman, 2002).

As part of the process of implementation of an innovation, prospective users are likely to think about what problems might be encountered and to seek resources for and support in putting the innovation into practice. Research studies often have focused on improving the self-efficacy and skills of adopters, and encouraging a trial of the innovation. The stages of maintenance and sustainability involve continued use of the program, and the final stage is institutionalization into communities, organizations, or other settings. Sometimes sustainability and institutionalization are combined into a single stage, although it is possible for an innovation to be sustained for a period of time but not ultimately institutionalized.

IMPORTANT FACTORS IN THE DIFFUSION PROCESS

A key premise of the Diffusion of Innovations model is that some innovations diffuse quickly and widely (like the Internet), whereas others are weakly or never adopted, and others are adopted but subsequently abandoned. Also, innovations are adopted by different individuals and spread at different rates in subgroups of individuals. Three groups of variables have been used to explain these different outcomes: (1) characteristics of the innovation, (2) characteristics of adopters, and (3) features of the setting or environmental context.

Characteristics of the Innovation

Rogers (1983, 1995, 2003) and others (for example, Greenhalgh and others, 2004; Wejnert, 2002) have comprehensively reviewed the attributes or characteristics of innovations most likely to affect the speed and extent of the adoption and diffusion process (see Table 14.2). The core attributes for which a strong body of evidence exists are: relative advantage, compatibility, complexity, trialability, and observability (Rogers, 2003; Greenhalgh and others, 2004).

TABLE 14.2. **Characteristics of Innovations That Affect Diffusion.**

Attribute	Key Question
Relative advantage	Is the innovation better than what was there before?
Compatibility	Does the innovation fit with the intended audience?
Complexity	Is the innovation easy to use?
Trialability	Can the innovation be tried before making a decision to adopt?
Observability	Are the results of the innovation visible and easily measurable?

1. *Relative advantage.* An innovation will only be adopted if it is seen as better than the idea, product, or program it supersedes. Advantages considered can be economic, social, utilitarian, and so on (Rogers, 2003). This is the sine qua non for adoption, and there is reasonably strong evidence for this (Greenhalgh and others, 2004). However, relative advantage alone does not guarantee widespread adoption (Denis and others, 2002; Fitzgerald, Ferlie, Wood, and Hawkins, 2002; Grimshaw and others, 2004).

2. *Compatibility.* Innovations that are compatible with the intended users' values, norms, beliefs, and perceived needs are more readily adopted (for example, Aubert and Hamel, 2001). These may be considered on the individual or organizational levels. The concept of *reinvention*, sometimes identified as a distinct feature of innovations (Greenhalgh, 2004), can also be thought of as an extension of compatibility. If potential adopters can adapt, change, and modify an innovation to suit their own needs and context, it will be adopted more easily.

3. *Complexity.* Innovations perceived as easy to use are more likely to be adopted, whereas more complex innovations are less successfully adopted. In addition, innovations that can be broken down into parts and adopted incrementally are more likely to be adopted.

4. *Trialability.* Innovations with which intended users can experiment on a limited basis are adopted and assimilated more easily.

5. *Observability.* If the benefits of an innovation are easily identified and visible to others, it will be adopted more easily.

Although these attributes of innovations have been extensively studied, others have been examined and proposed to help explain the uptake of complex innovations in organizations or other settings (Greenhalgh and others, 2004). These include the notion of *fuzzy* boundaries, where the distinction is made between the "hard core" (or irreducible elements) of a complex, multicomponent innovation and the "soft periphery," which includes the organizational structures and delivery systems required for full implementation. Elements of this concept clearly link with Rogers's (2003) concept of reinvention.

Characteristics of Individuals

Rogers (1995, 2003) described the process of innovation adoption by individuals as a normal, bell-shaped distribution, with five adopter categories: (1) innovators, (2) early adopters, (3) early majority adopters, (4) late majority adopters, and (5) laggards. He characterized the *early* and *late majority adopters* as being within one standard deviation on either side of the mean or midpoint of the curve, *adopters* and *laggards* as being two standard deviations away, and *innovators* as being three standard deviations on the positive side from the mean. He proposed that the identifying adopter categories could provide a strong basis from which to design and implement intervention strategies aimed at particular groups of individuals. As originally proposed, these adopter categories were to be used primarily for descriptive and planning purposes; however, there has been a tendency to use these categories as explanatory or predictor variables, despite little empirical support for this approach (Greenhalgh and others, 2004). The decision-making processes of potential adopters are influenced by many other factors in the context, environment, or system in which the process is taking place, several of which have been supported by some empirical evidence. These intra-individual factors include psychological antecedents (for example, learning style, tolerance of ambiguity), meaning, and concerns in the pre-adoption stage, early use, and once use is established (Greenhalgh and others, 2004).

Features of the Setting

Innovations may be disseminated successfully in some settings but not in others (Greenberg, 2006). Many different features of settings and organizations can influence the diffusion process. These can be categorized as (1) geographical settings, (2) societal culture, (3) political conditions, and (4) globalization and uniformity (Wejnert, 2002). Variables related to geographical location usually only have direct or personal consequences for individual adopters, whereas the other types of variables typically have consequences for both individual adopters and organization- or system-level adopters. Social network variables are especially important within the societal culture group of variables, in addition to relevant political and organizational variables.

THE ROLE OF SETTINGS AND ORGANIZATIONS IN DIFFUSION OF HEALTH BEHAVIOR INNOVATIONS

Most innovations in public health now consist of more complex, multicomponent programs, guidelines, policies, and legislation, where the unit of adoption is a group of implementers or a whole organization or system. In organizations such as workplaces, schools, and health care settings, successful uptake of an innovation may require the introduction of particular programs or services, changes in policies or regulations, and changes in the roles and functions of particular personnel. For issues being addressed at a broader communitywide or societal level, such as tobacco control, the dissemination process needs to involve the media, government policies and legislation, and coordination of a variety of other initiatives for individuals and groups. The field of tobacco control has become so complex globally that it is necessary to apply a systems approach to understand the diffusion of tobacco control measures and policies in both the developed and developing worlds (National Cancer Institute, 2007).

It has become increasingly clear that factors influencing diffusion are not just static features of the innovation or of the adopters. Rather, there is usually a dynamic interaction among features of the innovation, intended adopters, and the context or setting where the process is occurring. Indeed, most health behavior change programs take place in various settings, such as workplaces, schools, health departments, and international family planning organizations (see Chapter One). Recent examples from three studies on disseminating skin cancer prevention involved such diverse units of adoption as zoological parks (Lewis and others, 2005), public elementary schools and child-care facilities (Buller, Buller, and Kane, 2005), and swimming pools (Glanz, Steffen, Elliott, and O'Riordan, 2005).

Brownson and others (2007b) illustrate the interplay among these different groups of factors in their report on an evaluation of disseminating evidence-based guidelines to promote physical activity in state and local health departments across eight states. Dissemination strategies included conducting workshops, providing technical assistance, and distributing instructional CD-ROMs. Results showed that awareness increased more among local health department workers than among state health department participants. Intervention adoption and implementation showed a pattern of increase among state practitioners but mixed findings among local respondents.

Further analysis of the findings from this study showed that even though most respondents were aware of evidence-based guidelines to promote physical activity, decision making and adoption were heavily influenced by lack of resources, lack of authority to implement evidence-based programs and policies, and lack of support from state legislators and governors (Brownson and others, 2007b). The researchers concluded that dissemination strategies should be informed by a priori audience analysis and adapted on the basis of the information about the different adopter groups and individuals.

One strategy that has been demonstrated to improve the speed of uptake of HIV-prevention strategies is formation of active collaborations between researchers and community service organizations (Kelly and others, 2000). Similarly, the CDC's Diffusion of Effective Behavioral Interventions (DEBI) project found that the diffusion of evidence-based HIV/STD-prevention interventions to health departments and community-based organizations was enhanced by a coordinated and multilevel national strategy, consisting of strategic planning, marketing, training, technical assistance, capacity building, and evaluation (Collins, Harshbarger, Sawyer, and Hamdallah, 2006).

Much can be learned from public health programs that have been widely adopted, even though the evidence base in terms of outcomes may be poor. Des Jarlais and others' analyses of the adoption of programs for drug abuse prevention and syringe exchange programs underscored the importance of social and political context (Des Jarlais and others, 2006). They explored the apparent paradox between some programs that have been widely disseminated and adopted, despite an absence of effectiveness (the DARE [Drug Abuse Resistance Education] school-based drug abuse prevention program), and the limited diffusion of needle exchange programs to reduce transmission of HIV, despite their proven effectiveness. They observed that youth drug abuse prevention efforts were believed to address an important social problem with high political salience, whereas needle exchange programs were regarded as contrary to morals or standards. In this case, social and political values were stronger determinants of diffusion than any of the key attributes of innovations or adopters.

THE PRACTICE OF DISSEMINATION AND DIFFUSION OF HEALTH BEHAVIOR INTERVENTIONS

The most important practical implication from the previous section is the need to achieve a good fit between the attributes of an innovation, the adopting individual or organization, and the environment or context. Maximizing this fit requires consideration of the means used to communicate information about the innovation (*communication channels*), the collaboration between the developers and users of a system (*linkage agents*), and the characteristics of the systems or environment in which this process takes place (*diffusion context*). This can be achieved by using multiple formal and informal media to maximize the durability of an innovation. This process is more likely to be successful when communication occurs as an exchange process rather than merely persuading an audience to take action. Communication should also occur through both mass media and personal interactions. The two-step flow of communication, in which opinion leaders mediate the impact of mass media communications, further emphasizes the value of social networks and interpersonal channels, over and above mass media, for adoption decisions (Rogers, 1983).

Orlandi, Landers, Weston, and Haley (1990) conceptualized this process as involving a deliberate collaborative partnership between the group or individual promoting the program—the *resource system*—and the potential users of the program (the *user system*). *Linkage agents* can then be used to enhance the knowledge exchange and transfer between the resource system and the implementers or users. Recent research has examined this kind of approach with respect to program users, like school teachers, who are responsible for delivering health education and promotion programs to school students (Bartholomew, Parcel, Kok, and Gottlieb, 2006). Gatekeepers for delivery systems, such as school principals, are important program adopters, because their support for the program is likely to be critical for adoption of innovative curricula by teachers. In the school situation, the linkage might be a liaison group, including representatives of the user system, representatives of the resource system, and a linkage agent facilitating the collaboration. The critical point is that the innovation-development and dissemination planning processes should aim to improve the fit between the innovation and users, adapting and reinventing the innovation to the practical possibilities and constraints of the system where it is implemented and disseminated.

APPLICATIONS

The Pool Cool Skin Cancer Prevention Program

Pool Cool is a multicomponent skin cancer prevention program for use at swimming pool settings that was evaluated for its impact on sun-protection habits and swimming pool environments (Glanz and others, 2002a). The intervention includes staff training, sun-safety lessons, interactive activities, provision of sunscreen, shade, and signage, and promotion of sun-safe environments. The program is intended for children five to ten years of age (primarily those taking swimming lessons), their parents, and lifeguards and aquatic instructors. A cluster-randomized trial at twenty-eight swimming pools in Hawaii and Massachusetts tested the efficacy of this program, compared with an attention-matched injury-prevention control program. Participating pools included public municipal, suburban, YMCA, and military pools. Results showed significant changes in children's use of shade and sunscreen, overall sun-protection habits, and number of sunburns, and improvements in parents' hat use, sun-protection habits, and reported sun-protection policies and environments. These findings, based on self-report survey data, were corroborated by observations. Also, the program had a positive impact on audiences in two geographically and racially distinct regions (Glanz and others, 2002a).

During the Pool Cool efficacy trial, a thorough process evaluation provided information about the process and variations in implementation of the intervention (Glanz and others, 2002b). Pilot dissemination efforts involved partnering with a national organization of recreation and parks professionals, repackaging the program for wide distribution in tool kits, including a training DVD and Internet communication, and evaluating this dissemination in more than 300 pools across the United States.

The ensuing Pool Cool Diffusion Trial has been evaluating the effects of two strategies for diffusion of the Pool Cool skin cancer–prevention program in over 400 swimming pools across the United States and in Okinawa on (1) program implementation, maintenance, and sustainability, (2) improvements in organizational and environmental supports for sun protection at swimming pools, and (3) sun-protection habits and sunburns among children. The research also aims to identify organizational predictors of these outcomes (Glanz, Steffen, Elliott, and O'Riordan, 2005). In this four-year diffusion trial (with the field work occurring from 2003 to 2006), swimming pools have been the main organization-level unit of study and the unit of measurement for organization-level diffusion outcomes. Field coordinators throughout the program regions are linkage agents for the program, and the clusters of pools affiliated with each field coordinator are the main unit of randomization and intervention for the trial. Lifeguards and aquatic instructors are the potential mediators of the program effects on children. Children aged five to ten years taking swimming lessons at participating pools are the primary audience for the Pool Cool intervention, with their parents being a secondary audience.

The diffusion trial used an experimental design in which all participating swimming pools received an intervention package, with half the pools receiving additional strategies and resources. Both the basic and enhanced group pools received all the main components of the Pool Cool program, including a field coordinator training program and the program provided at swimming pools. In addition, the enhanced group pool sites received additional sun-safety resources for distribution, more ready-made environmental intervention resources, including a set of sun signs, and additional target goals and rewards for documenting high levels of implementation. The study approach and the interventions are grounded in three theories or models: (1) Social Cognitive Theory, (2) Diffusion of Innovations, and (3) theories of organizational change. Key constructs were derived from each of these theories, applied to the intervention, and then measured accordingly at each of the appropriate levels. The key theoretical constructs used, the application of the constructs in the study, and examples of related measures are summarized in greater detail in an article by Glanz and others (2005). Results of independent process evaluations at one and two years have demonstrated very good implementation and maintenance so far in a sample of 120 pools each year. However, according to the early process evaluation, there were few differences in implementation between the two conditions during the first two years (Escoffery, Glanz, and Elliott, 2007).

Comments on the Pool Cool Diffusion Trial

The Pool Cool Diffusion Trial is one of the most comprehensively conducted efforts to evaluate the process of diffusion and to compare two different approaches to promote dissemination on a wide scale throughout the United States. This program of research illustrates many of the issues and challenges involved in planning for program dissemination and conducting rigorous research in this field. Some of the key issues are discussed here.

Participation and Response Rates.   Even where initial participation is very high, attrition will always be a challenge when a program is disseminated widely in the "real world." It is important to build in substantial reminders and incentives to achieve good long-term program implementation, maintenance, and sustainability. Even so, high levels of participation in a program, even a well-received one, may not translate into equally high responses to data collection efforts over several years. Further, remote data collection in many locations involves unique challenges.

Program Implementation.   Data from this study demonstrated that sun-safety program implementation increased between the first and second years (Escoffery, Glanz, and Elliott, 2007). This provides encouraging evidence that it is possible to obtain an upward adoption curve with a health promotion intervention. However, the fact that the process evaluation did not reveal greater implementation among those in the enhanced study arm suggests that the basic program was already quite well implemented with a strong distribution system and easy adoption. Use of organizational theories of change that use stage theory and organizational development theory likely aided the high levels of implementation.

Study Design.   This study illustrates that design considerations for diffusion trials are not necessarily the same as those required in more traditional efficacy trials. In the Pool Cool efficacy trial, clustering occurred at the swimming pool level. In the diffusion trial, clustering was conducted at the level of field coordinators, who were the linkage agents in the Pool Cool diffusion trial. This provided a relatively efficient distribution system for the intervention and for encouraging pools to participate in data collection. The alternative design, in which individual pools in a multitude of locations would enroll in the study, was considered but abandoned because of its inefficiency and prohibitive cost to manage.

Measurement Issues.   This research shows the importance, but also the great complexity, of developing a sophisticated matrix of measurement that adequately addresses the measurement of program implementation, maintenance, and sustainability at each of the appropriate levels and with each of the required target groups. One key issue with such studies is the extent to which they typically rely on self-report measurement. Not only is this often the only feasible way to conduct most of the required measurement in community and other field settings, but if other kinds of "reactive" measurement were used, they could detract from the real-world applicability of an intervention. To address this concern, an ancillary study to validate self-reported sun exposure and sun-protection practices was conducted in four Pool Cool regions in 2006 (n = 16 pools and 541 participants). Findings from the validation study show that self-reports are significantly correlated with objective measures. For example, objective measures from skin swabbing (O'Riordan, Lunde, Urschitz, and Glanz, 2005) are associated with survey reports of sunscreen use (Glanz and others, forthcoming). In addition, observational measures of program implementation are being used in the process evaluation site visits to corroborate pool managers' survey reports (Escoffery, Glanz, and Elliott, 2007).

The Spread of Diabetes Prevention Programs from Finland to Australia

In Finland and Australia, as elsewhere in the world, the rapid increase in the incidence of type 2 diabetes became a major public health concern in the late 1990s. Efficacy trials have demonstrated that lifestyle modification can contribute to a significant reduction in diabetes risk (Knowler and others, 2002; Tuomilehto and others, 2001). However, these trials used very intensive individual counseling delivered by highly trained health professionals, potentially limiting their potential for wider uptake in other health care systems. Furthermore, the interventions were not strongly theory-based, and there was little information available about the determinants of individual and system uptake and diffusion.

GOAL Program in Finland. The context for the GOAL (Good Aging in Lahti Region) lifestyle implementation trial was the primary health care setting in the Päijät-Häme Region of Finland (Fogelholm and others, 2006; Absetz and others, 2007; Uutela and others, 2004). The region covers 14 municipalities and a total of 208,000 inhabitants (Fogelholm and others, 2006). The study involved the "real-world" evaluation of a group-based lifestyle change counseling program to prevent type 2 diabetes. The intervention program was adapted from the program and lifestyle change objectives used in a recently published Finnish efficacy trial, the Diabetes Prevention Study (DPS; Tuomilehto and others, 2001). The GOAL program was based on Social Cognitive Theory, the Health Action Process Approach (Schwarzer and Fuchs, 1996), and self-regulation theories (Gollwitzer and Brandstätter, 1997).

Program partners included municipalities and regional and local health care organizations as the eventual user system for the program. The National Public Health Institute, the UKK Institute for Health Promotion, the Lahti University of Applied Sciences, and the University of Helsinki were the developers of the program. To maximize the fit of the program with the local health care context, a group of user representatives from each municipality and relevant professional group was established to assist with planning. The program consisted of six two-hour group sessions with the first five sessions taking place over eight weeks and the last session delivered at eight months. Program content and design were adapted from the five key lifestyle change objectives that were the focus of the DPS and had been demonstrated to be sufficient to prevent type 2 diabetes (Tuomilehto and others, 2001): (1) less than 30 percent of total energy intake from fat, (2) less than 10 percent of total energy intake from saturated fat, (3) more than 15g of fiber/1,000 calories, (4) more than 4 hours per week of moderate-level physical activity, and (5) more than 5 percent weight reduction.

Intervention components included information provision, group discussions, self-monitoring of behavior, goal setting, and planning for behavior change and maintenance. Printed materials for facilitators and participants included existing health education leaflets, materials adapted from earlier studies, and materials developed for the intervention. Group facilitators were public health nurses, with nutritionists and municipal sports officers cofacilitating the relevant sessions on diet and physical activity. Nurses received a standardized two-day training program with written materials and practical exercises in group facilitation. To promote program sustainability, nurses who were currently employed in the region were trained to deliver the

GOAL program as part of their existing work situation. Participants were current primary health care patients (age fifty to sixty-five years) with identified risk factors (obesity, hypertension, elevated blood glucose or lipids). The intervention reached three times more women than men, and more people with low educational levels or who were retired, compared to the general population.

Comparing the results of the GOAL implementation trial to the original DPS efficacy trial, participants were almost as likely as those in the DPS to adopt the target lifestyle changes, with the exception of physical activity and weight loss. The program achieved favorable outcomes for several clinical risk factors. Diabetes risk, as measured by glucose tolerance at follow-up, was associated with attainment of the lifestyle objectives.

Diabetes Prevention Program in Australia. The Australian Diabetes Prevention Program (DPP) was adapted from the GOAL program as a result of collaborative links between senior researchers from the Finnish Public Health Institute and the Australian Greater Green Triangle (GGT) University Department of Rural Health in southeastern Australia. Drawing on evidence from the results of the earlier Finnish DPS and the short-term results from the GOAL implementation trial, the GGT department adapted and modified the GOAL program for the Australian Diabetes Prevention Program (DPP) implementation trial. Program materials required language and cultural translation, as well as changes to ensure alignment with Australian national physical activity and dietary guidelines.

Participants for the trial were screened by study nurses in reception areas of general practices in three rural areas. Using the same selection criteria as for the GOAL study, 343 individuals were identified and recruited for the trial. Participants improved significantly on all clinical indicators except systolic blood pressure. In contrast to the GOAL program, DPP participants achieved better weight loss, with 75 percent achieving some waist reduction and 68 percent achieving weight reduction. Significant positive changes were also observed in mental health functioning and quality of life (Laatikainen and others, 2007; Kilkkinen and others, 2007).

Building on the reported successes of the Finnish and Australian group-based lifestyle intervention programs for diabetes prevention, the *Life! Program* is currently commencing implementation in a number of urban and rural communities in the Australian state of Victoria. This program will use community-based facilitators who will receive four days of intensive training, along with support materials and self-learning tasks. The structure of the new *Life! Program* is similar to the previous programs, with the addition of screening for depression, modification of materials for persons with low education levels, and increased emphasis on motivational approaches and goal setting in the facilitator training.

Comments on GOAL and DPP Diabetes Education Programs in Finland and Australia

This example illustrates the process and steps by which programs based on groundbreaking behavioral clinical trials were translated into implementation trials in Finland and then Australia. They provide insights into some factors that inhibit and facilitate successful adoption of programs by individuals, as well as how the programs were refined to fit better into health services in different countries. As the Finnish GOAL program has become more refined over time and was adopted in another country, successive versions of the program aimed to improve the "fit" between characteristics of the innovation, the adopters, and the implementation environments. Changes have included some modifications to the "hard core" components of the intervention, as well as the "soft periphery," which includes the organizational structures for program development and program delivery systems. These systems become more salient as the emphasis shifts toward ensuring maintenance and sustainability of the program and uptake by the health services in Australia and Finland.

A key feature of this program, which facilitated the relatively quick transfer and adoption of the program between Finland and Australia, was the extensive interaction between research and program leaders from both countries. These leaders shared tacit knowledge that had not been published formally in peer-reviewed publications, and the interactions generated many of the recommendations that have been incorporated into subsequent iterations of the program. A new Finnish program being developed in 2008 will incorporate the training activities developed for the *Life! Program*, based on lessons learned from the Australian DPP.

Nevertheless, there are some important differences in outcomes of the two trials and between the implementation trials and the original intensive behavioral efficacy trials. Clearly, the implementation trials were less intensive. However, regarding different outcomes in the Finnish GOAL and Australian DPP implementation studies, it is not clear whether these were due to differences in the programs and their delivery, the participants, or cultural differences between Australia and Finland. The population in Australia is more culturally and ethnically diverse than in Finland, leading to a greater diversity in food habits and cultural beliefs about health and physical activity.

The GOAL and DPP studies also illustrate the importance of using study designs and measures that are relevant to the key questions being addressed. The completed efficacy trials had already established that lifestyle counseling was effective in reducing diabetes risk. So the key question being addressed in the GOAL and DPP implementation trials was how well the outcomes compared with those achieved in the earlier efficacy trials.

LIMITATIONS OF THE MODEL AND CHALLENGES FOR THE FUTURE

Although diffusion research has made many important contributions to improving public health, the Diffusion of Innovations model also has shortcomings (Haider and Kreps, 2004). Indeed, Rogers (1995, 2003) identified several.

Diffusion research has been criticized for its *pro-innovation bias*. An implicit assumption in much diffusion research is that a given innovation will be diffused and adopted by all members of a target group and will not be reinvented or rejected. Rogers urges researchers to recognize that some innovations should be re-invented and others should be rejected, and that we can learn much from studying these processes (Rogers, 2003).

Another often-cited criticism is that diffusion research perpetuates the *individual blame bias*—the tendency to hold individuals responsible for their problems, rather than the system of which the individual is a part (Rogers, 2003). Yet, much as public health has shifted to greater recognition of system- and policy-level determinants of health behavior (see Chapter Twenty), diffusion scholars and researchers should seek alternatives to using individuals as the sole unit of analysis. They should also keep an open mind about the causes of social problems and engage communities in defining both problems and assets (Peterson, Rogers, Cunningham-Sabo, and Davis, 2007; Yancey, Ory, and Davis, 2006; see Chapter Thirteen).

An increasing challenge to the productive application of diffusion theory, research, and practice is to balance complexity, specificity, and feasibility. Well organized and large-scale communitywide programs that involve multiple strategies and methods for dissemination will become more common in our efforts to improve population health outcomes (Owen, Glanz, Sallis, and Kelder, 2006). Widespread and multilevel diffusion strategies can lead to large benefits at the population level (Sorensen, Emmons, Hunt, and Johnston, 1998). As the emphasis on developing systemwide approaches to program diffusion increases, it becomes even more important to understand the workings of complex organizations and systems (see Chapter Fifteen).

Three specific areas of diffusion research warrant attention to enable us to better understand the process of adoption. The first area is more research into the complex interplay of variables associated with the diffusion of innovations and the relative weight of different variables, depending on the circumstances of the innovation and setting. The second area has been described as "the gating function of variables influencing adoption" (Wejnert, 2002). This is an important issue in workplaces and other organizations where authority structures and leaders' decision processes may determine adoption, regardless of the characteristics of the innovation itself. The third area is the further conceptual and empirical development of the determinants of success or failure of dissemination strategies in relation to implementation, maintenance, and sustainability. For example, relatively little is known about the mediators and moderators of dissemination (Brownson and others, 2007a). More research into interactions between programs and settings can also provide important information about mechanisms of success or failure.

Given the increasing opportunities to disseminate programs across regions and countries, more collaborative and coordinated approaches that compare and contrast methods and approaches between settings, regions, and countries are needed. For example, Green and colleagues (2006) reviewed the achievements of tobacco control measures in the United States and Canada over the last half century and explored the applicability of these lessons to societal attempts to increase physical activity globally. Because the global burden of disease is greatest in low- and middle-income countries, international research continues to need more attention in the future (Wright, 2005; Fajans, Simmons, and Ghiron, 2006), as it has in the historical development of diffusion research (Rogers, 2003). Some recent efforts to systematize dissemination processes between countries (Cuijpers, de Graaf, and Bohlmeijer, 2005) still need more testing and evaluation.

As with most health behavior research areas, diffusion study design and measurement issues require more systematic attention. It is important to use common definitions, measures, and tools to enable comparisons across studies. In particular, more valid and reliable indicators of organizational and policy change are needed, as well as giving more attention to economic measurement (Brownson and others, 2007a). Controlled and experimental study designs, as well as naturalistic and case study, can contribute designs that emphasize interpretive approaches. These types of study designs are now becoming more recognized as necessary and feasible for diffusion studies (Waterman and others, 2007).

Finally, as new information and communication technologies become more widely available, they will provide new and better opportunities for program dissemination and sharing of research tools. These include state-of-the-art Web sites for providing the most up-to-date information to researchers, practitioners, and the public about interventions (National Cancer Institute, 2007; Cancer Control PLANET [Plan, Link, Act, Network with Evidence-Based Tools], 2007) and interactive use of the Internet, handheld devices, and other technologies as methods for disseminating programs, materials, and research methods very quickly to very large numbers of individuals.

SUMMARY

If outcomes from decades of public health and health behavior intervention research are to be translated into major health improvements, we must understand factors that support and inhibit the uptake of effective programs and policies (Brownson and others, 2007a). Many well-evaluated interventions are effective in addressing health behaviors that contribute to the global burden of disease. However, knowledge and resources necessary to implement effective programs and interventions were lacking until recently.

The Diffusion of Innovations model has been used widely to understand these processes and as a foundation for dissemination strategies. Key constructs and concepts are defined in this chapter, and some of the most important methodological and research issues that need to be addressed in the future are discussed. There now is an increasing emphasis on and need to disseminate complex, multicomponent, and multilevel programs to address health behavior issues such as tobacco control, HIV/AIDS control, and increased physical activity. A major challenge for the future is more frequent and better application of the Diffusion of Innovations model to complex innovations and to use evaluation designs that are rigorous, feasible, and relevant to real-world settings. Probably the most important practical lesson arising from diffusion research in recent years has been the importance of achieving a good fit between the attributes of an innovation, the adopting individual or organization, and the environment or context where the process takes place.

REFERENCES

Absetz, P., and others. "Type 2 Diabetes Prevention in the 'Real World': One-Year Results of the GOAL Implementation Trial." *Diabetes Care*, 2007, 30(10), 2465–2470.
American Journal of Public Health, 2006, 96(8).

Aubert, B. A., and Hamel, G. "Adoption of Smart Cards in the Medical Sector: The Canadian Experience." *Social Science & Medicine*, 2001, 53(7), 879–894.

Bartholomew, L. K., Parcel, G. S., Kok, G., and Gottlieb, N. H. *Planning Health Promotion Programs: An Intervention Mapping Approach*. (2nd ed.) San Francisco: Jossey-Bass, 2006.

Bertrand, J. "Diffusion of Innovations and HIV/AIDS." *Journal of Health Communication*, 2004, 9(6), 113–121.

Brownson, R., and others. "The Effect of Disseminating Evidence-Based Interventions That Promote Physical Activity to Health Departments." *American Journal of Public Health*, 2007a, 97(10), 1900–1907.

Brownson, R., and others. "Evidence-Based Interventions to Promote Physical Activity: What Contributes to Dissemination by State Health Departments." *American Journal of Preventive Medicine*, 2007b, 33(1, Suppl 1), S66–S78.

Buller, D. B., Buller, M. K., and Kane, I. "Web-Based Strategies to Disseminate a Sun Safety Curriculum to Public Elementary Schools and State-Licensed Child-Care Facilities." *Health Psychology*, 2005, 24, 470–476.

Buller, D. B. (ed.). "Diffusion and Dissemination of Physical Activity Recommendations and Programs to Worldwide Populations." *American Journal of Preventive Medicine*, 2006, 31(4 Suppl 1).

Cain, M., and Mittman, R. *Diffusion of Innovation in Health Care*. Oakland: California HealthCare Foundation, May 2002.

Campbell, M. K., and others. "Process Evaluation of an Effective Church-Based Diet Intervention: Body and Soul." *Health Education and Behavior*, 2007, 34, 864–880.

Cancer Control PLANET. [http://cancercontrolplanet.cancer.gov]. Dec. 2007.

Collins, C., Harshbarger, C., Sawyer, R., and Hamdallah, M. "The Diffusion of Effective Interventions Project: Development, Implementation and Lessons Learnt." *AIDS Education and Prevention*, 2006, 18(4 Suppl A), 5–20.

Cuijpers, P., de Graaf, I., and Bohlmeijer, E. "Adapting and Disseminating Effective Public Health Interventions in Another Country: Towards a Systematic Approach." *European Journal of Public Health*, 2005, 15, 166–169.

Denis, J. L., and others. "Explaining Diffusion Patterns for Complex Health Care Innovations." *Health Care Management Review*, 2002, 27, 60–73.

Des Jarlais, D. C., and others. "Diffusion of the D.A.R.E and Syringe Exchange Programs." *American Journal of Public Health*, 2006, 96(8), 1354–1358.

Ellis, P., and others. "A Systematic Review of Studies Evaluating Diffusion and Dissemination of Selected Cancer Control Interventions." *Health Psychology*, 2005, 24, 488–500.

Escoffery, C., Glanz, K., and Elliott, T. "Process Evaluation of the Pool Cool Diffusion Trial for Skin Cancer Prevention Across 2 Years." *Health Education Research*, 2007. [http://her.oxfordjournals.org/cgi/content/full/cym060v1].

Fajans, P., Simmons, R., and Ghiron, L. "Helping Public Health Sector Health Systems Innovate: The Strategic Approach to Strengthening Reproductive Health Policies and Programs." *American Journal of Public Health*, 2006, 96, 435–440.

Fitzgerald, L., Ferlie, E., Wood, M., and Hawkins, C. "Interlocking Interactions, the Diffusion of Innovations in Health Care." *Human Relations*, 2002, 55, 1429–1449.

Fogelholm, M., and others. "Rural-Urban Differences in Health And Health Behaviour: A Baseline Description of a Community Health-Promotion Program for the Elderly." *Scandinavian Journal of Public Health*, 2006, 34(6), 632–640.

Gladwell, M. *The Tipping Point: How Little Things Can Make a Big Difference*. Boston: Little, Brown, 2000.

Glanz, K., and Oldenburg, B. "Relevance of Health Behavior Research to Health Promotion and Health Education." In D. S. Gochman (ed.), *Handbook of Health Behavior Research IV*. New York: Plenum Press, 1997.

Glanz, K., Steffen, A., Elliott, T., and O'Riordan, D. "Diffusion of an Effective Skin Cancer Prevention Program: Design, Theoretical Foundations, and First-Year Implementation." *Health Psychology*, 2005, 24, 477–487.

Glanz, K., and others. "A Randomized Trial of Skin Cancer Prevention in Aquatics Settings: The Pool Cool Program." *Health Psychology*, 2002a, 21(6), 579–587.

Glanz, K., and others. "Process Evaluation of Implementation and Dissemination of a Sun Safety Program at Swimming Pools." In A. Steckler and L. Linnan (eds.), *Process Evaluation for Public Health Interventions and Research*. San Francisco: Jossey-Bass, 2002b.

Glanz, K, and others. "Validity of Self-Reported Sunscreen Use by Parents, Children and Lifeguards," forthcoming.

Gollwitzer, P. M., and Brandstätter, V. "Implementation Intentions and Effective Goal Pursuit." *Journal of Personality and Social Psychology*, 1997, 73, 186–199.

Green, L.W., and Glasgow, R.E. "Evaluating the Relevance, Generalization, and Applicability of Research." *Evaluation and the Health Professions*, 2006, 29(1), 126–153.

Green, L. W., and others. "Inferring Strategies for Disseminating Physical Activity Policies, Programs, and Practices from the Successes of Tobacco Control." *American Journal of Preventive Medicine*, 2006, 31(4S), S66–S81.

Greenberg, M. R. "The Diffusion of Public Health Innovations." *American Journal of Public Health*, 2006, 96, 209–210.

Greenhalgh, T., and others. "Diffusion of Innovations in Service Organisations: Systematic Review and Recommendations." *Milbank Quarterly*, 2004, 82, 581–629.

Greenhalgh, T., and others. "Storylines of Research in Diffusion of Innovation: A Meta-Narrative Approach to Systematic Review." *Social Science and Medicine*, 2005, 61, 417–430.

Grimshaw, J. M., and others. "Effectiveness and Efficiency of Guideline Dissemination and Implementation Strategies." *Health Technology Assessment Report*, 2004, 8, 1–72.

Haider, M., and Kreps, G. "Forty Years of Diffusion of Innovations: Utility and Value in Public Health." *Journal of Health Communication*, 2004, 9, 3–11.

Institute of Medicine. *Crossing the Quality Chasm: A New Health System for the Twenty-First Century.* Washington: National Academy Press, 2001.

Kelly, J. A., and others. "Bridging the Gap Between the Science And Service of HIV Prevention: Transferring Effective Research-Based HIV Prevention Interventions to Community AIDS Service Providers." *American Journal of Public Health*, 2000, 90, 1082–1088.

Kerner, J., Rimer, B., and Emmons, K. "Dissemination Research and Research Dissemination: How Can We Close the Gap?" *Health Psychology*, 2005, 24, 443–446.

Kilkkinen, A., and others. "Prevention of Type 2 Diabetes in a Primary Health Care Setting Interim Results from the Greater Green Triangle (GGT) Diabetes Prevention Project." *Diabetes Research and Clinical Practice*, 2007, 76, 460–462.

Knowler, W. C., and others. "Reduction in the Incidence of Type 2 Diabetes with Lifestyle Intervention or Metformin." *New England Journal of Medicine*, 2002, 346(6), 393–403.

Laatikainen, T., and others. "Prevention of Type 2 Diabetes by Lifestyle Intervention in an Australian Primary Health Care Setting: Greater Green Triangle (GGT) Diabetes Prevention Project." *BMC Public Health*, 2007, 7, 249.

Lewis, E., and others. "Disseminating a Sun Safety Program to Zoological Parks: The Effects of Tailoring." *Health Psychology*, 2005, 24, 456–462.

Mosteller, F. "Innovation and Evaluation." *Science*, 1981, 211, 881–886.

"Moving Science into Practice: The Role of Technology Exchange for HIV/STD Prevention." *AIDS Education and Prevention*, 2006, 18(Suppl A):1–184.

National Cancer Institute. Greater Than the Sum: Systems Thinking in Tobacco Control. *Tobacco Control Monograph No. 18.* NIH Pub. No. 06-6085. Bethesda, Md.: U.S. Department of Health and Human Services, National Institutes of Health, National Cancer Institute, April 2007.

Oldenburg, B., Sallis, J., French, M., and Owen, N. "Health Promotion Research and the Diffusion and Institutionalization of Interventions." *Health Education Research*, 1999, 14(1), 121–130.

Oldenburg, B., and Parcel, G. "Diffusion of Health Promotion and Health Education Innovations." In K. Glanz, B. K. Rimer, and F. M. Lewis (eds.), *Health Behavior and Health Education: Theory, Research, and Practice.* (3rd ed.) San Francisco: Jossey-Bass, 2002.

O'Riordan, D. L., Lunde, K., Urschitz, J., and Glanz, K. "A Non-Invasive Objective Measure of Sunscreen Use and Reapplication." *Cancer, Epidemiology, Biomarkers and Prevention*, 2005, 14, 722–726.

Orlandi, M. A., Landers, C., Weston, R., and Haley, N. "Diffusion of Health Promotion Innovations." In K. Glanz, F. M. Lewis, and B. K. Rimer (eds.), *Health Behavior and Health Education: Theory, Research, and Practice.* San Francisco: Jossey-Bass, 1990.

Owen, N., Glanz, K., Sallis, J., and Kelder, S. "Evidence-Based Approaches to Dissemination and Diffusion of Physical Activity Interventions." *American Journal of Preventive Medicine*, 2006, 31(4 Suppl), S35–S44.

Peterson, J. C., Rogers, E. M., Cunningham-Sabo, L., and Davis, S. M. "A Framework for Research Utilization Applied to Seven Case Studies." *American Journal of Preventive Medicine*, 2007, 33(1 Suppl), S21–S34.

Ratzan, S. C. (ed.). "International Perspectives." *Journal of Health Communication*, 2004, 9(Suppl 1).

Resnicow, K., and others. "Body and Soul: A Dietary Intervention Conducted Through African American Churches." *American Journal of Preventive Medicine*, 2004, 27, 97–105.

Rogers, E. M. *Diffusion of Innovations.* New York: Free Press, 1962.

Rogers, E. M. *Diffusion of Innovations.* (3rd ed.) New York: Free Press, 1983.

Rogers, E. M. *Diffusion of Innovations.* (4th ed.) New York: Free Press, 1995.

Rogers, E. M. *Diffusion of Innovations.* (5th ed.) New York: Free Press, 2003.

Sallis, J. F., Owen, N., and Fotheringham, M. J. "Behavioral Epidemiology: A Systematic Framework to Classify Phases of Research on Health Promotion and Disease Prevention." *Annals of Behavioral Medicine,* 2000, 22, 294–298.

Schwarzer, R., and Fuchs, R. "Self-Efficacy and Health Behaviors." In M. Conner and P. Norman (eds.), *Predicting Health Behavior: Research and Practice with Social Cognition Models.* Buckingham: Open University Press, 1996.

Sorensen, G., Emmons, K., Hunt, M. K., and Johnston, D. "Implications of the Results of Community Intervention Trials." *Annual Review of Public Health,* 1998, 19, 379–416.

Strang, D., and Soule, S. "Diffusion in Organizations and Social Movements: From Hybrid Corn to Poison Pills." *Annual Review of Sociology,* 1998, 24, 265–290.

Tuomilehto, J., and others. "Prevention of Type 2 Diabetes Mellitus by Changes in Lifestyle Among Subjects with Impaired Glucose Tolerance." *New England Journal of Medicine,* 2001, 344(18), 1343–1350.

Uutela, A., and others. "Health Psychological Theory in Promoting Population Health in Päijät-Häme, Finland: First Steps Toward a Type 2 Diabetes Prevention Study." *Journal of Health Psychology,* 2004, 9(1), 73–84.

Waterman, H., and others. "The Role of Action Research in the Investigation and Diffusion of Innovations in Health Care: The PRIDE Project." *Qualitative Health Research,* 2007, 17(3), 373–381.

Wejnert, B. "Integrating Models of Diffusion of Innovations: A Conceptual Framework." *Annual Review of Sociology,* 2002, 28, 297–326.

Wright, M. T. "Homosexuality and HIV/AIDS Prevention: The Challenge of Transferring Lessons Learned from Western Europe to Central and Eastern European Countries." *Health Promotion International,* 2005, 20(1), 91–98.

Yancey, A. K., Ory, M. G., and Davis, S. M. "Dissemination of Physical Activity Promotion Interventions in Underserved Populations." *American Journal of Preventive Medicine,* 2006, 31(4 Suppl), S82–S91.

CHAPTER

15

MOBILIZING ORGANIZATIONS FOR HEALTH PROMOTION

Theories of Organizational Change

Frances Dunn Butterfoss
Michelle C. Kegler
Vincent T. Francisco

KEY POINTS

This chapter will

- Describe how organizational change theories have been and can be used in health promotion.
- Describe the key dimensions of organizational change.
- Discuss change *within* organizations and how stage and organizational development (OD) theories can be used to facilitate organizational change.

▪ Discuss change *across* organizations and how interorganizational relations and the Community Coalition Action Theory (CCAT) can be used to improve collaborations in health promotion.

▪ Present case examples illustrating how organizational change theories have been applied in health promotion projects.

INTRODUCTION TO THEORIES OF ORGANIZATIONAL CHANGE

An organization is a group of people intentionally organized to accomplish an overall, common goal or set of goals. An organization also is an integrated social system, often divided into smaller units, teams, or departments, that has various inputs or resources (such as raw materials, money, technologies, and people) that are used to produce certain outputs (such as products, services, and benefits). Together with feedback from employees, consumers, and the external environment, organizations accomplish their goals (McNamara, 2006). With technology and globalization, organizations are growing increasingly complex, and the boundaries between organizations and their environments are becoming harder to distinguish (Boonstra, 2004).

Understanding how to create change in organizations is a critical aspect of health promotion for both practitioners and researchers. Many health promotion programs take place in organizational settings. For example, schools offer sexuality education and substance abuse prevention programs, worksites offer smoking cessation classes, and clinics offer diabetes management and other patient education courses. Also, organizational environments may directly or indirectly influence health, through services and policies including, for example, whether they provide access to affordable healthy food, establish smoke-free office buildings, protect workers from occupational exposures, or provide attractive and convenient stairs as alternatives to riding the elevator.

Organizational change theories are not used as often in health promotion or public health programs as are the more familiar and perhaps easier-to-use social psychological theories of individual behavior change. Yet even when programs focus on individual behavior change informed by psychological theories, organizational theories are relevant. Organizational theories can provide insight into how to facilitate the adoption or institutionalization of a particular evidence-based intervention within an organization or help explain how an organization may actually discourage positive health behaviors.

Given how important organizations are in everyday life, organizational policies and practices are frequently the target of health promotion interventions. For example, health educators may encourage worksites to offer healthy foods in the cafeteria and vending machines, urge clinics to implement provider reminder systems to increase cancer screening, or advocate that schools expand the time for mandatory physical education classes. Moreover, health promotion practitioners and researchers recognize that today's organizations must plan and respond to the changing needs of their members, as well as individuals and groups with whom they interact or serve. Organizations must actually *embrace* change and innovation to successfully achieve their goals and objectives over the long haul. Ideally, the organizations that health education and health promotion experts work in should be flexible and responsive to innovative health promotion programs, services, and policies, and work with other organizations as necessary. Health educators and other practitioners who understand organizational change theories and principles will be able to analyze and facilitate successful policy and practice changes in organizations. In other words, understanding organizational change is critical to health promotion because organizations establish policies and environments that support or hinder healthy practices.

Change can occur at many levels within an organization. *Individual-level* behavior change focuses on intrapersonal factors such as knowledge, attitudes, beliefs, motivation, self-concept, past experience, and skills. Individuals are influenced by the opinions, behavior, advice, and support of friends, coworkers, supervisors, and influential others within organizational settings, such as worksites or schools. In addition, individuals, particularly organizational leaders, are in a position to either facilitate change or resist it. *Individual* behavior can be improved through coaching, training, goal setting, and obtaining performance feedback, whereas *team or workgroup* behavior change can be facilitated by effective communication and by the example set by role models; conflict management is another strategy. Organizations, like individuals, also operate in a larger social environment. As a result, broad change at the *organizational* level requires a complex set of complementary strategies that are responsive to internal and external cultural and environmental influences. Change strategies are most effective and likely to be sustained when they are directed at multiple levels of the organization, while simultaneously taking the external environment into account (Embry, 2004).

To successfully negotiate these complex changes, public health workers may first turn for guidance to the *social ecological model* (McLeroy, Bibeau, Steckler, and Glanz, 1988) and its applied translations (for example, Stokols, 1996). This model proposes that individual, interpersonal, community, organizational, and societal factors should be taken into account when planning and implementing health promotion interventions, because they have direct and indirect influences on lifestyle, behavior choices, and health (Israel, Checkoway, Schulz, and Zimmerman, 1994; McLeroy, Bibeau, Steckler, and Glanz, 1988). These interventions are directed at multiple levels but focus in important ways on organizational factors, such as organizational policies and practices, and the structure of programs and services, including their comprehensiveness, coordination, and linkages across organizations (McLeroy, Bibeau, Steckler, and Glanz, 1988). Public health and health promotion experts can also learn from experts in related fields such as organizational behavior and organizational psychology, whose work focuses on understanding and enhancing the way organizations operate and the results they achieve.

McNamara (2006) has identified four main dimensions of organizational change that are relevant to public health and health promotion: (1) organizationwide versus subsystem change, (2) transformational versus incremental change, (3) remedial versus developmental change, and (4) reactive versus proactive change. The organizational change theories covered in this chapter may be used to address any or all of these dimensions of change.

1. *Organizationwide versus subsystem change.* Organizationwide change usually involves major restructuring or new collaboration. Usually, organizations must undertake organizationwide change to evolve to a different level in their life cycle, such as moving from an informally organized interest group to becoming a nonprofit health coalition. Such change usually requires a change in culture, as would be needed if a health department developed a foundation to accept donations rather than relying on government contracts. Subsystem change, however, might include adding or removing a product or service, such as expanding clinic hours, creating a new leadership structure for a coalition, reorganizing a department to streamline health services, or implementing a new policy or process to deliver products or services, such as mail-order prescriptions.

2. *Transformational versus incremental change.* Transformational or radical change involves changing an organization's fundamental structure and culture—for example, moving from having a traditional top-down, hierarchical structure to self-directing teams. Incremental change is a series of small, often planned steps that take place over time. Such change often goes unnoticed and might include continuous quality improvement (CQI) or implementation of a new computer system to increase efficiency.

3. *Remedial versus developmental change.* Remedial change is intended to remedy current situations, for example, to improve performance of a product, reduce burnout and thus help the organization become more productive, or address a budget deficit. These changes seem more focused, urgent, and visible because they address current, major problems. Developmental change is more general and is intended to make an effective organization even more successful (for example, expanding services, products, or the number of patients served). If developmental changes are postponed, remedial changes may be needed. Organizations also may establish a developmental change process to address immediate, remedial issues.

4. *Reactive versus proactive change.* Reactive or unplanned change occurs when a major, sudden event in the organization causes its members to respond in highly disorganized ways (such as a leader's resignation or a major public relations problem). Proactive change occurs when leaders in the organization recognize the need for a major change and organize to accomplish the change, for example by engaging in strategic planning.

CHANGE *WITHIN* ORGANIZATIONS

The following section describes the origins and key constructs of two major organizational theories that focus on change *within* organizations: (1) Stage Theory and (2) organizational development (OD) theories.

Stage Theory of Organizational Change

Stage Theory is based on the idea that organizations pass through a series of steps or stages as they change. By recognizing those stages, strategies to promote change can be matched to various points in the process of change. Stage Theory explains how organizations develop new goals, programs, technologies, and ideas; it is not related to or derived from Prochaska and DiClemente's Stages of Change model (1983; see Chapter Five). According to Stage Theory of Organizational Change, adoption of an innovation by an organization, such as a school adopting an evidence-based intervention to prevent teen pregnancy, typically follows several stages. Each stage requires a specific set of strategies that are contingent on the organization's stage of adopting, implementing, and sustaining new approaches, as well as on socioenvironmental factors that may be outside the organization's control. For this reason, these organizational change theories are often referred to as *contingency* theories. To use Stage Theory effectively, the social environment and the innovation's stage of development must be carefully assessed before appropriate strategies are selected for each stage.

History of Stage Theory.   The foundation for action research and modern organizational change theories is Kurt Lewin's (1951) stage model. As the "father of organization development," Lewin is known for saying, "If you want truly to understand something, try to change it" (ThinkExist.com, 2007). He developed one of the earliest stage models (1951), which consisted of three stages: (1) unfreezing of past behavior and attitudes within the organization, (2) moving by exposure to new information, attitudes, and theories, and (3) refreezing through processes of reinforcement, confirmation, and support for the change. Modern stage theory is based on both Lewin's early work and Rogers's Diffusion of Innovations theory (2003), which focused initially on the adoption of innovations by individuals such as farmers and teachers (see Chapter Fourteen). Later research showed that individuals often adopt innovations as members of organizations and rarely adopt innovations unless they are first accepted by the organization (Steckler, Goodman, and Kegler, 2002).

Key Concepts of Stage Theory.   According to modern Stage Theory, the adoption of an innovation by an organization follows several stages. Beyer and Trice (1978) developed a comprehensive and well-defined seven-stage model that Kaluzny and Hernandez later condensed into four stages (1988). Table 15.1 outlines these stages and their application.

Application of Stage Theory.   Most research on Stage Theory has focused on the activities that occur within each stage rather than on the factors that influence how an organization moves from one stage to the next (Steckler, Goodman, and Kegler, 2002). However, we know that different leaders or "change agents" within the organization assume leading roles during different stages. For example, in a school environment, senior administrators (superintendents) are influential at the problem awareness and definition stage; mid-level administrators (principals, curriculum coordinators) at the adoption and early implementation stages; teachers at the implementation stage, and senior administrators are influential again during institutionalization (Huberman and Miles, 1984). Similarly, the strategies that organizations use depend on their stage of change and whether the social environment surrounding the innovation (for example, active parent-teacher or community involvement) is supportive (Smith, Steckler, McCormick, and McLeroy, 1995).

TABLE 15.1. **Organizational Change: Stage Theory.**

Concept			
Kaluzny & Hernandez (1988)	Beyer & Trice (1978)	Definition	Application
1. Define Problem (Awareness Stage)	1. Sense unsatisfied demands on system 2. Search for possible responses 3. Evaluate alternative 4. Decide to adopt course of action	Problems recognized and analyzed; solutions sought and evaluated.	Involve management and other personnel in awareness-raising activities.
2. Initiate Action (Adoption Stage)	5. Initiate action within system	Policy or directive formulated; resources for beginning change allocated.	Provide process consultation to inform decision makers and implementers about what is involved in adoption.
3. Implement Change	6. Implement the change	Innovation implemented; reactions occur, and role changes occur.	Provide training, technical, and problem-solving assistance.
4. Institutionalize Change	7. Institutionalize the change	Policy or program becomes entrenched in organization; new goals and values internalized.	Identify high-level champion, work to overcome obstacles to institutionalization, and create structures for integration.

Source: K. Glanz and B. K. Rimer, *Theory at a Glance*, Washington, D.C., National Cancer Institute, NIH Publication 05–3896,1995.

Organizational Development Theory

Organizational development (OD) is a field of research, theory, and practice dedicated to expanding the knowledge and effectiveness of people to accomplish more successful organizational change and performance. *OD* is defined as "a systemwide process of applying behavioral science knowledge to the planned change and development of the strategies, design components, and processes that enable organizations to be effective" (Cummings, 2004). *Organizational change* refers to the extent, rate, and overall nature of activities, led by a change agent, to enhance the overall performance of the organization. Organizations are viewed as complex social systems with multiple levels, including members, work teams, and the organization as a whole. OD addresses these organizational systems, as well as the relationships between organizations and the larger external environment. OD is a process of continuous diagnosis, action planning, implementation, and evaluation, with the goal of transferring knowledge and skills to organizations to improve their capacity for solving problems and managing future change (Cummings, 2004).

In OD, interventions are implemented to improve organizational effectiveness, performance, and the "quality of work life," as well as to enhance the ability of organization members to resolve a major problem or achieve a project goal or overall organizational goals (McNamara, 2006; Brown and Covey, 1987). An OD consultant is often employed to help the organization diagnose, evaluate, and address its perceived concerns. OD processes are grounded in participation and collective reflection in which organizational members and an outside change agent are co-learners (Levin, 2004).

History of Organizational Development Theory. OD Theory emerged out of human relations studies in the 1930s, when psychologists recognized that organizational structures and processes, such as large bureaucracies with authoritarian leadership, influence worker behavior and motivation, communication across work units, and the ability to solve problems within teams and across an organization (Cummings, 2004). The Hawthorne studies showed that increased attention to workers led to higher worker motivation and productivity (Roethlisberger and Dickson, 1939). Lewin's work in stage theory and action research in the 1940s and 1950s also influenced OD Theory, particularly with the observation that feedback was a valuable tool in addressing social processes in organizations.

Early OD interventions in the 1960s focused on organizational design, technologies, or human processes in an effort to make work more fulfilling and rewarding. The 1970s ushered in a focus on the impact of rewards in promoting performance (Cummings, 2004). More recently, OD has expanded its focus to align organizations with their rapidly changing and complex environments through organizational learning and knowledge management, as well transforming organizational norms and values (Brown and Covey, 1987; Cummings, 2004).

Key Concepts of Organizational Development Theory. Key concepts that are useful in understanding OD are summarized in Table 15.2 and explained more thoroughly in the paragraphs that follow.

TABLE 15.2. **Summary of Organizational Change Concepts.**

Concept	Definition	Application
Stage Theory		
Stages of change	Organizations pass through specific steps as they change.	Help organizations move through all the stages; do not stop at just adoption.
Problem definition* (Awareness stage)	Problems recognized and analyzed; solutions sought and evaluated.	Involve management and other personnel in awareness-raising activities.
Initiation of action* (Adoption stage)	Policy or directive formulated; resources for beginning change allocated.	Provide process consultation to inform decision makers and implementers of what adoption involves.
Implementation of change*	Innovation implemented, reactions occur, and roles change.	Provide training, technical assistance, and problem-solving aid.
Institutionalization of change*	Policy or program becomes entrenched in the organization; new goals and values are internalized.	Identify high-level champion, work to overcome obstacles to institutionalization, and create structures for integration.
Organizational Development Theory		
Organizational development	An approach that tries to improve the quality of worklife	Identify aspects of work life, through organizational diagnosis, that positively and negatively affect workers.
Organizational climate	The personality of an organization	Use existing measures as part of change efforts.
Organizational culture	Assumptions and beliefs that are shared by members of an organization; operate unconsciously	Requires an outsider to gauge culture; use deeper understanding to plan interventions.
Organizational capacity	Optimum functioning of an organization's subsystems	Identify an organization's strengths and weaknesses as part of program planning.

TABLE 15.2. **Summary of Organizational Change Concepts, Cont'd.**

Concept	Definition	Application
Organizational Development Theory, Cont'd.		
Action research	Four steps for improving organizations: diagnosis, action planning, intervention, and evaluation	Based on organizational diagnosis, develop and implement a plan for change.
Organizational development interventions	Specific techniques such as t-groups that are used to help improve organizations	Use techniques such as surveys, cultural inventories, t-groups, and process consultation.
Interorganizational Relations Theory		
Interorganizational relations	How organizations collaborate to solve problems of mutual interest	Determine which organizations in a community are concerned about a given health problem.
Stages of interorganizational collaboration	The steps that organizations go through as they attempt to collaborate	Develop strategies to help collaborating organizations overcome barriers at each stage; for example, process evaluation of coalition effectiveness.

Source: K. Glanz and B. K. Rimer, *Theory at a Glance,* Washington, D.C., National Cancer Institute, NIH Publication 05–3896, 1995.

Organizational Climate. *Organizational climate* is defined as the mood or unique "personality" of an organization (Forehand and Gilmer, 1964; Tagiuri, 1968). Attitudes and beliefs about organizational practices create organizational climate, and these perceptions influence members' collective behavior (Hoy and Miskel, 1987; Litwin and Stringer, 1968; Moos, 1986; Rousseau and McCarthy, 2007). Climate features such as leadership, openness of communication, participative management, role clarity, and conflict resolution are positively related to employee satisfaction and negatively associated with stress (Schneider, 1985). Organizational climate characteristics (such as leader support, leader control) in partnerships are related to satisfaction with the work, participation, costs and benefits, and implementation of action plans (Butterfoss, Goodman, and Wandersman, 1996; Kegler, Steckler, Malek, and McLeroy, 1998). The climate of an organization may also predict service quality and outcomes

(Glisson and Hemmelgarn, 1998) and influence whether new programs are successfully implemented (O'Keefe, 1999).

Organizational Culture. Closely related to climate, *organizational culture* involves the deep-seated values, norms, and behaviors that members share. The five basic elements of culture in organizations are assumptions, values, behavioral norms, behavioral patterns, and artifacts (symbols that express cultural messages, such as mission statements and logos). The subjective features of culture (that is, assumptions, values, and norms) reflect the way members unconsciously think about and interpret their organizations (Schein, 1985). They, in turn, shape the meaning that behaviors and artifacts take on within the organization. Culture, like climate, can exist at many levels and can be strong, weak, or transitory. Ashforth (1985) describes organizational climate as "shared perceptions" and organizational culture as "shared assumptions." Climate is dynamic and varies according to context, whereas culture forms slowly over time and is more comprehensive, stable, and resistant to change. Although differences between climate and culture are widely debated, Tagiuri (1968) offered a way to integrate them. He asserts that culture is one of four components of organizational climate, along with ecology, milieu, and structure (Owens, 2004).

From a health education and health promotion perspective, organizational culture and climate can affect an organization's willingness to integrate new scientific advances into practice, support interdepartmental collaboration, establish reward structures for exceptional performance or creativity, and involve many other practical dimensions of worklife that affect health education and promotion initiatives. Also, in health education, organizations such as schools and clinics are often the targets or recipients of an intervention, and organizational climate and culture affect adoption, implementation, and effectiveness of these kinds of change efforts.

Organizational Capacity. Both climate and culture influence an organization's capacity to function efficiently and effectively. Katz and Kahn's (1978) open systems framework showed how organizations function and maintain momentum as they interact with the surrounding environment. The framework proposed that organizations process resources obtained from the environment into products that affect that environment. Based on this work, Prestby and Wandersman (1985) developed an organizational viability framework that suggests four components of organizational capacity: (1) resource acquisition, (2) maintenance subsystem (organizational structure), (3) production subsystem (actions or activities), and (4) external goal attainment (accomplishments). Thus, any organization that fails to obtain adequate and appropriate resources, develop a structure for obtaining resources and conducting work, mobilize resources efficiently and effectively, and develop its products (for example, action, benefits to members) or accomplish something worthwhile will eventually cease to operate. More recently, Florin and colleagues (2000) applied an open systems framework to community coalitions. This adaptation defined *inputs* to include the following: information, external funding, staff, and technical assistance; *throughput* was defined as mobilization of members and community sectors, establishment of structure and functions, and building of member and organizational capacity; *outputs* was defined as action planning and implementation of programs.

Application of Organizational Development Theory. A typical OD strategy involves process consultation, in which an outside specialist helps identify problems and facilitates the planning of change strategies. Levin (2004) describes an experimentation-learning-reflection cycle as the "engine" of OD. Action research, inspired by Lewin, is a common OD approach that is used to help an organization negotiate change (Boonstra, 2004). The steps include diagnosis, action planning, intervention, and evaluation (Argyris, Putnam, and Smith, 1985; Lewin, 1946).

Diagnosis is similar to Lewin's *unfreezing.* It can help an organization identify problems that may interfere with its effectiveness and assess the underlying causes. The OD diagnosis is usually conducted by a consultant who helps the organization understand its problems by examining its mission, goals, policies, structures, and technologies, along with its climate and culture, environmental factors, desired outcomes, and readiness to take action (Porras and Robertson, 1987; Weisbord, 1988; Gregory, Armenakis, and Moates, 2007). Diagnostic methods range from informal key informant interviews to formal surveys of all organizational members (Cummings, 2004).

Action planning often follows diagnosis and involves developing strategic interventions for addressing the diagnosed problems. Selection of interventions should be based on the organization's readiness to adopt a proposed strategy (based on climate factors), how and where interventions can be leveraged within the organizations, and the skill of the OD practitioner in applying the chosen interventions (Porras and Robertson, 1987). Essentially, the organization is engaged in an action planning process to assess the feasibility of implementing different change strategies that lead to action (Hawe and Shiell, 2000).

Interventions may include management redesign, building and structural redesign, process consultation, and group development (Bradford, 1978; Lewin, 1946; Lippitt, Langseth, and Mossop, 1985; Schein, 1969). Change steps are specified and sequenced, progress is monitored, and stakeholder commitment is cultivated (Cummings, 2004). In all of these interventions, an OD consultant helps members of the organization identify barriers to a desired change and then facilitates problem solving among members to resolve them (Gregory, Armenakis, and Moates, 2007).

Evaluation assesses the planned change effort by tracking the organization's progress in implementing the change and by documenting its impact on the organization and whether additional alterations are needed (Goodman and Wandersman, 1994). For example, evaluation may show that a new health education curriculum has not been fully implemented due to a nonsupportive climate and, therefore, additional efforts are needed to strengthen stakeholder support.

CHANGE *ACROSS* ORGANIZATIONS

The following section describes the origins and key constructs of two theories that address change *across* organizations: Interorganizational Relations (IOR) Theory and the recently developed Community Coalition Action Theory (CCAT).

Interorganizational Relations Theory

Interorganizational Relations (IOR) Theory focuses on how organizations work together. Interorganizational networks may range from grassroots coalitions and partnerships for chronic disease management (Butterfoss, 2007) to hospital collaboratives that reduce competition and improve buying power (Zuckerman, Kaluzny, and Ricketts, 1995). IOR Theory is based on the premise that collaboration among community organizations leads to a more comprehensive, coordinated approach to a complex issue than can be achieved by one organization. Given the increasing complexity of health, social issues, economics, and politics, organizations that work together are likely to be more effective. Although IOR Theory was not developed for public health application per se, it can be useful in providing a foundation for understanding and enhancing community mobilization to address a range of public health issues, such as emergency preparedness response and tobacco control.

History of Interorganizational Relations Theory.   IOR research began in the 1960s with a growing interest in how the environment affected organizational behavior. Researchers were particularly interested in how organizations could decrease uncertainty in the environment through collaboration. Early research focused on the factors that influenced an organization's decision to enter into a collaborative relationship based on the relative balance of benefits and costs (Gray, 1989). Typical benefits of collaboration include access to new ideas, material, and other resources, reduced duplication of services, more efficient use of resources, increased power and influence, ability to address issues beyond a single organization's domain, and shared responsibility for complex or controversial issues (Alter and Hage, 1993; Butterfoss, Goodman, and Wandersman, 1993). Potential costs associated with collaboration include diversion of organizational resources or mission, incompatibility with partner organizations' policies or positions, and delays in taking action due to consensus building (Alter and Hage, 1993).

Several factors are critical to IOR formation, including recognition of the need for coordination and interdependence, available resources (time, staff, and expertise), mandates from a funding or regulatory agency, clear and mutually shared goals, values, interests, and norms, and positive previous experience in working together (Gray, 1989; D'Aunno and Zuckerman, 1987; Alter and Hage, 1993). Recent research on interorganizational relationships has shown that organizations that have similar resources (labor or technical competencies) tend to compete with one another, whereas those that have similar ideologies tend to have more positive, synergistic relationships (Freeman and Audia, 2006).

Key Concepts and Hypotheses of Interorganizational Relations Theory.   Stage Theory is often used to explain how interorganizational relations evolve over time. For example, one three-stage model of network development proposes a continuum from informal to formal linkages: (1) *exchange or obligational networks* are loosely linked organizations that exchange resources, engage in few joint activities, and are maintained by individuals who coordinate and integrate tasks across organizations; (2) *action or promotional networks* of organizations share and pool resources to accomplish concerted action that is secondary to member organizations' goals; and

(3) *systemic networks* of organizations are formally linked to jointly produce goods or services over the long term (Alter and Hage, 1993).

According to contingency theory, the design of an IOR, including its structure and processes, will reflect the degree of complexity of the environment in which the organization operates (Shortell and Kaluzny, 1988). For example, if an IOR depends on a single funding source (such as a funded coalition), its structure will tend to be centralized or dominated by a single or small group of organizations in order to enhance the funder's ability to regulate work and control costs (Alter and Hage, 1993). When funding comes from multiple sources and the work is voluntary, the resulting network is more likely to work through an interagency committee structure.

Community Coalition Action Theory

Many funded prevention initiatives over the past two decades required that a specific type of interorganizational relationship (IOR)—typically referred to as a community coalition—be used to build consensus and actively engage diverse organizations and constituencies in addressing community issues or problems. Community coalitions are formal, multipurpose and often long-term alliances that work locally or regionally and usually have paid staff (Butterfoss, Goodman, and Wandersman, 1993). State- and national-level coalitions are similar to community coalitions in purpose and structure, but they often recruit different types of organizational partners and implement more legislative and media advocacy strategies (Butterfoss, 2007).

The membership of community coalitions varies in size and diversity of professional and grassroots organizations and individual members. Working relationships and role expectations range from formal (for example, creating bylaws and contractual relationships) to informal (for example, using working agreements) and can change over time. A coalition can promote a health agenda or issue, prevent disease, or ameliorate a community problem by (1) analyzing the issue or problem, (2) assessing needs and assets, (3) developing an action plan, (4) implementing strategies, (5) accomplishing community-level outcomes, and (6) creating social change (Whitt, 1993). Building on the experiences of civic engagement and community and neighborhood building of the 1960s and 1970s, coalitions involve diverse members to ensure that interventions meet the needs of and are culturally sensitive to the community. Participation in coalitions facilitates ownership, which can increase the likelihood of successful institutionalization (Bracht, 1990). Coalitions can build capacity and competence among member organizations to address other community issues as well (Chavis, 2001; Goodman and others, 1998).

Because of the widespread use of coalitions among health educators and a common observation that they were atheoretical and lacked a research base, Butterfoss and Kegler (2002) developed Community Coalition Action Theory (CCAT), which can be thought of as a form of IOR Theory; CCAT builds on several earlier models for partnership building. Two of these focus on community building and community development, and others focus on the development and structure of collaborative organizational relationships within communities (Braithwaite, Murphy, Lythcott, and Blumenthal, 1989; Minkler and Wallerstein, 2005; Katz and Kahn, 1978; Prestby and Wandersman, 1985; Habana-Hafner and Reed & Associates,1989; Butterfoss, Goodman, and Wandersman, 1993; Francisco, Paine, and Fawcett, 1993; Francisco, Fawcett, Schultz, and Paine-Andrews, 2000; National Network for Collaboration, 1996; Lasker and Weiss, 2003). Each of these organizational models emphasizes important variables, but taken alone they do not provide a complete contextual understanding of interorganizational collaboration in a community health promotion context. That is the aim of the more comprehensive CCAT model.

CCAT describes the stages of coalition development, coalition functioning, development of coalition synergy, and creation of organizational and community changes that may lead to increased community capacity and improved health and social outcomes (Butterfoss and Kegler, 2002). The CCAT model is illustrated in Figure 15.1. The theory consists of testable propositions that focus on fourteen constructs, including coalition structure and processes, staffing and leadership, pooled resources, and member engagement. CCAT incorporates Stage Theory as coalitions progress from formation and implementation to maintenance and institutionalization, returning to earlier stages as new issues arise or planning cycles are repeated. The theory acknowledges that community contextual factors such as the sociopolitical climate, geography, history, and norms surrounding collaborative efforts affect each stage of development. The constructs are defined in Table 15.3. The outcomes that the theory seeks to explain or predict are these: improved organizational structure, function, and effectiveness; community changes such as environments, policies, and practices conducive to healthy living; increased community capacity (for example, enhanced assessment and planning skills among community members), and improved health and social outcomes (for example, fewer teen pregnancies or decreased prevalence of obesity).

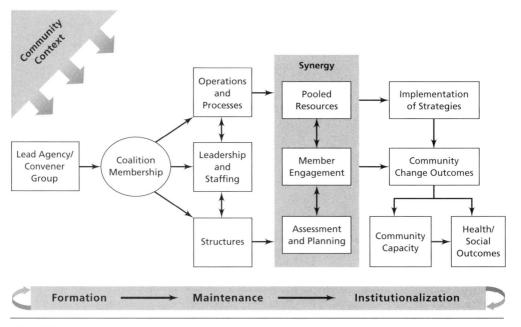

FIGURE 15.1. Community Coalition Action Theory (CCAT).

TABLE 15.3. Constructs of the Community Coalition Action Theory.

Constructs	Definition
Stages of Development	Stages or phases that a coalition progresses through from formation to implementation to maintenance to institutionalization
Community Context	Characteristics of a community that may enhance or inhibit coalition function and influence how the coalition develops, including geography, demographics, politics, social capital, trust between community sectors, community readiness
Lead Agency/Convener Group	Organization that agrees to convene the coalition; provide technical assistance, financial or material support; and provide valuable networks/contacts
Coalition Membership	Individuals who represent diverse interest groups and organizations that are committed to resolving a health or social issue and come together to do so
Operations and Processes	How business is conducted in the coalition setting; processes that facilitate staff and member communication, decision making, conflict management; influences organizational climate and member engagement
Leadership and Staffing	Volunteer leaders and paid staff who facilitate the collaborative process and coalition functioning
Structures	Formalized organizational arrangement, rules, roles, and procedures that are developed in a coalition, including vision or mission statements, goals and objectives, bylaws, organizational chart, steering committee, and work groups
Pooled Member and External Resources	Resources that are contributed or obtained as in-kind contributions, grants, donations, fundraisers, or dues.
Member Engagement	The extent of participation, commitment, and satisfaction of members in the work of the coalition
Assessment and Planning	Assessment and planning activities that precede implementation of strategies
Implementation of Strategies	Strategic actions that a coalition implements to help achieve changes in community policies, practices, and environments
Community Change Outcomes	Measurable changes in community policies, practices, and environments that may be associated with community capacity and health/social outcomes
Health/Social Outcomes	Measurable changes in health status/social conditions of a community that are the ultimate indicators of coalition effectiveness
Community Capacity	Characteristics of communities that affect their ability to identify, mobilize, and address social and public health problems

Source: Butterfoss and Kegler, 2002.

Complex IOR theories such as CCAT are difficult to test empirically. It is difficult to measure several of the core CCAT constructs due to their complexity. For example, "participation of coalition members," which is one component of the member engagement construct, can be measured in a variety of ways, ranging from time committed to coalition work to roles played by coalition members to meeting attendance. Similarly, coalition operations and processes encompass communication, decision making, and conflict negotiation, to name a few, each of which has multiple dimensions that could be measured. Other challenges to testing CCAT are similar to those applicable to other community-level theories: small sample sizes when considering the community or coalition as the unit of analysis, secular trends in health, and limitations to the feasibility of using experimental designs with randomization and control communities in the context of large-scale, multisite collaborations.

An important next step in developing CCAT and other IOR theories is to clearly define the major constructs and to operationalize them consistently across multiple studies. Until now, CCAT has been used to suggest variables to measure in evaluations and to organize descriptive evaluation data into meaningful categories (Kegler, Steckler, Malek, and McLeroy, 1998). Although selected associations have been tested, for example, between communication and member satisfaction, the theory has not yet been examined in a comprehensive manner. Efforts to do so are currently under way, using case study data from twenty California Healthy Cities and Communities coalitions, including member surveys, interviews, focus groups, and document reviews (Kegler, Norton, and Aronson, 2003).

APPLICATIONS OF ORGANIZATIONAL THEORY TO HEALTH PROMOTION

Organizational Development for Promoting Heart Health in Nova Scotia

This section illustrates how OD Theory was applied by researchers and practitioners to understand and influence health promotion efforts in a five-year heart health promotion change initiative in Nova Scotia, Canada. OD activities were conducted within twenty organizations (including provincial and municipal agencies and community-based organizations) involved in this initiative.

Project Overview. Risk factors for chronic disease include unhealthy diets, physical inactivity, tobacco use, and alcohol overuse, which are often attributed to underlying social, economic, and environmental determinants (Yach, Hawkes, Gould, and Hofman, 2004). Many public health systems address chronic disease prevention through fragmented prevention programs that are disease- or risk-factor-specific (such as cancer-prevention programs or tobacco control initiatives). Integrated approaches to address multiple chronic diseases and risk factors, improve health, increase patient satisfaction, and use limited health resources effectively may improve program sustainability and reduce duplication of effort (Robinson, Farmer, Elliott, and Eyles, 2007).

As part of the Canadian Heart Health Initiative, a federal and provincial partnership to combat cardiovascular disease (CVD), Heart Health Nova Scotia began in 1986 (Ebbesen, Heath, Naylor, and Anderson, 2004; Robinson, Farmer, Elliott, and Eyles, 2007). In its early years, Heart Health Nova Scotia developed community demonstration projects that addressed CVD using a public health approach that emphasized community mobilization, partnerships, and environmental change (MacLean and others, 2003). More recently, Heart Health Nova Scotia shifted its focus to building the capacity of organizations to plan, implement, and sustain heart health promotion efforts. By strengthening the organizational infrastructure of the province, dissemination and sustainability of heart health programs and policies could be more widespread and longer lasting, thus having a greater impact on population health (Ebbesen, Heath, Naylor, and Anderson, 2004).

OD was one of the main strategies used by Heart Health Nova Scotia to promote organizational capacity related to heart health policies and programs. MacLean and colleagues (2003) explain that OD was selected as an intervention strategy because it "would enhance health promotion knowledge and practices of organizational members and provide them with opportunities to assess and explore how health promotion could be facilitated through their organization." The OD intervention targeted twenty regional organizations in Nova Scotia from the health, education, and recreation sectors. Each had linkages to communities through chapters or local units, and either a mandate or a strong interest in health promotion.

The OD intervention (1996–2001) was multifaceted and included four specific strategies (MacLean and others, 2003). The first was technical support, which consisted of workshops on topics related to planning and implementing health promotion programs, such as health communication, advocacy, assessment, and evaluation. The technical support component also included establishing a health promotion clearinghouse, with a Web site that included resources on health promotion topics and a list of contact people willing to share their health promotion experiences. A second and related OD approach was to establish community heart health action teams to implement specific activities that addressed at least one modifiable CVD risk factor. This approach encouraged the organizations and their partners to apply the knowledge gained through technical support activities.

A third OD strategy was action research (MacLean and others, 2003), which involved cycles of assessment, action plan development, implementation, and monitoring and evaluation, followed by development of new action plans based on monitoring data. For example, organizational capacity profiles were developed to give feedback on policies, practices, supports, and challenges related to heart health promotion. These profiles encouraged each organization's leaders to reflect on how they could improve the heart health infrastructure within their setting. Multiple data collection tools were used in this action research initiative, including an organizational policies questionnaire, interviews on organizational practices, and learning opportunities logs. The approach used by Heart Health Nova Scotia included the OD stages of diagnosis, assessment, intervention, and evaluation.

Organizational consultation was the fourth OD strategy employed by Heart Health Nova Scotia. It focused on creating specific process and structural changes to support heart health infrastructure in participating organizations (MacLean and others,

2003). Examples include reallocating funds, broadening staff roles to encompass heart health, and increasing interdepartmental communication. Heart Health Nova Scotia staff played key roles in these consultations by developing model capacity-building strategies for organizations to implement and by facilitating learning across participating organizations.

Evaluation Methods and Results. The evaluation of the Heart Health Nova Scotia Initiative used qualitative and quantitative methods from managers, coordinators, and volunteers who participated in the initiative. Variables of interest included partnership and organizational development for heart health promotion; the number, type, and effectiveness of the capacity-building strategies, and factors that influenced capacity building, such as partner organizations' interest in heart health promotion, organizational readiness and leadership to engage in or support change, and competing work priorities. *Quantitative* methods included a network mapping questionnaire and technical support logs based on a tracking system (Fawcett and others, 1995), whereby partners monitored data related to partnership and organizational development (for example, number and type of learning opportunities, community activities, and consultation activities). *Qualitative methods* included (1) using organizational reflection logs that provided open-ended responses about participant reactions to policy changes, fund reallocations, and partnerships, and (2) semi-structured interviews to monitor the effectiveness of the organizational development process, the facilitators and barriers to capacity building, and the organizational change outcomes that resulted from capacity building.

Process evaluation results showed that OD strategies had significant reach (MacLean and others, 2003): 41 workshops reached over 140 organizations, and the community health action teams conducted 18 initiatives that involved 39 organizations. In addition, organizational representatives reported increased knowledge and skills related to heart health promotion as a result of the various OD strategies applied. Those interviewed described several ways they had disseminated their new knowledge and skills to their organizations—through application of the same tools and methods to new situations and through collaborative work with colleagues.

Based on case studies of six of the twenty participating organizations, OD contributed substantively to organizational change. MacLean and colleagues (2003) documented results from logs and interviews that detailed the creation of new staff positions for heart health promotion, new structures within organizations (such as committees), changes in organizational culture (such as increased communication and improved decision making), and new policies to support heart health promotion.

Impact of Rural Appalachian Cancer Coalitions in Pennsylvania and New York

This section illustrates how IOR Theory was applied by researchers and practitioners to understand and influence health promotion efforts across organizations that were involved in community coalition efforts. Eleven rural Appalachian cancer coalitions in Pennsylvania and New York based their development and community intervention on the CCAT.

Project Overview. The incidence of colorectal cancer in parts of rural Appalachia is higher than in much of the United States (Lengerich and others, 2005). Community cancer coalitions have been used to encourage cancer screenings, promote health awareness campaigns, disseminate educational materials to the public, and equip their members to serve as linking agents for wider adoption of innovative strategies to prevent and control cancer (Ward, Kluhsman, Lengerich, and Piccinin, 2006). One study found that counties with cancer coalitions recruited nearly three times as many local organizations to a cancer education intervention than did matched control counties without coalitions (Ward, Kluhsman, Lengerich, and Piccinin, 2006).

Eleven rural cancer coalitions were formed in New York and Pennsylvania during the Appalachia Leadership Initiative on Cancer from 1992–2000 and were members of the Appalachia Cancer Network from 2000–2005. These efforts comprised an academic-community partnership for community-based participatory research in cancer prevention and control, intended to address cancer-related health disparities. CCAT (Butterfoss and Kegler, 2002) served as a conceptual framework for coalition development activities, interventions, and analysis of change outcomes (Kluhsman and others, 2006).

Application of CCAT to Enhance Organizational Capacity. The goal of the evaluation of the coalitions and their initiatives was to determine whether cancer coalitions in rural Appalachia could (1) be linking agents to the community and (2) influence member organizations to be committed to and participate in disseminating materials to promote cancer awareness and screening. CCAT was used to identify the internal coalition factors and processes that lead to implementation of strategies and community change.

Methods. A computerized coalition data collection system was developed, based on an earlier system designed to monitor the activities and impact of CVD coalitions by Francisco, Paine, and Fawcett (1993). Field staff attended coalition meetings, followed up on coalition action plans, and recorded the relevant data electronically on nine forms: coalition background information, coalition meetings, coalition meeting attendees, coalition individual members, coalition organization members, coalition development activities, community interventions, proposals, and funders. Quality assurance was provided by the project director and data managers. Coalition activities were classified as either *coalition development* activities or *community interventions*. The objectives of community interventions were recorded, and interventions were categorized as education only, outreach only, education and outreach, and screening; each intervention could have more than one objective. A generalized estimating equations model was used to test for temporal trends in the proportion of each initiative for each of the eleven coalitions.

Organizational Capacity. The study categorized several factors as indicative of organizational capacity, corresponding to the CCAT constructs indicated here by bold typeface. They included descriptive factors of each coalition, such as their lead agency, coalition membership (individuals and organizations), governance (leadership and staffing), geographical area served (context), mission statements, bylaws, subcommittees, and cancer plans (structures).

Process. Several factors were characterized as coalition development activities or "a planned gathering of some or all coalition members primarily intended to educate, equip or enlarge coalition membership" (Kluhsman and others, 2006). These included meeting and agenda setting, assessment, implementation, and evaluation (referred to as operations and processes in CCAT). This category also includes intermediate change outcomes, such as partnering with new organizations or changes in practices and policies within a partner organization. In the CCAT model, these would be considered to be synergistic outcomes from member engagement or assessment and planning activities.

Outcome and Impact. These factors correspond to CCAT constructs and include intermediate outcomes such as funded proposals (pooled resources) and community interventions (implementation of strategies). Community interventions are defined as "planned events sponsored or cosponsored by the coalition and primarily intended to directly change behavior, detect risk or disease, or educate persons outside of the coalition" (Kluhsman and others, 2006). They also include more distal outcomes such as community changes, which included new or modified programs, policies, or practices that were likely to be sustained or occur without coalition in the future.

Results. From 2002 to 2004, the eleven Pennsylvania and New York coalitions conducted 1,369 activities; 16 percent were coalition development activities, and 84 percent were community interventions. The interventions were categorized according to type (outreach only, education only, outreach and education, or screening); colorectal (37 percent), breast cancer (33 percent), or other focus (30 percent), and demographic target priority by sex, age, income, profession, or other characteristic. During this period, of the 3,941 community residents reached through screening interventions, 49 percent completed the recommended behavioral change of being screened for cancer. In addition, three of the eleven coalitions reported fifteen sustainable community changes such as offering free breast and cervical cancer screening to underinsured persons, funding screening activities, and making space available for screening. Also, many restaurants became no-smoking facilities. The authors assert that they may not have captured all of the community changes, because some may have occurred after the data collection period.

The measures and observed results of coalition effectiveness in this study, including the increasing trend in interventions, the number of completed screenings, and documented community changes, are indicators of the success of the eleven coalitions over the three-year period. *Intermediate community changes* include changes in partnership structure, programs, or practices. *Long-term community changes* include sustained educational programs, screening practices, or health status changes resulting from community efforts. Community changes were likely underreported in the data system, because a substantial amount of time typically elapsed between an intervention and the resulting organizational or community change. CCAT was helpful as a guiding framework, as it proposes that the combined resources and intervention strategies of coalitions can improve health outcomes and lead to sustainable community change. The coalitions in this study reported that, together with their partners, they were able to achieve more than any one of them could have achieved alone.

CCAT proposes that attention to developmental activities that recruit, educate, and equip members to do coalition work (member engagement) will pay off later in the effectiveness of coalition interventions. Because the coalitions in this study were well established, only one in seven activities focused on coalition development, which meant that the coalitions truly focused on community interventions. This study also showed that the coalitions focused twice as often on activities that were more likely to result in community changes (such as education and screening), rather than merely outreach and awareness building. This achievement is attributed to the monthly training, technical assistance, and support that were provided by coalition staff and consultants. Researchers have proposed that coalition training and technical assistance is important (Butterfoss, Morrow, Webster, and Crews, 2003), though no benchmarks have been set for how much is optimal.

CCAT also proposes that *community context* is inextricably linked to coalition success. The Appalachia cancer coalition evaluators noted that the success of the interventions was possible because of the coalitions' long history and trusted relationships within their communities (Kluhsman and others, 2006). The coalitions continue as part of the Appalachian Community Cancer Network Initiative, which is funded through 2010.

This evaluation did not use or measure all of the constructs in the CCAT theory. For example, it did not characterize the role of Stage Theory that is inherent in CCAT, as it documents the coalition's progression through the stages of formation, maintenance, and institutionalization. This could be done in a retrospective analysis of these groups by looking at the development of structures, processes, and interventions that the coalitions developed. Similarly, specific processes such as communication, decision making, or conflict negotiation were not documented. However, most of these coalitions had already been functioning for more than five years and had reached a level of maturity where they had learned how to partner and work together effectively.

This evaluation adopted a theoretical foundation from CCAT. It also reported using planning models such as the Planned Action Toward Community Health (PATCH) (Shea and Basch, 1990) and PRECEDE-PROCEED (Green and Kreuter, 2005). This combination contributed to the evaluation findings showing that cancer coalitions could lead to sustainable changes in their own capacity and in individual health behavior and community capacity.

FUTURE RESEARCH TO INFORM ORGANIZATIONAL CHANGE THEORIES

Organizational change theories hold promise in guiding practitioners' efforts to nurture health promotion programs and use networks, strategic partnerships, and coalitions effectively. Several avenues of inquiry would improve the utility of the theories discussed in this chapter.

First, health educators should clearly define the stages that organizations progress through and then select appropriate strategies for each stage (Steckler, Goodman, and Kegler, 2002). Many stage models exist, but consensus on the expected duration of each stage, as well as tasks to be achieved, would help those practitioners who are responsible for building and maintaining these organizations. More studies of how organizations progress through these stages also are needed, as this process rarely occurs in a predictable, stepwise manner; stages are sometimes skipped and revisited later (Butterfoss and Kegler, 2002). Identifying such patterns would help organizations know when to seek training and technical assistance. Current organizational evaluations focus on programs implemented or outcomes achieved. Long-term studies of the life cycle of organizations are often beyond the scope of grant-funded evaluations that span three to five years. Moreover, incomplete organizational documents and turnover of staff and members provide further challenges.

Second, health educators often fail to understand the role that organizations play in adopting programs and therefore do not measure the environmental factors that help or hinder an organization's growth and maturity or minimize their contribution (Miller, Klotz, and Eckholdt, 1998; Miller, 2003). The influence of context on functioning at each stage deserves more attention, especially during maintenance and institutionalization (Butterfoss, 2007; Gray, 1996; Provan, Milward, and Brinton, 1995). To increase the likelihood of successful practice, organizational change strategies should be tailored to fit an organization's stage of development (Steckler, Goodman, and Kegler, 2002).

Third, future research should focus on the range and complexity of interorganizational relationships and clarify the types of collaborations that best fit the work to be accomplished. For example, networks may be most useful for information dissemination, strategic partnerships for program development and service delivery, and coalitions for advocacy efforts. By focusing on specific outcomes (for example, changes in systems and health status), we may understand the contributions that each kind of IOR can contribute (Roussos and Fawcett, 2000; Kreuter, Lezin, and Young, 2000).

Fourth, the theories, models, and methods described in this chapter attempt to deal with the dynamics of interorganizational networks and systems that are needed in a complex world. Researchers and practitioners are calling for a *systems approach* to health and health care issues that transcends traditional theory about how change occurs in and across organizations. New ways of framing public health may improve how we intervene to help organizations and communities understand their complex and recursive systems (Burnes, 2005) and navigate the change process more effectively. Systems thinking is concerned with "the interrelationships between parts and their relationships to a functioning whole, often understood within the context of an even greater whole" (Trochim and others, 2006).

Systems or complexity theory may presently be most useful as a metaphor; few empirical studies exist that inform the science at this point (Houchin and MacLean, 2005). It can help planners to understand and model the multiple dynamics at work in community health organizations (Lounsbury and Levine, 2001), workplaces, or communities. Systems theory is not yet organized well enough to allow for prediction of outcomes and control of variables that explain complex data sets with which we now struggle. However, it does suggest new ways of approaching those data sets to understand better the bi-directional interplay between broader organizational and social systems, policy change, physical environment variables, disease vectors, and individual behavior (Green, 2006; Leischow and Milstein, 2006).

SUMMARY

Few graduate education courses for health educators focus on the role of organizations in health behavior and promotion, and social-psychological theories of individual behavior change are certainly used more often in health promotion. Perhaps time and cost constraints may keep researchers and practitioners from considering complex organizational factors in assessment, planning, implementation, and evaluation processes (Steckler, Goodman, and Kegler, 2002). Alternatively, a lack of understanding of these theories and their relevance to the field may contribute to their underutilization in health behavior and health education.

This chapter illustrates the value of organizational change for health promotion and offers ideas on how to successfully facilitate theory-informed organizational change. Four theories of organizational change were presented: Stage Theory, Organizational Development (OD) Theory, Interorganizational Relationships (IOR) Theory, and Community Coalition Action Theory (CCAT). Stage Theory and OD Theory propose that different strategies are needed at different stages and have the greatest potential to produce positive changes in organizations when they are combined. IOR Theory and CCAT emphasize understanding how organizations work together and sustain their relationships.

Two community health examples illustrated how OD techniques can be used to intervene within organizations to build capacity for promoting community change, and how developmental activities can help collaboratives like coalitions recruit, educate, and equip members to do their work. Whether directing change strategies from within or outside an organization, health practitioners are presented with unique challenges. Organizational change theories suggest strategies to mediate such challenges and influence positive change.

REFERENCES

Alter, C., and Hage, J. *Organizations Working Together.* Newbury Park, Calif.: Sage, 1993.

Argyris, C. *Personality and Organization.* New York: McGraw-Hill, 1957.

Argyris, C., Putnam, R., and Smith, D. M. *Action Science: Concepts, Methods, and Skills for Research and Intervention.* San Francisco: Jossey-Bass, 1985.

Ashforth, S. J. "Climate Formations: Issue and Extensions." *Academy of Management Review,* 1985, 25(4), 837–947.

Beyer, J. M., and Trice, H. M. *Implementing Change: Alcoholism Policies in Work Organizations.* New York: Free Press, 1978.

Boonstra, J. Introduction. *Dynamics of Organizational Change and Learning.* West Sussex, England: Wiley, 2004.

Bracht, N. (ed.). *Health Promotion at the Community Level.* Newbury Park, Calif.: Sage, 1990.

Bradford, L. P. (ed.). *Group Development.* (2nd ed.) La Jolla, Calif.: University Associates, 1978.

Braithwaite, R., Murphy, F., Lythcott, N., and Blumenthal, D. S. "Community Organization and Development for Health Promotion within an Urban Black Community: A Conceptual Model." *Health Education,* 1989, 20(5), 56–60.

Brown, L. D., and Covey, J. G. "Development Organizations and Organization Development: Toward an Expanded Paradigm for Organization Development." In R. W. Woodman and W. A. Pasmore (eds.), *Research in Organizational Change and Development.* Vol. 1. Greenwich, Conn.: JAI Press, 1987.

Burnes, B. "Complexity Theories and Organizational Change." *International Journal of Management Reviews,* 2005, 7(2), 73–90.

Butterfoss, F. D. *Coalitions and Partnerships for Community Health.* San Francisco: Jossey-Bass, 2007.

Butterfoss, F. D., Goodman, R., and Wandersman, A. "Community Coalitions for Prevention and Health Promotion." *Health Education Research: Theory and Practice,* 1993, *8*(3), 315–330.

Butterfoss, F. D., Goodman, R., and Wandersman, A. "Community Coalitions for Prevention and Health Promotion: Factors Predicting Satisfaction, Participation and Planning." *Health Education Quarterly,* 1996, *23*(1), 65–79.

Butterfoss, F. D., and Kegler, M. C. "Toward a Comprehensive Understanding of Community Coalitions: Moving from Practice to Theory." In R. DiClemente, L. Crosby, and M. C. Kegler, (eds.), *Emerging Theories in Health Promotion Practice and Research.* San Francisco: Jossey-Bass, 2002.

Butterfoss, F. D., Morrow, A. L., Webster, J. D., and Crews, C. "The Coalition Training Institute: Training for the Long Haul." *Journal of Public Health Management and Practice,* 2003, *9*(6), 522–529.

Chavis, D. M. "The Paradoxes and Promise of Community Coalitions." *American Journal of Community Psychology,* 2001, *29*(2), 309–320.

Cummings, T. "Organizational Development and Change." In J. Boonstra (ed.), *Dynamics of Organizational Change and Learning.* West Sussex, England: Wiley, 2004.

D'Aunno, T., and Zuckerman, H. "A Life-Cycle Model of Organizational Federations: The Case of Hospitals." *Academy of Management Review,* 1987, *12*(3), 534–545.

Ebbesen, L., Heath, S., Naylor, P., and Anderson, D. "Issues in Measuring Health Promotion Capacity in Canada: A Multi-province Perspective." *Health Promotion International,* 2004, *19*(1), 85–94.

Embry, D. D. "Community-Based Prevention Using Simple, Low-Cost, Evidence-Based Kernels and Behavior Vaccines." *Journal of Community Psychology,* 2004, *32*(5), 575–591.

Fawcett, S. B., and others. *Work Group Evaluation Handbook: Evaluating and Supporting Community Initiatives for Health and Development.* Lawrence, Kan.: Work Group on Health Promotion and Community Development, University of Kansas, 1995.

Florin, P., Mitchell, R., Stevenson, J., and Klein, I. "Predicting Intermediate Outcomes for Prevention Coalitions: A Developmental Perspective." *Evaluation and Program Planning,* 2000, *23,* 341–346.

Forehand, G. A., and Gilmer, B. "Environmental Variation in Studies of Organizational Behavior." *Psychological Bulletin,* 1964, *62,* 361–381.

Francisco, V. T., Fawcett, S. B., Schultz, J. S., and Paine-Andrews, A. "A Model of Health Promotion and Community Development." In F. B. Balcazar, M. Montero, and J. R. Newbrough (eds.), *Health Promotion in the Americas: Theory and Practice.* Washington, D.C.: Pan American Health Organization, 2000.

Francisco, V. T., Paine, A. L., and Fawcett, S. B. "A Methodology for Monitoring and Evaluating Community Health Coalitions." *Health Education Research,* 1993, *8*(3), 403–416.

Freeman, J. H., and Audia, P. G. "Community Ecology and the Sociology of Organizations." *Annual Review of Sociology,* 2006, *32,* 145–169.

Glanz, K., and Rimer, B. K. *Theory at a Glance.* NIH Publication 05–3896. Washington, D.C.: National Cancer Institute, 1995.

Glisson, C., and Hemmelgarn, A. "The Effects of Organizational Climate and Interorganizational Coordination on the Quality and Outcomes of Children's Service Systems." *Child Abuse and Neglect,* 1998, *22*(5), 401–421.

Goodman, R. M., and Wandersman, A. "FORECAST: A Formative Approach to Evaluating the CSAP Community Partnerships." *Journal of Community Psychology,* 1994, CSAP special issue, 6–25.

Goodman, R. M., and others. "Identifying and Defining the Dimensions of Community Capacity to Provide a Basis for Measurement." *Health Education and Behavior,* 1998, *25*(3), 258–278.

Gray, B. *Collaborating: Finding Common Ground for Multi-Party Problems.* San Francisco: Jossey-Bass, 1989.

Gray, B. "Cross-Sectoral Partners: Collaborative Alliances Among Businesses, Government and Communities." In C. Husham (ed.), *Creating Collaborative Advantage.* London, England: Sage, 1996.

Green, L. W. "Public Health Asks of Systems Science: To Advance Our Evidence-Based Practice, Can You Help Us Get More Practice-Based Evidence?" *American Journal of Public Health,* 2006, *96,* 406–409.

Green, L. W., and Kreuter, M. Health Program Planning: An Educational and Ecological Approach. New York: McGraw-Hill, 2005.

Gregory, B. T., Armenakis, A. A., and Moates, K. N. "Achieving Scientific Rigor in Organizational Diagnosis: An Application of the Diagnostic Funnel." *Consulting Psychology Journal: Practice and Research,* 2007, *59*(2), 79–90.

Habana-Hafner, S., and Reed & Associates. *Partnerships for Community Development: Resources for Practitioners & Trainers.* Amherst: University of Massachusetts Center for Organizational and Community Development, 1989.

Hawe, P., and Shiell, A. "Social Capital and Health Promotion: A Review." *Social Science & Medicine,* 2000, *51,* 871–885.

Houchin, K., and McLean, D. "Complexity Theory and Strategic Change: An Empirically Informed Critique." *British Journal of Management,* 2005, *16,* 149–166.

Hoy, W. K., and Miskel, C. G. *Educational Administration: Theory, Research, and Practice.* (3rd ed.) New York: Random House, 1987.

Huberman, A. M., and Miles, M. B. *Innovation Up Close: How School Improvement Works.* New York: Plenum Press, 1984.

Israel, B. A., Checkoway, B., Schulz, A., and Zimmerman, M. "Health Education and Community Empowerment: Conceptualizing and Measuring Perceptions of Individual, Organizational and Community Control." *Health Education Quarterly,* 1994, *21*(2), 149–170.

Kaluzny, A. D., and Hernandez, S. R. "Organization Change and Innovation." In S. M. Shortell and A. D. Kaluzny (eds.), *Health Care Management: A Text in Organization Theory and Behavior.* (2nd ed.) New York: Wiley, 1988.

Katz, D., and Kahn, R. *The Social Psychology of Organizations.* (2nd ed.) New York: Wiley, 1978.

Kegler, M. C., Norton, B. L., and Aronson, R. E. *Evaluation of the Five-Year Expansion Program of California Healthy Cities and Communities (1998–2003). Final Report.* [http://www.civicpartnerships.org/docs/publications/ExecSummary.pdf]. September, 2003.

Kegler, M., Steckler, A., Malek, S., and McLeroy, K. "A Multiple Case Study of Implementation in 10 Local Project Assist Coalitions in North Carolina." *Health Education Research,* 1998, *13*(2), 225–238.

Kreuter, M., Lezin, N., and Young, L. "Evaluating Community-Based Collaborative Mechanisms: Implications for Practitioners." *Health Promotion Practice,* 2000, *1*(1), 49–63.

Kluhsman, B. C., and others. "Initiatives of 11 Rural Appalachian Cancer Coalitions in Pennsylvania and New York." *Preventing Chronic Disease (online),* October 2006, *3*(4), A122.

Lasker, R. D., and Weiss, E. S. "Broadening Participation in Community Problem Solving: A Multidisciplinary Model to Support Collaborative Practice and Research." *Journal of Urban Health,* 2003, *80*(1), 14–48.

Leischow, S. J., and Milstein, B. "Systems Thinking and Modeling for Public Health Practice." *American Journal of Public Health,* 2006, *96*(3), 403–405.

Lengerich, E. J., and others. "Cancer Incidence in Kentucky, Pennsylvania, and West Virginia: Disparities in Appalachia." *Journal of Rural Health,* 2005, *21*(1), 39–47.

Levin, M. "Organizing Change Processes: Cornerstones, Methods and Strategies." In J. Boonstra (ed.), *Dynamics of Organizational Change and Learning.* West Sussex, England: Wiley, 2004.

Lewin, K. "Action Research and Minority Problems." *Journal of Social Issues,* 1946, *2,* 34–36.

Lewin, K. *Field Theory in Social Science.* New York: Harper & Row, 1951.

Lippitt, G. L., Langseth, P., and Mossop, J. *Implementing Organizational Change.* San Francisco: Jossey-Bass, 1985.

Litwin, G. H., and Stringer, R. A. *Motivation and Organizational Climate.* Boston: Graduate School of Business Administration, Harvard University, 1968.

Lounsbury, D., and Levine, R. L. "Understanding the Dynamic Integration of Prevention, Care, and Empowerment: A Systems Approach to HIV/AIDS Policy Analysis." Proceedings of the International System Dynamics Society Meeting, Atlanta, Georgia, July, 2001.

MacLean, D. R., and others. "Building Capacity for Heart Health Promotion: Results of a 5-Year Experience in Nova Scotia, Canada." *American Journal of Health Promotion,* 2003, *17*(3), 202–212.

McLeroy, K. R., Bibeau, D., Steckler, A., and Glanz, K. "An Ecological Perspective on Health Promotion Programs." *Health Education Quarterly,* 1988, *15*(4), 351–378.

McNamara, C. "Clearing up the Language about Organizational Change and Development." In *Field Guide to Consulting and Organizational Development: A Collaborative and Systems Approach to Performance, Change and Learning.* Minneapolis, Minn.: Authenticity Consulting, LLC, 2006.

Miller, R. L. "Adapting Evidence Based Intervention: Tales of the Hustler Project." *AIDS Education and Prevention,* 2003, *15*(1), 127–138.

Miller, R. L, Klotz, D., and Eckholdt, H. M. "HIV Prevention with Male Prostitutes and Patrons of Hustler Bars: Replication of an HIV Preventive Intervention." *American Journal of Community Psychology,* 1998, *26*(1), 97–131.

Minkler, M., and Wallerstein, N. "Improving Health Through Community Organization and Community Building: A Health Education Perspective." In M. Minkler (ed.), *Community Organizing and Community Building for Health.* (2nd ed.) New Brunswick, N.J.: Rutgers University Press, 2005.

Moos, R. *Group Environment Scale Manual.* (2nd ed.) Palo Alto, Calif.: Consulting Psychologists Press, Inc., 1986.

National Network for Collaboration. *Collaboration Framework: Addressing Community Capacity.* Fargo, North Dakota: National Network for Collaboration, 1996.

Owens, R. G. *Organizational Behavior in Education: Adaptive Leadership and School Reform.* (8th ed.) Boston: Allyn & Bacon, 2004.

Porras, J. I., and Robertson, P. J. "Organization Development Theory: A Typology and Evaluation." In R. W. Woodman and W. A. Pasmore (eds.), *Research in Organization Change and Development.* Vol. 1. Greenwich, Conn.: JAI Press, 1987.

Prestby, J., and Wandersman, A. "An Empirical Exploration of a Framework of Organizational Viability: Maintaining Block Organizations." *The Journal of Applied Behavioral Science,* 1985, *21*(3), 287–305.

Prochaska, J. O., and DiClemente, C. C. "Stages and Processes of Self-Change of Smoking: Toward an Integrative Model of Change." *Journal of Consulting and Clinical Psychology,* 1983, *51,* 390–395.

Provan, K., Milward, H., and Brinton, H. "A Preliminary Theory of Interorganizational Network Effectiveness: A Comparative Study of Four Community Mental Health Systems." *Administrative Science Quarterly,* 1995, *40*(1), 1–33.

Robinson, K., Farmer, T., Elliott, S., and Eyles, J. "From Heart Health Promotion to Chronic Disease Prevention: Contributions of the Canadian Heart Health Initiative." *Preventing Chronic Disease* [serial online], *4*(2), 2007. [http://www.cdc.gov/pcd/issues/2007/apr/06_0076.htm].

Roethlisberger, F. J., and Dickson, W. J. *Management and the Worker.* Cambridge: Harvard University Press, 1939.

Rogers, E. M. *Diffusion of Innovations.* (5th ed.) New York: Free Press, 2003.

Rousseau, D. M., and McCarthy, S. "Educating Managers from an Evidence-based Perspective." *Academy of Management Learning & Education,* 2007, *6*(1), 84–101.

Roussos, S., and Fawcett, S. "A Review of Collaborative Partnerships as a Strategy for Improving Community Health." *Annual Review of Public Health,* 2000, *21,* 369–402.

Schein, E. H. *Process Consultation: Its Role in Organization Development.* Reading, Pa.: Addison-Wesley, 1969.

Schein, E. H. *Organizational Culture and Leadership.* San Francisco: Jossey-Bass, 1985.

Schneider, B. "Organizational Behavior." *Annual Review of Psychology,* 1985, *36,* 573–611.

Shea, S., and Basch, C. E. "A Review of Five Major Community-Based Cardiovascular Disease Prevention Programs: Part I. Rationale, Design and Theoretical Framework." *American Journal of Health Promotion,* 1990, *4*(3), 203–213.

Shortell, S. M., and Kaluzny, A. D. "Organization Theory and Health Care Management." In S. M. Shortell and A. D. Kaluzny (eds.), *Health Care Management: A Text in Organization Theory and Behavior.* (2nd ed.) New York: Wiley, 1988.

Smith, D. W., Steckler, A., McCormick, L. K., and McLeroy, K. R. "Lessons Learned About Disseminating Health Curricula to Schools." *Journal of Health Education,* 1995, *26,* 37–43.

Steckler, A., Goodman, R. M., and Kegler, M. C. "Mobilizing Organizations for Health Enhancement." In K. Glanz, B. K. Rimer, and F. M. Lewis (eds.), *Health Behavior and Health Education: Theory, Research, and Practice.* (3rd ed.) San Francisco: Jossey-Bass, 2002.

Stokols, D. "Translating Social Ecological Theory into Guidelines for Community Health Promotion." *American Journal of Health Promotion,* 1996, *10*(4), 282–298.

Tagiuri, R. "The Concept of Organizational Climate." In R. Tagiuri and G. W. Litwin (eds.), *Educator's Handbook: A Research Perspective.* New York: Longman, 1968.

ThinkExist.com. "Kurt Lewin Quotes." ThinkExist.com Quotations Online. Sept. 2007. [http://einstein/quotes/kurt_lewin].

Trochim, W. M., and others. "Practical Challenges of Systems Thinking and Modeling in Public Health." *American Journal of Public Health,* 2006, *96*(3), 1–9.

Ward, A. J., Kluhsman, B. C., Lengerich, E. J., and Piccinin, A. M. "The Impact of Cancer Coalitions on the Dissemination of Colorectal Cancer Materials to Community Organizations in Rural Appalachia." *Preventing Chronic Disease* [serial online]. Apr. 2006. [http://www.cdc.gov/pcd/issues/2006/apr/05_0087.htm].

Weisbord, M. R. "Towards a New Practice Theory of OD: Notes on Snap Shooting and Movie-making." In R. W. Woodman, and W. A. Pasmore (eds.), *Research in Organizational Change and Development.* Vol. 2. Greenwich, Conn.: JAI Press, 1988.

Whitt, M. *Fighting Tobacco: A Coalition Approach to Improving Your Community's Health.* Lansing, Mich.: Michigan Department of Public Health, 1993.

Yach, E., Hawkes, C., Gould, C. L., and Hofman, K. J. "The Global Burden of Chronic Diseases: Overcoming Impediments to Prevention and Control." *Journal of the American Medical Association,* 2004*, 291*(21), 2616–2622.

Zuckerman, H., Kaluzny, A., and Ricketts, T. "Strategic Alliances: A Worldwide Phenomenon Comes to Health Care." In A. Kaluzny, H. Zuckerman, and T. Ricketts (eds.), *Partners for the Dance: Forming Strategic Alliances in Health Care.* Ann Arbor, Mich.: Health Administration Press, 1995.

CHAPTER

16

COMMUNICATION THEORY AND HEALTH BEHAVIOR CHANGE

The Media Studies Framework

John R. Finnegan Jr.
K. Viswanath

KEY POINTS

This chapter will

- Provide an overview of how mass media influence individual and population health through routine and planned use.
- Discuss key organizational processes and occupational routines of media personnel and how they shape content.
- Review major theories and hypotheses at individual and societal levels that may explain the effects of media on public health.
- Describe examples of media effects on health.
- Present two applications of media to promote public health.

Human communication is about producing and exchanging information and meaning using signs and symbols (Gerbner, 1985). It takes place at various levels, including individual, group, organizational, and societal. It is composed of complex processes, including information encoding, transmitting, and receiving (decoding), as well as synthesizing meaning. Other processes include feedback and interaction at the individual level and generating, processing, and circulating information at the macro level. Key dimensions of communication include the sender (who encodes and transmits), the message (content), the channel (the medium used to transmit content), the receiver or audience (who decodes communication to derive meaning), and effect (some measurable outcome of the process). Communication captures the idea of interaction: effects may flow both ways from senders and receivers through various kinds of feedback and impact.

Communication attracts the attention of many in health education because of its perceived power and influence in shaping human affairs. Depending on the research interest, different models are available to assess communication impact: empirical, critical, or applied approaches. The purpose of this chapter is to describe communication theories especially relevant to public health and health behavior, review and critique their application in the study of health behavior, and provide examples of how communication theory informs health behavior change interventions. This chapter emphasizes communication theories in a media studies context (see Chapter Eleven for discussion of interpersonal communication).

ORGANIZATION OF COMMUNICATION STUDIES

Although communication studies could be organized in many ways, the framework of levels of analysis provides context for communication factors, processes, and outcomes from the "micro" to the "macro." For example, at the level of the individual we may study how a person processes information about health and converts it to action. At the interpersonal (dyadic) level, we may examine how two people interact and influence one another regarding some health behavior outcome. At the group or organization level, we may examine how communication among many people influences health behavior change, including the effective delivery of a health-related service. Finally, at the level of the community, society, or culture, we may examine how communication contributes to health behavior change within the constraints of social structure.

The impact of communication is everywhere and is central to understanding human behavior, but no single theory explains and predicts all communication outcomes (Bryant and Miron, 2004). The lack of grand unifying theory should not deter us from recognizing that communication processes and impact can operate simultaneously with synergy on different levels, however. Change at various levels may involve different dynamics, but they converge to shape behaviors. It is important to connect and integrate analyses of communication across levels (Parrott, 2004).

The applied emphasis of public health is at the root of questions addressed in this chapter. That is, how can communication theory and research be used to improve human health? How can we best understand health communication through the media and its large-scale effects? The media studies framework examines the conditions, processes, and structures that influence the development of media content and the effects of exposure to that content among individuals, institutions, and societies.

The "digitization" of information in the closing decades of the twentieth century and the emergence of the Internet and the Web have added a powerful new dynamic to communication. Many say that the Digital Revolution rivals the impact of the Industrial Revolution (Shapiro, 1999). The problem with revolutions is that when one is in the middle of them, it is difficult to fully comprehend their impact. One thing is for certain: since the invention of the World Wide Web beginning in about 1989, communication has never been the same. It has created global access to vast, growing reservoirs of information available every day and at any time (Internet Systems Consortium, 2007; Gulli and Signorini, 2005). It has blurred definitions of news, entertainment, advertising, journalists, intellectual property, and traditional mass media. It empowers the lonely pamphleteer and propels the global reach of multinational corporations (Croteau, 2006). It is not merely the Age of Information. It is also the Age of Interaction, and this provides extensive opportunities for health education and health behavior to achieve their full potential for behavior change. The Web increasingly enables building powerful social networks—Web-based "communities," simulated worlds, and online role-playing games. We are only beginning to comprehend what appears to be a huge and accelerating impact on economics, politics, culture, social norms, and human behavior (Bryant and Miron, 2004; Canton, 2006). As in any revolution, we wonder what the trade-offs will be between new freedom, creativity, and human progress and conformity, state control, and security (Lessig, 2001). There are great opportunities for researchers and practitioners to pioneer new uses of Web technology in creating health behavior interventions (Institute of Medicine, 2002).

The organization of technology into systems is of key importance. Today, media are interconnected organizations that systematically collect, process, and disseminate news, information, entertainment, and advertising worldwide and provide global platforms for interaction. Many are small operations like local TV stations, neighborhood newspapers, and city government Web sites. Others are global multimedia empires that own newspapers, television channels, books, magazines, films, and Web-based social networking sites like MySpace™. No matter the size or form of ownership, the media are all around us. From a public health perspective, advances in communication technology and the evolving influence of the media in our lives pose both great promise and worrisome perils.

MESSAGE PRODUCTION AND MEDIA EFFECTS

With such vast and accelerating change, there is widespread evidence that media have both positive and negative effects on health. To understand this, it is necessary to evaluate how, where, and with whom media interact and with what consequences. This is a large research agenda with many components and methods (Kamhawi and Weaver, 2003).

Under the organizing framework of levels of analysis, we will discuss two areas of research that are germane to health. One deals with message production. It asks the question, What are the social and organizational factors in media work that shape the creation of content that may influence health behavior? Here, we are interested particularly in *message production* processes for creating news, information, advertising, and entertainment.

The second area focuses on questions about the consequences of media exposure on individuals, groups, institutions, and social systems. These questions have been traditionally studied as *media effects*. Here, we are interested in some of the major hypotheses about media effects and the relevance of that work to health behavior change.

Media Message Production

Media organizations are bureaucracies in which tasks are specialized and routinized to create news, advertising, entertainment, and various combinations thereof. For example, journalists seek established or official sources routinely to gather information that is used to create news. The criteria for using sources are usually straightforward: they should be credible, available, and able to supply reliable information. Sources, in effect, subsidize the process of gathering news (Gandy, 1982). Sources may be spokespersons for government agencies, businesses, or other powerful groups and elites (Donohue, Tichenor and Olien, 1995; Gans, 2007). Journalists routinize their news-gathering process to ensure predictability in an idiosyncratic world. Before the digital era, reliance on a regular supply of information from established sources often meant that groups without social power were less likely to gain access to news making and therefore have less influence. Although this is still true for major media channels, the Web has made it possible for groups without social power to build a "work-around"—a public presence through vehicles such as blogs that can be leveraged to shape public influence, which may lead to greater acceptance in the mainstream (Reese and others, 2007).

What becomes news in mainstream media channels is the product of the interaction of news sources and media professionals, though nonprofessionals also are increasingly influencing the interpretation of news events. Sources perform the key role of identifying social problems and bringing them to the attention of the media. Whether representing campaigns, government agencies, advocacy groups, or other interests, sources compete for media and therefore also for public attention in seeking to define and to increase the public profile of an issue or problem. For example, the Centers for Disease Control and Prevention (CDC) is a major official source of public health information that regularly releases reports on the status of smoking and its effects on health. From year to year, the reports emphasize different aspects of the smoking problem that the CDC wishes to bring to the attention of news media and the general public (for example, increased smoking among young women). Despite their dependency on official sources, media professionals also enjoy some autonomy in defining a problem and in the way they construct news stories. The definition of a social problem is crucial to how the public understands it and influences the actions taken to ameliorate the problem, the attention different groups give to the problem, and the knowledge people acquire (Viswanath, Finnegan, Hannan, and Luepker, 1991). Here, too, the Web offers competing groups opportunities to provide alternative frames for social problems to those in the mainstream media. A marginalized viewpoint now may evolve into a social movement in opposition to the mainstream (Shapiro, 1999; Miroff, 2007).

Media Effects

The outcomes of media dissemination of images, ideas, themes, and stories are commonly discussed under the rubric of *media effects* (Bryant and Zillman, 1994). Media may shape an outcome (knowledge, opinion, attitude, behavior) among individuals, groups, institutions, or communities but also, in turn, be affected by the audience (McLeod, Kosicki, and Pan, 1991). Media research has a strong tradition of looking at audiences not as passive recipients but as active seekers and users of information.

Media studies vary in the level of analysis applied in research, from the individual to groups, communities, and social systems. Table 16.1 provides an overview of this variety in media studies and effects research. Major theories and concepts are organized by level of analysis. At each level, we provide a few key theories and concepts and also the disciplinary origin.

At the individual level of analysis, media studies emphasize effects on motivations, cognitions, involvement, attitudes, and behaviors from media exposure. In understanding the effects of media exposure at the individual level, research has drawn from often-used health behavior theories such as the Theory of Reasoned Action (TRA; Chapter Four), Health Belief Model (HBM; Chapter Three) and Social Cognitive Theory (SCT; Chapter Eight). Research has also drawn from theories that explain mechanisms of information processing such as the Elaboration Likelihood Model, and Message Effect theories such as sensation seeking and framing (Bryant and Zillman, 1994).

Since the 1960s, media effects research has changed its dominant focus from studying attitude change to studying cognitive impact and has also emphasized formation of community agendas and social systems levels of analysis (Beniger and Gusek, 1995; Bryant and Miron, 2004). Units of observation in this macro-level perspective have included populations in diverse community settings, groups, organizations, social institutions, and large-scale social systems, including communities and nation-states. It has an obvious connection to public health in which guided social change, social movements, and community-based health interventions have become important settings for testing communication strategies.

MAJOR MODELS AND HYPOTHESES AT THE INDIVIDUAL LEVEL

The impact of media on individuals' cognitions, affect, and behavior has dominated media studies mainly for historical and cultural reasons. Concerns about the impact of propaganda on soldiers and citizens during World War II led to a strong, sustained research program immediately after the war, looking at communication effects on individuals' attitudes. In parallel, concerns about the impact of movies and other media on the moral well-being of children (later, television, videogames, and the Internet) led to efforts to delineate mechanisms of how media content forms human behavior. Three broad groups of theories have influenced this work: (1) theories that explain

TABLE 16.1. Selected Communication Theories and Levels of Analysis.

Level of Analysis	Theory/Concept	Major Studies, Reviews	Disciplinary Origin
"Micro-level" analysis (for example, media effects on individuals)	Expectancy-Value Theories/Integrated Behavioral Model	Fishbein and Cappella, 2006 Bandura, 1994	Psychology Social Psychology
	Social Cognitive Theory	Bryant and Zillman, 1994	
	Information Processing Theories	Cappella and Rimer, 2006 Rothman, and others, 2006	
	Message Effect Theories and Persuasion	Zillman, 2006 Palmgreen and Donohew, 2002	
"Macro-level" analysis (for example media effects on and through communities and social systems)	Knowledge Gap	Tichenor, and others, 1980 Viswanath and Finnegan, 1996	Sociology Structural/ Functionalism Social Conflict
	Agenda Setting	Cho and McLeod, 2007 McCombs and Shaw, 1972	Sociology
	Definition, Framing of Social Issues	Kosicki, 1993 Bryant and Miron, 2004	Psychology Political Science
	Cultivation Studies	Reese, 2007	
	Risk Communication	Scheufele and Tewksbury, 2007 Gerbner, and others, 1994 Weimann, 2000 Hetsroni and Tukachinsky, 2006 Rimer, Glanz, and Rasband, 2001 Parrot, 2004 McComas, 2006	Sociology/Social Construction of Knowledge Sociology of Mass Society Sociology Psychology

the mechanisms that drive behavior such as Expectancy-Value theories and SCT, (2) theories of information processing, and (3) message effect theories.

Several theories that are often used in health behavior and health education offer explanations for media effects at the individual level. For example, several variants of Expectancy-Value theories, including the HBM, the TRA, and the TPB propose pathways of behavior change through changes in attitudes and beliefs. (These theories are discussed in greater detail in Chapters Three and Four; this section draws connections between those theories and media effects.)

The fundamental assumption of Expectancy-Value theories is that people's behavioral choices are driven by the beliefs or expectancies they have about outcomes of their choices and the value they place on those outcomes. New information may either modify the beliefs or reinforce existing beliefs. TRA proposes that a critical antecedent to behavior is behavioral intention, which is influenced by attitudes or feelings toward performing the behavior and the subjective norms about that behavior. These are assumed to be influenced by underlying beliefs that form them. Media communications may be targeted to either change these beliefs or to reinforce them.

In a similar vein, SCT, first proposed by Bandura (1994), offers a potent explanation for media effects (see Chapter Eight). The thrust of SCT, from a media effects perspective, is that people are active agents who are capable of self-regulation and who can learn by observation and model their own behavior after what they see. Even more, by virtue of the Web, people now create news, process it, and produce their own media. Mass media, such as characters in a TV drama, can provide models to emulate if their actions are perceived to lead to positive rewards. Sargent and others (2007) have argued that portrayal of smoking in movies provides models for youth to emulate, and watching movies that show smoking as glamorous or sexy is associated with smoking. The media also can reinforce or teach self-efficacy—a belief that one is capable of particular behavior and a key variable in SCT.

Fishbein and colleagues (Fishbein and Cappella, 2006; IOM Committee on Communication for Behavior Change in the 21st Century, 2002) attempted to bring these different theories together in the Integrative Behavioral Model (IBM) and applied it in the context of explaining media effects on marijuana use and sexual behavior (see Chapter Four). The argument of IBM is that human behavior is influenced by a core set of determinants: perceived susceptibility (risk), norms and beliefs of their social environment, attitudes toward the message, self-efficacy, and intentions to change. An understanding of how these factors are related to and influence each other can help predict behavior. The key proposition of this model, which has been used in just a few studies to date, is that media effects vary, depending on the behavior and population under study and the relative importance of the determinants. Also, media messages can be targeted, depending on which set of beliefs could most likely influence behavioral intentions.

Information processing theories focus on how media messages may lead to changes in attitudes or in reinforcing existing attitudes. There are several relevant theories. The most commonly used are the dual-process models such as the Elaboration Likelihood Model (ELM) or the Heuristic-Systematic Processing Model (HSM) (Bryant and Zillman, 1994). Both imply that persuasive messages, such as anti-smoking messages, may be processed in two possible ways. A central or a systematic processing route involves deliberate, thoughtful weighing of message arguments, and the changes accompanying such processing are likely to be more enduring. However, peripheral or heuristic processing occurs in low motivation conditions, and the recipient relies on peripheral cues, such as the celebrity status of a spokesperson pitching a product. Information processing theories provide explanations for how message elements are critical ingredients that interact with motivation and ability to influence information processing.

The so-called *elements of execution* in a message are the focus of a group of theories (*message effect theories*) that assume that formats and construction of messages interact with attitudes and abilities to influence information processing (Cappella and Rimer, 2006). The most commonly investigated elements include framing, exemplification, narratives, and sensation seeking. *Framing* has two meanings. It can refer to how messages frame an argument positively or negatively. For example, persuasive messages may encourage a person to quit smoking by describing the advantages of quitting or emphasizing the consequences of not quitting (Rothman and others, 2006). Framing has been used in a different way in sociology of communication, where framing refers to how a problem is defined. That definition is influenced by the power position of the frame sponsors and culture. For example, abortion has been framed either "pro-life" or "pro-choice," lending different interpretations to the same issue and having potentially different effects on the audience (Pan and Kosicki, 2001). *Exemplars* in messages are constructed to serve as illustrative of a general class of events. For example, a news story on bariatric surgery to reduce obesity may use the case of an obese person who is about to undergo the surgery or who has undergone the surgery to write about the surgery. The person serves as an exemplar for all who may undergo or who have gone through bariatric surgery. Some research shows that exemplars are more effective when they are simple, emotional, and concrete (Zillman, 2006).

Narratives are among the most powerful and visible message structures. Narratives are stories with a persuasive twist to them (Green, 2006). They have been used widely to promote family planning, AIDS education, and healthy lifestyles (Slater, 2002). Although it is widely believed that narratives have powerful effects on the audience, systematic evidence is only now beginning to accumulate. The mechanisms of how narratives work may be explained by SCT, where the characters and the situations in stories serve as models for emulation and learning. Narratives generate involvement, absorbing and transporting the audience and minimizing counterarguments (Green, 2006). Audience members who identify and empathize with the character will become more susceptible to the persuasive message.

Sensation seeking is a personality trait that is characterized by search for novelty, thrill seeking, and impulsive decision making and that influences the attention to, processing of, and comprehension of messages. Sensation seekers prefer intensity and stimulation in their experiences and are more likely to indulge in risky behaviors such as unprotected sex and illicit drug use (Palmgreen and Donohew, 2002). Messages with high sensation value are more likely to be effective among this audience and have been successfully used in discouraging drug use and promoting safe sex (Stephenson and Southwell, 2006).

In summary, a variety of communication theories focus on explaining how attitudes and behaviors could be changed at the individual level and the type of message formats that could lead to such changes. These theories draw extensively on other disciplines, such as social and cognitive psychology, and also contribute to their continuing refinement.

THEORIES AT THE MACRO LEVEL

Another group of theories that originated in media studies focus across multiple levels and have particular relevance for public health in relation to day-to-day interaction with media and strategic communication campaigns. Here we review and critique in greater detail four media effects perspectives: (1) the knowledge gap, (2) agenda setting, (3) cultivation studies, and (4) risk communication.

The Knowledge Gap

Conventional wisdom long held that persistent social problems could be resolved through public education. The assumption was that "if you tell them, they will know." However, studies examining public knowledge of a variety of topics and issues have shown that the public did not always know. Moreover, knowledge and information turned out not to be distributed equally across populations. Studies showed that people with more formal education learned and knew more about many issues than people with less formal education (Hyman and Sheatsley, 1947).

These findings were formally presented as the Knowledge Gap Hypothesis by Minnesota researchers Tichenor, Donohue, and Olien (1970). They proposed that an increasing flow of information into a social system (from a media campaign, for example) is more likely to benefit groups of higher socioeconomic status (SES) than those of lower SES. Increasing the information available in the system would only exacerbate already existing differences between these groups. They supported this proposition using studies of several topics, including health. The disturbing implications were, of course, that public campaigns would only perpetuate inequities. Because this called into question the entire basis of guided social change efforts, it attracted the attention of scholars and policymakers.

As a media studies perspective, knowledge gap research arises from a longstanding sociological tradition emphasizing how the structure and organization of communities and societies function as means of social control and conflict management. This tradition has long viewed mass media as important institutions of social control and conflict management. However, it also fits with public health's concern about socio-economically related health disparities (U.S. Department of Health and Human Services, 2000).

The Knowledge Gap Hypothesis advanced the idea of media effects in at least two important ways. It contradicted conventional wisdom that media campaigns are a simple panacea for resolving social problems, and it suggested that media have differential impact on audiences that can be traced to differences in social class and social-structural conditions in communities. It was thus one of the first media studies hypotheses to draw attention to the role of the social environment in shaping media impact on individuals (Viswanath and Finnegan, 1996).

Subsequent studies found that knowledge gaps were not intractable. Researchers discovered a variety of contingent and contributory conditions that could affect knowledge gaps and also present opportunities for applications in public health campaigns (Table 16.2): content domains, channel influence, social conflict and community mobilization, the structure of communities, and individual motivational factors (Viswanath and Finnegan, 1996).

TABLE 16.2. **Knowledge Gap Concepts, Definitions, and Applications.**

Concept	Definition	Application
Knowledge Gap	Difference in measured knowledge between groups of differing socioeconomic status (SES) over time.	Potential unintended consequence of public health interventions to increase SES-based differences over time.
Knowledge	Factual and interpretive information leading to understanding or usefulness for taking informed action.	Communication of factual and interpretive information about causes and prevention of disease and skills for health improvement.
Information Flow	Degree of availability of information on an issue or topic in a social system such as a community.	Increasing community opportunities (through multiple media and other channels) to encounter health information and knowledge.
Socioeconomic Status	Population units or subunits characterized on the basis of differing education, income, wealth, or occupation.	Emphasis on information of interest and use to differing SES groups; emphasis on channel strategies designed to reach especially low-SES groups.
Social Structure/ Pluralism	Differentiation and interdependence among community subsystems including social institutions, organizations, interest groups and other centers of power and influence that maintain the social system; often influenced by size of the community (the larger the community, the greater the differentiation).	Highly differentiated communities increase competition for public attention to health information. While level of communication activity required is often more intensive than in a smaller, less differentiated community, public health resources permit dominating the information flow but seldom; emphasis on targeting of media and other strategies to reach groups of interest.

TABLE 16.2. **Knowledge Gap Concepts, Definitions, and Applications, Cont'd.**

Concept	Definition	Application
Social Conflict	Opposition or disagreement over an issue or problem often representing a struggle for power and influence between social groups or leaders.	Controversy attracts media attention especially in highly differentiated communities; tends to increase public interest and may lead to equalizing information on a topic across SES groups.
Mobilization	Organized activity seeking to focus community power and influence to address a problem or issue.	Media publicity about a public health issue is frequently driven by the actions of social groups and leaders; increases public attention and may lead to equalizing information across SES groups.
Motivation	Factors influencing individuals to attend to, and act upon information and knowledge (for example, personal interest, involvement, self-efficacy).	Emphasis on strategies to increase motivational factors to acquire and act on information and knowledge.

Content and Channel Factors. Although studies have found SES-based knowledge gaps in the content domain of health, others have suggested that health information may appeal broadly to all SES groups (Ettema, Brown, and Luepker, 1983). That is, audiences may be more involved in the topic because, a priori, it affects everyone in some way. However, this does not account for other factors influencing knowledge gaps. For example, studies of channel influence show that people who obtain their news from print media are usually more knowledgeable than those who receive it from other media (Viswanath and Finnegan, 1996). There is a slight tendency for readers of newspapers to have more formal education than nonreaders. Television has the potential to be a knowledge equalizer among SES groups as the cost of access becomes more affordable. An additional modifiable aspect of channel influence has to do with the link between media and interpersonal communication. Tichenor, Donohue, and Olien (1980) have suggested that interpersonal discussion is helpful in narrowing knowledge gaps by reinforcing information received from the media.

Social Conflict and Mobilization. Media studies have also shown that significant knowledge gaps are less likely to be found where social conflict or community mobilization occur (Donohue, Tichenor, and Olien, 1975). Social conflict—an engine of social change—appears to increase public salience about issues encouraging greater interpersonal communication. Mobilization of community groups, institutions, and advocates to address a public problem has a similar effect, even if overt conflict is not present.

Community Structure and Pluralism.   An important though largely nonmodifiable factor affecting knowledge gaps is the structure of communities themselves. Large communities are characterized by greater specialization in interest groups, services, and institutions, including government, business, the media, and other organized centers of power. The potential for conflict is higher in these more pluralistic communities because of such diversity and specialization. Small towns are less specialized and differentiated across all these sectors. Thus, knowledge gaps are more likely in larger, more complex communities and less likely in smaller, less pluralistic communities (Shinghi and Mody, 1976; Ettema, Brown, and Luepker, 1983; Gaziano, 1988). Some studies, particularly in health communication, have reported findings counter to this: knowledge gaps were more likely to be found in smaller communities (Viswanath and others, 1994). It may be that in certain domains such as health, the greater availability of diverse sources may work to the advantage of residents of larger communities (Viswanath and Finnegan, 1996). However, research seeking to extend the knowledge gap to public participation as an outcome suggests that public participation in civic affairs is better predicted by community social cohesion, so smaller communities may have the advantage (Cho and McLeod, 2007). An evolving concept known as "communication infrastructure theory" is now examining the role of the media in building civic engagement (Kim and Ball-Rokeach, 2006).

Motivational Factors.   An important set of modifiable factors affecting knowledge gaps was proposed by Ettema and Kline (1977). They argued that gaps between higher- and lower-SES groups were not necessarily due to the effects of less formal education or economic deprivation but to differential levels of motivation, interest, and salience in specific topics. They shifted the focus in knowledge gap studies to the role of variables of individual difference. Support for this alternative explanation appeared in several studies reporting that the association between knowledge and individual variables such as interest, salience, motivation, and involvement was greater than the association between knowledge and education (Fredin, Monnett, and Kosicki, 1994). Contrary evidence has been reported by other studies (McLeod and Perse, 1994). In a study of a dietary health campaign, Viswanath and colleagues (1993) reported that among motivated people, the more educated knew more about diet and nutrition than did the less educated.

Despite conflicting evidence on the role of motivational factors, it is clear that both individual-level and social-structural variables are important in explaining knowledge gaps. However, future studies need to do a better job in linking these different levels of analysis (Viswanath and Finnegan, 1996).

The importance of these recent studies is that they have provided encouraging evidence about some potentially modifiable factors that, if appropriately understood and addressed, are cause for optimism about the use of media interventions to address public problems. However, unlike the unbounded optimism of the early days of public media campaigns, these studies urge attention to structural factors that pose barriers to effective campaigns. Public health regards it as an ethical precept to address problems of the whole population, both the information rich and the information poor.

Agenda Setting

Mass communication research has long been concerned with the influence of mass media on public opinion, especially as the media affect politics and policymaking. Early writers like Walter Lippman (1922) saw media's behavior as a "restless searchlight," panning from one issue to the next while seldom lingering long on any single issue. Later researchers like Bernard Berelson (1948) noted that while the media influence public opinion, the reverse is also true: public opinion influences what the media report. Researcher Paul Lazarsfeld and colleagues (1948) noted that media attention itself confers status on issues and raises their importance. These insights coalesced in the 1970s as a focus on the mass media's powerful role and influence in setting the public agenda of important issues and problems (Bryant and Miron, 2004).

Studies have shown high correlations between media coverage of issues and the public's opinion of the importance of those issues. The original hypothesis implied a strong if not direct link between the media's agenda of important issues (reflected in news coverage) and the public's opinion about what issues are important (the causal direction flows from the media to the public). Agenda setting attributes a "king-making" role to the media and presents a number of opportunities for applications in public health interventions (Table 16.3).

Kosicki (1993) identified three types of agenda-setting research: (1) public agenda setting, which examines the link between media portrayal of issues and their impact on issue priorities assigned by the public; (2) policy agenda setting, which examines the connection between media coverage and the legislative agenda of policymaking bodies, and (3) media agenda setting, which focuses on factors that influence the media to cover certain issues.

Recent research has suggested refinements to agenda-setting theory (Kosicki, 1993). Initial simple studies have given way to more empirically sophisticated designs with clearer causal links (Iyengar and Kinder, 1987). In addition, the approach is being further refined through several changes in the agenda-setting perspective. One has to do with the idea that the media not only tell us what's important in a general way, they also provide ways of thinking about specific issues by the signs, symbols, terms, and sources they use to define the issue in the first place. In this view, public problems are social constructions (Reese, 2007; Scheufele, 1999). That is, groups, institutions, and advocates compete to identify problems, to move them onto the public agenda, *and* to define the issues symbolically (Entman, 1993). This refinement is important because it suggests that the media's agenda-setting function is not completely independent but is built by various community groups, institutions, and advocates. It further suggests that the media are subject to numerous contingent factors that provide

TABLE 16.3. **Agenda-Setting Concepts, Definitions, and Applications.**

Concept	Definition	Application
Media agenda setting	Institutional roles, factors, and processes that influence "the definition, selection, and emphasis of issues in the media"	Work with media professionals to understand their work needs and routines ingathering and reporting news
Public agenda setting	The link between issues portrayed in the media and the public's issue priorities	Work with media professionals in advocacy or partnership context to build the public agenda for important health issues
Policy agenda setting	The link between issues developed in policymaking institutions and issues portrayed by the media	Work with community leaders and policymakers to build importance of health issues on the media's and public's agenda
Problem identification, definition	Factors and processes leading to identification of an issue by social institutions.	Community leaders, advocacy groups, organizations mobilized to define an issue and modes of solution or basis for action
Framing	Organized public discourse about an issue leading to the selection and emphasis of some characteristics and dimensions and the exclusion of others	Public health advocacy groups "packaging" an important health issue for the media and the public (for example, second-hand smoke framed as public's involuntary exposure to toxic pollutant, contrasted with "smokers' rights" emphasis of tobacco advocates)

broader context to predicting successful and unsuccessful outcomes by these actors working with the media (Walgrave and Van Aelst, 2006). These ideas have their basis in the sociology of knowledge that emphasizes processes involved in the social construction of reality (Van Gorp, 2007). This has applications for those in public health who seek to use the media to raise public salience and awareness of specific problems. Current research in this arena is bringing together agenda-setting theory with the concepts of framing and priming (Scheufele and Tewksbury, 2007). Framing is about how an issue is characterized, especially in the news, while priming encourages audiences to alter the standards they apply to evaluating outcomes related to an issue.

Cultivation Studies

Cultivation studies primarily concern the impact that mass media have on our perceptions of reality. The pervasive presence of television and visual media and their power to alter perception is the starting point of this approach. Simply stated, researchers proposed that heavy TV exposure often leads individuals to accept the world portrayed by television as real (Gerbner and others, 1980; Stossel, 1997). The more exposure to television, the more there is congruence between viewers' perception of reality and the mythical reality portrayed by television (Weimann, 2000; Hetsroni and Tukachinsky, 2006). In essence, television cultivates a stilted view of the world.

Cultivation studies have evolved into two types of research. The first—*message system analysis*—seeks to examine the world that television constructs. For example, in a long series of studies, Gerbner and colleagues (1980) tracked television's violent content. They defined *violence* as the overt expression of physical force by characters to compel victims to act against their will and measured the frequency of such acts. In an early report, they demonstrated an average of five violent acts per hour of prime-time programming and twenty acts of violence on weekend daytime television. They also tracked and recorded the gender, age, ethnic, and occupational composition of characters who frequent television dramas. They reported that in the TV world, men outnumber women, young people and senior citizens are underrepresented, and professional and law enforcement personnel are overrepresented.

The second type of research is *cultivation analysis*. Gerbner and his colleagues (1994) proposed that heavy exposure to television has a profound effect on viewers' perception of social reality. Heavy viewers were more likely to give "television answers" to opinion and knowledge questions, compared to light viewers. They were also more likely to perceive the world as violent and frightening out of proportion to reality, to be less trusting of others, to overestimate the number of people employed in law enforcement; and to fear that they are more likely than is statistically true to become victims of crime. They also are likely to be more accepting of violence as a means of dealing with social problems.

This cultivation of the television worldview is believed to occur through two distinct mechanisms: mainstreaming and resonance. Mainstreaming is the sharing of common of outlooks. It is interesting to note that, irrespective of their sociodemographic background, heavy viewers of television tend to share this worldview. As Gerbner and his colleagues (1980) asserted, heavy viewing "may serve to cultivate beliefs of otherwise disparate and divergent groups toward a more homogeneous 'mainstream' view."

Resonance is regarded as the more powerful mechanism. That is, for certain groups the reality seen on television programs may, in fact, be congruent with the reality of their lives. In such cases, they receive a double dose of the cultivation effect: television has stronger effects for these groups. At least one study has suggested that in some cases the source of resonance effects actually may be audience affinity. Some audience segments may identify so closely with crime victims in the news who resemble themselves that they then develop unreasonable fears about their own risk as victims (Chiricos, Eschholz, and Gertz, 1997).

Although other research has raised questions about the nature of evidence supporting the cultivation hypothesis, most researchers agree that television affects our perception of reality, depending on the level of exposure (Potter, 1999). Subsequent studies have added several contingent conditions that could affect cultivation. For example, some research suggests that the cultivation effects of television become weaker or disappear when controlled for other factors like age, gender, education, income, hours worked per week, social ties, and the size of one's community. More recent studies have found cultivation effects based solely on television exposure across demographic groups (Hetsroni and Tukachinsky, 2006). The fear of crime supposedly cultivated by heavy television viewing may be explained by heavy viewers living in high-crime areas, where they stay home watching more television. Some have also argued that cultivation effects could be nonlinear. That is, television viewing may lead to a cultivation of a television worldview only up to a point (Potter, 1999). Still others argue that entertainment programming is not the only culprit in the distortion of worldviews. The news media, politicians, government, and social and political advocacy groups often seek to further their ends by raising public fear and concerns out of proportion to reality (Glassner, 1999). Recent research has begun to focus on the cultivation effects of online games and the virtual world with mixed results that do not appear to carry over into real-world evaluations of risk and danger (Williams, 2006).

Risk Communication

Communication about risk is of special concern in public health, and it bridges individual and community levels of study. Risk in a health context is about dangers to be described, assessed, and managed for reduction or prevention of some negative outcome (McComas, 2006; Parrott, 2004). Research on risk communication concerns how individuals and groups perceive, process, and act on their understanding of risk. It also addresses how the media and other powerful institutions shape these processes for general or specific outcomes.

At the individual level, scholars have focused on understanding cognitive mechanisms and developing expert and mental models of communication (Fischoff, 1999; Weinstein, 2000), issues of confusion and misinformation (Weinstein, 2000), the efficacy of individualized counseling and tailoring (Rimer, Glanz, and Rasband, 2001), and the advantages to intensive, calibrated, and directed communication (Rimer and Glassman, 1999). Researchers also emphasize the cognitive mechanisms by which individuals are exposed to and attend to information about risk, how they interpret risk information in relation to themselves, and, finally, whether and how they act on risk information to alter their behavior (Glanz and Yang, 1996; Weinstein, 2000). This approach to the study of communication about risk owes much of its theoretical base to social-psychological models of behavior (discussed elsewhere in this volume), such as the Health Belief Model and the Theory of Reasoned Action and also to Social Cognitive Theory. This approach is a staple of communication research that examines media effects on knowledge, beliefs, and behavior.

Significant developments in the study of risk have also occurred at the community level of analysis. Recent work on social problems and the accompanying discourse in the public arena have attracted considerable attention. At the community level, studies of risk communication focus on the interaction of populations and social institutions such as government agencies, advocacy groups, and the mass media in the formation and management of public opinion and policymaking about risk. Here, risk communication studies owe much of their theoretical basis to the agenda-setting and agenda-building perspectives, as well as research on the definition and framing of public issues. Risk is seen as a social construction—a product of communication activity of social institutions, advocates, and the public (Sandman, 1987; Glanz and Yang, 1996).

Public definitions of risk usually include some form of scientifically assessed risk information (objective risk), mediated by the political and social context of the risk. Social conflict is a critical variable in drawing attention to social problems and leading to arousal and increased salience of the issue (Tichenor, Donohue, and Olien, 1980; Viswanath and Demers, 1999). This can have both negative and positive consequences, depending on whether the actual risk is low or high and whether public outrage is low or high. Outrage can have the effect of quickly propelling important information through the population at all socioeconomic levels. In such cases, there will be little difference in information holding among all socioeconomic groups (Viswanath and Finnegan, 1996). Where outrage is low, one might expect to find socioeconomic group differences in knowledge about risk. Either situation may have an impact on policymaking about risk where the public is well or ill informed. Further, a community's definition of risk can be crucial to social action by powerful actors, as can be seen in the case of AIDS in Africa. In the best case, strategic communication about risk accomplishes positive goals of adding social value (Palenchar and Heath, 2007). In the worst case, it is capable of destructive and dangerous unintended outcomes.

PLANNED USE OF MEDIA

This section presents applications of media use to promote public health, to illustrate how the perspectives described earlier can be used to understand and evaluate health promotion and disease prevention efforts. There are two main categories of research and action that apply communication theories to health behavior in the media studies framework. The first category focuses on effects of day-to-day interaction with media on health outcomes and has been covered earlier in this chapter with examples such as the impact of youth exposure to smoking in movies (Sargent and others, 2007) and concern about violence in the media (Gerbner and others, 1994; Potter, 1999; Smith, Nathanson, and Wilson, 2002). Here we focus on effects of the planned use of media to achieve health outcomes, usually in the context of media campaign interventions.

The planned use of media communications to accomplish health outcomes predates the founding of the United States and may have started as a uniquely American cultural phenomenon (Paisley, 1989). This American penchant for public campaigns continues unabated today but with a deeper understanding of, and a more systematic approach to, the role of planning.

Many of the media communication theories discussed in this chapter are relevant to public health communication campaigns. Media studies theories also are useful in the formative analysis and strategy development stages and in evaluating outcomes (see models presented in Part Five). This section gives examples of two such applications.

American Legacy Foundation's Counter-Marketing Campaigns

In considering *media effects*, the effects of exposure to media content on individuals and population groups, the "Truth" campaign, sponsored by the American Legacy Foundation (Healton, 2001), is lauded as an example of an effective planned-media strategy to reduce tobacco use among youth. The campaign uses counter-marketing (also called counter-advertising) to alert youth to deceptive and aggressive tobacco industry marketing practices (Healton, 2001). It has been found to be successful in changing tobacco-related beliefs, attitudes, and smoking prevalence among teens in the early Florida campaign (Sly, Heald, and Ray, 2001; Sly, Hopkins, Trapido, and Ray, 2001; Niederdeppe, Farrelly, and Haviland, 2004) and then in a national campaign (Farrelly and others, 2002; Farrelly and others, 2005). Further, evaluations that used school-based survey data linked to media tracking of exposure to the campaign, provided evidence of a dose-response relationship between exposure to the "Truth" antismoking ads and a lower youth smoking prevalence (Farrelly and others, 2005).

These impressive findings prompted researchers to seek a better understanding of how the "Truth" and similar counter-advertising campaigns operate to influence teen cognition and behavior. Hersey and colleagues (2005) used structural equation modeling to test a theory-based model that might provide insight into the mechanisms through which these campaigns may have affected receptivity to smoking and smoking behavior. They note that campaign effects were consistent with hypotheses derived from the Theory of Reasoned Action (TRA; Chapter Four) and social inoculation effects. Consistent with TRA, higher levels of exposure to the "Truth" campaign were associated with more negative beliefs about tobacco industry practices, negative attitudes toward the industry, and lower receptivity to tobacco advertising. In addition, negative industry attitudes were associated with lower likelihood of progression along a continuum of smoking intentions and behavior (Hersey and others, 2005), as would be predicted by the concept of social inoculation wherein media and peer influence help youth to increase resistance to persuasive communications (McGuire, 1974; Duryea, 1991).

Despite extensive campaign reach and impressive campaign success, there is evidence that a *knowledge gap* exists, resultant of exposure to the Truth campaign. Hersey and colleagues' results suggest that the campaign engendered stronger counter-industry beliefs and attitudes among African Americans than other groups, and that the direct relationship between industry attitudes and smoking status was stronger among African Americans and Hispanics than whites. Males also exhibited a stronger, direct association between industry attitudes and smoking status, compared to females (Hersey and others, 2005). Consistent with the previous discussion of the Knowledge Gap Hypothesis, even largely successful campaigns that set out to educate and influence behavior across gender and racial or ethnic groups may achieve different results in terms of learning, attitude effects, and behavior change.

News Frames of Childhood Nutrition and Obesity in California

Framing, discussed earlier in the chapter, is a critical part of the message production process (Rothman and others, 2006), as journalists and media organizations choose angles or frames in which to cast a given story. Public health professionals have an opportunity to influence the news frames around health issues and thus influence the public's routine exposure to health information. News frames can help to define a social problem and attribute responsibility for the problem and its solutions. As such, routine exposure to a particular news frame can establish a dominant dialogue and discourse among the public and policymakers.

To illustrate, we will discuss one example of how childhood obesity has been framed in the media and how public health professionals worked to influence the message production process by reframing the issue. In this case, the public health goal was to promote not just individual behavior change but also policy measures aimed at reducing childhood obesity.

Woodruff and colleagues conducted a content analysis of media coverage of childhood nutrition and obesity in major California newspapers from 1998 to 2000, to reveal the central arguments and perspectives used in stories about this issue (Woodruff, Dorfman, Berends, and Agron, 2003). They examined whether childhood nutrition and obesity were framed primarily as upstream public health problems requiring policy solutions or primarily as a problem of individual and family responsibility. They found that the problem of childhood obesity was attributed to both individual factors (such as too much television time, overeating) and environmental factors (such as school breakfast programs, the prevalence of fast-food outlets, and the availability of soda). In framing responsibility for *solutions* to the childhood obesity problem in California, however, the investigators found that attribution was almost entirely focused on individual behavior—for children and parents to change eating and exercise habits. Nearly one-third of the articles' proposed solutions included *only* an "individual responsibility" frame, despite attributing the problem to multiple levels of influence. Policy solutions such as improving school meals or simplifying food labeling were rarely discussed.

Building on this knowledge, the investigators published an article aimed at equipping public health practitioners and advocates with skills to reframe news coverage of public health issues, including childhood obesity. The authors pointed to values of social justice and collective responsibility as frames that could expand the discussion of solutions to public health problems (Dorfman, Wallack, and Woodruff, 2005). They sought to influence public agenda setting and policy agenda setting—issues discussed earlier in this chapter. They advocated reframing childhood obesity solutions as a shared responsibility among individuals, government institutions, and corporations in order to galvanize public support for policy-level interventions and persuade policymakers to pursue upstream solutions to the problem.

The authors suggest three key message components aimed at establishing core values that motivate people and institutions to act in support of large-scale change. Those questions, which they suggest should be limited to specifics and not to broad problems are, What's wrong? Why does it matter? What should be done?

They cite as an example the use of these message components to publicize a study of the prevalence of fast food in California high school cafeterias. The study revealed a high percentage of high schools with branded fast-food outlets on campus. The response by a coalition named Project LEAN (Leaders Encouraging Activity and Nutrition) called for institutional solutions at both the local school district and state government levels. Their core messages were

- Fast food is widespread on high school campuses. (What's wrong?)
- Fast food on campus contributes to youth obesity and endangers the health of the next generation. (Why does it matter?)
- There are two solutions: (1) schools must promote appealing, affordable healthy food options for students, and (2) the government must provide adequate funds for food service so that local school districts do not have to supplement their budgets by contracting with fast-food vendors. (What should be done?)

By using such a focused and strategic message statement, the coalition contributed to an increase in substantive news articles and opinion pieces in California newspapers, many of which reflected the frame of shared institutional responsibility for addressing the problem of youth obesity (Dorfman, Wallack, and Woodruff, 2005).

In order to influence the news frames used for public health problems and thus change the nature of the routine exposure people and policymakers have to health information, three lessons are offered for public health educators. Dorfman and others (2005) recommend that public health advocates (1) understand and be able to articulate the core values and beliefs motivating the desired change, (2) articulate the components of messages so they integrate those values with a concise description of the problem and corresponding, immediate solutions, and (3) develop media skills to deliver the message and compete effectively with adversaries, including the ability to make the (broad) landscape, or context, of the problem and solution visible to reporters.

FUTURE DIRECTIONS

There are several important issues in the application of media studies theory in health that will continue to influence research. Today, people are exposed to and use a variety of media—conventional media such as television and newspapers to content available through the World Wide Web, such as pod casts, networked or wired communities, blogs and such user-produced content as YouTube™ videos. What is only now beginning to be explored is how to refine current theories of media production and media effects to account for such radical shifts in the communication world. More germane, how do these developments influence population and individual health for both good and ill? For example, the World Wide Web has obviated the need for geographical proximity to allow users to congregate online to form patient support groups (Rimer and others, 2005; also see Chapter Ten) or offer tailored communications based on communication and health behavior theories (Rimer and Kreuter, 2006). At the same time, new media environments make it possible to market unhealthy products such as cigarettes through the Internet (Williams, Ribisl, and Feighery, 2006). These exemplar trends point to urgent needs for research on the role of mass and new media on public health.

One potentially important area for future research is continuing study of the media's influence on vulnerable audiences such as children and adolescents. Some areas that will continue to attract attention include the role of media and marketing in childhood obesity and entertainment media and adolescent health. Continuing and renewed interest in these issues is visible in recent reports on marketing of sugar-sweetened beverages and low-nutrient snacks to children (McGinnis, Gootman, and Kraak, 2006), portrayal of smoking in movies (Sargent and others, 2007, 2002), and media violence. The communication theories discussed earlier in this chapter will continue to be refined and expanded, or even abandoned, to account for changes in health behaviors as a result of media effects.

As advocate groups work to change the public and media agenda, communication theories will have a significant role to play. For example, there has been considerable pressure on movie producers to reduce depiction of tobacco use in movies (http://smokefreemovies.ucsf.edu/index.html). Efforts are also being made to influence the production process to introduce pro-health story lines (Valente and others, 2007). The success of these efforts in changing the media content and influencing behavior remains to be seen.

Another issue that warrants attention is the continuing problem of health disparities and how it relates to communication. *Healthy People 2010* (U.S. Department of Health and Human Services, 2000), which guides the nation's health objectives for the decade, declared elimination of racial- and socioeconomic-based health disparities as a major goal. Studies show that minorities and families with lower income and education suffer from a greater disease burden, compared to white Americans and those with higher income and education. Communication contributes to these circumstances and structural barriers of access and exposure are too frequently ignored or overlooked, a phenomenon that is beginning to be formalized as "communication inequality" (Viswanath and Emmons, 2006). While a great deal of creative and useful research is examining how to create more effective communication strategies and messages, some are now arguing for a more systematic examination of how social class and racial and ethnic status should influence communication strategies in health promotion (Viswanath and Emmons, 2006; Institute of Medicine, 2002).

Finally, in light of the current preference in public health for community-based interventions, is there a place for national media campaigns in public health? Some suggest that national campaigns are a waste of time and resources that could be better spent mobilizing local communities for health behavior change. Our judgment is that national media campaigns are important because they help build a national prevention agenda on specific issues. National programs create a foundation for local efforts. They can amplify local prevention efforts that are typically more targeted and intense, improving the development of social capital for health. National media campaigns are not a substitute for community prevention, nor should they be expected in themselves to accomplish widespread behavior change without local partnerships.

SUMMARY

The influence of the mass media cuts across individuals, groups, and societies. Media influence on public health may occur through routine, day-to-day use of media, such as exposure to advertising while watching a television program, and through planned use of the media, such as a campaign to promote safe sex or discourage teen smoking. A more refined understanding of how media work on public health requires the study of organizational norms, rules, and structures that lead to the production of media content. Media effects at the individual level are explained by a variety of theories that include expectancy-value, self-regulation, information processing, and message effects theories. Three major theories—the knowledge gap, agenda setting and framing, and cultivation—explain how media effects may cut across individuals and societies and influence individual and population health. These analytical and theoretical frameworks are important to help understand and appreciate the impact of communications.

The study of media and their influence on health cannot be done in isolation from other health behavior theories, and there is need to better integrate the media studies framework with other health behavior theories and relevant theories from psychology and sociology (Cappella and Rimer, 2006). Major theories such as the knowledge gap, agenda setting, and framing reviewed in this chapter, when used with other major health behavior theories discussed in the book, could prove to be helpful in understanding and promoting healthy behaviors.

REFERENCES

Bandura, A. "Social Cognitive Theory of Mass Communication." In J. Bryant and D. Zillman (eds.), *Media Effects: Advances in Theory and Research*. Hillsdale, N.J.: Erlbaum, 1994.

Beniger, J. R., and Gusek, J. A. "The Cognitive Revolution in Public Opinion and Communication Research." In T. L. Glasser and C. T. Salmon (eds.), *Public Opinion and the Communication of Consent*. New York: Guilford, 1995.

Berelson, B. "Communications and Public Opinion." In W. Schramm (ed.), *Communications in Modern Society*. Urbana, Ill.: University of Illinois Press, 1948.

Bryant, J., and Miron, D.. "Theory and Research in Mass Communication." *Journal of Communication,* 2004, *54*(4), 662–704.

Bryant, J., and Zillman, D. (eds.). *Media Effects: Advances in Theory and Research*. Hillsdale, N.J.: Erlbaum, 1994.

Canton, J. *The Extreme Future*. New York: Dutton, 2006.

Cappella, J. C., and Rimer, B. K. (eds.). "Integrating Behavior Change and Message Effects Theories in Cancer Prevention, Treatment and Care." *Journal of Communication,* 2006, *56*(s1), S1–S279.

Chiricos, T., Eschholz, S., and Gertz, M. "Crime, News and Fear of Crime: Toward An Identification of Audience Effects." *Social Problems,* 1997, *44*(3), 342–357.

Cho, J., and McLeod, D. M. "Structural Antecedents to Knowledge and Participation: Extending the Knowledge Gap Concept to Participation." *Journal of Communication,* 2007, *57*(2), 205–228.

Croteau, D. "The Growth of Self-Produced Media Content and the Challenge to Media Studies." *Critical Studies in Media Communication,* 2006, *23*(4), 340–344.

Donohue, G. A., Tichenor, P. J., and Olien, C. N. "Mass Media and the Knowledge Gap: A Hypothesis Reconsidered." *Communication Research,* 1975, *2*, 3–23.

Donohue, G. A., Tichenor, P. J., and Olien, C. N. "A Guard Dog Perspective on the Role of Media." *Journal of Communication,* 1995, *45*(2), 115–132.

Dorfman L., Wallack L., and Woodruff, K. "More Than a Message: Framing Public Health Advocacy to Change Corporate Practices." *Health Education and Behavior,* 2005, *32*, 320–326.

Duryea, E. J. "Principles of Non-Verbal Communication in Efforts to Reduce Peer and Social Pressure." *Journal of School Health*, 1991, *61*, 5–10.

Entman, R. M. "Framing: Toward Clarification of a Fractured Paradigm." *Journal of Communication*, 1993, *43*(4), 51–58.

Ettema, J. S., Brown, J., and Luepker, R. V. "Knowledge Gap Effects in a Health Information Campaign." *Public Opinion Quarterly*, 1983, *47*, 516–527.

Ettema, J. S., and Kline, F. G. "Deficits, Differences and Ceilings: Contingent Conditions for Understanding the Knowledge Gap." *Communication Research*, 1977, *4*, 179–202.

Farrelly, M. C., and others. "Getting to the Truth: Evaluating National Tobacco Countermarketing Campaigns." *American Journal of Public Health*, 2002, *92*(6), 901–907.

Farrelly, M. C., and others. "Evidence of a Dose-Response Relationship Between 'Truth' Antismoking Ads and Youth Smoking Prevalence." *American Journal of Public Health*, 2005, *95*(3), 425–431.

Fischoff, B. "Why Cancer Risk Communication Can Be Hard." *Journal of the National Cancer Institute Monographs*, 1999, *25, 7–13.

Fishbein, M., and Cappella, J. "The Role of Theory in Developing Effective Health Communication." *Journal of Communication*, 2006, *56*, S1–S17.

Fredin, E., Monnett, T. H., and Kosicki, G. M. "Knowledge Gaps, Social Locators, and Media Schemata: Gaps, Reverse Gaps, and Gaps of Disaffection." *Journalism Quarterly*, 1994, *71*, 176–190.

Gandy, O. H., Jr. *Beyond Agenda-Setting*. Norwood, N.J.: Ablex, 1982.

Gans, H. J. "Everyday News, Newsworkers, and Professional Journalism." *Political Communication*, 2007, *24* (2), 161–166.

Gaziano, C. "Community Knowledge Gaps." *Critical Studies in Mass Communication*, 1988, *5*, 351–357.

Gerbner, G. "Field Definitions: Communication Theory." In *1984-85 US Directory of Graduate Programs*, 1985.

Gerbner, G., Gross, L., Morgan, M., and Signorelli, N.. "Growing Up with Television: The Cultivation Perspective." In J. Bryant and D. Zillman (eds.), *Media Effects: Advances in Theory and Research*. Hillsdale, N.J.: Erlbaum, 1994.

Gerbner, G., Gross, L., Morgan, M., and Signorielli, N. "The "Mainstreaming" of America: Violence Profile no. 11." *Journal of Communication*, 1980, *30*, 10–29.

Glanz, K., and Yang, H. "Communicating About Risk of Infectious Diseases." *Journal of the American Medical Association*, 1996, *275, 3*, 253–256.

Glassner, B. *The Culture of Fear: Why Americans Are Afraid of the Wrong Things*. New York: Basic Books, 1999.

Green, M. C. "Narratives and Cancer Communication." *Journal of Communication*, 2006, *56*(s1), S163–S183.

Gulli, A., and Signorini, A. "The Indexable Web Is More Than 11.5 Billion Pages." 2005. [http://www.cs.uiowa.edu/~asignori/web-size].

Healton, C. "Who's Afraid of the Truth?" *American Journal of Public Health*, 2001, *91*(4), 554–558.

Hersey, J. C., and others. "The Theory of 'Truth': How Counterindustry Campaigns Affect Smoking Behavior Among Teens." *Health Psychology*, 2005, *1*, 22–31.

Hetsroni, A., and Tukachinsky, R. "Television-World Estimates, Real-World Estimates, and Television Viewing: A New Scheme For Cultivation." *Journal of Communication*, 2006, *56*(1), 133–156.

Hyman, H. H., and Sheatsley, P. B. "Some Reasons Why Information Campaigns Fail." *Public Opinion Quarterly*, 1947, *11*, 412, 423.

Institute of Medicine and Committee on Communication for Behavior Change in the 21st Century: Improving the Health of Diverse Populations. *Speaking of Health: Assessing Health Communication Strategies for Diverse Populations*, Washington, D.C.: National Academies Press, 2002.

Internet Systems Consortium. "ISC Internet Domain Survey." 2007. [http://www.isc.org/index.pl?/ops/ds].

Iyengar, S., and Kinder, D. R. *News That Matters*. Chicago: University of Chicago Press, 1987.

Kamhawi, R., and Weaver, D. "Mass Communication Research Trends from 1980 to 1999." *Journalism & Mass Communication Quarterly*, 2003, *80*, 7–27.

Kim, Y-C., and Ball-Rokeach, S. "Civic Engagement from a Communication Infrastructure Perspective." *Communication Theory*, 2006, *16*(2), 173–197.

Kosicki, G. M. "Problems and Opportunities in Agenda-Setting Research." *Journal of Communication*, 1993, *43*, 100–127.

Lazarsfeld, P., Berelson, B., and Gaudet, H. *The People's Choice*. New York: Columbia University Press, 1948.

Lessig, L. *The Future of Ideas: The Fate of the Commons in a Connected World*. New York: Random House, 2001.

Lippman, W. *Public Opinion*. New York: MacMillan, 1922.

McComas, K. A. "Defining Moments in Risk Communication Research: 1996–2005." *Journal of Health Communication,* 2006, *11*(1), 75–91.

McCombs, E. E. and Shaw, D. (1972). The agenda-setting function of the mass media. *Public Opinion Quarterly,* 1972, *36,* 176–187.

McGinnis, J. M., Gootman, J. A., and Kraak, V. I. (eds.). *Food Marketing to Children and Youth: Threat or Opportunity?* Washington, D.C.: National Academies Press, 2006.

McGuire, W. J. "Communication Persuasion Models for Drug Education: Experimental Findings." In M. Goodstadt (ed.), *Research Methods and Programmes of Drug Education.* Toronto: Addiction Research Foundation, 1974.

McLeod, J. M., Kosicki, G. M., and Pan, Z. "On Understanding and Misunderstanding Media Effects." In J. Curran and M. Gurevitch (eds.), *Mass Media and Society.* London: Edward Arnold, 1991.

McLeod, D. M., and Perse, E. M. "Direct and Indirect Effects of Socioeconomic Status on Public Affairs Knowledge." *Journalism Quarterly,* 1994, *71,* 433–442.

Miroff, N. "Muscling a Website into a Social Movement: Virginia Blogger Taps into Illegal-Immigration Ire." *Washington Post,* July 22, 2007, p. A01.

Niederdeppe, J., Farrelly, M. C., and Haviland, M. L. "Confirming 'Truth': More Evidence of a Successful Tobacco Countermarketing Campaign In Florida." *American Journal of Public Health,* 2004, *94*(2), 255–257.

Paisley, W. "Public Communication Campaigns: The American Experience." In R. E. Rice and C. K. Atkin (eds.), *Public Communication Campaigns.* (2nd ed.) Newbury Park, Calif.: Sage, 1989.

Palenchar, M. J., and Heath, R. L. "Strategic Risk Communication: Adding Value to Society." *Public Relations Review,* 2007, *33*(2), 120–129.

Palmgreen, P., and Donohew, L. "Effective Mass Media Strategies for Drug Abuse Prevention Campaigns." In Z. Sloboda and W. Bukoski (eds.), *Effective Strategies for Drug Abuse Prevention.* New York: Plenum Press, 2002.

Pan, Z., and Kosicki, G. "Framing as a Strategic Action in Public Deliberation." In S. D. Reese, O. H. Gandy, and A. E. Grant (eds.), *Framing Public Life: Perspectives on Media and Our Understanding of the Social World.* Mahwah, N.J.: Erlbaum, 2001.

Parrott, R. "Emphasizing 'Communication' in Health Communication." *Journal of Communication,* 2004, *54*(4), 751–787.

Potter, W. J. *On Media Violence.* Thousand Oaks, Calif.: Sage, 1999.

Reese, S. D. "The Framing Project: A Bridging Model for Media Research Revisited." *Journal of Communication,* 2007, *57*(1), 148–154.

Reese, S. D., and others. "Mapping the Blogosphere: Professional and Citizen-Based Media in the Global News Arena." *Journalism,* 2007, *8*(3), 235–261.

Rimer, B. K., Glanz, K., and Rasband, G. "Searching for Evidence About Health Education and Health Behavior Interventions." *Health Education and Behavior,* 2001, *28*(2), 231–248.

Rimer, B. K., and Glassman, B. "Is There a Use for Tailored Print Communications in Cancer Risk Communication?" *The Journal of National Cancer Institute Monographs,* 1999, *25,* 140–148.

Rimer, B. K., and Kreuter, M. W. "Advancing Tailored Health Communication." *Journal of Communication,* 2006, *56,* S184–S201.

Rimer, B. K., and others. "How New Subscribers Use Cancer-Related Online Mailing Lists." *Journal of Medical Internet Research,* 2005, *7*(3), e32.

Rothman, A. J., Bartels, R. D., Wlaschin, J., and Salovey, P. "The Strategic Use of Gain- and Loss-Framed Messages to Promote Healthy Behavior: How Theory Can Inform Practice." *Journal of Communication,* 2006, *56*(s1), S202–S220.

Sandman, P. M. "Apathy Versus Hysteria: Public Perception of Risk." In L. R. Batra and W. Klassen (eds.), *Public Perception of Biotechnology.* Bethesda, Md.: Agricultural Research Institute, 1987.

Sargent, J. D., and others. "Viewing Tobacco Use in Movies: Does It Shape Attitudes That Mediate Adolescent Smoking?" *American Journal of Preventative Medicine,* 2002, *22*(3), 137–145.

Sargent, J. D., and others. "Exposure to Smoking Depictions in Movies: Its Association with Established Adolescent Smoking." *Archives of Pediatrics and Adolescent Medicine,* 2007, *161,* 849–856.

Scheufele, D. A. "Framing as a Theory of Media Effects." *Journal of Communication,* 1999, *49,* 103–122.

Scheufele, D. A., and Tewksbury, D. "Framing, Agenda-Setting and Priming: The Evolution of Three Effects Models." *Journal of Communication,* 2007, *57*(1), 9–20.

Shapiro, A. *The Control Revolution: How the Internet Is Putting Individuals in Charge and Changing the World We Know.* New York: Century Foundation, 1999.

Shinghi, P., and Mody, B. "The Communication Effects Gap: A Field Experiment on Television and Agricultural Ignorance in India." *Communication Research,* 1976, *3*, 171–190.

Slater, M. D. "Entertainment Education and the Persuasive Impact of Narratives." In M. C. Green, J. F. Strange, and T. C. Brock (eds.), *Narrative Impact: Social and Cognitive Foundations.* Mahwah, N.J.: Erlbaum, 2002.

Sly, D. F., Heald, G. R., and Ray, S. "The Florida 'Truth' Anti-Tobacco Media Evaluation: Design, First Year Results, and Implications for Planning Future State Media Evaluations." *Tobacco Control,* 2001, *10*(1), 9–15.

Sly, D. F., Hopkins, R. S., Trapido, E., and Ray, S. "Influence of a Counteradvertising Media Campaign on Initiation of Smoking: The Florida 'Truth' Campaign." *American Journal of Public Health,* 2001, *91*(2), 233–238.

Smith, S. L., Nathanson, A. I., and Wilson, B. J. "Prime-Time Television: Assessing Violence During the Most Popular Viewing Hours." *Journal of Communication, 2002, 52*(1), 84–111.

Stephenson, M. T., and Southwell, B. "Sensation-Seeking, the Activation Model, and Mass Media Health Campaigns." *Journal of Communication,* 2006, 56, S38–S56.

Stossel, S. "The Man Who Counts the Killings." *Atlantic Monthly* (Atlantic Online), May 1997, pp. 86–104. [http://www.theatlantic.com/issues/97may/gerbner.htm].

Tichenor, P. J., Donohue, G. A., and Olien, C. N. "Mass Media Flow and Differential Growth in Knowledge." *Public Opinion Quarterly,* 1970, *34*, 159–170.

Tichenor, P. J., Donohue, G. A., and Olien, C. N. *Community Conflict and the Press.* Beverly Hills, Calif.: Sage, 1980.

U.S. Department of Health and Human Services. *Healthy People 2010: Understanding and Improving Health.* Washington, D.C.: Department of Health and Human Services, 2000. [http://www.healthypeople.gov/document/html/uih/uih_2.htm].

Van Gorp, B. "The Constructionist Approach to Framing: Bringing Culture Back In." *Journal of Communication,* 2007, *57*(1), 60–78.

Valente, T. W., and others. "Evaluating a Minor Storyline on ER About Teen Obesity, Hypertension, and 5 A Day." *Journal of Health Communication,* 2007, *12*(6), 551–566.

Viswanath, K., and Demers, D. "Mass Media from a Macrosocial Perspective." In D. Demers and K. Viswanath (eds.), *Mass Media, Social Control, and Social Change: A Macrosocial Perspective.* Ames: Iowa State University Press, 1999.

Viswanath, K., and Emmons, K. M. "Message Effects and Social Determinants of Health." *Journal of Communication,* 2006, *56*(S), S238–S264.

Viswanath, K., Finnegan, J. R., Hannan, P. J., and Luepker, R. V. "Health and Knowledge Gaps: Some Lessons from the Minnesota Heart Health Program." *American Behavioral Scientist,* 1991, *34*, 712–726.

Viswanath, K., and Finnegan, J. R. "The Knowledge Gap Hypothesis: Twenty-Five Years Later." In B. Burleson (ed.), *Communication Yearbook,* Vol. 19. Thousand Oaks, Calif.: Sage, 1996.

Viswanath, K., and others. "Motivation and the 'Knowledge Gap': Effects of a Campaign to Reduce Diet-Related Cancer Risk." *Communication Research,* 1993, *20*, 546–563.

Viswanath, K., and others. "Community Type and the Diffusion of Campaign Information." *Gazette,* 1994, *54*, 39–59.

Walgrave, S., and Van Aelst, P. "The Contingency of the Mass Media's Political Agenda Setting Power: Toward a Preliminary Theory." *Journal of Communication,* 2006, *56*(1), 88–109.

Weimann, G. *Communicating Unreality: Modern Media and the Reconstruction of Reality.* Thousand Oaks, Calif.: Sage, 2000.

Weinstein, N. D. "Perceived Probability, Perceived Severity, and Health-Protective Behavior." *Health Psychology,* 2000, *19*(1), 65–74.

Williams, D. "Virtual Cultivation: Online Worlds, Offline Perceptions." *Journal of Communication,* 2006, *56*(1), 69–87.

Williams, R. S., Ribisl, K. M., and Feighery, E. C. "Internet Cigarette Vendors' Lack of Compliance with a California State Law Designed to Prevent Tobacco Sales to Minors." *Archives of Pediatrics and Adolescent Medicine,* 2006, *160*(9), 988–989.

Woodruff, K., Dorfman L., Berends V., and Agron, P. "Coverage of Childhood Nutrition Policies in California Newspapers." *Journal of Public Health Policy,* 2003, *24*(2), 150–158.

Zillmann, D. "Exemplification Effects in the Promotion of Safety and Health." *Journal of Communication,* 2006, *56*(s1), S221–S237.

CHAPTER

17

PERSPECTIVES ON GROUP, ORGANIZATION, AND COMMUNITY INTERVENTIONS

Michelle C. Kegler
Karen Glanz

KEY POINTS

This chapter will

- Summarize and synthesize the four theoretical approaches to health behavior change through groups, organizations, and communities covered in Part Four of this book: (1) community organization and community building, (2) diffusion of innovations, (3) organizational change, and (4) mass media communications.
- Discuss similarities among the models and draw common themes.
- Critique the usefulness of the four approaches for research and practice in health promotion.
- Highlight new and emerging concepts and strategies for health behavior theories and models at the group, organization, and community levels.

The chapters in Part Four present four theoretical approaches to creating and supporting health behavior change through groups, organizations, and communities. The aim of these chapters is to demonstrate the utility and promise of each theory or framework in health behavior and health education. This chapter discusses similarities among the models, draws common themes, critiques their usefulness for research and practice in health promotion, and highlights the new concepts and strategies included in this fourth edition of *Health Behavior and Health Education.*

The central theme of Part Four is that we must understand, predict, and know how to influence the social systems and structures that provide the context for health behavior. We need models that increase the success of efforts to create healthier institutions and communities. Social networks, change within and among systems, organizational processes, and communication channels are apparent across each of the chapters.

NEW CONCEPTS AND STRATEGIES FOR MACRO-LEVEL CHANGE

Chapters in this section bring together longstanding ideas with new concepts and strategies to understand health behavior and facilitate positive changes. In Chapter Thirteen, Minkler, Wallerstein, and Wilson describe Rothman's (2001) models of community organization and explain how newer models emphasize community-building approaches. These newer models emphasize community assets and strengths rather than being solely problem-driven. They are not simply community-based but are community-driven. Minkler and colleagues define *empowerment, critical consciousness, community capacity,* and *social capital* and describe how leadership development is a strategy for building community capacity. Chapter Thirteen also discusses methods in issue selection, including dialogical problem solving, strategic action planning, and photovoice. The Internet has emerged as a major force in community building, making possible new modes of collecting data, disseminating tools for organizing, creating new linkages within disenfranchised communities, and connecting geographically dispersed advocates and activists. The chapter also notes concerns about the "digital divide," which may limit access and utility of online approaches to those who are poor, minorities, and less educated.

Chapter Fourteen, by Oldenburg and Glanz, analyzes diffusion theory—its main concepts, and implications for bridging the gap between health promotion research and practice. The chapter describes how earlier diffusion research and theory focused on individual adopters and individual innovations. Newer developments have shined more light on the implementation of innovations within specific contexts and on a blend of individual, organizational, and systems change. The authors examine diffusion as a multi-level change process and underscore the need to understand organizational context and culture.

Butterfoss, Kegler, and Francisco present and analyze four theories of organizational change in Chapter Fifteen: Stage Theory, Organizational Development (OD) Theory, Interorganizational Relations (IOR) Theory, and Community Coalition Action Theory (CCAT). Stage Theory has much in common with Diffusion of Innovations, in that they each describe similar steps through which change is created. IOR Theory overlaps with collaborative approaches to community organizing and community building, in which organizations and individuals come together to achieve mutual goals. CCAT is a relatively new theory that attempts to explain how coalitions create community change. This chapter raises intriguing questions about the dynamic organizational and community environments, where many aspects of public health practice occur, and what types of outcomes health promotion experts need to examine beyond individual behavior change.

In Chapter Sixteen, Finnegan and Viswanath use a media studies framework to synthesize the extensive literature on communication theories with special relevance to public health and health behavior change. They differentiate between research on message production and media effects and note that media can affect health both positively and negatively. Four media effects perspectives are introduced: (1) the knowledge gap, (2) agenda setting, (3) cultivation studies, which examine how mass media can affect our views of reality, and (4) risk communication. These models cut across a range of considerations about mass media: its differential impact on high- and low-socioeconomic status populations, its application in social action and advocacy, the impact of media on people's worldviews, and communication regarding health risks, especially those risks with broad public health implications.

These four chapters offer expanded and updated coverage of longstanding theory, research, and practice in health education, and introduce new concepts and strategies. Each chapter draws on multiple theoretical traditions that contribute to important areas of health behavior and health education, rather than presenting single or unified theories, such as those in Part Two of this book. The constraints of the present chapter preclude in-depth coverage of all the issues at hand. Rather, this synthesis focuses on similarities among the models, draws common themes, and critiques their usefulness for research and practice in health behavior and health education.

MULTIPLE LEVELS OF INFLUENCE AND ACTION

A central premise of this book is that improvements in health require both understanding the multi-level determinants of health behavior and a range of change strategies at the individual, interpersonal, and macro levels (Marmot, 2000). Critiques of the tendency for health education and health promotion programs to focus excessively on individuals abound in the literature (Orleans and others, 1999; Smedley and Syme, 2000). The view that societal-level changes and supportive environments are necessary to address major health problems successfully *and* to maintain individual-level behavior changes is now widely endorsed (Smedley and Syme, 2000; Emmons, 2000). The chapters in this section clearly exemplify a multi-level perspective, which builds on intrapersonal and interpersonal theories to explain or affect community change.

Minkler, Wallerstein, and Wilson describe the Youth Empowerment Strategies (YES!) project as drawing on youth development—a multi-level model, along with a strengths-based youth empowerment model. Oldenburg and Glanz review a skin cancer prevention intervention in swimming pools that targeted children, parents, lifeguards, and the pool environment and was based on a blend of SCT, Diffusion of Innovations, and organizational change theories. Butterfoss, Kegler, and Francisco begin with the premise that organizations have multiple levels or layers such as members, teams and departments, and carry through with the theme of the ecology of organizations. In the next chapter, Finnegan and Viswanath organize their review of communication studies according to multiple levels, from intrapersonal processes (for example, persuasion) and organizational (for example, news gatekeeping) to the level of community and macro social structure. They advance the central thesis that various levels of analysis are appropriate to considering various types of effects and aims of interventions.

An important message at the heart of these chapters is that the broader, community- or organization-level models and concepts are not intended to stand alone at the expense of neglecting the individuals who make up the groups, organizations, and communities. Although macro-level theories are invaluable for understanding the complex environments in which behavior takes place, creating change in these environments still often requires identifying and targeting individual change agents such as news gatekeepers, politicians, or school superintendents. In other words, understanding individual behavior will remain integral to the profession, even if the proximal behavior targeted is not health but, for example, an organizational policy. It is collectives of *individuals* who create organizational structures, provide leadership in communities, choose to participate—or not participate—in coalitions, and make decisions about local, state, and federal policies and priorities. Also, it is premature to assume that policy development, social action, and environmental change are sufficient for behavior change across various health topics and populations.

Research on the relative contribution of the environment to health behavior is just beginning to accumulate (see Chapter Twenty). Clearly, environments are important. For example, research on physical environments shows that people who live in neighborhoods with a mixture of land uses, connected streets, recreational facilities, and enjoyable scenery are more likely to be physically active than those who do not live in such neighborhoods (Humpel, Owen, and Leslie, 2002; Saelens, Sallis, Black, and Chen, 2003). Another study showed that different neighborhood features are associated with walking for transportation versus walking for recreation (Hoehner and others, 2005). The interplay between individuals and their environments is complex, and intervention strategies will need to address multiple levels *and* multiple types of determinants. Thus, when taking theoretically informed and research-based strategies to scale in community settings, each public health issue should be assessed with the specific population and local context taken into consideration; the most suitable and cost-effective approaches should be selected for health behavior change initiatives.

MODELS FOR CHANGE

The chapters in Part Four examine models for community activation, planned change, and collaboration. Here we discuss these models and cross-cutting themes.

Community Activation and Planned Change

Two general domains help define the scope of the models included in this section: (1) community activation and (2) planned processes for changing attitudes, behaviors, and policies. The former is usually characterized by internal or *intra*group stimuli for change, whereas the latter are more likely to be led by external change agents. None of the models is pure in this sense, but most break down roughly into these categories. These general approaches reflect implicit assumptions about power and social control versus empowerment and self-control.

Community activation is central to community building, organizational development, interorganizational relations, and media advocacy. As Minkler, Wallerstein, and Wilson note in Chapter Thirteen, several of the key principles of community organizing relate directly to creating the conditions for change: empowerment, community capacity, and the principles of participation and relevance. Newer models of community organization and community building, in particular, emphasize internal community activation. Locality (community) development and community building stress consensus, cooperation, group identity, and mutual problem solving.

Organizational Development (OD) Theory aims to improve organizational performance and the quality of worklife. It attempts to build capacity within organizations to negotiate change. Its roots are in human relations and humanistic psychology. It is concerned with members of organizations, and organizational problems are diagnosed by gathering information directly from the members or workers, often through formal surveys or key informant interviews. OD interventions include strategies such as management redesign, team building, group development, and process consultation. As Butterfoss, Kegler, and Francisco point out in Chapter Fifteen, participation and collective reflection are integral to this approach, as is a cycle of experimentation, learning, and reflection.

Agenda-setting approaches to media communication involve telling people *what to think about.* Media advocacy strategies are an extension of these techniques in which advocacy groups in the community define, identify, and frame a problem and stimulate media coverage of the problem as a public health issue (Wallack, 1990). Media advocacy activates forces in a social system (that is, media coverage) to help stimulate widespread public concern and action.

Processes for facilitating large-scale planned change can be informed by Diffusion of Innovations theory, Stage Theory of organizational change, and the branch of communication studies that emphasizes changes in cognitions, beliefs, and behavior. Each of these frameworks offers guideposts for professionals wishing to promote specific changes in individuals within organizations or in larger societies. The term *diffusion of innovations* describes the spread of ideas, products, and behaviors within a society or from one society or social system to another. It can help to understand a passive process in which an innovation spreads naturally through a social system, or a more structured and planned process (usually referred to as *dissemination*) to promote adoption and implementation of a particular innovation. Stage Theory is closely allied to diffusion of innovations because it focuses on understanding and matching the organizational stages of change with efforts to introduce or encourage organizational change.

These contrasting orientations to change—community activation and planned change—raise issues about power and control, who defines needs and problems, and the extent to which existing institutions (including the mass media) act as instruments of social control. In community activation, the impetus for change comes from *within* an organization or community. On the surface, this may seem like a relatively simple dichotomy—internal or external impetus for change. With deeper analysis, however, the complexity of any social system, with its multiple layers and factions, raises issues of power, control, and values. Of particular interest is the paradox suggested by Minkler, Wallerstein, and Wilson: that community needs and wants should be superseded by social justice concerns in cases where communities are mobilizing to restrict civil rights (such as anti-gay rights legislation). This underscores the dilemma faced by professionals whose personal values are not consistent with those of a given community. But even when community activation methods are used to promote social justice, there remains an exercise of power that may be disquieting to some audiences (Kipnis, 1994).

Collaboration

Collaboration, through partnerships of health promotion experts and other providers (such as educators, medical personnel, media producers), or through community coalitions with interorganizational representation, emerges as a strategy for change across the chapters of Part Four. The concepts of social support and social networks underpin these strategies (also see Chapter Nine). Oldenburg and Glanz, for example, discuss the importance of linking agents who facilitate implementation of an innovation through training and technical assistance. Dissemination researchers often describe the need for support systems that connect innovation developers with adopting organizations. In health behavior and health education, this would involve collaboration between researchers and practitioners (Wandersman and others, 2008). The planned use of media often requires collaboration between public health practitioners and media professionals. Partnerships between public health practitioners and low-SES communities are also useful in ensuring that the media are used in ways that do not exacerbate the knowledge gap described in Chapter Sixteen.

A major premise underlying collaborative approaches to health promotion is that partnerships can mobilize complementary and diverse material and human resources; the resulting synergy will lead to more effective solutions than could be achieved by an individual or organization working alone (Lasker and Weiss, 2003; Lasker, Weiss, and Miller, 2001). Collaborations have significant potential for community and systems change, too. They can achieve valued public health outcomes while also transforming power relations and revitalizing a sense of shared responsibility (Butterfoss and Kegler, 2002). Yet, collaborative efforts are complex, successful coalitions are not easy to develop, and the processes and outcomes of collaboration may be imperfectly correlated (Berkowitz, 2001). There is a small but growing literature that may reveal best practices in developing partnerships and helping them to succeed in achieving desirable changes (Foster-Fishman and others, 2001; Butterfoss, 2007; Zakocs and Edwards, 2006). Increasingly, the emphasis is on coalition *effectiveness,* not merely formation and maintenance of a broad-based and satisfied membership (Kegler and others, 2005; Feinberg, Greenberg, and Osgood, 2004; Hayes, Hays, DeVille, and Mulhall, 2000). Reviews of the literature have documented only modest evidence of effective partnerships with respect to environmental change, population-level outcomes, and communitywide behavior change (Roussos and Fawcett, 2000; Kreuter, Lezin, and Young, 2000). These findings remind us that a satisfied, active coalition with better linkages to other community organizations does not guarantee effective products or results any more than worker happiness ensures high productivity.

APPROACHES TO DEFINING NEEDS, PROBLEMS, AND AIMS

The roots of change efforts for health enhancement begin in the early phases of needs assessment or problem definition. Several philosophical and methodological questions for developing and implementing health promotion strategies are either explicitly decided or implicitly addressed when defining needs, problems, and program aims or objectives. *Who* will decide what is a problem? What is the balance of professional (outsider/change agent) definition of needs and the lay/community (insider/target audience) expression of needs? How are problems defined—as lack of knowledge and willpower, as living in an unhealthy environment, or a combination of the two? Concepts of felt ownership, participation, and relevance are shared in community organizing, organizational change, diffusion of innovations, and media communication studies, but their applications vary significantly.

Once needs or problems are defined (by whomever and by whatever methods), strategies are identified to achieve certain aims and objectives, usually to improve the situation or to prevent, reduce, or eliminate the problems. The way a problem is defined typically frames or limits the range of logical solutions. Take obesity, for example. If obesity is defined as a lack of will power, intervention strategies may focus on persuasive communication, motivation, applied behavioral analysis and self-monitoring to promote healthy eating and physical activity. If obesity is defined as environmentally determined, with factors such as living in an automobile- and fast-food-dominated society considered most important, solutions may involve urban planning, increasing mass transit options, and zoning regulations.

Questions that parallel these issues also involve defining the appropriate or desirable outcomes. Must we always aim for improvements in specific health behaviors, health risks, or health status outcomes, or are these effects compromised because of their narrow definition of physical health? Pressures for accountability for health improvement, and even cost savings, are growing at the same time that some health educators contend that these expectations may be inappropriately narrow and limiting. Is social capital or increased community capacity to solve problems valuable outcomes? Is adoption of an evidence-based health curriculum enough? Is it sufficient to accomplish change in health-related policies or environments, even if we are not certain these changes will translate into improved health behaviors? These questions are particularly challenging when disseminating evidence-based interventions. Can we assume that an intervention that was proven effective in an efficacy trial will achieve the same effects in a different context? When is an expensive and rigorous outcome evaluation necessary?

Indeed, a fundamental ideological tension about the goals of health education and health promotion has arisen: Should health promotion improve health status, serve as an instrument of social change, or both? Recently, increased public health attention on obesity has brought out critics who contend that this "health crisis" is being driven more by cultural and political factors than by real health threats (Campos and others, 2006). Robertson and Minkler (1994) noted that what appears as an ideological conflict may be best understood as boundary issues and that health promotion benefits by using multiple frameworks. They stress the importance of evaluating and demonstrating the benefits (or lack thereof) of whichever methods are chosen.

THE INFLUENCE OF TECHNOLOGY ON MACRO-LEVEL THEORY AND PRACTICE

Although the influence of the Internet was mentioned in earlier editions of this text, its impact and implications for macro-level theories is more pronounced in this edition. Butterfoss, Kegler, and Francisco discuss how communication technology and globalization are blurring the boundaries between organizations and their environments. With electronic communication, wireless technologies, telecommuting, and the Internet, it is no longer necessary for members of an organization to be in the same physical location. This has implications for the practice of organizational development in terms of how best to diagnose organizational problems and how to engage members in identifying, implementing, and evaluating solutions. Further, with increased globalization and out-sourcing of organizational functions, the lessons learned from interorganizational relations theory grow in relevance.

Minkler, Wallerstein, and Wilson review several ways in which the Internet affects community organizing and community building. One is through facilitating data collection. Access to secondary data, for example, from government Web sites, is markedly improved in recent years. Similarly, it has gotten easier to track media use through the Internet, and several community assessment and community-building toolkits are online. Minkler and colleagues note that the Internet facilitates the formation of new communities with shared interests, often dispersed geographically (also see Chapter Ten). These new communities can be tapped for community building and are also useful structures for policy advocacy and coalition building related to issues of common concern.

Finnegan and Viswanath's observation that the media can influence health both negatively and positively also applies to the Internet. As with television, the Internet can increase exposure to violence and encourage sedentary lifestyles. It differs from TV, however, in that the user has increased control over information exposure. Finnegan and Viswanath also discuss how technology has blurred boundaries between news and entertainment, media professionals, and the general public. They comment that it is too early to know how the Internet will influence society, and by implication, health behavior and the contexts in which it occurs. Last, Oldenburg and Glanz highlight the value of Web sites for program dissemination. Innovations, which in health promotion are often new programs and strategies for improving health, can be accessed through Web sites, such as the Community Guide (www.thecommunityguide.org) and Cancer Control P.L.A.N.E.T. (www.cancercontrolplanet.cancer.gov). Moreover, the Internet can provide tools for implementing and adapting evidence-based interventions to local contexts, and a vehicle through which researchers and practitioners can engage in two-way communication and begin to close the research-practice gap.

SIMILARITIES BETWEEN MODELS

Each theory and model in Part Four of *Health Behavior and Health Education* is distinctive in its perspective, emphasis, and research base. At the same time, there are many similarities between the models, as well as similarities to intrapersonal and interpersonal models of health behavior presented earlier in this book. This section highlights some similarities and the related differences in the models. It compares and contrasts (1) community organization and organizational change, (2) diffusion of innovations and organizational change, (3) diffusion of innovations and Social Cognitive Theory, and (4) diffusion of innovations and communication-persuasion models of attitude change. The question of stages, steps, and phases across models is also addressed. This chapter does not offer in-depth analyses of these related models because each comparison would require a chapter in itself (and these tasks have been accomplished in other books).

Community Organization and Organizational Change

Chapter Thirteen presents key principles and models of community organization and community building, along with the theoretical foundations that form a base for these activities. There is no single unifying theory of community organization that applies adequately to all health promotion work (Bracht, 1990) or other health applications. Rather, there are methods and approaches with theoretical underpinnings from other fields, such as political science, social work, and organizational and social psychology. Some of these theories are integral to the organizational change frameworks discussed in Chapter Fifteen. Theories of social support, community development, and network analysis are most pertinent to OD Theory as a component of organizational change. IOR Theory is consonant with coalition building as it is used in community organizing. Another important consideration relates to the final stage of Stage Theory that Butterfoss, Kegler, and Francisco present. That phase—institutionalization—is the adoption of an innovation (a new idea or practice) as an ongoing part of an organization's structure and activities. The relationship to community organization lies in the virtual necessity of considering community organization principles (such as participation, relevance, and community competence) if institutionalization is to occur.

Diffusion of Innovations and Organizational Change

Chapters Fourteen and Fifteen put forth concepts from diffusion theory and organizational change that bear remarkable resemblance to one another. A reason for this is that innovations in health promotion are often adopted by organizations such as schools and workplaces. Both chapters include multistage models (adoption, implementation, maintenance, and so on). Also, both describe trials of interventions to promote adoption, implementation, and institutionalization of health promotion strategies of demonstrated efficacy, with diffusion or organizational change occurring with varying degrees of success.

Diffusion of Innovations and Social Cognitive Theory

Albert Bandura's 1986 volume on Social Cognitive Theory (SCT) includes a chapter on social diffusion and innovation. In it, Bandura noted that "understanding how new ideas and social practices spread . . . has important bearing on personal and social change" (1986). Even before this relatively recent attention to diffusion, linkages between social learning (or cognition) and diffusion were set in place. The most apparent difference, which is reflected in the structure of this book, is that diffusion concepts and research emphasize the macro nature of social change, whereas social learning emphasizes intrapersonal and interpersonal factors, that is, the micro level. Similarities between diffusion and SCT include the focus on behavior change, the importance of interpersonal networks for behavior change, the essential role of information exchange, and the movement toward two-way influence processes. SCT and diffusion differ in their research traditions, as reflected in the dominant measurement methods and research designs. Historically, diffusion research has primarily involved naturalistic field surveys, whereas SCT research designs are primarily experimental and often conducted in the laboratory. However, these two traditions may be coming closer together, as suggested by some of Bandura's more recent writing that emphasizes agentic transactions and collective efficacy (Bandura, 1997; Bandura, 2001; also see Chapter Eight). The convergence of thinking and the increasing attention to people as both producers and products of social systems heralds an increasing tendency to conduct multi-level analyses of health behavior and to employ multi-level approaches for changing health-related behaviors and environments (Smedley and Syme, 2000).

Diffusion of Innovations and Communication-Persuasion

Diffusion frameworks are useful in understanding how mass media contribute to the spread of innovations in populations. Different communication channels may vary in their ability to communicate an innovation to various adopter groups. The phases of diffusion, especially the later stages, can also be examined as phases of psychological change in individuals, that is, adoption, implementation, and maintenance. The correspondence suggests parallels between models of communication and persuasion and information processing at the individual level, and the community framework of adoption and diffusion. Communications can be designed to promote effects on individuals at each stage of the individual models and disseminated to promote optimal diffusion in social systems (Rogers, 1983).

RESEARCH ISSUES

Each of the theories and action models presented in Part Four of *Health Behavior and Health Education* is complex and multimodal, and aims to influence not only large groups of individuals but organizational structures as well. An assessment of the impact of interventions based on these frameworks typically requires more complex and less controlled designs than those used at the intrapersonal or interpersonal levels (Merzel and D'Afflitti, 2003). Since organization, coalition, or community is usually the unit of randomization and analysis, statistical power is often lower due to the logistical and financial realities of designing a study with ten or more units per study condition. Moreover, when the numbers of organizations or communities is modest, identification of comparable communities is difficult, whether the design is randomized or not. A third challenge encountered by many of the large community trials to date are strong secular trends in the outcome of interest, such as smoking rates, cardiovascular disease risk, and teen pregnancy rates (Merzel and D'Affliti, 2003; COMMIT Research Group, 1995; Luepker and others, 1994; Carleton and others, 1995).

Measurement challenges also abound. Access to information at the organizational level may be difficult to obtain and even more difficult to validate, given the divergent perspectives of managers and workers or members and constituents/clients of an organization. In addition, valid and reliable environmental measures are still under development for many health behaviors. There also is a great need to examine the accuracy and completeness of archival, government, and commercial sources of data used as environmental indicators and used to define sampling frames for community observational studies, historical analyses, and Geographical Information Systems (GIS) analysis (Glanz, Sallis, Saelens, and Frank, 2007; Wang, Gonzalez, Ritchie, and Winkleby, 2006).

Action research and, more recently, community-based participatory research have been proposed as integral approaches to intervention and evaluation using a social ecological framework (Israel and others, 2003). These participatory research methods include active roles for community members in defining their own health needs, setting priorities, and evaluating health improvement efforts (Green and others, 1995; Israel, Eng, Schulz, and Parker, 2005; Minkler and Wallerstein, 2003). These methods are consistent with community participation, shared decision making, and the facilitation of ownership of change strategies. Community intervention research and evaluation require a balance of scientific rigor and dynamic community environments with ethical concerns (Glanz, Kegler, and Rimer, forthcoming). Partnership research models are not all-or-nothing phenomena; they are a continuum with varying degrees of community and scientist participation and control (Wallerstein, 1999). One end of the spectrum is characterized by "community-placed" interventions, and the other end is anchored in community-*driven* approaches. Their use reflects varied philosophical positions, as well as practical considerations.

The use of both quantitative, hypothesis-testing research methods and qualitative methodologies is illustrated in each chapter in this section. These methods complement each other, and both lend strength to our understanding of the processes and results of health behavior change efforts. A careful examination of how theory has been used in complex, multi-level interventions highlighted the lack of unified theory and methods to help understand the community change process (Merzel and D'Afflitti, 2003). New developments in measurement are increasing our tool box of community-level indicators (Goodman and others, 1998; Cheadle and others, 1992; Brownson and others, 2004; Glanz, Sallis, Saelens, and Frank, 2007), thus enabling better assessments of whether environments have changed and examination of the associations between individual- and community-level effects.

Additional research challenges involve the study of community change and societal change as two-way processes, the need to attend to personal influence, as well as the content of interventions, and the need to ensure that evaluation occurs prospectively, thus minimizing bias and ensuring that valuable information is not lost. We have an obligation to use our professional skills and resources for high-quality evaluation, even in the most process-driven change efforts. Models that work warrant wide dissemination, and models and strategies that are ineffective need to be improved or discarded (Rimer, Glanz, and Rasband, 2001). It is a disservice to the field of health education and health behavior to promulgate models based on ideology alone if they are not useful in achieving worthwhile aims.

SUMMARY

Societal, community, and institutional factors are critical to promoting health behavior changes. They can provide a fertile environment for health enhancement, as well as directly shape individuals' health behavior. The power of policy is evident in health education settings such as workplaces and schools. Both broad social changes and specific organizational and governmental policies have been linked to individual behavior and perceptions. Macro-level approaches complement intrapersonal and interpersonal methods of health education and health behavior. Blended models suggest integrated strategies for reaching various units of practice in communitywide programs. Some health issues, for example, environmental protection through control of hazardous waste and infectious disease, cannot be influenced through individual-level efforts alone. However, they may be affected positively through methods based on individual behavior analysis frameworks, combined with two-way communication with public health leaders and media efforts to promote wide awareness and prompt community action (Glanz and Yang, 1996; Weinstein and Sandman, 1993; Kegler and Miner, 2004).

Integration of group, organization, and community intervention frameworks with individual and interpersonal models of health behavior has potential impact that exceeds the use of any one approach. Our most challenging public health problems require increased attention to organizational and environmental factors. Because behavior is highly influenced by settings, rules, organizational policy, community norms, and opportunities for action, changes in these factors are promising targets for change. Individual change will follow successful organizational and environmental changes, provided that these changes are both intensive enough and sustained over time.

Ideally, comprehensive health education efforts build on strategies that have been tried and found effective for reaching health and health behavior goals. However, while strategies have been shown to be effective in many behavioral arenas (for example, marketing, political), there are currently few health issues for which a variety of demonstrably effective strategies is known. Tobacco prevention and control is one of the few areas for which effective interventions have been developed and evaluated at each level of change (Warner, 2000; Green and others, 2006). Hopefully, the armamentarium of effective strategies for other health behaviors will grow to the same level.

Theories and methods of community organization and community building, diffusion of innovations, organizational change, and media communication provide a strong foundation for understanding and positively influencing health behavior. Advances in research will clarify the mechanisms of these theories' and models' operation and refine our understanding of how best to use them. Health education and health behavior change strategies will achieve greater success through informed application of these frameworks for social activation and community attitude and behavior change.

REFERENCES

Bandura, A. *Social Foundations of Thought and Action: A Social Cognitive Theory.* Englewood Cliffs, N.J.: Prentice Hall, 1986.

Bandura, A. *Self-Efficacy: The Exercise of Control.* New York: Freeman, 1997.

Bandura, A. "Social Cognitive Theory: An Agentic Perspective." *Annual Review of Psychology,* 2001, *52,* 1–26.

Berkowitz, B. "Studying the Outcomes of Community-Based Coalitions." *American Journal of Community Psychology,* 2001, *29*(2), 213–227.

Bracht, N. (ed.). *Health Promotion at the Community Level.* Newbury Park, Calif.: Sage, 1990.

Brownson, R., and others. "Measuring the Environment for Friendliness Toward Physical Activity: A Comparison of the Reliability of 3 Questionnaires." *American Journal of Public Health,* 2004, *94,* 473–483.

Butterfoss F., and Kegler, M. "Toward a Comprehensive Understanding of Community Coalitions: Moving From Practice to Theory." In R. DiClemente, R. Crosby, and M. Kegler (eds.), *Emerging Theories in Health Promotion Practice and Research.* San Francisco: Jossey-Bass, 2002.

Butterfoss, F. *Coalitions and Partnerships in Community Health.* San Francisco: Jossey-Bass, 2007.

Campos, P., and others. "The Epidemiology of Overweight and Obesity: Public Health Crisis or Moral Panic?" *International Journal of Epidemiology,* 2006, *35,* 55–60.

Carleton, R., and others, for The Pawtucket Heart Health Program Writing Group. "The Pawtucket Heart Health Program: Community Changes in Cardiovascular Risk Factors and Projected Disease Risk." *American Journal of Public Health,* 1995, *85,* 777–785.

Cheadle, A., and others. "Environmental Indicators: A Tool for Evaluating Community-Based Health-Promotion Programs." *American Journal of Preventive Medicine,* 1992, 8(6), 345–350.

COMMIT Research Group. "Community Intervention Trial for Smoking Cessation (COMMIT) Changes in Adult Cigarette Smoking Prevalence." *American Journal of Public Health,* 1995, *85,* 193–200.

Emmons, K. "Health Behaviors in Social Context." In L. F. Berkman and I. Kawachi (eds.), *Social Epidemiology.* New York: Oxford University Press, 2000.

Feinberg, M., Greenberg, M., and Osgood, D. "Readiness, Functioning, and Perceived Effectiveness in Community Prevention Coalitions: A Study of Communities That Care." *American Journal of Community Psychology,* 2004, *33*(3/4), 163–176.

Foster-Fishman, P., and others. "Building Collaborative Capacity in Community Coalitions: A Review and Integrative Framework." *American Journal of Community Psychology,* 2001, *29*(2), 241–261.

Glanz, K., Kegler, M. C., and Rimer, B. K. "Ethical Issues in the Design and Conduct of Community-Based Intervention Studies." In S. Coughlin, T. Beauchamp, and D. Weed (eds.), *Ethics in Epidemiology*. (2nd ed.) New York: Oxford University Press, forthcoming.

Glanz, K., Sallis, J. F., Saelens, B. E., and Frank, L. D. "Nutrition Environment Measures Survey in Stores (NEMS-S): Development and Evaluation." *American Journal of Preventive Medicine,* 2007, *32,* 282–289.

Glanz, K., and Yang, H. "Communicating About Risk of Infectious Diseases." *Journal of the American Medical Association,* 1996, *275*(3), 253–256.

Goodman, R. M., and others. "Identifying and Defining the Dimensions of Community Capacity to Provide a Basis for Measurement." *Health Education and Behavior,* 1998, *25,* 258–278.

Green, L., and others. "Inferring Strategies for Disseminating Physical Activity Policies, Programs, and Practices from the Successes of Tobacco Control." *American Journal of Preventive Medicine,* 2006, *31*(4 Suppl), S66–81.

Green, L.W., and others. *Study of Participatory Research in Health Promotion: Review and Recommendations for the Development of Participatory Research in Health Promotion in Canada.* Vancouver: University of British Columbia, 1995.

Hayes, C., Hays, S., DeVille, M., and Mulhall, P. "Capacity for Effectiveness: The Relationship Between Coalition Structure and Community Impact." *Evaluation and Program Planning,* 2000, *23,* 373–379.

Hoehner, C., and others. "Perceived and Objective Environmental Measures and Physical Activity Among Urban Adults." *American Journal of Preventive Medicine,* 2005, *28*(2 Suppl2), 105–116.

Humpel, N., Owen, N., and Leslie, E. "Environmental Factors Associated with Adults' Participation in Physical Activity: A Review." *American Journal of Preventive Medicine,* 2002, *22*(3), 188–199.

Israel, B., Eng, E., Schulz, A., and Parker, E. *Methods in Community-Based Participatory Research for Health.* San Francisco: Jossey-Bass, 2005.

Israel, B., and others. "Critical Issues in Developing and Following Community-Based Participatory Research Principles." In M. Minkler and N. Wallerstein (eds.), *Community-Based Participatory Research for Health.* San Francisco: Jossey-Bass, 2003.

Kegler, M., and Miner, K. "Environmental Health Promotion Interventions: Considerations for Preparation and Practice." *Health Education and Behavior,* 2004, *31*(4), 510–525.

Kegler, M., and others. "Mobilizing Communities for Teen Pregnancy Prevention: Associations Between Coalition Characteristics and Perceived Accomplishments." *Journal of Adolescent Health,* 2005, *37*(3S); S31–S41.

Kipnis, D. "Accounting for the Use of Behavior Technologies in Social Psychology." *American Psychologist,* 1994, *49*(3), 165–172.

Kreuter, M., Lezin, N., and Young, L. "Evaluating Community-Based Collaborative Mechanisms: Implications for Practitioners." *Health Promotion Practice,* 2000, *1*(1), 49–63.

Lasker, R., and Weiss, E. "Broadening Participation in Community Problem Solving: A Multidimensional Model to Support Collaborative Practice and Research." *Journal of Urban Health,* 2003, *80*(1), 14–47.

Lasker, R., Weiss, E., and Miller R. "Partnership Synergy: A Practical Framework for Studying and Strengthening the Collaborative Advantage." *The Milbank Quarterly,* 2001, *79*(2), 179–205.

Luepker, R., and others. "Community Education for Cardiovascular Disease: Risk Factor Changes in the Minnesota Heart Health Program." *American Journal of Public Health,* 1994, *84,* 1383–1393.

Marmot, M. "Multilevel Approaches to Understanding Social Determinants." In L. F. Berkman and I. Kawachi (eds.), *Social Epidemiology.* New York: Oxford University Press, 2000.

Merzel, C., and D'Afflitti, J. "Reconsidering Community-Based Health Promotion: Promise, Performance, and Potential." *American Journal of Public Health,* 2003, *93,* 557–574.

Minkler, M., and Wallerstein, N. (eds.). *Community-Based Participatory Research for Health.* San Francisco: Jossey-Bass, 2003.

Orleans, C. T., and others. "Rating Our Progress in Population Health Promotion: Report Card on Six Behaviors." *American Journal of Health Promotion,* 1999, *14,* 75–82.

Rimer, B. K., Glanz, K., and Rasband, G. "Searching for Evidence About Health Education and Health Behavior Interventions." *Health Education and Behavior,* 2001, *28,* 231–248.

Robertson, A., and Minkler, M. "New Health Promotion Movement: A Critical Examination." *Health Education Quarterly,* 1994, *21*(3), 295–312.

Rogers, E. M. *Diffusion of Innovations.* (3rd ed.) New York: Free Press, 1983.

Rothman, J. "Approaches to Community Intervention." In J. Rothman, J. Erlich, and J. Tropman (eds.), *Strategies of Community Intervention.* Itasca, Ill.: Peacock, 2001.

Roussos, S., and Fawcett, S. "A Review of Collaborative Partnerships as a Strategy for Improving Community Health." *Annual Review of Public Health,* 2000, *21,* 369–402.

Saelens, B., Sallis, J., Black, J., and Chen, D. "Neighborhood-Based Differences in Physical Activity: An Environment Scale Evaluation." *American Journal of Public Health,* 2003, *93*(9), 1552–1448.

Smedley, B. D., and Syme, S. L (eds.). *Promoting Health: Intervention Strategies from Social and Behavioral Research.* Washington, D.C.: National Academies Press, 2000.

Wallack, L. "Media Advocacy: Promoting Health Through Mass Communication." In K. Glanz, F. M. Lewis, and B. K. Rimer (eds.), *Health Behavior and Health Education: Theory, Research, and Practice.* (1st ed.) San Francisco: Jossey-Bass, 1990.

Wallerstein, N. "Power Between Evaluator and Community: Research Relationships Within New Mexico's Healthier Communities." *Social Science and Medicine,* 1999, *49,* 39–53.

Wandersman, A., and others. "Bridging the Gap Between Prevention Research and Practice: The Interactive Systems Framework for Dissemination and Implementation." *American Journal of Psychology,* Feb. 27, 2008 (eJournal).

Wang, M. C., Gonzalez, A. A., Ritchie, L. D., and Winkleby, M. A. "The Neighborhood Food Environment: Sources of Historical Data on Retail Food Stores." *International Journal of Behavioral Nutrition and Physical Activity,* 2006, *3*(15) (eJournal).

Warner, K. "The Need for, and Value of, a Multi-Level Approach to Disease Prevention: The Case of Tobacco Control." In B. D. Smedley and S. L. Syme (eds.), *Promoting Health: Intervention Strategies from Social and Behavioral Research.* Washington, D.C.: National Academies Press, 2000.

Weinstein, N. D., and Sandman, P. M. "Some Criteria for Evaluating Risk Messages." *Risk Analysis,* 1993, *13,* 103–114.

Zakocs, R., and Edwards, E. "What Explains Community Coalition Effectiveness? A Review of the Literature." *American Journal of Preventive Medicine,* 2006, *30*(4), 351–361.

PART

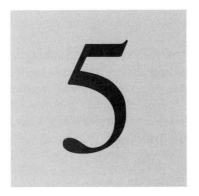

Using Theory In Research and Practice

Karen Glanz

One of the greatest challenges to public health professionals is to learn to analyze the "fit" of a theory or model for issues and populations with whom one is working. A working knowledge of a handful of theories and how they have been applied is a first step. Mastering the challenges of using theories appropriately and effectively is the logical next step. Effective practice depends on marshaling the most appropriate theory or theories and practice strategies for a given situation. Theory-based research and evaluation further require appropriate designs, measures, and procedures for the health problem, organization, and unique population at hand, as well as the development of appropriate interventions.

No one theory or model will be right in all cases. Depending on the unit of practice and type of health behavior or issue, different theoretical frameworks will be appropriate, practical, and useful. Often, more than one theory is needed to adequately address an issue. For comprehensive health promotion programs, this is almost always true. It is also evident in the use and description of applied theories in the professional literature. However, using too many theories may be counterproductive.

The preceding sections of this book make clear that theories often overlap and that some fit easily within broader models. Generally, theories can be used most effectively if they are integrated within a comprehensive planning framework. Such a system assigns a central role to research as input to determine the situation and needs of the population to be served, the resources available, and the progress and effectiveness of the program at various stages. Planning is a continuous process in which new information is gathered to build or improve the program.

Part Five gives specific examples of how theories can be combined for greater impact. PRECEDE-PROCEED—a well-developed planning model that can be used to integrate and apply diverse theoretical frameworks—is discussed in this section. In Chapter Eighteen, Gielen and associates describe the PRECEDE-PROCEED Model for health promotion planning and present two case studies of theory-driven program planning that used the PRECEDE-PROCEED planning model for a child safety program and a diabetes management program.

In Chapter Nineteen, Storey and colleagues describe the purpose, key components, and methods of social marketing. They illustrate the application of social marketing in a family health program in Egypt and an HIV-testing promotion program in Baltimore. These examples illustrate diverse approaches and issues that arise in U.S.-based and international social marketing programs.

In Chapter Twenty, Sallis and colleagues describe the current status of ecological models for health promotion and propose principles that should be followed if these models are to contribute substantially to health promotion research and practice. Ecological models are comprehensive multi-level frameworks for health promotion. This chapter clarifies how ecological models have been advanced and how they are being used for health behavior and health education, and emphasizes the need for greater clarity, precision, and understanding of how these models operate. The authors provide examples, applying ecological models to physical activity behavior, tobacco use, and diabetes self-management.

Chapter Twenty-One describes the rationale for and benefits of evaluating theory-based interventions and examining them in a broader public health perspective. In this chapter, Glasgow and Linnan describe the key components of leading evaluation models, such as the RE-AIM Model, and offer tools and perspectives that are potentially valuable for planning, implementing, evaluating, and interpreting the results of studies of health behavior change interventions.

Using theory thoughtfully and appropriately is not simple, but it can be rewarding. Our aim in Part Five is to bring together many constructs and models and equip readers to work effectively with them in their own practice settings.

CHAPTER

18

USING THE PRECEDE-PROCEED MODEL TO APPLY HEALTH BEHAVIOR THEORIES

Andrea Carlson Gielen

Eileen M. McDonald

Tiffany L. Gary

Lee R. Bone

The SAFE Home Project was funded by the Maternal and Child Health Bureau (MCJ-240638), with additional support provided by the Johns Hopkins Center for Injury Research and Policy, which is funded by the Centers for Disease Control and Prevention, National Center for Injury Prevention and Control (R49/CCR302486). The needs assessment for the SAFE Home project was supported by the Faculty Development Fund of the Johns Hopkins University. Project Sugar was funded by grants from the National Institutes of Health (R01-DK48117 and R00052). We acknowledge the Project Sugar investigators, staff, and the Johns Hopkins General Clinical Research Center (GCRC). We also acknowledge the Project Sugar participants, whose cooperation and support made this research possible.

KEY POINTS

This chapter will

- Provide an overview of the PRECEDE-PROCEED Model.
- Explain the phases of the PRECEDE-PROCEED Model for health promotion program planning.
- Illustrate the use of PRECEDE-PROCEED for choosing and applying behavior change theories and constructs during the intervention planning process.
- Provide two case studies of the application of PRECEDE-PROCEED, using a child safety program (SAFE Home Project) and a diabetes program (Project Sugar 1).

The health professional's ability to apply theories of health behavior is one of the most critical skills needed in designing programs to address contemporary public health problems, virtually all of which address important underlying behavioral risk and protective factors. The PRECEDE-PROCEED planning model can help to put these skills in action. Although the emphasis in PRECEDE-PROCEED has been on its utility for programs delivered in practice settings, the framework has also been useful to researchers conducting health behavior change intervention trials, which we will illustrate in the case studies presented in this chapter.

Individual-level theories, community-level theories, interpersonal communication, printed materials, interactive computer technologies, media campaigns, grassroots organizing—these represent but a few of the tools available to health professionals for designing, implementing, and evaluating health behavior change programs. The appropriate selection and application of these tools can mean the difference between program success and failure. Typically, a problem affecting a particular population has been identified, and the health professional must *do something* to fix the problem, whether it is high rates of obesity among young children in a community or inappropriate use of emergency departments for nonurgent care. A planning model like PRECEDE-PROCEED, which has been a cornerstone of health promotion practice for more than three decades, can help guide this process (Green, Kreuter, Deeds, and Partridge, 1980; Green and Kreuter, 2005).

OVERVIEW OF THE PRECEDE-PROCEED MODEL

PRECEDE-PROCEED can be thought of as a *road map* and behavior change theories as the specific *directions* to a destination. The road map presents all the possible avenues, whereas the theory suggests certain avenues to follow. Unlike the theories described in previous chapters, the main purpose of the PRECEDE-PROCEED Model is not to *predict or explain* the relationship among factors thought to be associated with an outcome of interest. Rather, its main purpose is to provide a structure for *applying theories* and concepts systematically for planning and evaluating health behavior change programs. In Green and Kreuter's most recent version of the model (Green and Kreuter, 2005), they make the point that the numerous applications and validations of PRECEDE-PROCEED support calling it a model and qualifying it as a theoretical or causal model in some of its applications. The authors also distinguish between causal theory that seeks to identify the determinants of an outcome and action theory that attempts to explain how interventions affect the determinants and outcomes. Together, causal and action theories make up program theory, depicted as logic models. PRECEDE-PROCEED is an example of a logic model, in that it links the causal assessment and the intervention planning and evaluation into one overarching planning framework. We will use the terms *model* and *framework* interchangeably in reference to PRECEDE-PROCEED and reserve the use of the term *theory* for causal theories such as the Theory of Planned Behavior (TPB) and the Health Belief Model (HBM).

The PRECEDE framework was developed in the 1970s by Green and colleagues (Green, Kreuter, Deeds, and Partridge, 1980). The acronym stands for Predisposing, Reinforcing, and Enabling Constructs in Educational/Environmental Diagnosis and Evaluation. PRECEDE is based on the premise that, just as medical diagnosis precedes a treatment plan, so should educational diagnosis precede an intervention plan. This approach addressed a concern among some professionals that health education was focused too much on implementing programs and too little on designing interventions that were strategically planned to meet demonstrated needs (Bartholomew, Parcel, Kok, and Gottlieb, 2001).

In 1991, PROCEED (Policy, Regulatory, and Organizational Constructs in Educational and Environmental Development) was added to the framework to recognize the importance of environmental factors as determinants of health and health behaviors. As appreciation of the impact of "lifestyle" (that is, patterns of health-related behaviors) on health grew (McGinnis and Foege, 1993; Mokdad and others, 2004), so did recognition that these behaviors, such as smoking and drinking, are influenced by powerful forces outside the individual, such as industry, media, politics, and social inequalities. Thus, more ecological approaches to health promotion were needed to understand and address these larger contextual determinants of health and health behavior (McLeroy, Bibeau, Steckler, and Glanz, 1988; Institute of Medicine, 2001).

In 2005, PRECEDE-PROCEED was revised again, this time (1) to respond to growing interest in ecological and participatory approaches that have become more widely appreciated as essential elements of public health programs broadly, not only health behavior change programs, and (2) to incorporate rapidly growing new knowledge from the field of genetics (Institute of Medicine, 2001, 2003). This version of PRECEDE-PROCEED is also more streamlined, consisting of four planning phases, one implementation phase, and three evaluation phases (see Figure 18.1). The new version offers a more efficient planning model that (1) merges two phases (that is, epidemiological assessment and behavioral, and environmental assessment) and (2) provides options for skipping phases when appropriate evidence already exists (for example, on community engagement, on specific health objectives). In addition, the new version explicitly discusses the role of genetic factors in addition to the behavioral and environmental determinants of health that must be considered in program planning. Readers are referred to the most recent textbook for more detailed information on the PRECEDE-PROCEED Model (Green and Kreuter, 2005).

The model has not changed in its fundamental principle of participation, which states that success in achieving change is enhanced by the active participation of the

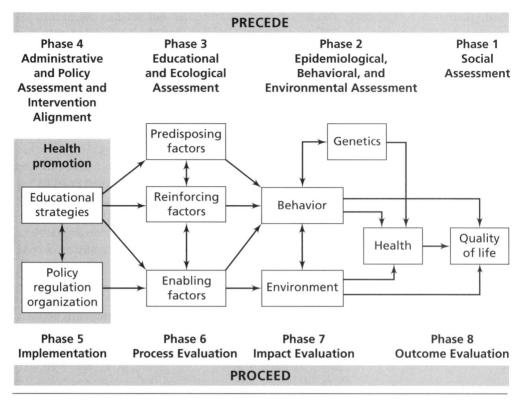

FIGURE 18.1. PRECEDE-PROCEED Planning Model.

intended audience in defining their own high-priority problems and goals and in developing and implementing solutions (Green and Kreuter, 2005; Minkler, 2004; Minkler and Wallerstein, 2002; Israel, Eng, Schulz, and Parker, 2005; see also Chapter Thirteen). Accordingly, at each step in a PRECEDE-PROCEED assessment and planning, efforts should be made to include input from the program's intended audience and stakeholders. The planning process offered by the PRECEDE-PROCEED framework also involves prioritizing the targets for intervention by choosing to address those factors that are most important and most changeable. Finally, measurable objectives are specified throughout the process (for example, Who will do how much of what by when? How much of what—for instance, conditions, circumstances, policies—will be changed by when?).

Phase 1: Social Assessment, Participatory Planning, and Situation Analysis

A social assessment is the "application, through broad participation, of multiple sources of information, both objective and subjective, designed to expand the mutual understanding of people regarding their aspirations for the common good" (Green and Kreuter, 2005). At this stage, the planners expand their understanding of the community in which they are working by conducting multiple data collection activities, such as interviews with key opinion leaders, focus groups with members of the community, observations, and surveys. The term *community* is typically used to mean a geographical area with defined boundaries; more generally, it may be used to describe a group with shared characteristics, interests, values, and norms (see Chapter Thirteen). Today, *virtual communities* exist through the Internet, which, as defined by Demiris (2006), are social units "that involve members who related to one another as a group and interact using communication technologies that bridge geographic distance." In peer-to-peer virtual communities, people with common interests can share experiences and provide social support (Eysenbach and others, 2004), making the Web a potentially useful venue for health promotion programs.

The social assessment articulates the community's needs and desires and considers the community members' problem-solving capacity, their strengths and resources, and their readiness to change. Focusing on community strengths in addition to problems allows the planners and community members to form more effective and meaningful partnerships that will help to support both initial and sustained commitment to the program (Bartholomew, Parcel, Kok, and Gottlieb, 2006). Although programs are often predetermined with regard to audience, health problem, or health behavior problem, the planner should still engage the community in partnership to build the program and link the community's concerns about quality-of-life issues to the program objectives. Developing a planning committee, holding community forums, and conducting focus groups or surveys are all examples of helpful activities to engage the audience in planning and are necessary, regardless of where a planner begins in the PRECEDE-PROCEED process.

An innovative method that may be particularly appropriate for this phase in the planning process is concept mapping (Burke and others, 2005; O'Campo and others, 2005). Concept mapping is a participatory method that allows the planner to obtain a conceptual model of how people understand or feel about a particular topic or issue. It is a structured group activity that allows participants to generate a large number of ideas that are then subjected to quantitative analysis in real time. This analysis results in cluster maps that show participants' ideas in relation to one another, and, with input from the participants, final agreement is reached on the concept maps that best reflect the participants' views.

Theory and Phase 1.   At this phase in the program planning process, community organizing theories and principles are relevant (Table 18.1). Community organization is a process by which community groups are helped to identify common problems or goals, mobilize resources, and develop and implement strategies for reaching the goals they have set collectively (Minkler and Wallerstein, 2002). Minkler's (1985) work in the Tenderloin Project with low-income older adults and Eng and Blanchard's (1991) work conducting a community action diagnosis in a rural county are classic examples of the importance of social assessment and the use of community organizing strategies.

Related to "community organization" but not necessarily as focused on a process that is heavily participant-driven is "community mobilization"—a process that involves community members in activities ranging from defining prevention needs (problem identification, needs assessment, program design) to obtaining community support for a pre-designed program; by definition, it may be "bottom-up" or "top-down" planning or a combination of both (Treno and Holder, 1997). Holder and colleagues (2000) demonstrated the effectiveness of this approach in their community alcohol and trauma program.

Phase 2: Epidemiological, Behavioral, and Environmental Assessments

This phase of the needs assessment identifies the health priorities and their behavioral and environmental determinants.

Epidemiological Assessment. This analysis (1) identifies the health problems, issues, or aspirations on which the program will focus, (2) uncovers the behavioral and environmental factors most likely to influence the identified priority health issues, and (3) translates those priorities into measurable objectives for the program being developed (Green and Kreuter, 2005). Planners can conduct secondary data analysis using existing data sources (for example, vital statistics, state and national health surveys, medical and administrative records). Data necessary for the epidemiological assessment are increasingly available electronically, and health promotion planners should be aware of the various online databases that can provide national, state, and local health data: (1) the National Health Information Center (http://www.health.gov/nhic/), (2) National Library of Medicine Databases and Electronic Resources (http://www.nlm.nih.gov/databases/), and the (3) National Center for Health Statistics (http://www.cdc.gov/nchs/). Sometimes, it is inappropriate to extrapolate from national data to a smaller region, and original data collection on health problems will be necessary. In that case, time and resources will need to be allotted for this planning activity.

Genetics has taken on an increasingly important role in understanding health problems. Although genetic factors are not changeable through a health promotion program, they may be useful to identify high-risk groups for intervention. For example, a program to promote breast cancer screening might include special efforts to reach women with a family history of the disease. As more is learned about the interactions of genes with behavior and the environment, health promotion planners will have much more information with which to target their interventions, and they may be called upon to communicate this new knowledge in ways that help people make informed personal decisions.

Behavioral Determinants. The behavioral determinants of a health problem can be understood on three levels. Most proximal are those behaviors or lifestyles that contribute to the occurrence and severity of a health problem (for example, a teen smoker's tobacco use). The second, more distal determinant is the behavior of others who can directly affect the behavior of the individuals at risk (such as the teen smoker's parents keeping cigarettes in the home). The third and most distal behavioral determinant

TABLE 18.1. PRECEDE-PROCEED Model as an Organizing Framework for Application of Theory and Principles.

Change Theories and Principles by Level of Change	Phase 1: Social Assessment	Phase 2: Epidemiological, Behavioral, and Environmental Assessments	Phase 3: Educational and Ecological Assessment	Phase 4: Administrative and Policy Assessment and Intervention Alignment
Community level:				
Participation and relevance	X	X	X	X
Community organization	X	X	X	X
Community mobilization	X	X	X	X
Organizational change				X
Diffusion of innovation				X
Interpersonal level:				
Social Cognitive Theory		X	X	
Adult learning			X	
Interpersonal communication			X	
Individual level:				
Health Belief Model		X	X	
Stages of Change		X	X	
Theory of Reasoned Action			X	
Theory of Planned Behavior			X	
Information processing			X	

Source: Adapted from Glanz and Rimer, 1995.

is the action of decision makers whose decisions affect the social or physical environment that influences the individuals at risk (for example, actions by police to enforce laws that restrict youth access to cigarettes). By thinking about these three levels of behavioral determinants of the health problem, the program planner increases the likelihood that comprehensive and effective interventions will be created.

Environmental Determinants. Environmental factors are those social and physical factors external to the individual, often beyond his or her personal control, that can be modified to support the behavior or influence the health outcome. Modifying environmental factors usually requires strategies other than education. For example, poor nutritional status among school children is a function of poor dietary habits (most proximal behavioral factor), which in turn may be partly affected by the availability of unhealthy foods in schools (environmental factor). Although an educational program could effectively teach students about healthy diets, it would not change institutional policies about making healthy foods available in schools. Other strategies, including influencing the behaviors of school decision makers such as food service managers (a more distal behavioral factor), would be required.

Theory and Phase 2. Using theory, literature, and the planning group's input, an inventory should be made of behavioral and environmental influencing factors. Interpersonal theories of behavior change can be useful at this stage of the PRECEDE-PROCEED framework because of the emphasis on the interaction between individuals and their environment (Table 18.1). Social Cognitive Theory (SCT) posits that behavior, cognition, and other personal factors have reciprocal relationships with environments, so they continually influence one another, and that behavior is influenced by observing others and by receiving reinforcement (see Chapter Eight). Planners should consider how these constructs can be used to help specify behavioral and environmental factors that contribute to the health problem of interest. For example, in the assessment for a program to reduce low birth weight, consideration should be given to whether there are women in the community who model appropriate use of prenatal care and whether community leaders and health professionals reinforce it.

Organizational change theories are particularly relevant when the policies and practices of formal organizations have been identified as environmental factors to be changed (Erlich, Rothman, and Teresa, 1999; see Chapter Fifteen). For example, in a worksite, policies restricting smoking may need to be strengthened; planners need to understand how organizational policy can be changed if they are to make a reasonable estimate of the changeability of this environmental factor. Community mobilization may be used to change environmental conditions that directly affect individuals' health or that influence health behaviors (Treno and Holder, 1997). Similarly, diffusion of innovations theory describes and predicts the process by which new ideas are adopted in a community (Rogers, 2003; see Chapter Fourteen). If, for example, the assessment at this point suggests that an important behavioral factor is bicycle helmet use, then evaluating its changeability according to diffusion theory would consider such features of helmets as their observability by others, perceptions of their relative advantage, and how compatible their use is with existing norms.

Phase 3: Educational and Ecological Assessment

After selecting the relevant behavioral and environmental factors for intervention, the framework directs planners to identify the antecedent and reinforcing factors that should be in place to initiate and sustain the change process. These factors are classified as *predisposing, reinforcing,* and *enabling,* and they collectively influence the likelihood that behavioral and environmental change will occur. "*Predisposing factors* are antecedents to behavior that provide the rationale or motivation for the behavior" (Green and Kreuter, 2005); they include individuals' knowledge, attitudes, beliefs, personal preferences, existing skills, and self-efficacy beliefs. "*Reinforcing factors* are those factors following a behavior that provide continuing reward or incentive for the persistence or repetition of the behavior" (Green and Kreuter, 2005). Examples include social support, peer influence, significant others, and vicarious reinforcement. "*Enabling factors* are antecedents to behavioral or environmental change that allow a motivation or environmental policy to be realized" (Green and Kreuter, 2005). Enabling factors can affect behavior directly or indirectly through an environmental factor. They include programs, services, and resources necessary for behavioral and environmental outcomes to be realized and, in some cases, the new skills needed to enable behavior change.

Theory and Phase 3. All three levels of change theories—individual, interpersonal, and community—can be useful at this stage of the planning process (Table 18.1). Individual-level theories generally are most appropriate for addressing predisposing factors. They help planners identify messages for direct communication methods such as mass media and face-to-face education, as well as for newer technologies such as computer tailoring of health messages (Kreuter, Farrell, Olevitch, and Brennan, 2000). Interpersonal-level theories are most appropriate for reinforcing factors, and they suggest indirect communication channels (for example, through significant others, social networks) and methods (for example, train-the-trainer models, social support enhancement). Community-level theories are most appropriate for enabling factors, and they suggest environmental changes (for example, organization and delivery of services; availability of products; policies, laws, and regulations that govern products and behaviors,) and methods such as grassroots organizing and advocacy (Clark and McLeroy, 1995).

For example, in a community with high teen pregnancy and sexually transmitted disease (STD) rates, community norms and teen attitudes may support the use of contraception, but teens may not have access to confidential reproductive planning services. In this case, organizational change theories can provide more effective guidance, as they would suggest ways to enable the delivery of services through on-site school-based clinics or other structures. In another example, planners of a program to promote bicycle helmet use might learn that children find helmets uncomfortable, fear "looking nerdy," and believe they won't get hurt on their bikes. These unfavorable attitudes might be best addressed, from a diffusion theory perspective, by emphasizing the relative advantage, compatibility, and observability attributes of helmet use that would be meaningful to children in the community. Drawing also on SCT, these findings would suggest that social influence plays an important role in both predisposing and reinforcing helmet use. Finally, if children's personal beliefs are that bike riding is not dangerous, application of a theory such as the HBM (Chapter Three) will help. The model includes the construct of perceived susceptibility, which would be an important predisposing factor for helmet use in this hypothetical example.

Phase 4: Administrative and Policy Assessment and Intervention Alignment

In Phase 4, the planner selects and aligns the program's components (that is, interventions) with the priority determinants of change previously identified. Its purpose is to identify resources, organizational barriers and facilitators, and policies that are needed for program implementation and sustainability.

When creating the program plan, it is important to look at two levels of alignment between the assessment of determinants and the selection of interventions (Green and Kreuter, 2005). First, at the macro level, the organizational and environmental systems that can affect the desired outcomes should be considered. These are interventions that affect enabling factors for environmental change, which in turn support the desired health behavior or health outcome. Second, at the micro level, the focus is on individual, peer, family, and others who can influence the intended audience's health behaviors more directly. Interventions at the micro level are specifically directed at changing the predisposing, reinforcing, and enabling factors. There are many available strategies, such as mass and small media, counseling, and advocacy, and the "best" strategy is the one that matches the context of the program, the audience's needs, and the theory of the problem that the PRECEDE-PROCEED diagnosis has uncovered. Typically, successful programs use multiple strategies to have an effective impact on complex health issues.

Green and Kreuter (2005) have drawn on a body of literature about program development to offer recommendations for "intervention matching, mapping, pooling and patching" at this stage of planning (Simons-Morton, Greene, and Gottlieb, 1995; D'Onofrio, 2001). Specifically, building a comprehensive program requires (1) *matching* the ecological levels to broad program components; (2) *mapping* specific interventions based on theory and prior research and practice to specific predisposing, enabling, and reinforcing factors, and (3) *pooling* prior interventions and community-preferred interventions that might have less evidence to support them, and if necessary, (4) *patching* those interventions to fill gaps in the evidence-based best practices.

Theory and Phase 4.   The mapping of interventions to predisposing, reinforcing, and enabling factors is influenced by theoretical considerations similar to those described in Phase 3, focusing mainly on community-level theories (Table 18.1). Organizational change theory addresses the processes and strategies for creating and sustaining changes in health policies and procedures that influence the success of health promotion programs.

Phases 5–8: Implementation and Evaluation

At this point, the health promotion program is ready for implementation (Phase 5). Data collection plans should be in place for evaluating the process, impact, and outcome of the program, which are the final three phases in the PRECEDE-PROCEED planning model (Phases 6–8). Typically, process evaluation determines the extent to which the program was implemented according to protocol. Impact evaluation assesses change in predisposing, reinforcing, and enabling factors, as well as in the behavioral and environmental factors. Finally, outcome evaluation determines the effect of the program on health and quality-of-life indicators. Generally, the measurable objectives that are written at each step of the PRECEDE-PROCEED planning model serve as milestones against which accomplishments are evaluated. Because the emphasis in this chapter is on the application of behavior change theory to program planning, the details of these phases will not be reviewed. Rather, their application will be described in two case studies that follow.

ISSUES TO CONSIDER IN USING PRECEDE-PROCEED

Despite its wide adoption and considerable success, potential users of PRECEDE-PROCEED should be aware of some of the challenges in applying the model. The model is heavily data-driven, and its application may require greater financial and human resources, technical skill, and time than are available in some situations (Bertera, 1990; Orenstein and others, 1992), thus frustrating community planning teams interested in taking immediate action to address a problem. Green and Kreuter (2005) describe situation analysis within the context of the social assessment as a way toward a balanced approach to planning—that is, one that neither shortcuts nor belabors the process. It may be possible to shorten some of the model's intermediate assessment phases by using the growing body of literature on frequently identified community priorities, determinants, and targets for change.

The PRECEDE-PROCEED planning process also does not emphasize the specifics of intervention development and methods in detail. Planners may find it helpful to incorporate Bartholomew and colleagues' (2006) *intervention mapping* process at this stage. This approach guides planners to select theory-based intervention methods that are then operationalized and organized as specific strategies. For example, a PRECEDE-PROCEED assessment may determine that the absence of role models for a particular behavior is a reinforcing factor to be addressed in a program. Intervention mapping would identify role modeling as a theory-based *method* (derived from SCT) to be used in the program; a *strategy* for implementing this method could be the development and distribution of printed role-model stories.

Another set of methods for the contemporary health promotion planner is the use of computers and the Internet (van den Berg and others, 2007; Cline and Haynes, 2001). Computer-tailored health communication has demonstrated its effectiveness across a range of behavioral outcomes, and methods for developing and implementing tailored messages have been well articulated (Kreuter, Jacobsen, McDonald, and Gielen, 2003; Gielen and others, 2007; McDonald and others, 2005; Kroeze, Werkman, and Brug, 2006). Wantland and colleagues (2004) noted that from 1996–2003, there was a twelve-fold increase in MEDLINE citations for "Web-based therapies." Their meta-analysis of the effectiveness of Web-based interventions for behavior change concluded that Web-based interventions often had better knowledge and behavior change outcomes than non-Web-based interventions. Powell and colleagues' (2005) review concludes, however, that there remains much to learn about how consumers are actually using the Internet as a health information resource. Virtual reality technology has an emerging body of literature in both the rehabilitation and physical medicine field (Chuang, Sung, and Lin, 2005; Crosbie, Lennon, Basford, and McDonough, 2007), as well as in the injury-prevention field (Thomson and others, 2005; Ku and others, 2002), although much more work is needed to fully understand both its potential and limitations as an intervention method for health promotion.

CASE STUDY: THE SAFE HOME PROJECT

The SAFE Home Project was an intervention trial aimed at reducing in-home childhood injury risk among low-income, urban families. It was conducted between 1994 and 1999. The project took place in a pediatric continuity clinic that provided medical care to children living in one of the most impoverished areas of Baltimore City. This case study describes the application of PRECEDE-PROCEED to the planning, implementation, and evaluation of the project. Results of the study have been published elsewhere (Gielen and others, 2001, 2002; McDonald and others, 2003); readers should consult those sources for additional information.

Social and Epidemiological Assessment (Phases 1 and 2)

Injuries occurring in the home and their associated impact on quality of life were defined at the outset (Figure 18.2). This injury focus was driven, in part, by the availability of evidence supporting an injury initiative, professional interest and expertise of the research team, data to support home injuries as a significant public health problem, and the availability of known, effective safety products to minimize injuries.

The first two phases of PRECEDE-PROCEED—the social and epidemiological assessment—relied heavily on a review of the literature and data on injuries among the intended audience. The prevalence of injuries among children in the local area was documented with a one-year analysis of the hospital database. Input from parents was solicited to confirm that injury prevention was an important topic to families. Informal surveys in the clinic waiting room were used to ask parents about "things that concern you as a parent," and child health and safety issues were frequently mentioned. When asked specifically to rank childhood injury in terms of its overall importance, about half the parents identified it as among their "most important" concerns.

These two phases in the process were conducted without drawing on any specific behavior change theory. However, the principles of *participation* and *relevance* were used. Parents were engaged in the program planning process through the informal survey in this phase, as well as in subsequent phases, as described next.

Behavioral, Environmental, Educational, and Ecological Assessment (Phases 2 and 3)

Based on the literature and advice from pediatricians, the most important and most changeable behavioral factors associated with in-home injuries in preschool-age chil-

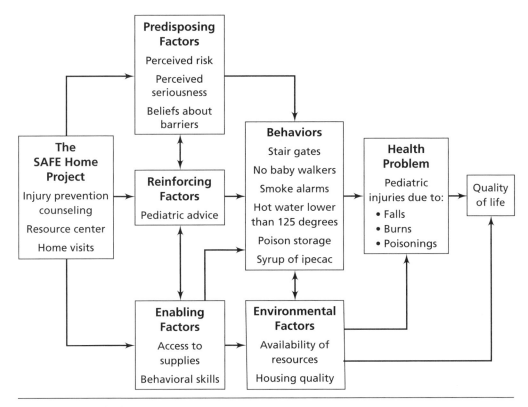

FIGURE 18.2. Application of PRECEDE-PROCEED to Injury Prevention.

dren were found to be a cluster of behaviors, commonly referred to as "childproof-ing" (Wilson and others, 1991). For falls, burns, and poisonings, this included six safety practices: using stair gates, not using baby walkers, having working smoke alarms, turning down the hot water temperature to less than 125 degrees, keeping poi-sonous substances locked away, and having syrup of ipecac in the home. (At the time this research was conducted, syrup of ipecac was recommended as a poison-preven-tion strategy for homes with young children. The American Academy of Pediatrics [1994] and other professional groups have since withdrawn this recommendation.) At the time, the literature offered little guidance about the relevant environmental factors associated with childproofing or with children's in-home injury experience. Therefore, additional data collection was needed, and parent interviews and analy-sis of audiotaped well-child visits were conducted (Gielen and others, 1995, 1997).

Data from Parents. Parent interviews were guided by the Theory of Planned Behav-ior (TPB; see Chapter Four) and examined the roles of personal beliefs about the con-sequences of childproofing, general attitudes toward childproofing, subjective norms, and barriers and facilitators of childproofing, including environmental factors. A con-venience sample of 150 parents in the clinic (Gielen and others, 1995) were inter-viewed to provide quantifiable data on parents' injury-prevention practices (*behavioral* *factor)* and associated *environmental factors,* as well as *predisposing, reinforcing, and enabling* determinants. Only 5 percent of respondents reported doing all six child-proofing practices, although virtually all respondents expressed favorable *personal beliefs and attitudes* about childproofing, and the majority reported positive *subjective norms* favoring childproofing. In terms of environmental factors, housing quality, income, and *barriers* to childproofing—such as not having help from others and moving often—were significantly associated with the number of childproofing practices reported.

Constructs from the TPB were helpful in demonstrating the importance of barriers to parents but did not help to identify key beliefs that distinguished parents who practiced childproofing from those who did not. The HBM (see Chapter Three) and the Precaution Adoption Process Model (PAPM; see Chapter Six) suggest that parents' perceptions of the *risk of injury* and the *salience of this threat* might help to explain their adoption of safety practices.

These data demonstrate that disadvantaged living conditions, including a lack of resources and skills, interfere with parents' ability to implement safety practices, and uniformly favorable attitudes and norms suggest that a risk-oriented theory may be more useful for developing an intervention that would influence parents' safety practices.

Data from Pediatricians.   One of the reinforcing factors suggested by the parent interviews was routine injury-prevention counseling by pediatricians. Theoretical and empirical support for their role was bolstered by evidence that the communication style of physicians has an impact on patient outcomes and that adherence to principles of adult learning in counseling increases the chances of behavior change (Roter, 1989; U.S. Preventive Services Task Force, 1996; Green and Kreuter, 1999). To better understand pediatricians' potential role in the intervention, an analysis of 214 audiotaped pediatric visits collected as part of another study in the same clinic (Wissow, Roter, and Wilson, 1994) was used to determine the types of injury topics discussed and the communication skills used (Gielen and others, 1997). The majority (61 percent) of visits did not include any discussion of injury prevention, and among those that did, the average length of time spent on injury topics was 1.08 minutes per child. The most common communication pattern used by physicians was information giving, with little involvement of parents in any discussion. These data indicated that injury-prevention counseling was not a routine component of pediatric well-child care, potentially effective behavior change counseling skills were not widely evident, and prioritizing injury topics and enhancing communication skills should help pediatricians use limited time effectively and efficiently.

Predisposing, enabling, and reinforcing factors were derived from the assessments described earlier. For *predisposing factors,* parents had extremely favorable attitudes toward childproofing, and it was hypothesized that their perceptions about the likelihood and seriousness of the risk of injury would be important determinants of their childproofing behaviors. With regard to *reinforcing factors,* mothers reported that their social support networks felt childproofing the home was important. Professional associations endorsed injury-prevention counseling by pediatricians during well-child visits. One potentially important reinforcing factor was clearly missing:

effective pediatric advice regarding childproofing. Finally, in terms of *enabling factors,* access to safety supplies and the skills or assistance to use them effectively were identified as important and missing. The next step in the process was translating these findings into effective intervention strategies.

Administrative and Policy Assessment and Implementation (Phases 4 and 5)

Three distinct yet related interventions were identified: (1) enhancing pediatricians' injury-prevention counseling, (2) developing a clinic-based safety resource center, and (3) conducting home visits. Administrative and policy aspects of implementing these interventions are described here.

Enhanced Pediatric Counseling. Pediatric residents completed five hours of training that covered developmentally appropriate injury-prevention topics (falls, burns, poisonings) to discuss with parents, as well as specific communication skills to use for greater success in improving parents' adoption of safety behaviors. As a result of the training, residents were expected to provide enhanced anticipatory guidance on injury prevention as a routine part of well-child care.

A number of theories were useful in the development and implementation of the enhanced pediatric counseling component. The primary objective was to enable pediatricians to heighten parents' perceptions about the risk and seriousness of childhood injuries and to help them overcome specific barriers to injury prevention that are associated with living conditions in the inner city. In addition to drawing on these issues identified in the parent interview, constructs from Stages of Change and Information Processing were included in the training. Pediatricians were educated about the notion that behavior change is a process and that individuals are at different levels of readiness to change (Prochaska, DiClemente, and Norcross, 1992; see Chapter Five). Incorporating ideas about information processing capacity—specifically that people are limited in the amount of information they can use and remember—we taught pediatricians how to select the most important injury-prevention advice to communicate. Principles of adult learning and SCT were used to implement the enhanced pediatric counseling training successfully. Because residents brought to the training a considerable amount of experience communicating with parents, these experiences were drawn out in discussions during the training. Experiential teaching techniques were used, such as "skills stations" for hands-on practice with safety supplies (for example, smoke detectors, stair gates), shopping trips (for example, to purchase syrup of ipecac), and demonstrations (for example, walker falling down stairs). Role-playing opportunities were provided for residents to both observe and model effective communication and counseling skills. As residents practiced integrating new communication skills and safety messages into their counseling repertoire in the role plays, faculty trainers observed them and provided immediate feedback and critiques.

On-Site Safety Resource Center. The safety resource center was intended to reduce barriers of access to and costs of safety supplies—the enabling factors identified in earlier diagnostic phases. However, predisposing factors were also addressed because education was provided by a trained health educator at the center. The objectives of the center were to increase the accessibility and affordability of home safety supplies for low-income families; to provide personalized, skills-oriented education that reinforces and supplements pediatric advice about child safety, and to elevate the priority given to injury prevention in medical care settings. Parents who came to the Children's Safety Center received personalized home safety risk assessments and education, and could purchase safety products at reduced cost.

Many administrative and organizational constraints surfaced during the planning for this intervention component: space in the clinic for the center; renovation costs for the space, staffing, selecting, and stocking of supplies and educational materials, and access to the center by families who did not receive care in the clinic. A full year of planning was devoted to these issues before the center opened in March 1997 (McDonald and others, 2003).

The principles of participation and relevance were high priorities for developing the Children's Safety Center. Focus groups with parents were conducted to obtain their ideas about the role of the center, the supplies it should carry, and its operating policies and procedures. The notion of "empowerment" also influenced this component of the project. The clinic's Parent Advisory Board was consulted about plans for the center, and also for the home visit component (described next). Because pediatric residents made referrals to the center, their input was solicited to shape the policies and procedures of the center.

Home Visits. The third intervention—home visits—addressed another recognized enabling factor: skills to adopt childproofing practices. Home visits were conducted by community health workers (CHW), who described and demonstrated appropriate safety practices (such as changing a smoke alarm battery, testing the water temperature) and then allowed mothers to practice and master these skills. The CHWs did not actually install products, due to liability concerns. Throughout the visit, efforts were made to emphasize predisposing factors, such as perceptions of injury risk and seriousness. The CHWs also reinforced education that may have been provided by the pediatrician or health educator in the Children's Safety Center.

The administrative and organizational aspects of implementing this intervention were challenging. Time and commitment from administrative staff were required for training, supervising, and providing for the safety of the CHWs. It was especially important to develop a mechanism to make referrals for housing code violations, because poor housing quality had been identified by parents as a barrier to implementing safety practices.

Community empowerment and capacity building were supported by employing health workers from the community where the families lived. Moreover, the tasks of the CHW were informed by the SCT constructs of role modeling and self-efficacy.

Process, Impact, and Outcome Evaluation (Phases 6–8)

Process evaluation data were collected to document how well program components were implemented as planned and how well the intended audiences were reached. Enhanced injury-prevention counseling was documented by audiotaping all pediatric visits with families enrolled in the project. Data were collected and monitored throughout the project to document completion of the home visits and use of the Children's Safety Center.

Impact evaluation was conducted, using a randomized controlled trial of two cohorts of pediatricians and their patients' parents (Gielen and others, 2001, 2002; McDonald and others, 2003; see Figure 18.3). In both cohorts, parents were enrolled when they brought their 0- to 6-month-old child to a clinic visit, and families were followed until the child was 12 to 18 months old. Baseline and follow-up surveys of parents' knowledge, beliefs, and barriers (predisposing, reinforcing, enabling factors) were completed, and home observations were used to document safety practices and household hazards (behavioral and environmental factors). Cohort 1 pediatricians (and their patients' parents) were randomized to either a control or intervention group. Pediatricians in both groups attended a one-hour seminar on pediatric injuries, provided by the director of general pediatrics, as part of their routine pediatric education. Pediatricians in the intervention group also participated in the more intensive

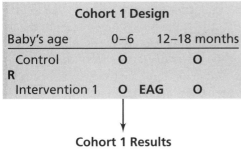

Cohort 1 Results
Training physicians in EAG significantly increased pediatric injury prevention counseling and parent satisfaction with safety information.

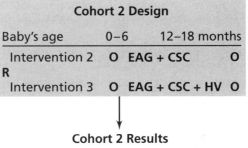

Cohort 2 Results
Adding a single HV to EAG and CSC had no effect on parents' safety behaviors. Families in both intervention groups who visited the CSC adopted significantly more safety behaviors compared to those who did not, controlling for selected confounders.

Key

R = Random assignment

Interventions:
EAG = Enhanced Anticipatory Guidance
CSC = Children's Safety Center
HV = Home Visit

Observations:
O = Baseline and follow-up interviews, audiotapes of pediatric visits from enrollment to follow-up; home observations of safety behaviors at follow-up

FIGURE 18.3. Safe Home Case Study Design and Results.

training. Before the start of Cohort 2 enrollment, the on-site Children's Safety Center was opened, and Cohort 2 pediatricians (and their patients' parents) were recruited and randomly assigned to one of two intervention groups. Pediatricians in both intervention groups in Cohort 2 received the same intensive training that was used in Cohort 1, and all parents had access to the Children's Safety Center. One-half of Cohort 2 parents were randomized to receive a home visit when their babies were 6 to 9 months old.

In Cohort 1, physicians who received the intensive training provided significantly more injury-prevention counseling, compared to those who did not receive the training, and patients' families were more satisfied with the information they received. However, there were no differences between the groups on their home safety knowledge, beliefs, and self-reported practices, or on observed safety practices (Gielen and others, 2001). In Cohort 2, the home visit intervention had no effect on observed safety practices, although families who visited the Children's Safety Center (n = 75), compared to those who did not (n = 74), were using significantly more safety products and practices, even after adjusting for their exposure to the other intervention components (that is, counseling and home visits) and for potential selection biases (Gielen and others, 2002). The results of these evaluation activities suggest that short-term improvements in physician counseling practices, parent satisfaction, and home safety were achieved. Also, of the theoretical constructs used to guide program design, the enabling factors were paramount for the issue of home safety in this low-income, urban sample. It was not feasible to conduct an outcome evaluation because it would have required a much longer follow-up period and larger sample.

CASE STUDY: PROJECT SUGAR 1

Project Sugar 1 was a randomized controlled trial of community outreach and primary-care-based interventions to improve diabetic control in adults. The study population consisted of 186 African American adults with type 2 diabetes living in East Baltimore. This case study highlights the application of the PRECEDE-PROCEED model to the program. The design and details of the study have been described in two publications (Gary and others, 2003; Gary and others, 2001), and readers who want more information should refer to those articles.

Social and Epidemiological Assessment (Phases 1 and 2)

An informal social assessment for this project was based on the investigators' understanding of the community, acquired while providing diabetes care and conducting intervention projects with community members for more than twenty years. Complications from diabetes can have a significant detrimental effect on individuals' quality of life; health problems to address with diabetics include their HbA1c levels, blood pressure, lipids, weight, and other general health status factors (see Figure 18.4).

The literature was used to define the burden of diabetes among African Americans. The prevalence and incidence of type 2 diabetes is higher in African Americans than in whites (Tull and Roseman, 1995; Carter, Pugh, and Monterrosa, 1996; Brancati and others, 2000). Further, the rate of diabetic retinopathy is twice as high com-

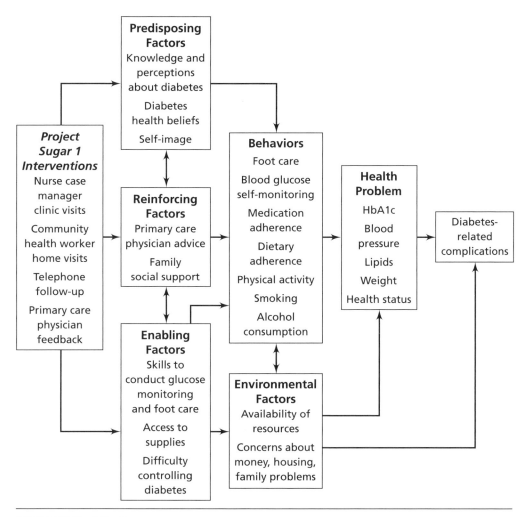

FIGURE 18.4. Application of PRECEDE-PROCEED to Diabetes Care and Self-Management Interventions.

pared to whites, and severe visual impairment is 40 percent higher among African Americans than whites. The excess risk of diabetic nephropathy, including end stage renal disease (ESRD), is 2–5 times greater in African Americans than in whites, and the amputation rate is 1.2 times higher (Tull and Roseman, 1995). The excess risk of complications in African Americans may be due to potentially modifiable factors, including individual and physician behaviors, and interactions with the health care system (Brown and others, 2004). Interventions to promote foot care, blood glucose self-monitoring, medication adherence, and physical activity while reducing smoking and alcohol consumption may substantially reduce the excess burden of medical complications of diabetes in African Americans.

As medical care providers active in the East Baltimore community, the program planners were well aware of environmental factors contributing to the problem. Few culturally competent programs were available to assist community members interested in secondary prevention measures to minimize complications. Moreover, planners were familiar with community members' concerns about their lack of financial resources, housing issues, and family problems.

Behavioral, Environmental, Educational, and Ecological Assessment (Phases 3 and 4)

PRECEDE-PROCEED guided intervention development by focusing planners on consideration of multiple factors. For diabetes care this includes recognition of factors at the individual, provider, and health care system levels. Individuals may have limited knowledge, as well as beliefs and attitudes that prevent them from remaining in care, modifying their lifestyle, or taking medications and following the treatment regimen.

Important reinforcing factors may not be available. Primary care providers, who are generally responsible for providing care for most individuals with diabetes, may not adhere to clinical recommendations or may lack the time or skills to provide effective health education. Social support provided by family members can be another important reinforcing factor that is not fully realized. Finally, systems issues such as the discontinuity of care within the health care system and lack of access to adequate health care may hinder the supportive relationship between the individual, provider, and health care system. Additional important enabling factors identified included patients' lack of skills to conduct glucose monitoring and foot care, and problems with access to necessary supplies. All of these factors contribute to poor metabolic control (HbA1c, as well as blood pressure and lipid control), which in turn, leads to diabetes complications.

Administrative and Policy Assessment and Implementation (Phases 5 and 6)

Recent evidence from the Diabetes Control and Complications Trial (1993) and the United Kingdom Prospective Diabetes Study (UK Prospective Diabetes Study, 1998) suggests that achieving low HbA1c levels, or tight glycemic control, can substantially reduce the risk of complications. However, the translation of this evidence into clinical practice is still uneven. The adoption of proven practice patterns is inconsistent. Nurses have generally been used to supplement diabetes care by providing case management and education (Norris and others, 2002). Also, community health workers (CHW) have served as liaisons between the patient, health care system, and the family, in addition to providing diabetes education and social services (Norris and others, 2006). Previous intervention studies in diabetes care have not evaluated combinations of enhanced medical practice and community outreach (that is, home visits), and few have developed and evaluated culturally sensitive interventions for African Americans (Sarkisian and others, 2003; Gary and others, 2003).

Four intervention components were developed to address the multiple determinants that can positively or negatively affect individual and environmental factors related to preventing medical complications of type 2 diabetes. These include nurse case manager (NCM) clinical visits, CHW home visits, telephone follow-up, and primary care physician feedback. NCM interventions were forty-five-minute face-to-face clinic visits or telephone contacts. These providers coordinated care by assessing and monitoring diabetes status between clinic visits, and intervening as necessary for all participants assigned to the enhanced practice and the combined group. They conducted diabetes monitoring, and provided direct patient care, management, education, counseling, follow-up, and referrals. They also played key roles to complement the physician feedback and prompting (described next), by advising regimen changes and implementing changes under the physician's orders. The goal was to conduct visits at least three times per year, plus additional contacts as needed. The NCM also was available to the patient between visits.

The CHW, a woman recruited from the community, was a local high school graduate who was enrolled in college part-time and had no formal training in health care before the study (Hill-Briggs and others, 2007). CHW interventions were forty-five–sixty-minute-minute face-to-face home visits or telephone contacts. Unlike the NCM, the CHW did not directly execute therapeutic strategies (for example, changing medication doses). The CHW encouraged preventive care by addressing barriers to patients' adherence to treatment regimens. Her main responsibility was to assess patient and family behavior related to diabetes care and to reinforce adherence to treatment recommendations, mobilize support, and provide feedback to physicians, including reporting on identifiable problems such as high blood pressure readings or dietary habits. The goal was to conduct visits approximately three times per year, plus additional contacts as needed. Like the NCM, the CHW was available to the patient between visits as needed.

The two remaining program components—telephone follow-up and physician feedback—were provided as needed by both the NCM and CHW. Participants were encouraged to contact their interventionist (NCM or CHW, depending on which study group they were assigned to), and the interventionists were encouraged to report relevant patient findings to primary care providers.

Process, Impact, and Outcome Evaluation (Phases 7–9)

The evaluation of Project Sugar 1 was completed using a randomized controlled trial in which participants were randomized to one of four parallel study arms for a period of three years: (1) usual medical care (control); (2) usual medical care + Nurse Case Manager Intervention (NCM); (3) usual medical care + Community Health Worker Intervention (CHW), or (4) usual medical care + NCM + CHW Combined Intervention. Participants assigned to the usual medical care (control) group received ongoing care from their own health professionals. In addition, they received a quarterly newsletter that contained information on various diabetes-related health topics and ongoing trial results (for example, baseline demographic profile of all participants). The combined intervention group received visits from both the NCM and CHW.

All initial intervention visits focused on multiple domains: diet, physical activity, foot care, vision care, glucose self-monitoring, blood pressure control, medication and appointment adherence, referrals, and smoking cessation (Batts and others, 2001). Participants were asked to choose three priority areas from this list for attention at future visits. Interventionists (either NCM or CHW) completed a baseline assessment of each participant, and subsequent visits were tailored to address the overlapping areas between patient priorities and baseline assessment. Interventionists attended one- to two-hour weekly meetings initially with project investigators. Cases were presented at these meetings to address barriers related to the predisposing, enabling, and reinforcing factors featured in the PRECEDE-PROCEED framework. Both types of interventionists maintained ongoing charts of each intervention interaction and documented all interactions with participants. Clinical flow sheets and summaries of intervention visits, including phone interventions, were documented for the study, as well as for providers. In addition to intervention visits, yearly follow-up study visits were conducted to track the participants' diabetes progress. Questions were asked about behaviors and attitudes related to diabetes, and clinical measurements were also obtained.

The main results of the Project Sugar 1 interventions are presented in Table 18.2. Overall, the trial had good intervention participation and led to modest improvements

TABLE 18.2. Main Results of Project Sugar 1 Interventions.

Intervention Participation	25% in the NCM groups and 62% in the CHW groups received at least three visits
	50% of participants had at least one telephone intervention
	Overall, more individuals were seen in the CHW groups
Intention-to-Treat Analyses	Modest improvements in HbA1c (0.8%) for the combined NCM/CHW group compared to controls
	Statistically significant declines in triglycerides and diastolic blood pressure for the combined NCM/CHW group compared to controls
	Statistically significant improvements in health-related quality of life (SF-36 scale); higher scores on the vitality subscale for the NCM only and the CHW-only group
	Within-group changes were statistically significant for many outcomes
On-Treatment Analyses (at least one face-to-face intervention visit)	Similar to intention-to-treat analyses
	Within-group declines in HbA1c for the CHW only and the combined NCM/CHW group

NCM = Nurse Case Manager, CHW = Community Health Worker

Sources: Gary and others, 2003; Hill-Briggs, Gary, Baptiste-Roberts, and Brancati, 2005.

in clinical parameters and health-related quality of life (Gary and others, 2003; Hill-Briggs, Gary, Baptiste-Roberts, and Brancati, 2005). The most noted improvements were shown for the combined NCM-CHW group. Over all, intervention groups showed greater improvements in metabolic control than did controls. This pattern was also found for the study's main outcome, HbA1c. Although clinically significant improvements were shown, they did not reach statistical significance. The sample size (n = 186 across 4 groups) had limited statistical power. After adjustment for covariates, the effect on triglycerides and diastolic blood pressure in the combined group was statistically significant. However, these significant results should be interpreted with caution because no adjustments were made for comparisons on several different outcome measures.

One surprise surfaced from the results: the CHW and the NCM individual groups produced similar effects. In fact, changes in the NCM and CHW groups were comparable for all parameters of metabolic control except systolic and diastolic blood pressure, in which the CHW group had a greater effect (Gary and others, 2003). The CHW group also had better improvements in dietary risk scores and leisure time physical activity than the NCM group. One explanation for this similarity may be the differential intervention participation. Intervention participation was much higher in the CHW groups, with 62 percent of the participants in the CHW groups completing at least three visits, compared to only 25 percent of participants in the NCM groups. Not surprisingly, the combined NCM-CHW group had the largest effect for all parameters except HDL cholesterol and systolic blood pressure. These results suggest that the CHW role may be an essential component of the diabetes care team. In other analyses of the intervention data, we found that 77 percent of the intervention visits addressed needs outside the defined intervention diabetes-specific focus areas, including social systems, insurance, and other health concerns (Batts and others, 2001), providing evidence that CHWs can provide comprehensive care regarding social and some medical needs. The findings suggest that for the best results, a NCM-CHW team may be most effective.

SUMMARY

PRECEDE-PROCEED is a widely used planning model that has guided the design of programs in a varied array of settings and for numerous health problems (for example, Morisky and others, 1983; Bertera, 1993; Gielen, 1992; Wright and others, 2006; Chiang, Huang, and Lu, 2003; Zimmerman and others, 2001; Gary and others, 2003; see also http://www.lgreen.net for an extensive bibliography). The model has also been incorporated into national policy documents for community health (Centers for Disease Control, 1992) and injury control (National Committee, 1989). An interactive computerized version of the model, called EMPOWER, has been developed for community-level cancer prevention and control interventions.

Following the sequential phases of PRECEDE-PROCEED helps ensure that program development can be replicated and that phases in the process can be documented for later critique. It also provides touch points for applying health behavior theories. At each phase it is wise to consider the impact of new analyses on previous decisions. Program planning is usually an iterative process in which prior decisions are constantly being evaluated in light of new data, resources, and other decisions, as was illustrated in the case studies. The PRECEDE-PROCEED Model can be used to enhance evaluation of health problems, health behaviors, and desired changes and can serve as a guide for intervention planning and evaluation. This model provides a structured framework for applying health behavior theories at all levels. Consistent with principles of community-based participatory research, this model emphasizes community participation in selecting priority behaviors or issues to be addressed. Finally, the framework encourages a multidisciplinary approach and a comprehensive assessment of the multiple factors that contribute to today's public health problems.

In this chapter, we have presented an overview of the history and current conceptualization of the PRECEDE-PROCEED framework, focusing on its utility for integrating theory into health promotion program planning. The two case studies demonstrate the flexibility of the framework for developing different types of programs, both for primary and secondary prevention and in response to injury as well as chronic disease. PRECEDE-PROCEED provides a systematic approach for priority setting among the myriad determinants of many of today's complex health problems and the options for interventions.

REFERENCES

American Academy of Pediatrics. *TIPP: The Injury Prevention Program: A Guide to Safety Counseling in Office Practice.* Chicago, Ill.: American Academy of Pediatrics, 1994.

Bartholomew, L. K., Parcel, G. S., Kok, G., and Gottlieb, N. H. *Planning Health Promotion Programs: An Intervention Mapping Approach.* San Francisco: Jossey-Bass, 2006.

Batts, M. L., and others. "Patient Priorities and Needs for Diabetes Care among Urban African American Adults." *The Diabetes Educator,* 2001, *27,* 405–412.

Bertera, R. L. "Planning and Implementing Health Promotion in the Workplace: A Case Study of the Dupont Company Experience." *Health Education Quarterly,* 1990, *17*(3), 307–327.

Bertera, R. L. "Behavioral Risk Factor and Illness Day Changes with Workplace Health Promotion: Two-Year Results." *American Journal of Health Promotion,* 1993, *7*(5), 365–373.

Brancati, F. L., and others. "Incident Type 2 Diabetes Mellitus in African Americans and White Adults: The Atherosclerosis Risk In Communities Study." *Journal of the American Medical Association,* 2000, *283,* 2253–2259.

Brown, A. F., and others. "Socioeconomic Position and Health Among Persons with Diabetes Mellitus: A Conceptual Framework and Review of the Literature." *Epidemiologic Reviews,* 2004, *26,* 63–77.

Burke, J. G., and others. "An Introduction to Concept Mapping as a Participatory Public Health Research Methodology." *Qualitative Health Research,* 2005, *15*(10), 1392–1410.

Carter, J. S., Pugh, J. A., and Monterrosa, A. "Non-Insulin Dependent Diabetes Mellitus in Minorities in the United States." *Annals of Internal Medicine,* 1996, *125,* 221–232.

Centers for Disease Control, National Center for Chronic Disease Prevention and Health Promotion. "PATCH: Planned Approach to Community Health." *Journal of Health Education,* 1992, *23*(3), 129–192.

Chiang, L. C., Huang, J. L., and Lu, C. M. "Educational Diagnosis of Self Management Behaviors of Parents with Asthmatic Children by Triangulation Based on PRECEDE-PROCEED Model in Taiwan." *Patient Education and Counseling,* 2003, *49*(10), 19–25.

Chuang, T. Y., Sung, W. H., and Lin, C. Y. "Application of Virtual Reality-Enhanced Exercise Protocol in Patients After Coronary Bypass." *Archives of Physical Medicine and Rehabilitation,* 2005, *86*(10), 1929–1932.

Clark, N. M., and McLeroy, K. R. "Creating Capacity through Health Education: What We Know and What We Don't." *Health Education Quarterly,* 1995, *22*(3), 273–289.

Cline, R. J., and Haynes, K. M. "Consumer Health Information Seeking on the Internet: The State of the Art." *Health Education Research,* 2001, *16*(6), 671–692.

Crosbie, J. H., Lennon, S., Basford, J. R., and McDonough, S. M. "Virtual Reality in Stroke Rehabilitation: Still More Virtual Than Real." *Disability and Rehabilitation,* 2007, *29*(14), 1139–1146.

Demiris, G. "The Diffusion of Virtual Communities in Health Care: Concepts and Challenges." *Patient Education and Counseling,* 2006, *62,* 178–188.

Diabetes Control and Complications Trial Research Group. "The Effect of Intensive Treatment of Diabetes on the Development and Progression of Long-Term Complications in Insulin-Dependent Diabetes Mellitus." *New England Journal of Medicine,* 1993, *329,* 978–985.

D'Onofrio, C. N. "Pooling Information About Prior Interventions: A New Program Planning Tool." In S. Sussman (ed.), *Handbook of Program Development for Health Behavior Research and Practice.* Thousand Oaks, Calif.: Sage, 2001.

Eng, E., and Blanchard, L. "Action-Oriented Community Diagnosis: A Health Education Tool." *International Quarterly of Community Health Education,* 1991, *11*(2), 93–110.

Erlich, J. L., Rothman, J., and Teresa, J. G. *Taking Action in Organizations and Communities.* (2nd ed.) Dubuque, Iowa: Eddie Bowers Publishing, 1999.

Eysenbach, G., and others. "Health Related Virtual Communities and Electronic Support Groups: Systematic Review of the Effects of Online Peer to Peer Interactions." *British Medical Journal,* 2004, *328,* 1–6

Gary, T. L., and others. "Randomized Controlled Trial of the Effects of Nurse Case Manager and Community Health Worker Interventions on Risk Factors for Diabetes-Related Complications in Urban African Americans." *Preventive Medicine,* 2003, *37,* 23–32.

Gary, T. L., and others. "Meta-Analysis of Randomized Controlled Trials of Educational and Behavioral Interventions in Type 2 Diabetes." *The Diabetes Educator,* 2003, *29,* 488–501.

Gielen, A. C. "Health Education and Injury Control: Integrating Approaches." *Health Education Quarterly,* 1992, *19*(2), 203–218.

Gielen, A. C., and others. "In-Home Injury Prevention Practices for Infants and Toddlers: The Role of Parental Beliefs, Barriers, and Housing Quality." *Health Education Quarterly,* 1995, *22*(1), 85–95.

Gielen, A. C., and others. "Injury Prevention Counseling in an Urban Pediatric Clinic: Analysis of Audiotaped Visits." *Archives of General Pediatrics and Adolescent Medicine,* 1997, *151,* 146–151.

Gielen, A. C., and others. "Randomized Trial of Enhanced Anticipatory Guidance for Injury Prevention." *Archives of General Pediatrics and Adolescent Medicine,* 2001, *155,* 42–49.

Gielen A.C., and others. "The Effects of Improved Access to Safety Counseling, Products and Home Visits on Parents' Safety Practices." *Archives of General Pediatrics and Adolescent Medicine,* 2002, *156,* 33–40.

Gielen, A. C., and others. "Using a Computer Kiosk to Promote Child Safety: Results of a Randomized, Controlled Trial in an Urban Pediatric Emergency Department." *Pediatrics,* 2007, *120*(2), 330–339.

Green, L. W., and Kreuter, M. W. *Health Promotion Planning: An Educational and Environmental Approach.* (2nd ed.) Mountain View, Calif.: Mayfield, 1999.

Glanz, K., and Rimer, B. K. "Theory at a Glance: A Guide for Health Promotion Practice." *National Institutes of Health Publication Number 95–2896, 1995* [http://oc.nci.nih.gov/services/Theory_at_glance/HOME.html].

Green, L. W., and Kreuter, M. W. *Health Promotion Planning: An Educational and Ecological Approach.* (4th ed.) New York: McGraw-Hill, 2005.

Green, L. W., Kreuter, M. W., Deeds, S. G., and Partridge, K. B. *Health Education Planning: A Diagnostic Approach.* Mountain View, Calif.: Mayfield, 1980.

Hill-Briggs, F., Gary, T. L., Baptiste-Roberts, K., and Brancati, F. L. "Thirty-Six-Item Short-Form Outcomes Following a Randomized Controlled Trial in Type 2 Diabetes." *Diabetes Care,* 2005, *28,* 443–444.

Hill-Briggs, F., and others. "Training Community Health Workers as Diabetes Educators for Urban African Americans: Value Added Using Participatory Methods." *Progress in Community Health Partnerships: Research, Education, and Action,* 2007, *1*(2), 185–193.

Holder, H. D., and others. "Effect of Community Based Interventions on High Risk Drinking and Alcohol Related Injuries." *Journal of the American Medical Association,* 2000, *284*(18), 2341–2347.

Israel, B. A., Eng, E., Schulz, A. J., and Parker, E. A. (eds.). *Methods in Community-Based Participatory Research for Health.* San Francisco: Jossey-Bass, 2005.

Institute of Medicine Committee on Health and Behavior. *The Interplay of Biological, Behavioral and Societal Influences, Executive Summary.* Washington, D.C.: National Academy Press, 2001.

Institute of Medicine. *The Future of the Public's Health in the 21st Century.* Washington, D.C.: The National Academies Press, 2003.

Kroeze, W., Werkman, A., and Brug, J. "A Systematic Review of Randomized Trials on the Effectiveness of Computer-Tailored Education on Physical Activity and Dietary Behaviors." *Annals of Behavioral Medicine,* 2006, *31*(3), 205–223.

Kreuter, M. W., Farrell, D., Olevitch, L., and Brennan, T. *Tailoring Health Messages: Customizing Communication with Computer Technology.* Mahwah, N.J.: Erlbaum, 2000.

Kreuter, M. W., Jacobsen, H. A., McDonald, E. M., and Gielen, A. C. "Developing Computerized Tailored Health Messages." In R. J. Bensley and J. Brookins-Fisher (eds.), *Community Health Education Methods: A Practical Guide.* (2nd ed.) Boston: Jones and Bartlett, 2003.

Ku, J., and others. "The Development and Clinical Trial of a Driving Simulator for the Handicapped." *Studies in Health Technology and Informatics,* 2002, *85,* 240–246.

McDonald, E. M., and others. "Evaluation Activities to Strengthen an Injury Prevention Resource Center for Urban Families." *Health Promotion Practice,* 2003, *4*(2), 129–137.

McDonald, E. M., and others. "Evaluation of Kiosk-Based Tailoring to Promote Household Safety Behaviors in an Urban Pediatric Primary Care Practice." *Patient Education and Counseling,* 2005, *58,* 168–181.

McGinnis, J. M., and Foege, W. H. "Actual Causes of Death in the United States." *Journal of the American Medical Association,* 1993, *270*(18), 2207–2212.

McLeroy, K. R., Bibeau, D., Steckler, A., and Glanz, K. "An Ecological Perspective on Health Promotion Programs." *Health Education Quarterly,* 1988, *15*(4), 351–377.

Minkler, M. "Building Supportive Ties and Sense of Community among the Inner-City Elderly: The Tenderloin Senior Outreach Project." *Health Education Quarterly,* 1985, *12,* 303–314.

Minkler, M. (ed.). *Community Organizing and Community Building for Health.* New Brunswick, N.J.: Rutgers University Press, 2004.

Minkler, M., and Wallerstein, N. *Community-Based Participatory Research for Health.* New York: Wiley, 2002.

Mokdad, A. H., and others. "Actual Causes of Death in the United States, 2000." *Journal of the American Medical Association,* 2004, *291*(10), 1238–1245.

Morisky, D. L., and others. "Five-Year Blood Pressure Control and Mortality Following Health Education for Hypertensive Patients." *American Journal of Public Health,* 1983, *73*(2), 153–162.

National Committee for Injury Prevention and Control. *Injury Prevention: Meeting the Challenge.* New York: Oxford University Press, 1989.

Norris, S. L., and others. "Self-Management Education for Adults with Type 2 Diabetes: A Meta-Analysis of the Effect on Glycemic Control." *Diabetes Care,* 2002, *25,* 1159–1171.

Norris, S. L., and others. "Effectiveness of Community Health Workers in the Care of Persons with Diabetes." *Diabetic Medicine,* 2006, *23,* 544–556.

O'Campo, P., and others. "Uncovering the Neighborhood Influences on Intimate Partner Violence Using Concept Mapping." *Journal of Epidemiology and Community Health,* 2005, *59,* 603–608.

Orenstein, D., and others. "Synthesis of the Four PATCH Evaluations." *Journal of Health Education,* 1992, *23*(3), 187–193.

Powell, J. A., Lowe, P., Griffiths, F. E., and Thorogood, M. "A Critical Analysis of the Literature on the Internet and Consumer Health Information." *Journal of Telemedicine and Telecare,* 2005, *22*(Suppl 1), 41–43.

Prochaska, J. O., DiClemente, C. C., and Norcross, J. C. "In Search of How People Change: Applications to Addictive Behaviors." *American Psychologist,* 1992, *47*(9), 1102–1114.

Rogers, E. M. *Diffusion of Innovations.* (5th ed.) New York: Free Press, 2003.

Roter, D. "Which Facets of Communication Have Strong Effects on Outcome—A Meta-Analysis." In M. Stewart and D. Roter (eds.), *Communicating with Medical Patients.* Newbury Park, Calif.: Sage, 1989.

Sarkisian, C. A., and others. "A Systematic Review of Diabetes Self-Care Interventions for Older, African American, or Latino Adults." *The Diabetes Educator,* 2003, *29,* 467–479.

Simons-Morton, B. G., Greene, W. H., and Gottlieb, N. H. *Introduction to Health Education and Health Promotion.* (2nd ed.) Prospect Heights, Ill.: Waveland Press, 1995.

Smedley, B. D., and Syme, S. L. (eds.). *Promoting Health: Intervention Strategies from Social and Behavioral Research. Introduction.* Washington, D.C.: Institute of Medicine, National Academy Press, 2000.

Thomson, J. A., and others. "Influence of Virtual Reality Training on the Roadside Crossing Judgments of Child Pedestrians." *Journal of Experimental Psychology: Applied,* 2005, *11*(3), 175–186.

Treno, A. J., and Holder, H. D. "Community Mobilization: Evaluation of an Environmental Approach to Local Action." *Addiction,* 1997, *92*(Suppl 2), S173–S187.

Tull, E. S., and Roseman, J. M. "Diabetes in African Americans." In National Institutes of Health, National Diabetes Data Group, National Institute of Diabetes and Digestive and Kidney Diseases (eds.), *Diabetes in America.* (2nd ed.) NIH Publication No. 95–1468. Bethesda, Md.: National Institutes of Health, 1995.

UK Prospective Diabetes Study (UKPDS) Group. "Intensive Blood-Glucose Control with Sulphonylereas or Insulin Compared with Conventional Treatment and Risk of Complications in Patients with Type 2 Diabetes (UKPDS 33)." *The Lancet,* 1998, *352,* 837–853.

U.S. Preventive Services Task Force. *Guide to Clinical Preventive Services.* (2nd ed.) Baltimore, Md.: Williams and Wilkins, 1996.

Van den Berg, M. H., Shoones, J. W., and Vliet Vlieland, T. P. "Internet-Based Physical Activity Interventions: A Systematic Review of the Literature." *Journal of Medical Internet Research,* 2007, *9*(3), e26.

Wantland, D. J., and others. "The Effectiveness of Web-Based Vs. Non Web-Based Interventions: A Meta-Analysis of Behavioral Change Outcomes." *Journal of Medical Internet Research,* 2004, *6*(4), e40.

Wilson, M.E.H., and others. *Saving Children: A Guide to Injury Prevention.* New York: Oxford University Press, 1991.

Wissow, L. S., Roter, D. L., and Wilson, M.E.H. "Physician Interview Style and Mothers' Disclosure of Psychosocial Issues Important to Child Development." *Pediatrics,* 1994, *93,* 289–295.

Wright, A., and others. "Development and Evaluation of a Youth Mental Health Community Awareness Campaign: The Compass Strategy." *BMC Public Health,* 2006, *22*(6), 215–237.

Zimmerman, R. K., and others. "A Comprehensive Investigation of Barriers to Adult Immunization: A Methods Paper." *Journal of Family Practice,* 2001, *50*(8), 1–9.

CHAPTER

SOCIAL MARKETING

J. Douglas Storey
Gary B. Saffitz
Jose G. Rimón

KEY POINTS

This chapter will

- Define social marketing, its basic principles, and how they can be applied within a strategic health communication framework.
- Link commonly used theories of health communication and health behavior to the effective practice of social marketing.
- Describe the uses of research in designing, monitoring, and evaluating social marketing programs.
- Provide examples of social marketing programs that illustrate how principles and processes can come together to achieve behavioral and social change.

In the more than half a century since Wiebe (1951–1952) posed his famous question—"Why can't you sell brotherhood like soap?"—the concept of social marketing has had enormous appeal for health promotion and social change programs, in part, because it evokes the image of ubiquitous and successful commercial advertising. The reality, however, is complicated. Not only is commercial marketing, of which advertising is an important component, a highly sophisticated and complex undertaking, it is also hugely expensive (albeit not always successful). Marketers of soap typically have much larger budgets than marketers of brotherhood, as well as much larger infrastructures dedicated primarily to the marketing function. They also are most often focused on selling a specific brand rather than generating demand for a product category. Nevertheless, key perspectives, principles, and tactics adapted from commercial marketing for social change programs can improve the strategic value of health communication and increase the likelihood that people will make healthy behavioral choices.

The influence of social marketing perspectives has been such that, in the early twenty-first century, most health promotion programs that operate at scale use multiple, mutually reinforcing tactics, including some aspects of social marketing. So what distinguishes social marketing from other health promotion and health communication approaches? And why should one consider social marketing as a strategy for influencing health behavior? The rest of this chapter will address these questions, starting with a definition of *social marketing*.

DEFINITION OF SOCIAL MARKETING

Some of the earliest applications of social marketing may have occurred in the field of public health, specifically family planning campaigns in India in the 1960s (Harvey, 1999). But the term itself is usually attributed to Kotler and Zaltman (1971), who defined it as "a social influence technology involving the design, implementation and control of programs aimed at increasing the acceptability of a social idea or practice in one or more groups of target adopters" (Kotler and Roberto, 1989). Since then, it has evolved through widespread application and extensive scholarship. Journals, Web sites, textbooks, institutes, university courses, and funding from the nonprofit sector and from foreign assistance donors continue to drive this evolution.

Andreasen's definition continues to be one of the clearest and most concise summaries of social marketing's essential features: "Social marketing is the *application of commercial marketing technologies* to the analysis, planning, execution and evaluation of programs *designed to influence the voluntary behavior* of target audiences in order *to improve their personal welfare and that of their society*" (Andreasen, 1994; emphasis added). These three highlighted aspects—the use of a marketing perspective to influence behavior for individual and social good—lie at the heart of all social marketing efforts. The focus on outcomes that improve personal and social welfare is the primary distinction between social and commercial marketing.

To the features noted by Andreasen (1994) and Maibach and colleagues (2002), we add another one, derived from Bagozzi (1974, 1978) and Rothschild (1999): the mutual fulfillment of self-interest through voluntary exchange. *Voluntary exchange,* from a consumer's point of view, means that interaction fulfills some felt need or desire, the perceived cost—social, economic, physical—of which does not outweigh the perceived gain. In economic terms, the return on investment (ROI)—the need or desire fulfilled at some expense—is judged to be net positive. *Voluntary exchange,* from the marketers' point of view, means providing a good or service that is also in *their* best interest—that is, not provided at a loss. In commercial settings this means that the cost of providing and promoting a product or service is more than offset by what consumers pay in exchange for it. In the case of social marketing, consumers and marketers presumably share the same goal, namely increasing benefits to society as a whole, so the ROI is a combined sum of consumer and marketer costs and benefits. This way of calculating ROI can be problematic for marketing organizations and funding agencies. Because the marketing organization operates as an agent of the public-at-large, it may tolerate a financial loss if the larger social benefit to society is judged to offset institutional costs.

It is likely that debate over the definitions of social marketing will continue, but it seems clear that social marketing as an approach to social and behavioral change is here to stay. The Centers for Disease Control and Prevention (CDC) has thrown its institutional weight behind social marketing for health in the form of a new National Center for Health Marketing, which their Web site describes as an approach that "draws from traditional marketing theories and principles and adds science-based strategies to prevention, health promotion and health protection" (Bernhardt, 2006; Centers for Disease Control and Prevention, 2007).

A summary of some key distinctions between social and commercial marketing and health education in general is provided in Table 19.1.

TABLE 19.1. **Comparisons Between Social Marketing, Commercial Marketing, and Health Education.**

	Social Marketing	Commercial Marketing	Health Education
Primary Locus of Benefit	Individuals Social and political leaders Professionals Society at large	Marketing organization Producer of marketed goods	Individuals
Types of Outcomes	Behaviors that increase personal and social welfare Knowledge, attitudes, norms, values, and consumer self-image addressed to the extent that they inform behavioral decisions Gratifications more likely to be delayed Benefits tend to be longer term	Purchasing behaviors Attitudes toward & image of product Consumer self-image Norms and values addressed to the extent that they affect purchases Gratifications may be more immediate Benefits tend to be shorter term	Knowledge Attitudes Skills Practice of skills

TABLE 19.1. **Comparisons Between Social Marketing, Commercial Marketing, and Health Education, Cont'd.**

	Social Marketing	Commercial Marketing	Health Education
Characteristics of Audiences	Tend to be less affluent, more diverse, more in need of social services, harder to reach Audience typically segmented by psychographic attributes and relationship or involvement with product	Tend to be more affluent, more connected to media, easier to reach Audience typically segmented by psychographic and demographic attributes and relationship or involvement with product	Tend to be less well-educated with regard to featured health issues Audience segmented by education or skill level
Voluntary Exchange	Includes weighing of economic and non-economic social costs and benefits More emphasis on non-monetary exchange Costs of marketing organizations usually subsidized Expectation that information about the social product is complete and that choices are fully informed	More emphasis on monetary exchange May include weighing of social costs and benefits, mostly for consumer Expectation that information about the commercial product is true, but biased in favor of the product	Education sometimes mandated (non-voluntary), sometimes volitional "Value" of content usually determined by educators
Market Perspective	Products tend to be less tangible and more complex Competition tends to be more varied and less tangible Economic factors (for example, purchasing power) tend to be less important	Products tend to be more tangible Competition tends to be more tangible and categorical Economic factors (for example, purchasing power) tend to be more important	Economic factors tend to be less important except as they affect health literacy or ability to process information

BASIC PRINCIPLES OF SOCIAL MARKETING

What are some of the basic principles that have made social marketing popular and effective as a health promotion strategy? In this section, we describe five principles: (1) focusing on behavioral outcomes, (2) prioritizing consumers' rather than marketers' benefits, (3) maintaining an ecological perspective, (4) developing a strategic "marketing mix" of communication elements according to the Four Ps, and (5) using audience segmentation to identify meaningful differences among consumers that affect their responses to the product or service being offered.

Focusing on Behavior

Whereas in earlier eras social "products" were defined broadly to include ideas (for example, family planning, environmental conservation, cardiovascular health), attitudes (for example, preference for small family size, approval of recycling, fear of heart disease), services (for example, family planning clinics, recycling centers, health clubs) and behaviors (for example, use of hormonal contraceptives, recycling glass bottles, thrice-weekly vigorous exercise), Andreasen (1994, 2006) and others argue that the proper objective of social marketing is to influence behavior. It is not enough to promote products or services; people must obtain and use them. In the commercial world, soft drink manufacturers would fail if their business goal was merely to promote awareness of or positive attitudes toward their products; consumers must act to purchase them. Yet, in most cases, the marketing organization is indifferent as to how the product is used or if it is used at all, as long as this does not negatively affect future sales; it doesn't matter if a customer drinks the beer or pours it down the drain, as long as he buys it again. In social marketing, the *use* of the product is of much greater importance because the use usually confers the benefit. A condom marketing campaign would have to be judged unsuccessful, even if millions of condoms were distributed, if they were not used as they were meant to be—to prevent disease and pregnancy. In other words, the focus on behavior is inextricably linked to the second principle—consumer benefit.

Prioritizing Consumer Benefits

A general dimension of communication campaigns—*locus of benefit* (Rogers and Storey, 1987)—refers to whether successful achievement of program objectives primarily benefits the program designers, in this case the marketing organization or the program audience. Social marketing programs properly focus on the benefit of the consumer and not on the benefit of the organization marketing the product or the service. Although consumers *may* benefit from commercial advertising and marketing campaigns, an important focus also includes the benefit for the producers of consumer goods and their stockholders. In contrast, social marketing campaigns benefit members of the audience or society-at-large in the form of better health or a cleaner and more stable environment. For example, little if any direct benefit may accrue to the designers of a health campaign in a government agency if consumers change their health behavior, except in the sense that a healthier populace means a lower burden of disease and fewer demands on public health resources.

Maintaining a Market Perspective

Another principle of social marketing that sets it apart from other forms of purposive communication is the concept of the market itself. First, a market perspective implies adoption of a *consumer orientation*; that is, markets revolve around consumer needs and desires and the ways in which decisions are made to satisfy those needs. Second, the functioning of markets is dependent on the *communication of information* about available products, what they cost, how they can be used, what benefits they provide, and where to obtain them. Third, promoted products always face *competition* for the consumer's attention and resources in a dynamic marketplace of ideas, priorities, and choices. Therefore, marketing communication explicitly acknowledges the environment within which decisions are made and develops strategies to increase the desirability or perceived relative value of particular decisions within that context, so that the product can compete favorably with consumers' other options.

Some social marketing approaches (Andreasen, 2006) refer to strategies addressing different levels of communication in terms of an *upstream* focus on infrastructural change (such as policy or regulatory change) or a *downstream* focus on individual change (such as knowledge, attitudes, or practices). Often, upstream and downstream strategies need to be coordinated in order to change upstream structural conditions that pose downstream barriers to individual change. Paisley (1989), for example, described the interrelated "Three Es: of public communication campaign strategy: Engineering, Enforcement, and Education. The upstream engineering of safety features such as seat belts and airbags into automobiles helps prevent traffic accident injuries. But engineering approaches must be supported by the upstream enforcement of seatbelt laws, as well as the downstream education of the public about those laws, about the penalties that can result from noncompliance, and about the effectiveness of seat belts in reducing death and injury.

Determining Marketing Mix with the Four Ps

Another distinguishing characteristic of social marketing approaches is consideration of the proper marketing mix (or combination of strategic elements), often described in terms of the "Four Ps:" Product, Price, Place, and Promotion. These are closely interwoven in an effective strategy, but each draws attention to different aspects of the market environment.

Product. Rather than thinking of products as physical objects (for example, antiretroviral AIDS drugs, hygiene products, seat belts, recycling centers), marketers think of them as a constellation of benefits that can be offered to consumers to make using those products (behaviors) enticing. To identify the most important bundle of benefits to offer, social marketers conduct research to understand the current behaviors of consumer groups and how a new or alternative behavior can be made more attractive or valuable. For example, consider a campaign to make it easier for restaurant patrons to identify and choose healthier foods on the menu. By labeling such menu items as "heart healthy" or "light" to distinguish them from other choices, the perceived package of benefits associated with a particular food choice is enhanced ("the Greek salad not only looks tasty, it has lower fat content"). The attributes or benefits that define a product in the mind of the consumer may be physical, economic, social, psychological, or some combination thereof.

Price. *Price* refers to the perceived costs or barriers associated with the product being offered and is an essential aspect of the voluntary exchange dynamic. Costs can be monetary, social, or psychological. Will maintaining a low-fat diet cost more in terms of monthly food expenditures? Will a program of exercise cut into time spent with family or friends? Will trying to reduce alcohol consumption result in higher levels of stress? Consumers weigh the perceived costs of a behavior against its perceived benefits, sometimes casually and sometimes with great care and attention, before making a decision to purchase a product or adopt a behavior (see Chapter Three). Social marketers try to set an attractive price or influence the perceived cost-benefit ratio in order to tip the balance in favor of the promoted behavior.

Consider a campaign to increase the practice among backyard poultry farmers in Indonesia of caging their chickens to prevent the birds and people who work with them from becoming infected with the H5N1 virus that causes avian influenza. Free ranging of chickens is generally cheaper than keeping birds caged because it costs less to feed them and because building cages, although not highly expensive, requires some investment of time and materials. But in a country where the H5N1 virus is endemic in wild birds, where laws allow the culling of entire poultry flocks if infection is suspected, and where roughly 80 percent of the people who contracted the virus from their chickens died as a result, it may be wise to keep one's chickens separated from other people's flocks, from contact with wild birds, and from contact with one's family and neighbors. Therefore, social marketing efforts in Indonesia promote, among other things, low-cost caging using local materials as a behavior that not only protects the farmer's economic investment in her chickens but protects her health and the health of her family as well. By encouraging the use of local materials such as split bamboo rather than more expensive wire fencing, the anticipated price of caging is lowered, thereby making the marketing offer appear more affordable. Furthermore, by pairing the idea of lower cost with the desirable benefits of protecting one's investment and the health of one's family, the cost-benefit ratio associated with the behavior is more favorable.

Place. *Place* refers to where the consumer is reached with the product and information about it and where the voluntary exchange takes place. Distribution channels for the product being promoted (if there is a physical object to be used, such as oral contraceptives, exercise equipment, diet aids, water purification compounds, or vaccines) or for information about how to enact the promoted behavioral product must be chosen to maximize the convenience of the "buying" experience for the consumer.

Convenience may include such things as the product's location in physical or virtual space, the times at which it is available, and the time and effort it takes to find and access the product. In the case of commercial products, place might include a retail outlet, door-to-door delivery through outreach workers (or sales force), and nontraditional social networks. Products, services, and the opportunities to take action must be placed in outlets that intended consumer groups patronize and must be located conveniently within those outlets to maximize attention and favorable comparison with other product or service options.

For example, the placement of condom vending machines and messages about the prevention of sexually transmitted diseases in the restrooms of nightclubs, gas stations, and twenty-four-hour convenience stores increases the likelihood that the idea of, as well as the means to practice, safer sex will be available at a convenient place and at a time of elevated risk for some consumers. Or consider the *Mindset* satellite broadcasting system in South Africa that delivers information about antiretroviral drugs, treatment adherence, and other health topics directly to television monitors in the waiting rooms of health clinics (Mindset, 2007).

A multitude of placement options are available to social marketers, from point-of-purchase opportunities (like the condom vending machine example or in-store signage or packaging labels that provide nutritional content information about food products), to Web-based delivery, advertisements in popular entertainment programs or magazines, local and national broadcast media, interpersonal channels in the community or at service delivery sites, message placement at public sporting or holiday events, outdoor media, direct mail, and telemarketing. In short, any placement options may be considered, with the choice being determined by up-to-date information about which ones reach and are used by the greatest numbers of the intended audience. The growth of Internet technologies has dramatically expanded the virtual space within which consumers can access and choose from a nearly unlimited range of products and personalize the purchasing experience. This, in turn, extends the lifetime of product placement and the "long tail" (Anderson, 2006) of profit or social benefit.

The importance of place was discussed by Maibach, Abroms, and Marosits (2007), who describe the social marketing perspective in terms of a social ecological "people and places" framework that situates audiences and choices within geographical, economic, and cultural spaces that determine access to, and relevance and value of, the product. The "people and places" perspective highlights the importance of a situated behavioral approach to social marketing. This requires a thorough understanding, obtained through systematic research, of the individual-level factors (such as outcome expectancy, self-efficacy, motivations, demographic characteristics, social relationships, media habits, skill levels, and emotions), as well as the characteristics of the place within which decisions are made (such as availability of products and services, physical features of the environment, social structures, laws and regulations, and the content of the symbolic environment provided by mediated and interpersonal communication).

Promotion. *Promotion* refers to the communication and messaging elements of a social marketing program, to the forms and content of information provided and the ways in which they are formatted, sequenced, reinforced, and complemented by other elements of the marketing mix. Promotional strategies typically provide information about the other Ps, such as the salient features of the product and the costs and benefits the consumer can expect, how barriers to product use can be overcome or minimized, where the product can be obtained or practiced, and so on.

Different consumer groups may respond better to one promotional strategy than to another. For example, high-sensation-seeking teenagers may respond better to anti-marijuana messages that feature dramatic depictions of drug use consequences than to messages that emphasize health statistics or social disapproval of drug use (Palmgreen and others, 2007). Whatever the issue may be, promotional approaches must be selected to correspond with audience preferences and information processing styles. An enormous catalog of message strategies is available to chose from, including the use of emotional or rational appeals, one-sided or two-sided messages, the use of humor, visual or graphic presentations versus more text-based presentations, interactive messages delivered through electronic media or through live events in a community, mass appeal versus highly tailored individualized messages, messages that emphasize social values or norms versus messages that emphasize individual benefits or purely personal considerations, and many others. (For additional discussion of message strategies, see Chapter Sixteen).

Using Audience Segmentation

The principle of audience segmentation refers to the identification of relatively homogeneous subgroups and the development of marketing strategies customized to the unique characteristics of each subgroup. Different subgroups require different strategies because they may value different benefits associated with a product, prioritize price considerations differently, seek and obtain product information or social support for behavior change through different channels, and respond more readily to some kinds of message strategies than others.

Consider an adolescent reproductive health campaign focused on reducing teenage pregnancy. Teenagers are a diverse group of people representing many different socioeconomic, cultural, geographical, psychographic, and age cohorts. Within the age range of fourteen to eighteen years, for example, some individuals are sexually active and some are not, suggesting that different products and different promotional strategies are necessary to meet different needs. Some might argue that sexual abstinence messages are appropriate for all teenagers, yet for those who are already sexually active, educating about contraceptive use may be essential, whereas for those who are not sexually active, encouraging continued abstinence may be appropriate. Therefore, an audience segmentation strategy for teenage pregnancy prevention, based on sexual activity status, might focus on condom use for teens who are sexually active and delay of sexual debut for teens who are not sexually active. Each product would have its own bundle of benefits, product and message placement, description of costs and benefits, and promotional strategy (perhaps using different types of role models) appropriate for the target audience.

THE ROLE OF SOCIAL MARKETING WITHIN A STRATEGIC COMMUNICATION FRAMEWORK

Ideal marketing strategies do not just implore people to change, but they help them make appropriate health decisions by fostering healthy, engaged communities and effective health care delivery systems, supported by enlightened health policy. This is not a new idea. As early as the late 1950s, the World Health Organization pushed efforts to define health and well-being away from a narrow disease-prevention perspective to, "a state of complete mental, physical, and social well-being and not merely the absence the disease" (World Health Organization, 1958). The problem with these earlier models is that they made no explicit mention of communication, even though many of the influence pathways implied in the model (for example, via education or family processes) would be impossible without communication.

Consistent with this view, social marketing communication must be grounded in underlying social, political, and economic conditions, which together define the market. In all societies, health communication occurs within three principal domains: (1) the social political environment, (2) health service delivery systems, and (3) among individuals within communities (United States Agency for International Development, 2001; Storey, Figueroa, and Kincaid, 2005). Communication within these domains motivates and facilitates a variety of changes in audiences and institutions over time. In turn, these changes facilitate behavioral outcomes that make the environment more supportive of healthy practices, improve the performance of health services, and improve the likelihood of preventive health practices. Changes in behavioral outcomes at the different levels reinforce each other, resulting in improved health status at the population level. To the extent that these changes are durable, improved health outcomes can be sustained. (For more discussion of how communication works at the three levels, see Chapter Sixteen.)

Obviously, not all levels of the market environment will be engaged in every social marketing program, but within this larger framework, specific social marketing approaches can be selected, depending on the type of product, the nature of demand, and the factors that constrain behavior. We can think of these as *product-driven* approaches, *consumer- or demand-driven* approaches, and *market-driven* approaches.

Product-Driven Approaches

Product-driven approaches naturally focus on the first of the Four Ps—product—and aim to increase its appeal and differentiate it positively from alternatives. Product differentiation is often accomplished through the promotional practice of *branding*. In commercial marketing, branding creates a product category and associates it with desirable product attributes. *Coca-Cola* soft drinks, *Shell* petroleum products, *Nike* athletic gear, the *International Committee of the Red Cross, Smokey Bear,* and (unfortunately), *Marlboro* cigarettes are just some examples of popular, internationally recognized brands. Marketers offer such products with a consistent bundle of promised benefits (for example, good times, reliable quality, social status, compassion, environmental protection, good taste). Consumers come to expect those benefits and return to the products again and again in anticipation of predictable outcomes. Social marketers use similar branding tactics.

For example, Indonesia's highly successful 1988 national family planning program originally introduced the Blue Circle (*Lingkaran Biru*; see Figure 19.1) as the brand image for services provided by private sector doctors and midwives. This original program, focused in urban areas, was designed to expand family planning services into the private sector in recognition of changing economics and the need to shift responsibility for family planning from the government to the people. The program was designed under the umbrella of *KB Mandiri*—an expression of "individual self sufficiency and personal choice." Two years later, the Blue Circle was extended to an array of private sector contraceptive products (Piotrow, Kincaid, Rimón, and Rinehart, 1997; Mize and Robey, 2006). Eventually, the Blue Circle was featured in an enormous variety of ways: with the letters KB (*Keluarga Berencana* or family planning) inside to denote the concept of "making your own choice" about contraception; as signs indicating hospitals, clinics, pharmacies, and other facilities where contraceptive services and supplies were available; on contraceptive packaging; on posters, billboards, and televised public service announcements promoting health care providers who offered value-added Blue Circle services; on car wheel covers, and as decoration on village gates to indicate the community's support for families choosing to practice family planning. Even old tires were painted blue and mounted on fence posts lining country roads.

The use of Blue Circle branding was part of an integrated national social marketing campaign at a time when Indonesia was trying to move from subsidizing supply-side approaches to focusing on demand generation. The campaign helped break through old beliefs that family planning was the responsibility of and belonged to the government, by repositioning family planning as a personal choice and social norm, and fueled the rise in the use of modern contraceptive methods from 23 percent of married women in 1977 to nearly 60 percent in 2006 (Mize and Robey, 2006). Not only did the contraceptive prevalence rate increase, but the share of the private sector in 2003 increased to 65 percent, with 95 percent of hormonal contraceptive users paying market price for their supplies, whether they bought them from public or private sector sources (Rimón, Negrette, and Storey, 2006).

Consumer-Driven Approaches

Consumer-driven approaches go beyond pushing the product itself to building demand for the product, so that maintaining behavioral momentum shifts from the marketing organization to consumers. Such approaches may be more sustainable than product-driven ones, due to the nonprofit nature of social marketing. In commercial

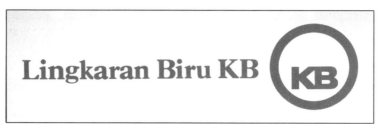

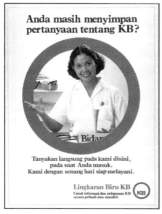

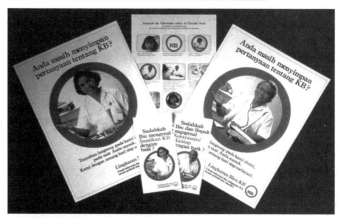

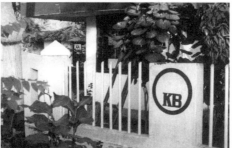

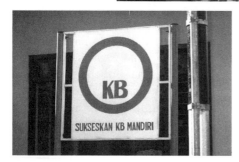

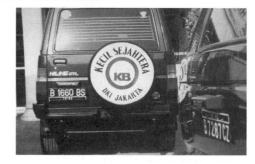

Images: courtesy of the Media/Materials Clearinghouse at Johns Hopkins Bloomberg School of Public Health/Center for Communication Programs

FIGURE 19.1. The Blue Circle (Indonesia).

marketing programs, the more product sold, the greater the profit and ROI for the marketing organization. But in social marketing programs where products are often subsidized or free, the greater the success, the more it costs the marketing organization to provide the product.

One strategy for achieving and sustaining consumer demand is to target social norms (Haines, 1998; Linkenbach, 1999). This approach is based on the theory that much behavior is influenced by perceptions of what is "normal" or "typical" and the perceived sanctions or rewards that result from deviating from or complying with those norms (Perkins and Berkowitz, 1986; Cialdini and Goldstein, 2004). Unfortunately, the misperception of norms, even among one's peers, is common, especially when the behaviors are less publicly visible, as in the case of taboo or illegal behaviors like sex or drug use, or visible behaviors like alcohol use. Perception usually trumps reality, so if a teenager believes that the majority of his peers smoke marijuana, then he is more likely to try it himself. If a married woman believes that few of her peers use contraception, she is less likely to seek family planning services or methods for herself. Social norms marketing can be used to inform people about the actual frequency of behaviors among groups they care about, in order to create salient social pressure. Or a program might even introduce and promote a new norm and reinforce its practice by creating visible symbols in the environment, increasing perceived social support (Kincaid, 2004).

Consider again the example of the family planning program in Indonesia. In a departure from traditional social marketing of condoms or oral contraceptives, the National Family Planning Coordinating Board chose to focus on making small family size a new social norm with the introduction of the theme *"Dua anak cukup"* (Two Children Are Enough) (Mize and Robey, 2006), with the use of contraception being promoted as a way to achieve that goal. National campaigns facilitated family planning practice by providing a full range of branded products and services from which couples could choose, at first primarily through government health service outlets, then later through Blue Circle private sector hospitals, clinics, pharmacies, and health service providers. Almost nonstop national and local campaigns during the 1980s and 1990s contributed to a rapid increase in the contraceptive prevalence rate, as noted earlier, and to a drop in the total fertility rate from 5.6 to 2.6 average number of births in a woman's lifetime between 1971 and 2006 (BPS and ORC Macro, 2003). By the late 1990s, family planning and small family size had become so deeply engrained that even the economic crisis and political instability that Indonesia suffered from 1998 to 2002 had little effect on contraceptive use rates, even though commodities became more expensive and harder to obtain (Storey and Schoemaker, 2006; Frankenberg, Sikoki, and Suriastini, 2003).

Market-Driven Approaches

An extension of consumer-driven (or demand-driven) approaches are market-driven ones. Consumer demand operates in a world of options, where behavioral choices are made in light of other possibilities, many of which have their own champions and promoters. For example, responsible consumption of alcoholic beverages, especially around holiday periods, competes with the allure of drinking portrayed in a flood of seasonal advertising that emphasizes the social benefits and camaraderie of alcohol consumption. Does *not* drinking with friends mean a less active and fulfilling social life?

A market-driven approach to responsible drinking must position its product (one aspect of which is alcohol-free social interaction) as an attractive alternative to the competition. Accordingly, a growing number of communities in the United States sponsor "First Night" events on New Year's Eve—a time when alcohol abuse is common. For example, the City of Williamsburg, a popular history-themed tourist destination in Virginia, hosts and heavily promotes a celebration of the performing arts every New Year's Eve. In 2007, members of the public could purchase a single ticket that allowed entrance to more than sixty venues offering all types of performances from classical, folk, and popular music to dances, drama, and art shows as alternatives to public events, clubs, restaurants, and bars where alcohol is served.

THE ROLE OF THEORY AND RESEARCH IN SOCIAL MARKETING

The Use of Theory

Many theories are available to guide the planning and evaluation of social marketing programs (for more extensive discussion of health behavior theories, see Parts Two and Three in this book). In this chapter, we highlight four health behavior theories that are commonly used in large international health interventions: (1) the Integrated Model of Behavioral Prediction (Kasprzyk, Montano, and Fishbein, 2001; Fishbein and Yzer, 2003; see Chapter Four), which focuses primarily on cognitive or rational processes around decision making; (2) the *extended parallel processing model* (Witte, 1994), sometimes referred to as fear or threat management theory, which focuses on emotional response and its effects on motivations and behavior and is particularly relevant for some health issues like HIV/AIDS or avian influenza prevention; (3) *observational (or social) learning theory* (Bandura, 1986; see Chapter Eight), which focuses on how people learn to behave by observing others; and (4) *diffusion of innovations* (Rogers, 2003; see Chapter Fourteen)—in some ways the most "social" of these theories, which focuses on the flow of information about a new product or practice within the social environment (for example, neighborhoods and networks) and how these influence access to information and response to it.

Key ideas and applications of these four theories in social marketing research and design are summarized in Table 19.2.

Such theories offer insights into characteristics of a product that may be of interest to consumers and that can be confirmed through formative research. For example, the adoption of a new behavior tends to be more rapid if it (1) is perceived to have a relative advantage over current behavior, (2) is compatible with one's daily routine, sociocultural values, and priorities, (3) does not seem overly complex to adopt or practice, (4) can be tried without great risk before committing to it, and (5) can be observed in action to see what outcomes others experience before trying it oneself (Rogers, 2003). By evaluating the perceived characteristics of a product among potential consumers,

TABLE 19.2. **Applications of Major Theories and Research in Social Marketing.**

Theoretical Framework	Applications of Framework		
	Identify Motives for Action	Identify Message Strategies	Identify Target Audiences
Reasoned Action/ Planned Behavior	What are the advantages (benefits) and disadvantages (costs), both personal and social, of a health behavior?	Change beliefs about and evaluations of consequences (costs and benefits) of action Change perceptions of subjective norms Change motivations to comply with subjective norms	Define primary audiences (those who would benefit from attitude change) Define secondary audiences (significant others of those to be influenced)
Extended Parallel Processing Model	To what extent is the health issue thought to pose a serious and personal threat (costs of inaction)? To what extent are proposed actions perceived to be effective (response efficacy or benefit of action)? How do people perceive their ability to enact the behavior (personal efficacy)?	Create messages that increase understanding of the threat and explain or demonstrate how responses can effectively reduce the threat Create messages that explain how to do the recommended response Explain how to overcome barriers to recommended response	Segment audiences into categories representing levels of perceived threat and efficacy
Observational Learning	What perceived personal and social incentives or reinforcements (benefits) affect learning and action? What perceived personal and social barriers (costs) affect learning and action?	Provide models of effective action that are appealing and compelling Encourage rehearsal and trial of the behavior Provide feedback and reinforcement for behavioral attempts Provide incentives for performance of the proposed behavior	Define primary audiences (those who would benefit from attitude change) Define secondary audiences (potential role models and advocates)

TABLE 19.2. **Applications of Major Theories and Research in Social Marketing, Cont'd.**

	Applications of Framework		
Theoretical Framework	**Identify Motives for Action**	**Identify Message Strategies**	**Identify Target Audiences**
Diffusion of Innovations	How do members of the audience perceive the behavioral innovation?	Show and explain the benefits of the proposed action	Segment audience according to perceptions of the behavior
	What relative advantage (benefits) does it offer?	Explain how to do it in simple terms	Target people who are key network members (opinion leaders)
	How complex or risky is it (costs)?	Show how new behavior fits with or grows out of current practices	
	Can consequences (costs and benefits) of the behavior be observed?	Encourage those who already practice the behavior to advocate it to others	
	Is the behavior compatible with current practices (costs)?		
	What social influences or networks exist in the environment that encourage or discourage the action (social costs and benefits)?		

marketers can determine which positive perceptions to reinforce and which negative perceptions to change through their message strategy.

Theory, too, can help social marketers segment audiences in meaningful ways. For example, the Extended Parallel Processing Model (EPPM) describes the interaction between emotion (perceived threat) and rationality (perceived efficacy) in behavioral decision making (Witte, 1994). Splitting each of these dimensions into low and high categories creates a 2 × 2 typology of audience segments. Consider the backyard poultry farmer in Indonesia again, who has heard that mortality is high among humans infected with the avian influenza virus. If the farmer believes that avian flu poses a real and present threat to his health (higher fear) but feels confident that the use of protective equipment and hygienic poultry handling practices are both effective and feasible (higher efficacy), he is more likely to take protective action, compared to another farmer who is neither concerned about the disease (lower fear) nor is confident in the proposed solutions or in his ability to implement them (lower efficacy). A communication strategy for the lower fear/lower efficacy segment might focus on raising realistic risk perceptions and educating about or modeling possible actions that are known to mitigate the threat. For the higher fear/higher efficacy segment, a communication strategy might focus simply on cueing them to action during the season when avian flu outbreaks are more likely to occur. Multiple audience segments may be addressed within an integrated marketing strategy through the use of multiple models representing distinct segments, tailored persuasive strategies, or personalized channels of communication (Kalyanaraman and Sundar, 2006).

Various stage theories of behavior change are also applied widely to market health behaviors in general (Prochaska and DiClemente, 1992; see Chapter Five), family planning (Piotrow, Kincaid, Rimon, and Rinehart, 1997), fertility behavior (Coale and Watkins, 1986; Kincaid, 2000; Lesthaeghe and Vanderhoeft, 1998), and attitude change (McGuire, 1989). These are often also used to identify different segments of the overall audience who may be at different stages; some are barely aware of a health issue while others are knowledgeable and capable of responding but lack motivation to act, requiring strategies tailored to the needs of each group.

The Use of Research

Because consumer decision making and behavior are complex and situational, systematic investigation into the conditions and dynamics of targeted behaviors, rather than inspired guesswork, helps validate program planning decisions and increases the likelihood that social marketing programs will succeed. Because research plays an essential role across the entire lifespan of a social marketing program, researchers should be involved in program planning from the beginning, rather than brought in only at the end to evaluate outcomes.

During the design phase of a program, research helps planners determine the prevalence of the problem overall and among specific sub-audiences; select audiences to target in order to achieve maximum individual and social benefit; identify the unique communication needs, media habits, and preferences of the different audience segments; catalog the social, cultural, and structural/environmental factors that positively or negatively influence behavior; and identify sources of personal influence over the behavior of intended audience members. At a more structural level, research helps identify organizations and social structures that influence the intended audiences and might be engaged to support the program and be available as communication and media channels.

Concept testing and pretesting are essential research steps in the design process that help planners explore the Four Ps and determine an optimum marketing mix. What attributes of a product are valued? What perceived costs are associated with the desired behavior? Where can or must the exchange take place and how can it be made most convenient? What promotional strategies, formats, presentations, and placement channels will reach and appeal to targeted audiences and are likely to motivate the desired behaviors?

During implementation, research helps track progress by providing answers to such questions as these: Is the program being implemented as designed? Are activities and materials reaching the audience? What is the level of exposure within the intended audience? Is the timing of activities and message distribution going as planned? Is the program beginning to have an impact? Does the program need adjustment and fine-tuning at midcourse?

Finally, *during the evaluation phase* of the program, research helps determine how well a program met its objectives. It can explain why a program was effective (or not), including the effects of different activities on different audience segments. Did anything change during the program? What did the program contribute to those changes? Which parts of the program explain the most change? How much did it cost to achieve specific outcomes or effects? Which parts of the program should be continued or strengthened?

INTERNATIONAL AND DOMESTIC (U.S.) SOCIAL MARKETING EXPERIENCES

In this section, we profile two health communication programs from a social marketing perspective: the integrated Communication for Healthy Living (CHL) family health program in Upper Egypt and the Red Ribbon Question Mark (RRQ) HIV-testing promotion program in Baltimore, Maryland, USA. We describe how each program reflects the five principles of social marketing (focus on behavior, not products; focus on consumer benefits; maintain an ecological market perspective; optimize market mix through the use of the Four Ps, and audience segmentation), as well as how each effectively used theory and research to guide decision making. We also describe some of the impact data from each program to illustrate how social marketing programs can be evaluated.

Case Study 1: Communication for Healthy Living, 2002–2009 (Egypt)

Communication for Healthy Living (CHL) is a seven-year integrated health communication program in Egypt, funded by the United States Agency for International Development (USAID). Begun in 2002, CHL builds on 25+ years of USAID-supported partnership between Egypt's Ministry of Health and Population (MOHP) and the Ministry of Information-State Information Services (MOI-SIS).

Focus on Behavior. Because funding for the project prioritizes family planning as an outcome, contraceptive use is a primary behavioral goal. However, CHL positions contraceptive use within a larger array of family health behaviors, using marriage as an entry point for the communication strategy. Newlywed couples immediately face health issues related to reproduction, including the decision to have children right away or to delay the first pregnancy. When the first pregnancy does occur, new behaviors become relevant: protecting the prenatal health of the mother and the fetus, preparing for a safe delivery, and delivery itself with the assistance of a doctor or trained midwife. After delivery, immediate postpartum care for the mother and post-natal care for the infant, initiation of breastfeeding, and postpartum initiation of con-traceptive use to delay a subsequent pregnancy become relevant, followed by infant feeding practices and immunization. Then, as the family matures, other lifestyle prac-tices assume greater importance. Routinely washing hands and preventing infectious diseases such as hepatitis, HIV/AIDS, and avian influenza are examples; exercise, smoking, and the avoidance of secondhand smoke are others.

CHL publicizes the availability of health services and promotes the purchase and use of health products such as oral contraceptives, hand soap, feminine hygiene prod-ucts, and disposable syringes but positions these as products that can be used to achieve behavioral goals, not as consumer products per se.

Focus on Consumer Benefit. The signature theme that brands all CHL messages and activities is "*Sahetak Sarwetak*" (Your Health is Your Wealth). Achieving and main-taining one's own health and that of one's family is the overall benefit communicated to target audiences, but each of the lifestage behaviors is described in terms of the ben-efits it conveys: better maternal and child health as a result of longer spacing between births, improved mental and physical development of infants through immunization and breastfeeding, reduced risk of cardiovascular disease and cancer through avoid-ance of secondhand smoke, and so on. Each of these behaviors is positioned as an in-formed choice that people make in order to protect their greatest asset—good health—a deeply held value that emerged strongly in pre-campaign formative research.

Maintain a Market Perspective. CHL reflects a market perspective in several ways, most notably through its private sector pharmacy initiative, known as *Isaal Istashir* (Ask-Consult). As of mid-2007, Ask-Consult had built a national network of 16,000 private sector neighborhood pharmacists who associate with the project in order to improve the level of the services and products they provide and to increase their sales. As donor funds begin to phase out, a small membership fee will help support brand-ing and generic marketing of Ask-Consult services and products, as well as members' access to customer service and health information materials and training. The sig-nature campaign invites consumers to "ask and consult" for family health informa-tion and appropriate products where they see the Ask-Consult logo.

Ask-Consult competes for consumer attention through national television adver-tising, public relations activities, point-of-sale promotions, direct mail, and contests. Messages promote positive behaviors and appropriate health products for family plan-ning, safe injection, hygiene, and maternal and child health. By expanding and sup-porting this network, CHL attempts to affect the market structure itself by improving access to and quality of local sources of information and health care products people need in order to protect their greatest asset—their family's health.

Beyond the Ask-Consult initiative, CHL also works with potential competitors for consumer attention and advertising expenditures by leveraging the support of health industry manufacturers. CHL has attracted corporate partners such as Procter & Gamble, Shering, Organon, Vodafone, and Durex, who participate in and fund activities such as pharmacy contests, distribution of health information and promotional materials, direct corporate support of training and events, product promotions, and prizes at public events and on health-related television game shows.

Focus on the Four Ps.

Product. As noted earlier, CHL products are a set of lifestage-appropriate behaviors bundled together under the *Sahetak Sarwetak* umbrella. Together, the individual benefits of family planning, maternal and child health, and healthy lifestyle practices add up to a lifetime of family health and well-being but are broken down into manageably small but concrete actions that can be taken at various points in time. Associating each behavior with a particular lifestage also makes it easier to contextualize. For example, less than half of Egyptian women first use contraceptives after the birth of their first child, even though delaying the second pregnancy has health benefits for both the mother and the newborn child. CHL messages position this decision in the context of pressures newlyweds face from in-laws to have more children, the economic pressures that more children create, and the health benefits of a longer time between pregnancies.

Price. CHL attempts to reduce the real and perceived cost of everyday health behaviors, in part by increasing access to quality health information and products at conveniently located local pharmacies. Messaging also attempts to explain the negative costs associated with inaction (for example, failing to protect pregnant women and infants from secondhand smoke can result in lower birthweight and lower growth rates) in order to influence the perceived cost-benefit ratio.

Place. Outreach activities promoting healthy lifestyles and behaviors include community events, home visits, contests, and birth preparedness and infant feeding classes at public health clinics. Print materials covering priority health messages for both health service providers and clients are distributed nationwide to 5000+ public sector clinics, private sector pharmacies, a network of nongovernmental organizations (NGOs), and in birthing hospitals along with product sampling packs for new mothers.

Promotion. CHL messaging is extremely varied and tailored to different audience segments and different topics. On issues where baseline knowledge is limited, messages are more informational. For example, many Egyptians purchase medical supplies such as syringes from pharmacies and take them to hospitals when they need treatment because such commodities are sometimes in short supply. Few people know about the link between hepatitis C infection and the reuse of syringes, so CHL messages on this topic feature pharmacists explaining the importance of using disposable syringes to prevent the transmission of blood-borne diseases. In the case of avian influenza, television and radio spots clearly model simple behaviors that people can take (for example, avoiding wild birds, regular hand washing, hygienic handling of poultry for

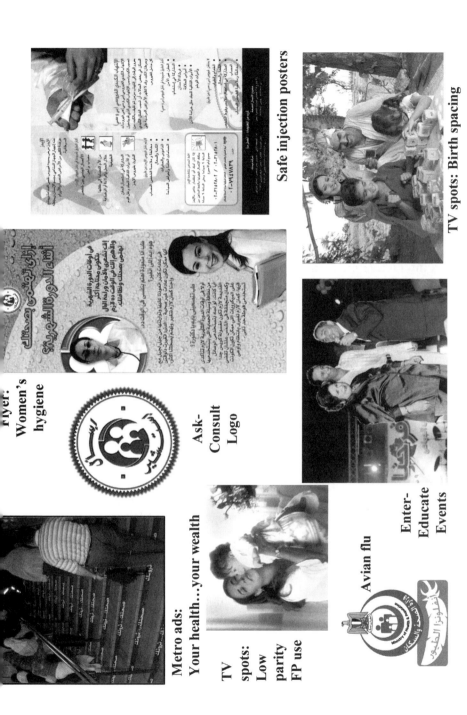

Images: courtesy of the Media/Materials Clearinghouse and Photoshare at Johns Hopkins Bloomberg School of Public Health/Center for Communication Programs

FIGURE 19.2. Communication for Healthy Living (Egypt).

food, thorough cooking of poultry and eggs). And entertainment-education events and media programming embed health messages within game shows, children's shows like *Alam Simsim* (the Egyptian Sesame Street), and wedding celebrations to maximize attention and emotional appeal. Some examples of CHL messages are provided in Figure 19.2.

The messages were spread through multiple channels, including national and regional TV, radio, and the press, as well as telephone hotlines, the Internet, performing arts, publicity events, community meetings, home visits, and clinic-based counseling. CHL cultivates relationships with print, TV, and radio journalists to encourage accurate and timely reporting of health news supporting the national health agenda. Large-scale publicity events, such as regional "Newlywed Celebrations" for hundreds of local couples and guests, receive extensive national media coverage. Press inserts on special topics are produced for national distribution in popular magazines. Popular television game shows are used to reach a national audience of 15 million with information for newlywed couples to help them get their families off to a good start. Finally, various interactive media are used, such as national telephone hotlines on HIV/AIDS and avian influenza, a CHL Web site, and an online database of health communication materials in Arabic and English (http://www.healthcom-egypt.info).

Audience Segmentation. CHL segments its audience primarily by lifestage, as well as by urban-rural differences and gender. Newlywed couples are a primary target audience, as are pregnant women, postpartum and breastfeeding women, couples with one or two children, and children between the ages of four and six years. As noted earlier, key behaviors are associated with each family lifestage and promoted to the appropriate audience segment. In addition, different versions of the same television spot are tailored, for example, to rural audiences and urban audiences with the featured characters reflecting appropriate dress, language, and other cultural characteristics but delivering the same message about birth spacing.

Use of Theory and Research. CHL research was comprehensive and systematic. During the design phases of CHL, in-depth audience segmentation and trend analysis were conducted using publicly available Egyptian Demographic and Health Survey data (MOHP and ORC Macro, 1995, 2000, 2003, 2005) and commercially available pharmaceutical marketing and media monitoring data. After the program launched in 2002, CHL continued to mobilize a diverse set of data sources, some specially commissioned and some publicly available. These data provided trend indicators at a national level, while commissioned national surveys in 2005 and 2006 (Communication for Healthy Living, 2005, 2006a) measured national exposure and response to specific CHL messages among adult audience segments. The commissioned surveys were able to include measures of key theoretical constructs such as social norms, perceived threat and efficacy, and perceived benefits of specific behaviors, as well as measures of various knowledge, attitudes, and self-reported behaviors related to CHL health issues. Commercially purchased data on media ratings and pharmaceutical sales helped the project track the reach of CHL's mass media offerings and the impact of the Ask-Consult promotions. Finally, NGOs working as outreach partners at the community level in focal project areas collected extensive monitoring data on maternal and child health, including infant birth weights, immunization coverage, and malnutrition.

According to PARC Media Monitoring reports, CHL TV spots reached an estimated 32 million adults between the ages of fifteen and forty-nine in 2004 (Communication for Healthy Living, 2006b). A national health communication survey, fielded in August 2005, found recognition and recall of *Sahetak Sarwetak* to be 67 percent and of Ask-Consult to be 70 percent (Communication for Healthy Living, 2005). The same survey in 2006 found that 71 percent of Egyptian adults over the age of fifteen had initiated at least one new behavior to protect themselves from avian influenza as a result of a national campaign coordinated by CHL and that the mean number of protective behaviors increased with the number of CHL messages recalled (Communication for Healthy Living, 2006a). Other national survey data showed that the use of contraception after the birth of the first child increased from 35 percent of married women in 2000 to 50 percent in 2005 (MOHP and ORC Macro, 2000, 2005). Finally, 2005 monitoring data at the village level showed that the percentage of malnourished infants in focal villages had declined from 26 percent to 16 percent (Communication for Healthy Living, 2006b).

The CHL project will continue at least through 2009. Due to the extensive involvement of stakeholder organizations from the highest levels of government, the public sector, and private sector service delivery systems and civil society at the community level, it is likely that many parts of the program will be sustained beyond the end of the current phase of donor funding.

Case Study 2: Red Ribbon Question Mark HIV-Testing Campaign 1999–2003 (Baltimore, Maryland)

The Red Ribbon Question Mark (RRQ) campaign in Baltimore, Maryland was a four-year HIV-testing promotion program, funded by the Maryland AIDS Administration (MAA) and the state Department of Health and Mental Hygiene. Its ultimate goal was to reduce HIV infection rates in Baltimore City, where African Americans, twenty-five to forty-four years old, are at particularly high risk. The CDC estimate that at least 25 percent of HIV-infected individuals in the Unites States are unaware of their positive serostatus (Centers for Disease Control, 2003), and from this it is estimated that Baltimore could have over four thousand undiagnosed HIV-positive individuals.

Focus on Behavior. The behavioral goals of the RRQ campaign were to increase HIV testing in Baltimore City by 10 percent during the intervention period; to encourage at-risk individuals to seek out services by raising awareness and creating a supportive environment, and to motivate prenatal caregivers to encourage HIV testing among their clients.

Focus on Consumer Benefits. Although increased HIV testing would benefit public health in general, the campaign focused primarily on the benefits individuals would gain from knowing their HIV status under the banner "Live Long. Live Strong. Get Tested. Get Treatment." In the case of pregnant women who test negative, the benefits include peace of mind that their children would be born free of HIV. To counteract fears of testing positive, the described benefits also include access to treatments that reduce the risk of mother-to-child transmission and increase a woman's own chances of living a normal life and surviving to care for her child. For men, the benefits included access to treatment (if someone tests positive) that can increase vitality and allow a return to normal life as long as the treatment regimen is followed.

Maintaining a Market Perspective. It was important for the RRQ to operate within the context of the African American culture and community structure. This meant working closely with faith-based organizations, popular local media, and annual community events that provided access to audiences that are stigmatized, marginalized, and fearful of the consequences of knowing their HIV status. The campaign also acknowledged the critical role of communication processes within the community—not just information delivery—about HIV testing, testing and treatment facilities, and the positive consequences of treatment in supporting decisions to seek testing. By providing information about testing, treatment, and support options, the campaign sought to affect market conditions by reducing physical and psychological barriers to testing and increasing incentives for someone to come forward to be tested.

Focus on the Four Ps.

Product. As in all good social marketing programs, the main product in the RRQ was a behavior and the benefits associated with it: getting an HIV test and the hope for a healthier life that is possible for HIV-positive individuals who get treatment. A number of other associated actions, such as calling an HIV-testing hotline, contacting referral networks, communicating with health workers about HIV testing, and more open public discussion with family and friends about HIV/AIDS and testing also were promoted to increase knowledge about testing and treatment.

Place. The RRQ used a wide variety of distribution points to deliver information and to encourage and support testing. Hotlines, outreach events, and HIV-testing centers provided clients with ways to contact testing services and access information about testing. The campaign promoted the United Way's "First Call for Help" telephone referral hotline and featured the number prominently on campaign advertisements and giveaways. In addition, the campaign tapped into local community outreach activities such as health fairs, heritage festivals, church events, and block parties that offered opportunities for broad community participation. Radio station 92Q, the most popular local station among African Americans in Baltimore, aired spots and announcements featuring the campaign slogan and sponsored events such as the 92Q Stone Soul Picnic, attended by over 100,000 people annually, where materials, referrals, and on-site testing were available.

Price. The campaign attempted to reduce the perceived material and psychological costs of getting tested by facilitating access to testing facilities and to counseling, increasing the acceptability of public discussion of testing and treatment, and reducing stigma associated with HIV/AIDS by creating a more supportive social environment within communities and community organizations. In addition, by emphasizing the health benefits of treatment for people who test positive for HIV, the cost-benefit ratio of the marketing offer and of the voluntary exchange was enhanced.

Promotion. Posters on buses and in subways, outdoor billboards, direct mail to health care providers about how to talk with patients about voluntary HIV testing, additional posters in health facilities and community centers, and radio and television advertising all delivered messages citywide but with concentrated distribution in three postal zones with the highest HIV infection rates. Over 550,000 promotional items, such as calendars, coffee mugs, T-shirts, and lapel pins with messages were distributed to service providers, their clients, and members of the target populations.

The campaign slogan ("Live Long. Live Strong. Get Tested. Get Treatment.") was designed to reduce the anxiety and stigma common in the African American community, which pose major barriers to testing and treatment. Messages addressing pregnant women who may not be aware that mother-to-child transmission can be reduced with proper treatment showed pictures of a mother and baby with such captions as, "HIV is one thing you don't have to pass along to your baby," "My baby's healthy. I'm glad I got tested for HIV," and "What kind of mother could give her baby HIV? An untested one." Other ads spoke directly to African American men who might be skeptical or fearful of being tested for HIV. One ad showed a basketball player with the caption, "11 years with HIV. And he can still dunk in your face," indicating that being infected does not mean a death sentence. The campaign logo—a red ribbon in the shape of a question mark—immediately evoked recall of the almost universally recognized red ribbon AIDS-prevention symbol, but with a twist that made it unique and easily associated with testing to resolve the question of one's HIV status (see examples of campaign materials in Figure 19.3).

Audience Segmentation. Three main audience segments were targeted by the campaign: (1) women of childbearing age, (2) their at-risk male partners, and (3) prenatal caregivers and service providers. Messaging for each group, as described earlier, was developed on the basis of focus group research that revealed unique sources of concern or skepticism about testing or, in the case of service providers, uncertainty about how to broach the subject and discuss testing and treatment with their patients. Because a significant proportion of at-risk women speak Spanish, some materials were produced in Spanish and featured Hispanic women.

Use of Theory and Research. As noted earlier, valuable insights were gathered during focus group discussions with health care providers, community members, and individuals at risk for HIV infection; these insights were used to develop messages that reflected the ethnic background and identity of the neighborhoods in Baltimore most affected by HIV/AIDS. Resulting message concepts were pretested for comprehension, appeal, and emotional impact in additional focus groups with representatives of the primary audience segments.

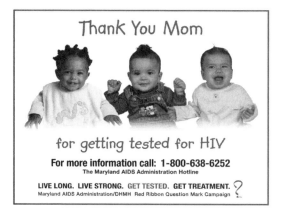

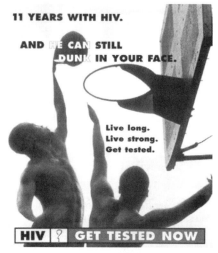

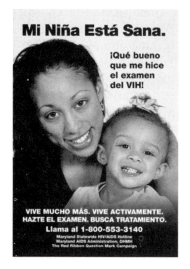

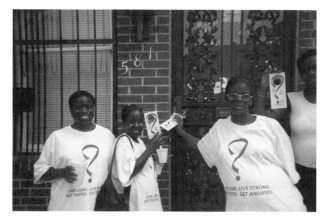

Images: courtesy of the Media/Materials Clearinghouse at Johns Hopkins Bloomberg School of Public Health/Center for Communication Programs

FIGURE 19.3. Red Ribbon Question Mark Campaign (Baltimore, Md.).

Message strategies drew on elements of the integrative model of behavioral prediction (Kasprzyk, Montano, and Fishbein, 2001; Fishbein and Yzer, 2003) regarding the weighing of beliefs about the consequences of an action, in this case what could happen as a result of HIV testing and the determination of one's HIV status. It also drew on elements of social learning theory (Bandura, 1986, 1997) related to learning from modeled behavior to help determine what types of models would most likely be appealing to the targeted audiences.

Results of the campaign were assessed using a variety of data sources. Call logs from the United Way "First Call for Help" hotline showed that the average monthly number of calls increased to fifteen times what they were in the three months prior to the campaign. Sixty-two percent of callers cited the RRQ messages as the reason for their call.

Questions about RRQ message recall, knowledge of HIV testing, and discussion of testing with others were purchased on random sample commercial omnibus surveys conducted by WB&A/MarketTrak in 2002 and 2003 (n = 306 male and female heads of households, age eighteen to fifty, in the Baltimore metropolitan area). Results in 2003 showed 88 percent recall of at least one RRQ message, while the percentage of respondents who reported talking to friends or family about HIV testing increased from 29 percent in 2002 to 59 percent in 2003.

In addition, the Maryland AIDS Administration (MAA) provided RRQ researchers with clinical data about HIV infection rates and testing rates. These data indicated that between 2001 and 2003, HIV testing increased by 61 percent throughout the City of Baltimore and by 68 percent in the campaign's three targeted postal zones, compared to the previous three-year period. Data also indicated a reversal in HIV infection rates. From 1994 to 1999, HIV infections increased by 35 percent annually in the targeted postal zones. However, during the first three years of the campaign, from 1999 to 2002, the MAA reported that the rate of new HIV cases declined by 24 percentage points, representing approximately 619 new HIV cases averted.

SUMMARY

This chapter has introduced the reader to the core principles and some examples of the social marketing of health behaviors. Social marketing should not be considered— any more than other approaches described in this book—as a panacea for overcoming public health challenges. Nevertheless, in its systematic approach to understanding and strategically responding to audience characteristics and the context or market structure surrounding behavioral decisions, social marketing offers powerful guidelines for communication planning.

More than some other approaches at least, social marketing draws our attention to factors beyond individual behavior change and toward ways that communication can affect the market structure itself through policy (fluoridation of water, iodization of salt), legislative (seat-belt use), and social normative (reduced HIV/AIDS stigma) change, thereby facilitating voluntary exchange and the uptake of beneficial health behaviors. Even so, social marketing strategies necessarily work backwards from the existing needs and conditions of consumers' lives to reduce barriers to beneficial behavior. In both commercial and social marketing, it is sometimes necessary to build or create value, but in social marketing it is always important to identify and fulfill demand. The social marketing perspective also demands that planners seek the optimum marketing mix or balance among the "Four Ps." Creating appealing messages about the product is important, but this must be filtered through considerations of the cost-benefit ratio, where the exchange is likely to take place, and what forces compete against the product for attention and resources.

One of the enduring appeals of social marketing is its family resemblance to commercial advertising, which is both widely loathed and widely admired. This resemblance should not be discounted or rejected with the best of high-minded intentions. Commercial advertising can be highly imaginative and often has its finger on the pulse of popular culture. So, although creativity and cultural resonance may not be enough—by themselves—to sell brotherhood or achieve other highly desirable social improvements, their combination with the systematic application of the social marketing principles described in this chapter may be.

REFERENCES

Anderson, C. *The Long Tail: Why the Future of Business Is Selling Less of More.* New York: Hyperion, 2006.

Andreasen, A. "Social Marketing: Definition and Domain." *Journal of Public Policy & Marketing,* 1994, *13*(1), 108–114.

Andreasen, A. *Social Marketing in the 21st Century.* Thousand Oaks, Calif.: Sage, 2006.

Bagozzi, R. P. "Marketing as an Organized Behavioral System of Exchange." *Journal of Marketing,* 1974, October, 77–81.

Bagozzi, R. P. "Marketing as Exchange." *American Behavioral Scientist,* 1978, March-April, 535–556.

Bandura, A. *Social Foundation of Thought and Action: A Social Cognitive Theory.* Upper Saddle River, N.J.: Prentice Hall, 1986.

Bandura, A. *Self-Efficacy: The Exercise of Control.* New York: Freeman, 1997.

Bernhardt, J. M. "Improving Health Through Health Marketing," *Preventing Chronic Disease,* 2006, *3*(3), 1–3.

BPS and ORC Macro. *Indonesian Demographic and Health Survey.* Ministry of Health (Indonesia). Calverton, Md.: Macro International, 2003.

Cialdini, R. B., and Goldstein, N. J. "Social Influence: Compliance and Conformity." *Annual Review of Psychology,* 2004, *55,* 591–621.

Centers for Disease Control and Prevention. "Advancing HIV Prevention: New Strategies for a Changing Epidemic—United States 2003." *MMWR, Morbidity and Mortality Weekly Report,* 2003, *52,* 329–332.

Centers for Disease Control and Prevention. "What Is Health Marketing?" [http://www.cdc.gov/health marketing/whatishm.htm]. 2007.

Coale, A. J., and Watkins, S. *The Decline of European Fertility.* Princeton: Princeton University Press, 1986.

Communication for Healthy Living. *Egypt Health Communication Survey.* Cairo, Egypt: Zanaty & Associates and the Health Communication Partnership, 2005.

Communication for Healthy Living. *Egypt Health Communication Survey.* Cairo, Egypt: Zanaty & Associates and the Health Communication Partnership, 2006a.

Communication for Healthy Living. *Year Three Progress Report.* Baltimore, Md.: Johns Hopkins Center for Communication Programs, 2006b.

Fishbein, M., and Yzer, M. "Using Theory to Design Effective Health Behavior Interventions." *Communication Theory,* 2003, *2,* 164–183.

Frankenberg, E., Sikoki, B., and Suriastini, W. "Contraceptive Use in a Changing Service Environment: Evidence from Indonesia During the Economic Crisis." *Studies in Family Planning,* 2003, *34*(2), 103–116.

Haines, M. P. "Social Norms: A Wellness Model for Health Promotion in Higher Education." *Wellness Management,* 1998, *14*(4), 1, 8.

Harvey, P. D. *Let Every Child Be Wanted: How Social Marketing is Revolutionizing Contraceptive Use Around The World.* Westport, Conn.: Auburn House, 1999.

Kalyanaraman, S., and Sundar, S. "The Psychological Appeal of Personalized Content in Web Portals: Does Customization Affect Attitudes and Behavior?" *Journal of Communication,* 2006, *56*(1), 110–132.

Kasprzyk, D., Montano, D., and Fishbein, M. "Application of an Integrated Behavioral Model to Predict Condom Use: A Prospective Study Among High HIV Risk Group." *Journal of Applied Social Psychology,* 2001, *28,* 1557–1583.

Kincaid, D. L. "Mass Media, Ideation, and Contraceptive Behavior: A Longitudinal Analysis of Contraceptive Change in the Philippines." *Communication Research,* 2000, *27*(6), 723–763.

Kincaid, D. L. "From Innovation to Social Norm: Bounded Normative Influence." *Journal of Health Communication,* 2004, *9*(1), 37–57.

Kotler, P., and Roberto, E. L. *Social Marketing Strategies for Changing Public Behavior.* New York: Free Press, 1989.

Kotler, P., and Zaltman, G. "Social Marketing: An Approach to Planned Social Change." *Journal of Marketing,* 1971, *35,* 3–12.

Lesthaeghe, R., and Vanderhoeft, C. "Ready, Willing, and Able: A Conceptualization of Transitions to New Behavioral Forms." Paper presented at the National Academy of Sciences meeting on the Social Dynamics of Fertility Change in Developing Countries, Washington, D.C., January 29–30, 1998.

Linkenbach, J. W. "Application of Social Norms Marketing to a Variety of Health Issues." *Wellness Management,* 1999, *15*(3) [entire issue].

Maibach, E., Abroms, L., and Marosits, M. "Communication and Marketing as Tools to Cultivate the Public's Health: A Proposed 'People and Places' Framework." *BMC Public Health,* 2007, *7*(88) [http://www.biomed central.com/1471–2458/7/88].

Maibach, E. W., Rothschild, M. L., and Novelli, W. D. "Social Marketing." In K. Glanz, B. K. Rimer, and F. M. Lewis (eds.), *Health Behavior and Health Education.* (3rd ed.) San Francisco: Jossey-Bass, 2002.

McGuire, W. J. "Theoretical Foundations of Campaigns." In R. Rice, and C. Atkin (eds.), *Public Communication Campaigns.* (2nd ed.) Newbury Park, Calif.: Sage, 1989.

Mindset. "About Mindset." [http://www.mindset.co.za/corporate/templates/about.htm]. 2007.

Mize, L., and Robey, B. *A 35 Year Commitment to Family Planning in Indonesia: BKKBN and USAID's Historic Partnership.* Baltimore, Md.: Johns Hopkins Bloomberg School of Public Health/Center for Communication Programs, 2006.

MOHP and ORC Macro. "Egypt Demographic and Health Survey." Ministry of Health and Population (Egypt). Calverton, Md.: Macro International, 1995.

MOHP and ORC Macro. "Egypt Demographic and Health Survey." Ministry of Health and Population (Egypt). Calverton, Md.: Macro International, 2000.

MOHP and ORC Macro. "Egypt Demographic and Health Survey." Ministry of Health and Population (Egypt). Calverton, Md.: Macro International, 2003.

MOHP and ORC Macro. "Egypt Demographic and Health Survey." Ministry of Health and Population (Egypt). Calverton, Md.: Macro International, 2005.

Paisley. W. "Public Communication Campaigns: The American Experience." In R. E. Rice and C. K. Atkin (eds.), *Public Communication Campaigns.* (2nd ed.) Newbury Park, Calif.: Sage, 1989.

Palmgreen, P., and others. "Effects of the Office of National Drug Control Policy's Marijuana Initiative Campaign on High-Sensation-Seeking Adolescents." *American Journal of Public Health,* 2007, *97*(9), 1644–1649.

Perkins, H. W., and Berkowitz, A. D. "Perceiving the Community Norms of Alcohol Use Among Students: Some Research Implications for Campus Alcohol Education Programming." *International Journal of the Addictions,* 1986, *21,* 961–976.

Piotrow, P. T., Kincaid, D. L., Rimon, J. G., and Rinehart, W. *Health Communication: Lessons from Family Planning and Reproductive Health.* Westport, Conn.: Praeger, 1997.

Prochaska, J., and DiClemente, C. "The Transtheoretical Approach." In J. C. Norcross and M. R. Goldfield (eds.), *Handbook of Psychotherapy Integration.* New York: Basic Books, 1992.

Rimon, J. G., Negrette, J. C., and Storey, J. D. "The Family Planning Program in Indonesia: Addressing Critical Problems." Working Paper. Baltimore, Md.: Johns Hopkins Bloomberg School of Public Health/Center for Communication Programs, 2006.

Rogers, E. M. *Diffusion of Innovations.* (5th ed.) New York: Free Press. 2003.

Rogers, E. M., and Storey, J. D. "Communication Campaigns." In C. R. Berger and S. H. Chaffee (eds.), *Handbook of Communication Science.* Thousand Oaks, Calif.: Sage, 1987.

Rothschild, M. L. "Carrots, Sticks, and Promises: A Conceptual Framework for the Management of Public Health and Social Issue Behaviors." *Journal of Marketing,* 1999, *63,* 24–37.

Storey, J. D., Figueroa, M. E., and Kincaid, D. L. "Health Competence Communication: A Systems Approach to Sustainable Preventive Health." Technical Report. Baltimore, Md.: Johns Hopkins Bloomberg School of Public Health/Center for Communication Programs, 2005.

Storey, J. D., and Schoemaker, J. "Communication, Normative Influence and the Sustainability of Health Behavior Over Time: A Multilevel Analysis of Contraceptive Use in Indonesia, 1997–2003." Paper presented at the Annual Conference of the International Communication Association, Dresden, Germany, May 2006.

United States Agency for International Development. Communication Activity Approval Document. Draft Concept Paper. Washington, D.C.: United States Agency for International Development, Office of Population and Reproductive Health, 2001.

Wiebe, G. D. "Merchandising Commodities and Citizenship on Television." *Public Opinion Quarterly,* 1951–1952, *15,* 679–691.

Witte, K. "Fear Control and Danger Control: A Test of the Extended Parallel Processing Model (EPPM)." *Communication Monographs,* 1994, *61,* 113–134.

World Health Organization. The First Ten Years of WHO. Geneva: World Health Organization, 1958.

CHAPTER

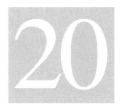

ECOLOGICAL MODELS OF HEALTH BEHAVIOR

James F. Sallis

Neville Owen

Edwin B. Fisher

KEY POINTS

This chapter will

- Provide a brief history of ecological models as applied to health promotion.
- Propose four core principles of ecological models of health behavior: (1) there are multiple levels of influence on specific health behaviors; (2) influences on behaviors interact across these different levels; (3) ecological models should be behavior-specific; and (4) multi-level interventions should be most effective in changing behavior.
- Describe applications of ecological models for health behavior research related to understanding influences on physical activity behavior and to comprehensive, multi-level interventions for tobacco control and diabetes self-management.
- Review strengths and limitations of ecological models, along with the challenges of applying them.

Ecological models of health behavior emphasize the environmental and policy contexts of behavior, while incorporating social and psychological influences. Ecological models lead to the explicit consideration of multiple levels of influence, thereby guiding the development of more comprehensive interventions.

In the past two decades, there has been a dramatic increase in interest in, and application of, ecological models in research and practice, due in part to their promise for guiding comprehensive populationwide approaches to changing behaviors that will reduce serious and prevalent health problems. The combination of environmental, policy, social, and individual intervention strategies is credited with the major reductions in tobacco use in the United States since the 1960s (Institute of Medicine, 2001), and this experience has stimulated the application of multi-level models and interventions to many health problems.

The core concept of an ecological model is that behavior has multiple levels of influences, often including intrapersonal (biological, psychological), interpersonal (social, cultural), organizational, community, physical environmental, and policy. Ecological models are believed to provide comprehensive frameworks for understanding the multiple and interacting determinants of health behaviors. More important, ecological models can be used to develop comprehensive intervention approaches that systematically target mechanisms of change at each level of influence.

Four core principles of ecological models of health behavior are proposed:

1. There are multiple influences on specific health behaviors, including factors at the intrapersonal, interpersonal, organizational, community, and public policy levels.

2. Influences on behaviors interact across these different levels.

3. Ecological models should be behavior-specific, identifying the most relevant potential influences at each level.

4. Multi-level interventions should be most effective in changing behavior.

The ultimate purpose of ecological models of health behavior is to inform the development of comprehensive intervention approaches that can systematically target mechanisms of change at several levels of influence. Behavior change is expected to be maximized when environments and policies support healthful choices, when social norms and social support for healthful choices are strong, and when individuals are motivated and educated to make those choices.

BACKGROUND, HISTORY, AND PRINCIPLES OF ECOLOGICAL MODELS

The term *ecology* is derived from biological science and refers to the interrelations between organisms and their environments. Ecological models, as they have evolved in behavioral sciences and public health, focus on the nature of people's transactions with their physical and sociocultural surroundings, that is, environments (Stokols, 1992). The environmental levels of influence distinguish ecological models from behavioral models and theories that emphasize individual characteristics, skills, and proximal social influences such as family and friends, but do not explicitly consider the broader community, organizational, and policy influences on health behaviors. Ecological models can incorporate constructs from models that focus on psychological, social, and organizational levels of influence to provide a comprehensive framework for integrating multiple theories, along with consideration of environments and policy in the broader community.

Healthy behaviors are thought to be maximized when environments and policies support healthful choices, and individuals are motivated and educated to make those choices (Ottawa Charter for Health Promotion, 1986). Educating people to make healthful choices when environments are not supportive can produce weak and short-term effects, which are common. Yet just providing plentiful vegetables, sidewalks, or accessible condoms is no guarantee that people will make use of those resources. Thus, a central conclusion of ecological models is that it usually takes the combination of *both* individual-level and environmental/policy-level interventions to achieve substantial changes in health behaviors.

A general acceptance of, and enthusiasm for, ecological models as applied to health behavior is reflected in authoritative documents that guide public health programs nationally and internationally. These documents include *Healthy People 2010* (U.S. Department of Health and Human Services, 2000a), Institute of Medicine (IOM) reports on health behaviors (Institute of Medicine, 2001) and childhood obesity prevention (Koplan, Liverman and Kraak, 2005), the World Health Organization's (WHO) strategy for diet, physical activity, and obesity (World Health Organization, 2004), and the WHO Framework Convention on Tobacco Control (World Health Organization, 2003).

Historical and Conceptual Background of Ecological Models

The proliferation of contemporary ecological models is based on a rich conceptual tradition in the behavioral and social sciences. The contributions of many of these authors were described in a previous version of the present chapter (Sallis and Owen, 2002), and they are summarized in Table 20.1. Early on, there was a progression from the concept that only *perceptions* of environments were important (Lewin and Cartwright, 1951) to an emphasis on *direct effects* of environments on behavior (Barker, 1968). Many models were meant to apply broadly to behaviors, but more recent models were created for application to health behaviors and health promotion, such as those proposed by McLeroy and others (1988), Stokols and others (1992, 2003), Flay and Petraitis (1994), Cohen, Scribner, and Farley (2000), Fisher and others (2005), Glanz and others (2005), and Glass and McAtee (2006). Categories and hierarchies of behavioral influences have been described in numerous ways, from Bronfenbrenner's (1979) micro, meso, and exo environment approach to McLeroy and others' (1988) five sources of influence: intrapersonal, interpersonal, institutional, community, and policy. The first part of Table 20.1 describes models mainly designed to help explain behavior, and the second part contains models primarily intended to guide interventions. Some of the newer models are designed to be applicable to many health behaviors (Cohen, Scribner, and Farley, 2000; Glass and McAtee, 2006; Stokols, 1992; Stokols, Grzywacz, McMahan, and Phillips, 2003), while others are tailor-made for specific categories of behaviors (Flay and Petraitis, 1994; Fisher and others, 2005; Glanz, Sallis, Saelens, and Frank, 2005). This diversity illustrates the adaptability and robustness of ecological models.

TABLE 20.1. **Historical and Contemporary Ecological Models.**

Author, Citation, Model	Key Concepts
Models designed mainly to explain behavior	
Kurt Lewin (1951) Ecological Psychology	"Ecological psychology" is the study of the influence of the outside environment on the person.
Roger Barker (1968) Environmental Psychology	"Behavior settings" are the social and physical situations in which behaviors take place; concludes that behaviors could be predicted more accurately from the situations people are in than from their individual characteristics.
Rudolph Moos (1980) Social Ecology	Four categories of environmental factors: (1) physical settings—features of the natural (weather) and built environment (building); (2) organizational settings—size and function of worksites and schools; (3) the "human aggregate"—sociocultural characteristics of the people in an environment; and (4) "social climate"—supportiveness of a social setting for a particular behavior.
Urie Bronfenbrenner (1979) Systems Theory	Three levels of environmental influences: (1) "microsystem" is interactions among family members and work groups; (2) "mesosystem" is physical family, school, and work settings; and (3) "exosystem" is the larger social system of economics, culture, and politics.
Thomas Glass and Matthew McAtee (2006) Ecosocial Model	Conceptualizes hierarchies of influences on behavior within biology and society, which has social and physical environment dimensions. Structural contingencies provide opportunities and constraints, and biological processes regulate expression of behavior.
Models designed mainly to guide behavioral interventions	
B. F. Skinner (1953) Operant Learning Theory	Primary model is Environment→Behavior. Reinforcers and cues in the environment directly control behavior. Recently, Hovell and colleagues (2002) proposed a behavioral ecological model that draws heavily on Skinner.
Albert Bandura (1986) Social Learning and Social Cognitive Theories	Proposes environmental and personal influences on behavior. Bandura referred mainly to social environments and rarely addressed the role of physical, community, or organizational environments. (See Chapter Eight.)

TABLE 20.1. **Historical and Contemporary Ecological Models, Cont'd.**

Author, Citation, Model	Key Concepts
Models designed mainly to guide behavioral interventions, Cont'd.	
Kenneth McLeroy and others (1988) Ecological Model of Health Behavior	Five sources of influence on health behaviors: intrapersonal factors, interpersonal processes and primary groups, institutional factors, community factors, and public policy.
Daniel Stokols (1992, 2003) Social Ecology Model for Health Promotion	Four assumptions: (1) health behavior is influenced by physical environments, social environments, and personal attributes; (2) environments are multidimensional, such as social or physical, actual or perceived, discrete attributes (spatial arrangements) or constructs (social climate); (3) human-environment interactions occur at varying levels of aggregation (individuals, families, cultural groups, whole populations); and (4) people influence their settings, and the changed settings then influence health behaviors.
Deborah Cohen and others (2000) Structural-Ecological Model	Four categories of structural influences: (1) availability of protective or harmful consumer products, (2) physical structures (or physical characteristics of products), (3) social structures and policies, and (4) media and cultural messages.
Brian Flay and J. Petraitis (1994) Theory of Triadic Influence	Genes and environment are assumed to affect all behaviors, and the three streams of influence on behavior are intrapersonal, social, and sociocultural.
Karen Glanz and others (2005) Model of Community Food Environments	Proposes key constructs that affect eating behaviors: availability, price, placement, and promotion of foods, as well as nutrition information. Applies to restaurants and food stores.
Edwin Fisher and others (2005) Resources and Skills for Self-Management Model	Based on integration of individuals' skills and choices with support they receive from the social environment, as well as physical and policy environments of communities.

Principles of Ecological Perspectives on Health Behavior Change

Four core principles of ecological perspectives are proposed.

1. *Multiple levels of factors influence health behaviors.* Ecological models specify that factors at multiple levels, often including intrapersonal, interpersonal, organizational, community, and public policy, can influence health behaviors. Concepts that cut across these levels include sociocultural factors and physical environments, which may apply to more than one level. Inclusion of all these levels of influence distinguishes ecological models from theories that primarily focus on one or two levels.

2. *Influences interact across levels.* The interaction of influences means that variables work together. For example, individuals with high motivation to avoid weight gain may react differently than those with lower motivation to driving past a strip of fast-food restaurants. Education to be physically active may work better when policies support physician counseling and insurance discounts for engaging in regular activity. Because ecological models specify multiple levels of influence, and there are likely to be multiple variables at each level, it may be difficult to discern which of the possible interactions are most important. Thus, a challenge for research is to expand understanding of these interactions across levels.

3. *Multi-level interventions should be most effective in changing behavior.* A direct implication of ecological models is that single-level interventions are unlikely to have powerful or sustained populationwide effects. Many examples of interventions targeting individuals have shown short-term effects. Educational interventions designed to change beliefs and behavioral skills are likely to work better when policies and environments support the targeted behavior changes. Similarly, environmental changes by themselves may be insufficient to change behavior. Putting more fruits and vegetables in all convenience stores may have little impact unless the environmental change is supported by communication, education, and motivational campaigns.

4. *Ecological models are most powerful when they are behavior-specific.* Ecological models appear most useful to guide research and intervention when they are tailored to specific health behaviors. Often, environmental and policy variables are behavior-specific. The availability of condoms in nightclubs has little relevance to dietary behaviors, the presence of cycling trails in suburban neighborhoods is unlikely to affect alcohol intake, and policies related to food subsidies have little relevance to sun protection behaviors. The need to identify environmental and policy variables that are specific to each behavior is a challenge in the use of ecological models, because lessons learned with one behavior, for example, promoting jogging, may not translate to an apparently similar behavior, for example, promoting walking to work. Of course, some lessons learned in one can apply to others. General ecological models can be used as the basis of behavior-specific models that are needed for application to research and interventions.

APPLICATION OF ECOLOGICAL MODELS TO HEALTH BEHAVIOR

The following sections describe examples of ecological models applied to understanding influences on health behavior and guiding interventions for health behavior change.

The first example describes the recent emergence of ecological models to understand physical activity. The second and third applications illustrate the impact of multi-level interventions for tobacco control and diabetes management that were guided by ecological models.

Application to Understanding Influences on Physical Activity

Physical inactivity is one of the most significant health challenges, because of its effects on risk of major chronic diseases, mental health, quality of life, and early mortality (U.S. Department of Health and Human Services, 1996). The physical activity field has advanced from a broad recognition of the importance of environmental influences to development and testing of specific multi-level ecological models. For example, Giles-Corti and colleagues (2005) and Saelens and colleagues (2003) proposed models to highlight the different influences on recreational versus transportation physical activity, while Owen and others' (2004) model was specific to walking for different purposes. Matsudo and colleagues (2004) developed an ecological model to guide community interventions in a Latin American context.

Sallis and coauthors (2006) synthesized findings and concepts from the fields of health, behavioral science, transportation and city planning, policy studies and economics, and leisure sciences to create the ecological model shown in Figure 20.1. The model has a commonly used layered or "onion" structure to represent the multiple levels of influence, but with three distinguishing features. First, the model is organized around four domains of physical activity, reflecting the principle that behavior-specific ecological models are useful. Second, some types of relevant influences are not tied to settings where the behavior takes place. For example, information environments are ubiquitous, and counseling in health care settings can influence physical activity done elsewhere. A third key feature is that social and cultural environments operate at multiple levels. Other ecological models can be developed for specific physical activity behaviors (for example, walking to school, use of parks) and population subgroups (for example, racial-ethnic minority groups, rural residents).

It is important to test empirically the principles of ecological models and the propositions and hypotheses derived from these principles. Studies based on ecological models have recently addressed a major gap in understanding community environmental attributes. In the health and behavioral sciences field, a review by Humpel, Owen, and Leslie (2002) identified that access to physical activity facilities, and the aesthetic qualities of those places were consistently related to recreational physical activity. Saelens, Sallis, and Frank (2003) reviewed studies from the transportation and urban planning fields and found consistent evidence of more walking (and possibly cycling) for transportation among adults living in "walkable neighborhoods." In walkable neighborhoods, land uses are mixed, with homes near commercial and institutional destinations, and streets are highly connected, providing direct routes from place to place.

Most studies of environmental correlates of physical activity have not distinguished the relative importance of personal, social, and environmental influences on physical activity (Biddle and Mutrie, 2001). A few studies have examined correlates

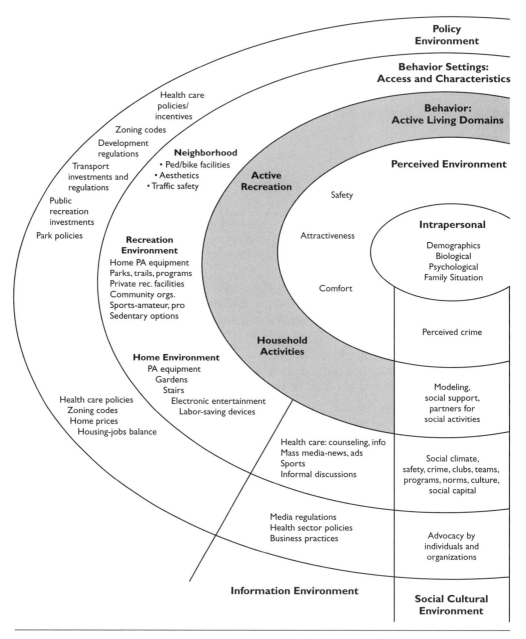

FIGURE 20.1. Ecological Model of Four Domains of Active Living.

Source: Sallis, J. F., Cervero, R. B., Ascher, W., Henderson, K. A., Kraft, M. K., and Kerr, J. (2006). "An Ecological Approach to Creating More Physically Active Communities." *Annual Review of Public Health, 27,* 297–322. Reprinted, with permission, from the *Annual Review of Public Health*, Volume 27, ©2006 by Annual Reviews (www.annualreviews.org).

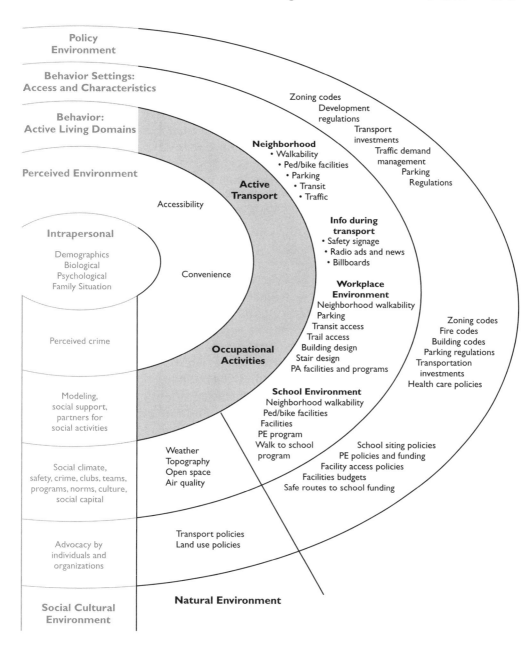

Policy
Environment

Behavior Settings:
Access and Characteristics

Behavior:
Active Living Domains

Perceived Environment

Intrapersonal

Demographics
Biological
Psychological
Family Situation

Perceived crime

Modeling,
social support,
partners for
social activities

Social climate,
safety, crime, clubs, teams,
programs, norms, culture,
social capital

Advocacy by
individuals and
organizations

Social Cultural
Environment

Accessibility

Convenience

Active
Transport

Neighborhood
• Walkability
• Ped/bike facilities
• Parking
• Transit
• Traffic

Zoning codes
Development
regulations
Transport
investments
Traffic demand
management
Parking
Regulations

Info during
transport
• Safety signage
• Radio ads and news
• Billboards

Occupational
Activities

Workplace
Environment
Neighborhood walkability
Parking
Transit access
Trail access
Building design
Stair design
PA facilities and programs

Zoning codes
Fire codes
Building codes
Parking regulations
Transportation
investments
Health care policies

School Environment
Neighborhood walkability
Ped/bike facilities
Facilities
PE program
Walk to school
program

School siting policies
PE policies and funding
Facility access policies
Facilities budgets
Safe routes to school funding

Weather
Topography
Open space
Air quality

Transport policies
Land use policies

Natural Environment

of physical activity at multiple levels and found that built environment variables, such as the presence of sidewalks and nearby destinations, accounted for the least variance (De Bourdeaudhuij, Sallis, and Saelens, 2003; Burton, Turrell, Oldenburg, and Sallis, 2005; Giles-Corti and Donovan, 2002). An Australian study showed that built environment factors accounted for a modest amount of variation in walking for transport, and that such environmental factors (that is, objectively assessed neighborhood walkability) remained significant after controlling for personal attributes, such as individuals' reasons for choosing to live in their neighborhoods (Owen and others, 2007). Although recent physical activity studies appropriately focused on previously understudied built environment attributes, it is now time to examine correlates and interactions across multiple levels.

Testing hypotheses derived from ecological models presents particular study design challenges. A central problem is that there may be too little variation in social, environmental, and policy variables across units of study (Giles-Corti and Donovan, 2002). For example, a random sample from a U.S. city might yield few adults who value active transport (walking and bicycling), limited social support for walking for transportation, and few high-walkable neighborhoods. A random sample in many European cities would likely produce few participants with negative attitudes, widespread social support for active transportation, and few low-walkable neighborhoods. Within a study region, there may be no variation at all in policies related to park resources or zoning laws. Lack of variation leads to underestimation of effect sizes and inability to test some hypotheses. Thus, studies that include assessments of environmental and policy variables must be designed to ensure variation in those factors.

In summary, the rapidly growing literature on built environment correlates of physical activity complements a large literature on intrapersonal and interpersonal correlates. The next priority is to improve understanding of multi-level correlates and interactions across levels of influence, then use the findings to guide development of more effective interventions.

Application to Health Behavior Interventions: Tobacco Control

Ecological Models and Cigarette Smoking.   Influences on smoking range from the brain physiology of nicotine addiction to peer pressure to smoke, household smoking restrictions, and taxation policy. At the individual level, addiction to nicotine and genetic factors contribute to persistence of smoking. These add to the effects of substantial psychological conditioning—the average smoker of a pack a day for twenty years has inhaled over a million times, establishing conditioned associations of smoking with work, relaxation, drinking coffee, and moods like anxiety and depression (Fisher and others, 2004). At the social level, parents' and peers' smoking are predictors of youth smoking (U.S. Department of Health and Human Services, 1994). Cigarettes are one of the most heavily marketed products in the United States. In 2005, tobacco companies spent $13.1 billion in advertising and marketing—over $35 million a day (American Lung Association, 2007). Youth with greatest exposure to tobacco marketing are more likely to start smoking and to become frequent smokers (Pierce and others, 1998).

Influences at different ecological levels can interact with each other. For example, the genetics of nicotine metabolism and the addictive nature of smoking create strong markets for cigarettes. Profitability of selling cigarettes drives advertising and marketing campaigns that promote the mood-elevating benefits of tobacco, as well as political contributions by companies that oppose restrictions on tobacco products. The cycle continues as success in attracting new smokers and keeping them addicted ensures the profitability of the cigarette business.

Individual-Level Interventions for Smoking Cessation. Parallel to the many levels of influences on smoking are the levels of interventions. Brief advice to quit in individual medical encounters is effective in promoting cessation (U.S. Department of Health and Human Services, 2000b). Ample evidence supports the helpfulness of nicotine replacement and other pharmacological quitting aids (U.S. Department of Health and Human Services, 2000b). Telephone counseling (Task Force on Community Preventive Services, 2005), self-help pamphlets, books, videotapes, and Web resources (Fisher and others, 2004) also work at an individual level but can more readily reach large numbers of smokers.

Organizational, Community, and Policy Approaches At the organizational level, reductions in smoking have been documented through programs restricting smoking at the workplace (Brownson, Hopkins, and Wakefield, 2002). Programs that emphasize community participation in program development have been successful in several settings, including low-income neighborhoods (Fisher and others, 2004).

Policy interventions—for example, promoting smoke-free environments, limiting access, and increasing tobacco prices through excise taxes—were the focus of the American Stop Smoking Intervention Study (ASSIST) program. ASSIST was implemented in seventeen states through grants to state departments of health and local steering committees. Policies promoting not smoking (for example, proportion of smoke-free workplaces) increased more in ASSIST states than in other states, and smoking prevalence fell from 25.2 percent to 22.2 percent, significantly more than the decline from 24.4 percent to 22.3 percent in the non-ASSIST states (Stillman and others, 2003). The strength of local coalitions and extent of focus on policy change predicted statewide improvements. Internationally, tobacco policy initiatives include the World Health Organization's (2003) Tobacco Free Initiative and Framework Convention on Tobacco Control. Tobacco control policies play an especially important role in prevention. In the United States, states with the most extensive array of tobacco control policies have significantly lower youth smoking prevalence (U.S. Department of Health and Human Services, 1994).

Importance of Multiple Intervention Approaches. Research on smoking cessation is consistent with ecological models' emphasis on the interplay among influences on health behaviors. At the individual level, the likelihood of success of an intervention is not as strongly influenced by the specific form of treatment (for example, self-help, individual counseling) as by the *number of different forms* of treatment used (U.S. Department of Health and Human Services, 2000b). This importance of combining interventions is also reflected in benefits of simultaneously educating health

care workers about smoking cessation and creating systems to remind them to counsel patients about quitting or combining telephone counseling with mass media (Task
Force on Community Preventive Services, 2005).

At the state level, comprehensive multi-level programs have created substantial
reductions in smoking. Multicomponent campaigns of public education, including
"counter-marketing" TV advertisements and billboards, increased taxes on cigarettes,
support services for cessation, smoking prevention programs for youth, and multicultural approaches are often coordinated by community coalitions. Evaluations support the importance of the combination of multiple components in comprehensive
campaigns (Siegel, 2002).

Comprehensive Interventions at the National Level. The combination of efforts
at all levels of the ecological model contributed to a marked drop in smoking rates
among adults in the United States, from 42 percent in 1965 to 21 percent in 2005
(Centers for Disease Control and Prevention, 2006). This has been achieved through
the best example of an array of multi-level population-based health behavior interventions to date. Highlights at several ecological levels include wide dissemination
of individualized smoking cessation programs, nicotine replacement therapy, counseling by health professionals (individual level), workplace and community-based
programs, as well as programs tailored to reach different groups (social/cultural and
organizational levels), news coverage, government reports, anti-smoking campaigns
of various health agencies (population-level mass communication), clean indoor air
restrictions (physical environment and policy levels), and restrictions on access to
cigarettes and tax increases on their sale (policy level) (Fisher and others, 2004; Task
Force on Community Preventive Services, 2005). Interactions among levels are likely
to be important. For example, worksite smoking restrictions have motivated employees to seek help in quitting smoking, mass communication and social marketing have
promoted individual cessation interventions such as quitline-based telephone counseling, and increased excise taxes have probably helped to reduce youths' initiation
of smoking and to increase the acceptability of policy changes, such as restrictions
on where people can smoke.

In summary, multiple, varied, and sustained interventions are responsible for the
massive decline in smoking in the United States. Tobacco use is now widely recognized as a social and public health problem, not just an individual behavior. To explain the population changes in smoking *requires* an ecological perspective, and
population-level changes reflect the aggregate of the many interventions promoting
not smoking, not a single-level "magic bullet."

Application to Health Interventions: Diabetes Self-Management

Diabetes is a major cause of mortality through cardiovascular and other diseases. Substantial evidence indicates that self-management training enhances diabetes management (Norris and others, 2002). It may seem surprising to examine *self*-management
from an ecological perspective. Self-management is often conceptualized as an individual responsibility in which "only the patient can be responsible for his or her

day-to-day care over the length of the illness" (Lorig and Holman, 2003). However, research does not support the contention that self- management interventions make individuals self-sufficient or autonomous in managing their disease. Rather, a meta-analysis of diabetes self-management programs found sharp declines in benefits a few months after the interventions ended (Norris and others, 2002). These findings are congruent with an ecological perspective in which the long-term success of "self-management" depends on the contexts that surround the individual.

An ecological approach to diabetes self-management guided program development in fourteen ethnically and economically diverse primary care and community settings of the Robert Wood Johnson Foundation's Diabetes Initiative (http://www.di-abetesinitiative.org). From an ecological perspective, people with diabetes need diverse resources and supports for self- management to manage the disease in their daily lives. These include (1) individualized assessment, (2) collaborative goal-setting, (3) opportunities to learn skills specific to diabetes (for example, measuring blood sugar) and for addressing challenges, including negative emotions, that may interfere with management, (4) ongoing follow-up and support, (5) community resources, such as for regular physical activity and healthy diet, and (6) continuity of quality clinical care. As indicated in Figure 20.2, several of the Resources and Supports for Self Management (RSSM), such as individualized assessment and collaborative goal setting, are most often addressed at the individual level while others, such as access to resources and continuity of quality clinical care, must be addressed at the group, health system, community, or policy levels. Consistent with ecological models' emphasis on interactions among levels, policies influence the resources and choices available to the individual, and individuals learn skills to access resources.

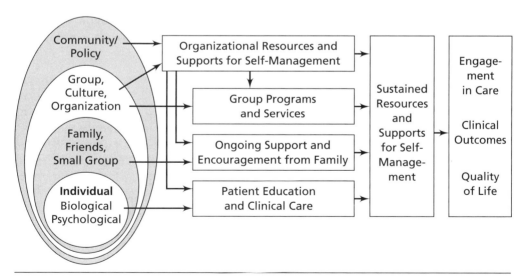

FIGURE 20.2. Illustrative Model of Relationships among Organizational Factors and Supports for Diabetes Self-Management. (*Reprinted with permission.*)

There is a substantial literature on evaluations of individual and group approaches to this intervention model of RSSM (Fisher and others, 2005). To highlight the contributions of an ecological framework, the following sections review ongoing follow-up and support, community resources, and organizational and system approaches to continuity of quality clinical care.

Ongoing Follow-Up and Support. The goals of follow-up include continued assistance in refining problem-solving plans and skills, encouragement in the face of challenges, and assistance in responding to problems that emerge in the course of a chronic disease. Several approaches to providing follow-up and support can be used, including phone calls with nurses and contacts with community health workers, lay health workers, and *Promotores de Salud* (Health Coaches).

The structure of clinical care may contribute to ongoing support through group medical visits (Trento and others, 2004). In these visits, patients with diabetes are scheduled for two- to three-hour group visits that include medical appointments, education (for example, reviews of self-management plans or cooking classes), and supportive discussions. As one example of this type of strategy, the Open Door Health Center in Homestead, Florida expanded group medical visits to a weekly open group that included cooking demonstrations, physical activity, group support, opportunities to ask questions of health care staff, and, when scheduled, physician appointments.

Diabetes is "for the rest of your life," and the meta-analytic review by Norris and colleagues (2002) points to the critical role of duration of follow-up and support. However, most of the U.S. health care system and most intervention research are oriented toward time-limited treatment. Few diabetes intervention studies include follow-up periods longer than one or two years, yet many with diabetes live thirty or forty years with the disease. One health center secured state funding for Health Coaches for diabetes, but the funding was time-limited and restricted to newly diagnosed cases and those whose disease had gotten worse. *Ongoing* follow-up and support for *good self-management* are among the effective and recommended components of diabetes self-management, but they are infrequently provided.

Continuity of Quality Clinical Care. Self-management and quality clinical care are dependent on each other. Without sound clinical care, the individual's efforts may be misdirected. An example would be frustration over failure of dietary changes to lower cholesterol when cholesterol-lowering medications are indicated. Without self-management, clinical care will fall short of its potential, through failure to achieve healthful behavior patterns (for example, increased physical activity or healthy diet), nonadherence to recommended use of prescribed medications, or both.

A comprehensive approach to improving diabetes care services developed in one health system included handouts and manuals, out-patient programs, Web-based programs, telephone/nurse case management, financial incentives for physicians' meeting testing guidelines, and patient incentives for annual eye exams. The multi-level intervention led to improvements in a variety of outcomes (Larsen, Cannon, and Towner, 2003). As only 30 percent to 40 percent of patients with diabetes report receiving self-management interventions (Austin, 2006), there is a need to better disseminate integrated comprehensive clinical and self-management services.

Access to Resources in Daily Life. Recent studies demonstrate the connections between health behaviors and access to healthy food outlets in neighborhoods (Glanz, Sallis, Saelens, and Frank, 2005) and resources for physical activity (Humpel, Owen, and Leslie, 2002). It makes little sense to teach someone about physical activity and healthy diet while ignoring her neighborhood, where it is dangerous to walk alone, food sellers offer little healthy food, and there is limited public transportation to access health resources. Deprivation of community resources is more common in low-income and minority neighborhoods and may contribute to the disproportionate burden of diabetes in low-income and minority communities. Research-based approaches to increasing community resources for diabetes management include community approaches to enhancing resources for physical activity and healthy eating (Nasmith and others, 2004), as well as Web-based discussion groups (Goldberg and others, 2003) and training pharmacists to support self-management (Cranor, Bunting, and Christensen, 2003).

Diabetes self-management illustrates the potential for ecological models to address a complex array of health behaviors. Ecological models can be used to reframe behavior often seen as the "responsibility" of the individual to include required change at the clinical (organizational) and community levels. Finally, because diabetes is an excellent model of chronic disease care in general, the ecological RSSM model may also be applied in the management of other chronic diseases.

CRITICAL EXAMINATION OF ECOLOGICAL MODELS OF HEALTH BEHAVIOR

Ecological models have been central to health promotion for several decades now. Health policy groups rely increasingly on multi-level interventions to solve the most pressing health problems. Based in part on the success in reversing the epidemic of tobacco use, there are high expectations that interventions based on ecological models can reverse the obesity epidemic by improving environments and policies that drive physical activity and nutrition behaviors. The Institute of Medicine (2001; Koplan, Liverman, and Kraak, 2005) and the World Health Organization (2004) propose solutions to obesity that require policy and environmental change. The increasing emphasis on applications of ecological models creates a need for a critical examination of their strengths and weaknesses. Enthusiasm for the potential of ecological models does not reduce the need to understand the benefits and limitations of multi-level interventions, test hypotheses derived from ecological models, and continue to refine the concepts and methods used in research and practice informed by ecological models.

A key strength of ecological models is their focus on multiple levels of influence that broadens options for interventions. Policy and environmental changes are expected to affect virtually entire populations, in contrast to interventions that reach only individuals who choose to participate (Glanz and Mullis, 1988). Policy and environmental interventions establish settings and incentives that can persist in sustaining behavior changes, helping to solve the problem that the effects of many individually directed interventions are poorly maintained.

A weakness of many general ecological models of health behavior is their lack of specificity about the most important hypothesized influences. This puts a greater burden on health promotion professionals to identify critical factors for each behavioral application. A related weakness—even for behavior-specific ecological models—is the lack of information about how the broader levels of influence operate or how variables interact across levels. Thus, the models broaden *perspectives* without identifying specific variables or providing guidance about how to use ecological models to improve research or interventions. By contrast, individual-level psychosocial theories of health behavior are more likely to specify the variables and mechanisms by which those variables are expected to influence behavior (see chapters Three through Six). A major challenge for those working with ecological models is to develop more sophisticated operational models that lead to testable hypotheses and useful guidance for interventions. Other key challenges of ecological models of health behavior also warrant attention.

Are the Principles of Multi-Level Influences and Interactions Across Levels Supported?

Physical activity researchers have begun to test principles of ecological models by developing testable behavior-specific and study-specific hypotheses. Though the number of studies is small and many have important methodological limitations, there is consistent support for the principle of multi-level influences but inconsistent support for interactions across levels. Giles-Corti and Donovan (2002) compared the ability of psychological, social, and physical environment variables to explain exercise. Each category of variables was significantly related to exercise, but associations were strongest for individual variables and weakest for physical environment variables. This study provides some support for the multi-level principle but found no significant interactions across levels.

Two studies examined the combined and interactive effects of the Theory of Planned Behavior (TPB) and perceived physical environment variables to explain walking (Rhodes, Brown, and McIntyre, 2006) and overall physical activity (McNeill and others, 2006). McNeill and colleagues (2006) found both social and physical environment factors were related to physical activity, but Rhodes and colleagues (2006) reported the effects of physical environment factors were completely explained by psychosocial variables. Rhodes and colleagues (2006) tested an interaction based on the hypothesis that mixed land use would make it easier for people to follow through on their intentions. The interaction was significant and of moderate strength, supporting the principle of interactions across levels. All of these studies relied on self-report measures and examined only a few variables, so they cannot be considered definitive.

Studies from diverse fields also support the principle of multi-level influences. For example, a study of youth smoking (Leatherdale and others, 2006) found that smoking of significant others and the broader social environment variable of school smoking rate helped to explain youth smoking. In an international study of alcohol abuse (Cherpitel and others, 2006), perceptions of harmful effects of drinking differed in low- and high-consumption countries. Improved understanding of the multi-level and interactive influences could lead to more targeted and effective interventions.

Methodological Challenges of Multi-Level Interventions

Ecological principles point to complex interactions of personal, social, and community characteristics that are difficult to manipulate experimentally. The goal of experimental designs—to isolate an intervention from the effects of its context—may be conceptually at odds with the ecological emphasis on studying how intervention components are influenced by their context. Although controlled experiments with multi-level interventions are challenging to design and conduct, rigorous analytical strategies can be applied productively (Bull, Eakin, Reeves, and Riley, 2006). For example, a community program to promote childhood asthma management intervened on personal, social, and community factors (Fisher and others, 2004). The program was evaluated with a nonrandomized design using structural equation modeling. Individual-level factors like parents' attitudes toward asthma predicted children's medical utilization. In addition, social support from lay asthma workers and asthma management classes predicted reduced emergency and hospital care. Thus, interventions targeted at multiple levels predicted outcomes.

With the application of multi-level analytic approaches, evaluations could be expanded to examine the impact on outcomes of further individual-level factors like genetic predispositions, neighborhood features measured objectively with Geographic Information Systems, variability in multiple intervention components, and contextual factors at organizational, community, and policy levels. With sufficient numbers, multi-level analyses can yield estimates not only of the contributions of interventions to outcomes but also of the extent to which those contributions are influenced by moderating factors. Multi-level statistical models are increasingly accessible, and their use is increasing in evaluations of multi-level interventions and observational studies of the multi-level etiology of health behaviors and diseases (Bingenheimer and Raudenbush, 2004).

Logistical Challenges of Conducting Research and Interventions Based on Ecological Models

Research based on ecological models is, by definition, more demanding than behavioral research at a single level. Developing and collecting measures of influences at multiple levels, expanding the number of disciplines represented in investigative teams, conceptualizing and implementing interventions at multiple levels, and using more sophisticated statistical strategies place substantial demands on investigators and program evaluators. However, multi-level studies are the only way to generate knowledge that will lead to effective multi-level interventions.

Of equal importance, the difficulty of implementing multi-level interventions should not be underestimated. The length of time required to change policies and environments is a deterrent to program directors who are called on to make changes to meet legislators' schedules or within grant timelines. Most environmental variables and policies of interest are not controlled by health professionals, and change requires a political process. To implement multi-level interventions, public health professionals must become more skilled in advocacy and political change, or partner with those who have such skills.

Ecological Models, Individual Responsibility, and Human Dignity

The reframing of health behavior as the result of influences across diverse ecological layers rather than the responsibility of individuals raises interesting issues about the role of individual responsibility for change. Consider how cigarette smoking has become widely viewed as an addiction with biological, behavioral, social, and economic determinants rather than simply an "individual choice." One could view ecological models as "robbing the individual of dignity" by attributing their behaviors to such a range of forces. Alternatively, one could view the ecological perspective as removing an unreasonable attribution of responsibility to the individual—a sort of victim blaming—by recognizing the many forces that shape each individual's behavior. Ecological models transcend philosophical and political polarization over individual versus external influences. From an ecological perspective, individual level and many levels of external influence are integrated in a single framework, making it clear that causation of behavior is widely distributed, not lodged in one or another source. Ecological models can enhance human dignity by moving beyond explanations that hold individuals responsible for, and even blame them for, harmful behaviors.

SUMMARY

Ecological models help us to understand how people interact with their environments. That understanding can be used to develop effective multi-level approaches to improve health behaviors. The basic premise of the ecological perspective is simple. Providing individuals with motivation and skills to change behavior cannot be effective if environments and policies make it difficult or impossible to choose healthful behaviors. Rather, we should create environments and policies that make it convenient, attractive, and economical to make healthful choices, and then motivate and educate people about those choices. The challenge for health promotion researchers and practitioners is to be creative and persistent in using ecological models to generate evidence on the roles of behavioral influences at multiple levels, and on the effectiveness of multi-level interventions on health behaviors, and to translate that evidence into improved health.

REFERENCES

American Lung Association. "Smoking 101 Fact Sheet." [http://www.lungusa.org/site/pp.asp?c=dvLUK9O0E&b=39853#fourteen]. June 2007.

Austin, M. M. "Diabetes Educators: Partners in Diabetes Care and Management." *Endocrinology Practice*, 2006, *12*(Suppl 1), 138–141.

Bandura, A. "Social Foundations of Thought and Action: A Social Cognitive Theory." Englewood Cliffs, N.J.: Prentice Hall, 1986.

Barker, R. G. *Ecological Psychology*. Stanford, Calif.: Stanford University Press, 1968.

Biddle, S., and Mutrie, N. *Psychology of Physical Activity: Determinants, Well-Being and Interventions.* London: Routledge, 2001.

Bingenheimer, J. B., and Raudenbush, S. W. "Statistical and Substantive Inferences in Public Health: Issues in the Application of Multilevel Models." *Annual Review of Public Health*, 2004, *25*, 53–77.

Bronfenbrenner, U. "The Ecology of Human Development." Cambridge, Mass.: Harvard University Press, 1979.

Brownson, R. C., Hopkins, D. P., and Wakefield, M. A. "Effects of Smoking Restrictions in the Workplace." *Annual Review of Public Health*, 2002, *23*, 333–348.

Bull, S., Eakin, E., Reeves, M., and Riley, K. "Multi-Level Support for Physical Activity and Healthy Eating." *Journal of Advanced Nursing*, 2006, *54*, 585–593.

Burton, N. W., Turrell, G., Oldenburg, B., and Sallis, J. F. "The Relative Contributions of Psychological, Social, and Environmental Variables to Explain Walking, Moderate-, and Vigorous-Intensity Leisure-Time Physical Activity." *Journal of Physical Activity and Health*, 2005, *2*, 181–196.

Centers for Disease Control and Prevention. "Tobacco Use Among Adults—United States, 2005." *MMWR, Morbidity and Mortality Weekly Report*, 2006, *55*(42), 1145–1148.

Cherpitel, C. J., and others. "Multi-Level Analysis of Causal Attribution of Injury to Alcohol and Modifying Effects: Data from Two International Emergency Room Projects." *Drug and Alcohol Dependence*, 2006, *82*, 258–268.

Cohen, D. A., Scribner, R. A., and Farley, T. A. "A Structural Model of Health Behavior: A Pragmatic Approach to Explain and Influence Health Behaviors at the Populations Level." *Preventive Medicine*, 2000, *30*, 146–154.

Cranor, C. W., Bunting, B. A., and Christensen, D. B. "The Asheville Project: Longterm Clinical and Economic Outcomes in a Community Pharmacy Diabetes Care Program." *Journal of the American Pharmaceutical Association*, 2003, *43*, 173–184.

De Bourdeaudhuij, I., Sallis, J. F., and Saelens, B. E. "Environmental Correlates of Physical Activity in a Sample of Belgian Adults." *American Journal of Health Promotion*, 2003, *18*, 83–92.

Fisher, E. B., and others. "Cigarette Smoking." In J. Raczynski, L. Bradley, and L. Leviton (eds.), *Health Behavior Handbook*, Vol. 2. Washington, D.C.: American Psychological Association, 2004.

Fisher E. B., and others. "Ecologic Approaches to Self Management: The Case of Diabetes." *American Journal of Public Health*, 2005, *95*(9), 1523–1535.

Flay, B. R., and Petraitis, J. "The Theory of Triadic Influence: A New Theory of Health Behavior with Implications for Preventive Interventions." In G. S. Albrecht (ed.), *Advances in Medical Sociology,* Vol. IV: *A Reconsideration of Models of Health Behavior Change*. Greenwich, Conn.: JAI Press, 1994.

Giles-Corti, B., and Donovan, R. J. "The Relative Influence of Individual, Social and Physical Environment Determinants of Physical Activity." *Social Science and Medicine*, 2002, *54*, 1793–1812.

Giles-Corti, B., Timperio, A., Bull, F., and Pikora, T. "Understanding Physical Activity Environmental Correlates: Increased Specificity for Ecological Models." *Exercise and Sport Sciences Reviews*, 2005, *33*, 175–181.

Glanz, K., and Mullis, R. M. "Environmental Interventions to Promote Healthy Eating: A Review of Models, Programs, and Evidence." *Health Education Quarterly*, 1988, *15*, 395–415.

Glanz, K., Sallis, J. F., Saelens, B. E., and Frank, L. D. "Healthy Nutrition Environments: Concepts and Measures." *American Journal of Health Promotion*, 2005, *19*, 330–333.

Glass, T. A., and McAtee, M. J. "Behavioral Science at the Crossroads in Public Health: Extending Horizons, Envisioning the Future." *Social Science and Medicine*, 2006, *62*, 1650–1671.

Goldberg, H. I., and others. "Using an Internet Comanagement Module to Improve the Quality of Chronic Disease Care." *Joint Commission Journal on Quality & Safety*, 2003, *29*, 443–451.

Hovell, M. F., Wahlgren, D. R., and Gehrman, C. A. "The Behavioral Ecological Model: Integrating Public Health and Behavioral Science." In R. J. DeClemente, R. A. Crosby, and M. Kegler (eds.), *Emerging Theories in Health Promotion Practice and Research: Strategies for Improving Public Health*. San Francisco: Jossey-Bass, 2002.

Humpel, N., Owen, N., and Leslie, E. "Environmental Factors Associated With Adults' Participation in Physical Activity: A Review." *American Journal of Preventive Medicine*, 2002, *22*, 188–199.

Institute of Medicine. *Health and Behavior: The Interplay of Biological, Behavioral, and Societal Influences.* Washington, D.C.: National Academies Press, 2001.

Koplan, J. P., Liverman, C. T., and Kraak, V. I. (eds.). *Preventing Childhood Obesity: Health in the Balance*. Washington, D.C.: National Academies Press, 2005.

Larsen, D. L., Cannon, W., and Towner, S. "Longitudinal Assessment of a Diabetes Care Management System in an Integrated Health Network." *Journal of Managed Care Pharmacy*, 2003, *9*, 552–558.

Leatherdale, S. T., and others. "A Multi-Level Analysis Examining How Smoking Friends, Parents, and Older Students in the School Environment Are Risk Factors for Susceptibility to Smoking Among Non-Smoking Elementary School Youth." *Prevention Science*, 2006, *7*, 397–402.

Lewin, K., and Cartwright, D. *Field Theory in Social Science.* New York: Harper, 1951.

Lorig, K. R., and Holman, H. "Self-management Education: History, Definition, Outcomes, and Mechanisms." *Annals of Behavioral Medicine*, 2003, *26*, 1–7.

Matsudo, S. M., and others. "Physical Activity Promotion: Experiences and Evaluation of the Agita Sao Paulo Program Using the Ecological Mobile Model." *Journal of Physical Activity and Health*, 2004, *1*, 81–97.

McLeroy, K. R., Bibeau, D., Steckler, A., and Glanz, K. "An Ecological Perspective on Health Promotion Programs." *Health Education Quarterly*, 1988, *15*, 351–377.

McNeill, L. H., and others. "Individual, Social Environmental, and Physical Environmental Influences on Physical Activity Among Black and White Adults: A Structural Equation Analysis." *Annals of Behavioral Medicine*, 2006, *31*, 36–44.

Moos, R. H. "Social-Ecological Perspectives on Health." In G. C. Stone, F. Cohen, and N. E. Adler (eds.), *Health Psychology: A Handbook.* San Francisco: Jossey-Bass, 1980.

Nasmith, L., and others. "The Challenge of Promoting Integration: Conceptualization, Implementation, and Assessment of a Pilot Care Delivery Model for Patients with Type 2 Diabetes. *Family Medicine*, 2004, *36*, 40–50.

Norris, S. L., and others. "Self-Management Education for Adults with Type 2 Diabetes: A Meta-Analysis of the Effect on Glycemic Control." *Diabetes Care*, 2002, *25*, 1159–1171.

Ottawa Charter for Health Promotion. Ottawa: Canadian Public Health Association, 1986.

Owen, N., and others. "Understanding Environmental Influences on Walking: Review and Research Agenda." *American Journal of Preventive Medicine*, 2004, *27*, 67–76.

Owen, N., and others. "Neighborhood Walkability and the Walking Behavior of Australian Adults." *American Journal of Preventive Medicine,* 2007, *33*, 387–395.

Pierce, J. P., and others. "Tobacco Industry Promotion of Cigarettes and Adolescent Smoking." *Journal of the American Medical Association*, 1998, *279*, 511–515.

Rhodes, R. E., Brown, S. G., and McIntyre, C. A. "Integrating the Perceived Neighborhood Environment and the Theory of Planned Behavior When Predicting Walking in a Canadian Adult Sample." *American Journal of Health Promotion*, 2006, *21*, 110–118.

Saelens, B. E., Sallis, J. F., and Frank, L. D. "Environmental Correlates of Walking and Cycling: Findings from the Transportation, Urban Design, and Planning Literatures." *Annals of Behavioral Medicine*, 2003, *25*, 80–91.

Sallis, J. F., and Owen, N. "Ecological Models of Health Behavior." In K. Glanz, B. K. Rimer, and F. M. Lewis (eds.), *Health Behavior and Health Education: Theory, Research, and Practice.* (3rd ed.) San Francisco: Jossey-Bass, 2002.

Sallis, J. F., and others. "An Ecological Approach to Creating More Physically Active Communities." *Annual Review of Public Health*, 2006, *27*, 297–322.

Siegel, M. "The Effectiveness of State-Level Tobacco Control Interventions: A Review of Program Implementation and Behavioral Outcomes." *Annual Review of Public Health*, 2002, *23*, 45–71.

Skinner, B. F. *Science and Human Behavior.* New York: Macmillan, 1953.

Stillman, F. A., and others. "Evaluation of the American Stop Smoking Intervention Study (ASSIST): A Report of Outcomes." *Journal of the National Cancer Institute*, 2003, *95*(22), 1681–1691.

Stokols, D. "Establishing and Maintaining Healthy Environments: Toward a Social Ecology of Health Promotion." *American Psychologist*, 1992, *47*, 6–22.

Stokols, D., Grzywacz, J. G., McMahan, S., and Phillips, K. "Increasing the Health Promotive Capacity of Human Environments." *American Journal of Health Promotion*, 2003, *18*, 4–13.

Task Force on Community Preventive Services. "The Guide to Community Preventive Services: What Works to Promote Health?" New York: Oxford University Press, 2005.

Trento, M., and others. "A 5-year Randomized Controlled Study of Learning, Problem Solving Ability, and Quality of Life Modifications in People with Type 2 Diabetes Managed by Group Care." *Diabetes Care*, 2004, *27*, 670–675.

U.S. Department of Health and Human Services. "Preventing Tobacco Use Among Young People: A Report of The Surgeon General." Atlanta: U.S. Department of Health and Human Services, Public Health Service, Centers for Disease Control, Center for Chronic Disease Prevention and Health Promotion, Office on Smoking and Health, 1994.

U.S. Department of Health and Human Services. "Physical Activity and Health: A Report of the Surgeon General." Atlanta: Centers for Disease Control, 1996.

U.S. Department of Health and Human Services. "Healthy People 2010." Washington, D.C.: U.S. Department of Health and Human Services, 2000a.

U.S. Department of Health and Human Services. "Treating Tobacco Use and Dependence." Washington, D.C.: Public Health Service, 2000b.

World Health Organization. *Framework Convention on Tobacco Control.* [http://www.who.int/tobacco/frame work/WHO_FCTC_english.pdf]. Geneva: World Health Organization, 2003.

World Health Organization. *Global Strategy on Diet, Physical Activity, and Health.* [http://www.who.int/gb/ebwha/pdf_files/WHA57/A57_R17-en.pdf] Geneva: World Health Organization, 2004.

CHAPTER

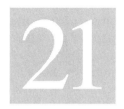

EVALUATION OF THEORY-BASED INTERVENTIONS

Russell E. Glasgow
Laura A. Linnan

KEY POINTS

This chapter will

- Discuss the rationale for and benefits of evaluating theory-based programs.
- Describe different types of validity.
- Identify key components of thorough evaluations and leading evaluation models.
- Illustrate the use of evaluation with two theory-based intervention examples.
- Describe challenges to conducting meaningful evaluations and provide recommendations for addressing these issues.

BENEFITS AND CHALLENGES OF EVALUATING THEORY-BASED INTERVENTIONS

According to Weiss (1998), two overarching and important reasons for evaluating interventions are to contribute to (1) improvements in programs and (2) improvements in policy. Evaluations that help improve programs may clarify the dose or intensity of intervention required to produce change, specify the methods that produce the most powerful change, identify (better) strategies for increasing participation or adherence in programs, identify subgroups for whom the intervention is particularly effective (or ineffective), and change program content to improve outcomes. Evaluation that leads to improvements in policy may clarify the costs and resources required, as well as the benefits and return on investments. Such evaluation may also mobilize public support or increase political will to take needed action, remove support for ineffective programs, and provide accountability to funders and stakeholders.

Finally, and particularly relevant for this chapter, evaluation results may contribute to the development of new knowledge that creates new theory, refines existing theory, or contributes to the evidence base for intervention effectiveness. Specifically, strong theoretical foundations are the hallmark of carefully constructed interventions that emerge from strategic planning efforts. Thus, a benefit of evaluating *theory-guided* interventions is that one is able to measure specified intervention outcomes, as well as the change in the theoretical constructs that were expected to lead to the change in outcomes. This is clearly an "added value" of evaluating theory-based interventions.

Researchers and practitioners are typically most interested in the outcomes or results of their study or program. If they have thoughtfully designed the intervention, it is likely that theory has guided the effort. Conceptual and logic models can be used to depict how intervention activities or "inputs" are expected to produce desired outcomes by way of changes in intermediate factors that are often theoretically linked. For example, changes in colorectal cancer screening behavior are more likely to occur when there are subsequent changes in knowledge, attitudes, perceived susceptibility to colon cancer, and reduced barriers to obtaining screening. If there is a theory behind the design of intervention activities, one can measure change in the theoretical constructs along the pathway of change, as well as the intended outcomes. If we find that colorectal screening (the outcome of interest) increases without a change in perceptions about the risk of colon cancer, perhaps there is a need to modify the guiding theory hypothesizing that perceived risk of, or susceptibility to, was important. Alternatively, the intervention strategy may need to change to affect risk perceptions. Improvements in theory based on the results of an evaluation of theory-based interventions create new knowledge that may improve theory and lead to the development of more effective interventions.

Conceptual and logic models depict the specific activities or interventions of an overall intervention plan designed for a particular population and setting, as well as the intermediate and final outcomes intended by the planned interventions. They make explicit the assumptions about theoretically guided determinants of behavior change and how intervention strategies are hypothesized to affect them. An example of a conceptual model depicting intervention components, hypothesized change mechanisms (mediators), and intended primary outcomes associated with a multi-level intervention guided by Social Cognitive Theory (SCT) and the Transtheoretical Model (TTM) of behavior change is shown in Figure 21.1. This conceptual model depicts three levels of intervention activities (stylist training workshops, in-salon educational displays, and health magazines for customers), and the hypothesized influences on the stylists, the salon environment, and the interactions that occur between the stylist and

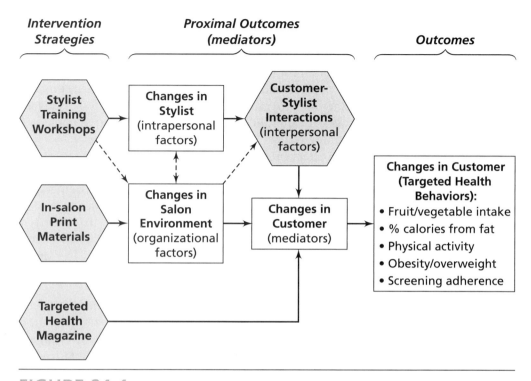

FIGURE 21.1. BEAUTY Conceptual Model.

customers from those intervention activities. These activities are hypothesized to lead to changes in cognitions among customers (self-efficacy, stage of readiness, and re-duced barriers to change), and ultimately to changes in each targeted behavioral out-come. Conceptual and logic models are often used in program planning and evaluation, but they often have been under-utilized when designing comprehensive evaluations of theory-based interventions.

TYPES OF EVALUATION

Several key types of evaluation should be considered. *Formative evaluation* typically occurs prior to the development of an intervention. In this context, formative evalu-ation is designed to help refine and assess the strengths and limitations of theoreti-cally based ideas or materials before full-scale implementation. Formative evaluation should be conducted with members of the intended audience, may be qualitative or quantitative, and may use a variety of data-gathering tools such as focus groups, ob-servations, surveys, and interviews, as well as emerging data collection methods such as photovoice and storytelling. For example, later in this chapter, formative research is described that helped develop culturally and contextually appropriate interven-tion strategies for the BEAUTY Project, summarized in Figure 21.1. (See also Chap-ter Eighteen on the PRECEDE-PROCEED Model for program planning.)

Process evaluation measures the extent to which an intervention was delivered or implemented as intended. Process evaluation is essential for answering "how" and "why" interventions may have been effective (or ineffective) (Linnan and Steckler, 2002). Process evaluation is essential for understanding how well the program or policy was delivered as originally planned and how it may have been modified. Process evaluation also measures whether the program was received, how much was received, and by which subgroups. Process evaluation can help tease out negative outcomes and can help expand understanding of positive outcomes.

In our ongoing beauty salon intervention research (Linnan and others, 2007), we are documenting the extent to which participating stylists attended each of seven four-hour stylist training workshops that were offered over the eighteen-month intervention period. Some stylists attended all seven workshops; others attended less than half. This information can be used to document the extent to which stylists received a "dose" of training that might produce expected effects (for example, increased number of health conversations between stylists and customers in the salons). The variation among stylists in training attendance may help explain outcomes for specific salons and their customers.

Impact (secondary outcomes) and *outcome* (primary outcomes) *evaluations* seek to document program effects, both proximal (impact) and more distal (outcome). Again, a logic model can help to depict the theoretically expected outcomes. Impact evaluation assesses the shorter-term changes in perceptions or attitudes that lead to behavior change. In this case, behavior change may be the most distal outcome measured. In the beauty salon example, we expected educational materials in the salon environment, workshops for stylists, and magazines for customers to produce change in stylists' motivational readiness and self-efficacy to be more physically active among salon customers. As depicted in Figure 21.1, the changes in stylist behaviors, salon environments, and customer cognitions were evaluated as part of an impact evaluation; one of the primary outcomes evaluated was customer change in physical activity behavior.

In some cases, impact evaluation may focus on behavior change, and outcome evaluation may be even more distal—for example, changes in morbidity, mortality, or quality of life. A continuum of outcomes is often the reality in many public health projects and research studies. The decision about what to measure as outcome/impact evaluation depends on the type and intensity of the intervention, timeframe to assess results, and the stated, measurable objectives of the intervention components.

PHASES OF RESEARCH

The question of how to evaluate interventions should also take into account the phase of research or investigation that is intended (Greenwald and Cullen, 1985). Several research groups have proposed a series of "phases of research" that should guide the development of health behavior interventions and evaluations. Some of these, especially those of Greenwald and Cullen (1985) and Flay (1986), have been widely adopted and have been used by the National Cancer Institute, the National Heart, Lung, and Blood Institute, and other influential funding agencies and organizations concerned with advancing the science of health promotion. The Greenwald and Cullen model of five phases of research is summarized in Table 21.1, along with a health education example of each phase. The basic point shared by these conceptualizations is that research should evolve in a preferred sequence, beginning with basic laboratory research and literature reviews to explore initial hypotheses, followed by "efficacy" studies designed to assess interventions under ideal or optimal conditions. These efficacy studies maximize internal validity, to firmly establish the scientific basis of interventions, before proceeding to later "effectiveness" studies. Effectiveness studies then determine the impact of the intervention when conducted under more representative or applied field conditions and when applied to more representative or "defined populations," rather than the highly screened and motivated, self-selected volunteers who are studied in efficacy research (Rohrbach, Grana, Sussman, and Valente, 2006; Sussman and others, 2006).

A final phase, but one which has received much less attention until recently, is that of translation and dissemination research. Such research investigates ways to enhance, and factors that influence, the widespread adoption of interventions proven to be efficacious and effective in previous stages of research. Several authors have contrasted the different goals, assumptions, and issues studied in efficacy research, which is concerned primarily with internal validity, with those of translation/dissemination research, which is more concerned with external validity and public health impact issues (Lichtenstein and Glasgow, 1992; Flay, 1986; McKinlay, 1996; Glasgow, Lichtenstein,

TABLE 21.1. **Model of Phases of Research (Greenwald and Cullen, 1985).**

Phase		Health Behavior Example
Phase 1	Hypothesis development	Identification of link in existing literature between sedentary behavior and obesity among adolescents
Phase 2	Methods development	Pilot testing of intervention to increase adolescent physical activity and validation of measures
Phase 3	Controlled intervention trials (efficacy studies)	Small-scale randomized trial of physical activity intervention for adolescents
Phase 4	Defined population studies (effectiveness)	Larger-scale trial of physical activity intervention when applied to all adolescents in participating middle schools
Phase 5	Demonstration (dissemination)	Evaluation of results when physical activity program provided to all middle schools in a given state

Source: Greenwald and Cullen, 1985.

and Marcus, 2003). It is generally agreed that the broadest public health impact will occur when effective interventions are disseminated widely and that this should occur as often as possible.

TYPES OF VALIDITY

The types of validity emphasized vary at different stages of research and are discussed next. In general, *validity* refers to the degree to which a study accurately reflects or captures what the researchers set out to measure. In this discussion, we refer to the validity of research designs and execution, as contrasted with validity as a characteristic of measures.

Internal and Construct Validity

Internal validity refers to the extent to which outcomes can be attributed to an experimental factor (for example, an intervention) rather than to extraneous or confounding factors. *Construct validity* refers to the ability to attribute differences between conditions (usually an intervention versus a control or comparison condition) to the "active ingredient" or factor of theoretical interest. (Again, this is different from the construct validity of a measure [Shadish, Cook, and Campbell, 2002]). Many of these issues involve research design and methodological procedures to ensure that the differences between conditions are restricted (1) to those about which one wants to make interpretive statements and (2) to collection of appropriate process measures of the hypothesized theoretical mechanisms of change. A subset of process measures especially relevant to this chapter is the measurement of intervention delivery, or consistency of implementation. Such measures assess the extent to which the intervention(s) are actually delivered as intended. This is important for avoiding "Type III errors," or concluding that an intervention is ineffective when in fact it was not delivered or implemented as intended (Basch, Sliepcevich, and Gold, 1985).

External Validity

External validity refers to the extent to which it is possible to generalize or apply the results of a study to other populations, contexts, settings, and situations outside the specific situations studied in a given investigation (Shadish, Cook, and Campbell, 2002). External validity also concerns the representativeness of the intervention settings, intervention agents, and participants in a study. External validity is especially important for translation of research to practice (that is, will this program be likely to work with this population, here, and under these conditions?) and is of particular concern to clinicians, practitioners, and policymakers.

Balancing Internal and External Validity

Finding the right balance between internal and external validity can be challenging. Evaluation designs that produce higher internal validity often lead to lower external validity. This is because enhanced internal validity is usually accomplished by re-

stricting the conditions or populations being studied, and such decisions, by definition, make the study results less broadly applicable. To assess an intervention's efficacy, internal validity should be maximized. But to enhance relevance and
disseminability, external validity is critical. Fortunately, there are strategies that can
be used to enhance external validity without sacrificing internal validity, and these
are discussed later in this chapter.

The ultimate goal of evaluation is to gain sufficient knowledge about a theory-
based intervention to answer the key question phrased so well over thirty years ago
by Gordon Paul: "What treatment, for what population, delivered by whom, under
what conditions, for what outcome, is most effective, and how did it come about?"
(Paul, 1969).

INTERVENTION CONTEXTS AND INTERMEDIATE OUTCOMES

To assess the impact of an intervention, it is necessary to understand the conditions
under which it works and for whom it works. For most health behavior and education interventions, especially those delivered within a setting such as a worksite,
school, medical clinic, or community organization, it is also important to understand
contextual issues at both the setting and the individual levels. To facilitate understanding and to place the results of a study in appropriate context, it is often helpful to create a visual representation of the steps involved in recruiting for, delivering, and
evaluating a program. For randomized controlled trials (RCTs), such a figure is referred to as a CONSORT flow diagram (Moher, Schulz, Altman, and CONSORT
Group, 2001). For nonrandomized trials, related criteria that enhance the transparency
of reporting are summarized in the TREND statement (Des Jarlais, Lyles, Crepaz,
and TREND Group, 2004).

This type of information often includes or reflects specification of inclusion or
exclusion criteria to clarify the population targets: intervention settings), participation rates, and reasons for nonparticipation or dropout. Figure 21.2 shows an example of such a diagram. Such schematics are now standard requirements for publishing
the results of RCTs, so that reviewers and readers can understand the flow of participation in a study. The diagrams can also give a quick "at-a-glance" view of what was
expected from the intervention and how the population was recruited and retained
over time.

When evaluating theory-based interventions, it is also important to include process
variables and to conduct analyses to evaluate the effects of mediating variables. Mediating variables typically represent hypothesized pathways or processes through which
an intervention is expected to achieve its effects and should be specified in the study's
conceptual or logic model (see Figure 21.1). Theory is fundamental to identifying such
mediating mechanisms. For example, a program based on SCT that aims to reduce
recreational drug use might be expected to achieve change by increasing participants'
self-efficacy to resist peer pressure; thus, "self-efficacy" is a hypothesized mediator.
In-depth discussions of analytical procedures to evaluate mediating variables can be
found elsewhere (Kraemer, Wilson, Fairburn, and Agras, 2002; MacKinnon, Fairchild,
and Fritz, 2007). The point, however, is that it is important to identify how health

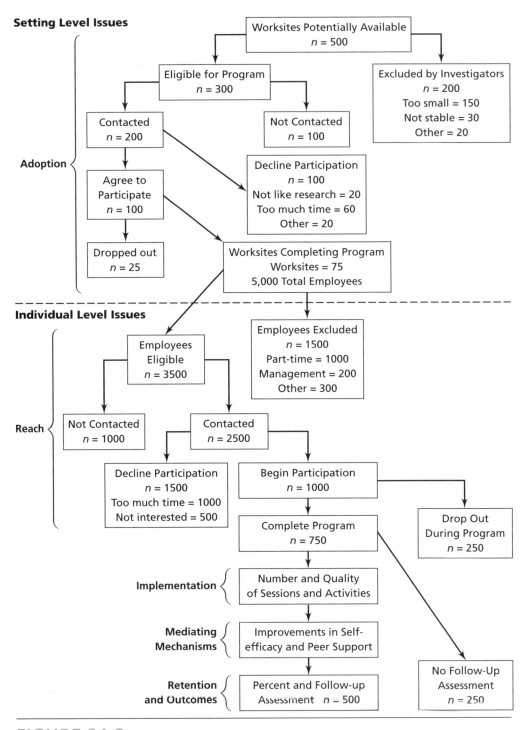

FIGURE 21.2. Hypothetical Worksite Intervention Participation Flow Diagram.

behavior interventions work, both to increase our understanding of theoretical mechanisms and to create more efficient and effective interventions.

EVALUATION MODELS

Several separate but related models and frameworks have been proposed to help guide theory-based evaluation of health promotion interventions. Although this chapter does not provide an exhaustive list of all potential evaluation models, a few of particular relevance are noted. Some models are designed to help both develop and evaluate interventions (Green and Kreuter, 2005; Shediac-Ritzkallah and Bone, 1998; Viswanathan and others, 2004; Klesges, Estabrooks, Glasgow, and Dzewaltowski, 2005), and others are intended only to help frame evaluation issues (Lomas, 1997). For practitioners, evaluation models identify key factors to consider when developing or selecting health behavior programs and when reading the research literature. For researchers, evaluation models identify important dimensions to be included in program evaluations and to assess theoretical contributions. Two of the most comprehensive models are the PRECEDE-PROCEED planning model (Green and Kreuter, 1999; see also Chapter Eighteen) and diffusion of innovations (Rogers, 2003; Nutbeam, 1996; see Chapter Fourteen).

In addition to strategic planning models, other lines of research have stressed the importance of considering factors that determine the "real-world" impact of research and applicability in a variety of settings. Several reports have examined the availability of research on diffusion, dissemination, and institutionalization and have questioned the almost exclusive preoccupation of health promotion research with efficacy studies that emphasize internal validity (Glasgow and Emmons, 2007; Oldenburg, Sallis, French, and Owen, 1999; Oldenburg, French, and Sallis, 2000).

Important work by Goodman, Steckler, and colleagues (Goodman and Steckler, 1987) identified and measured factors to assess the extent to which interventions are sustained or become "institutionalized." More recently, Shediac-Ritzkallah and Bone (1998) proposed a conceptual model that clarifies factors associated with the program, community or larger context, and the organization or group where the program is to be sustained, as a basis for discussing how to plan for the possibility of sustaining effective interventions. This work is impressive in suggesting that not all interventions should be sustained, so that another important role of evaluation is to consider factors a priori that will help with decision making about whether or not theory-based interventions *should* be sustained and considered for dissemination. Another line of research that has helped focus development of practical and feasible interventions has been that of Abrams and colleagues (Abrams and others, 1996), who proposed that the impact of interventions should not be determined solely by their efficacy (effects and magnitude of change related to internal validity) but also by their reach—or the percentage of potentially eligible persons who participate in an intervention. They suggested that the impact of an intervention is a multiplicative function of its reach times efficacy (Abrams, Emmons, and Linnan, 1997)—an idea that was incorporated into the development of the RE-AIM evaluation framework described in the following section.

THE RE-AIM FRAMEWORK

RE-AIM is an acronym for Reach, Effectiveness, Adoption, Implementation, and Maintenance (Glasgow, Vogt, and Boles, 1999; Glasgow, McKay, Piette, and Reynolds, 2001). *Reach* refers to the percentage of potential participants who are exposed to an intervention and how representative they are. Reach and Effectiveness (see Table 21.2) relate to individuals or intended end users. *Effectiveness* concerns both the intended or positive impacts of an intervention on targeted outcomes and the possible negative or unintended consequences of the intervention on quality-of-life and nontargeted outcomes.

In the context of the RE-AIM evaluation framework, *Adoption* and *Implementation* operate at the setting or contextual level. Adoption refers to the participation rate

TABLE 21.2. **RE-AIM Dimensions and Questions in Evaluating Health Education and Health Behavior Programs.**

RE-AIM Dimension	Questions for Assessment
Reach (individual level)	What percentage of potentially eligible participants will take part and how representative are they?
Effectiveness (individual level)	What impact did the intervention have on all participants who began the program, on process and primary outcomes, and on both positive and negative (unintended) outcomes, including quality of life?
Adoption (setting level)	What percentage of settings and intervention staff (such as worksites, schools/educators, medical offices/physicians), will participate and how representative are they?
Implementation (setting/staff level)	To what extent are the various intervention components delivered as intended (in the protocol), especially when conducted by regular (nonresearch) staff in applied settings? To what extent and how was the program modified over time?
Maintenance (both individual and setting level)	1. *Individual level:* What are the long-term effects (minimum of six to twelve months following intervention)?
	2. *Setting level:* To what extent are different intervention components modified, continued, or institutionalized?

and representativeness of both the settings in which an intervention is conducted (such as worksites, medical offices, schools, communities) and the intervention agents who deliver the intervention (for example, teachers, physicians, health educators). Although Adoption is as important as Reach (at the individual level), far less attention has been devoted to it. Implementation refers to the extent to which an intervention is delivered consistently across different components and staff, and over time. Implementation is often problematic, especially when conducted in applied settings by staff who have many other responsibilities beyond implementation of an intervention protocol.

Maintenance—the final dimension of the RE-AIM model—has indices at both the individual and setting levels. At the individual level, it refers to the long-term results of an intervention (a minimum of six months following the last intervention contact). For most behaviors, long-term maintenance has proven challenging, and the factors that influence maintenance may be different than those that influence initial behavior change (Orleans, 2000). An important issue when evaluating maintenance is to follow and characterize results for all participants who begin a program, not just those who are present for follow-up. Attrition can often be substantial or differential across conditions or participant subgroups.

At the setting level, Maintenance refers to the continuation (short-term) or institutionalization (long-term) of a program (Goodman and Steckler, 1987). This is the extent to which intervention settings will continue a program (and which of the original components of the intervention are retained or modified), once the formal research project and supports are withdrawn. As Patterson, Kristal, Biener, and colleagues (Patterson and others, 1998) found in their follow-up study of a worksite nutrition intervention, even well-designed and effective interventions are unlikely to be maintained if resources are not allocated for this purpose. This leads to one of the key conclusions of this chapter: if sustainability and dissemination are key goals of a project, planning for them needs to start at project inception, not when program results become available, at which point it will be too late.

The relationships among various RE-AIM dimensions are as important as the results on any given dimension. Expanding on the work of Abrams and colleagues (Abrams, Emmons, and Linnan, 1997), who proposed that Impact = Reach × Efficacy, RE-AIM hypothesizes that the overall public health impact of an intervention is a function of all five RE-AIM dimensions. Glasgow and colleagues (Glasgow and others, 2006a; Glasgow, Nelson, Strycker, and King, 2006) have proposed RE-AIM summary indices for use in determining overall impact. All five RE-AIM dimensions are important and equally in need of evaluation. The implication is that, to have a substantial impact at the population level, an intervention must do reasonably well on all or most RE-AIM dimensions. It is not enough to have a highly efficacious intervention if that intervention has poor reach, is not likely to be adopted by many settings, and can only be implemented by a handful of highly trained specialists. Few current health behavior programs are strong on all five RE-AIM dimensions.

The RE-AIM framework can be helpful to decision makers in clarifying outcomes that are most important to them and in considering the pros and cons of different alternatives (Glasgow and others, 2006a). For example, one may need to choose between a program that has high Effectiveness but is unlikely to be adopted by many practitioners and one that has demonstrated high Reach but appears to have only modest Effectiveness.

In summary, readers are encouraged to use theory to guide intervention development and to describe specifically how the theory is expected to work through use of a logic or conceptual model. It is also helpful to consider the sequence of steps and factors influencing participation at each step (as illustrated in Figure 21.2) to include the information recommended in the CONSORT (Moher, Schulz, Altman, and CONSORT Group, 2001) or TREND (Des Jarlais, Lyles, Crepaz, and TREND Group, 2004) statements, and to articulate (a priori) if and how dissemination and translation is expected. Use of a systematic evaluation model can help in all stages of this process from planning through implementation, assessment, analysis, and reporting. It is important that process (theoretical mechanisms), impacts, and outcomes be reported clearly and in sufficient detail, so that they can be included in evidence-based reviews such as those conducted by the Cochrane Collaboration and the Guide to Community Preventive Services, and so that questions such as those in Table 21.2 can be answered.

EVALUATION METHODS AND ANALYTICAL STRATEGIES FOR THEORY-BASED INTERVENTIONS

Choosing an evaluation design requires a balance between internal and external validity considerations, as well as state of the literature, cost, resources, time, and potential burden to participants for data collection. Ideally, evaluation design should be matched to the evaluation questions to be answered. For example, an evaluation design to test the feasibility of a new idea, theory, or intervention approach does not demand a large, multi-site, randomized controlled design—a one-group, pre/post-test design, or two groups (one intervention and one comparison/control) may be sufficient to explore feasibility. However, a large-scale dissemination trial may benefit from an RCT or quasi-experimental design that thoroughly addresses external validity and contextual issues. Some of the most exciting recent analytical advances include strategies for assessing mediating mechanisms of change via hierarchical modeling, path analysis, latent growth curves, and related techniques (Kraemer, Wilson, Fairburn, and Agras, 2002; Reynolds and others, 2006).

Data collection methods vary with the type of design and evaluation questions asked. For example, typical data collection methods for outcome evaluations include surveillance and monitoring systems. Changes in populationwide behavioral outcomes can be monitored at the state level with Behavioral Risk Factor Surveillance System results gathered by most state health departments. Like formative evaluation, process evaluation data are gathered using a wide range of methods—both qualitative and quantitative. Focus groups, interviews, photovoice, storytelling narratives, and observation are also possible process evaluation methods.

Excellent resources to guide process evaluation are now available, including a book edited by Steckler and Linnan (2002) that includes detailed examples, sample instruments, and lessons learned about process evaluation for public health interventions and research in a wide range of settings (including schools, worksites, churches, and more). Also, Tashakkori and Teddlie (1998) offer a useful guide to mixing methods (qualitative and quantitative) at all stages of the evaluation process, from developing evaluation questions through data collection and reporting.

COST ISSUES

Data on costs and cost-effectiveness are one of the least frequently reported types of data in health program evaluations (Glasgow and others, 2004). This is a major barrier to translation and dissemination of theory-based programs into practice settings, because program cost is one of the first questions that decision makers and policymakers ask. Part of the reason there have not been more cost analyses in health promotion is that program developers and researchers often have felt overwhelmed by the complexity and magnitude of the task, and the time and costs involved in evaluating cost-effectiveness.

Fortunately, recent advances and simpler methods are now available that do not attempt to answer every economic issue but restrict their focus to issues of the costs of program implementation (or replication) and the cost per unit of behavior change. Such models are practical for most research (Ritzwoller, Toobert, Sukhanova, and Glasgow, 2005), answer the questions that decision makers usually have, and do not require a great deal of health economist time (unlike more complicated issues such as determining cost-benefit or impact on health care utilization).

EXAMPLES OF EVALUATING THEORY-BASED INTERVENTIONS

The first example illustrates formative evaluation results that were used to guide the development of a multi-level intervention for a large community-based participatory research study attempting to address cancer disparities among African American beauty salon customers. The second example uses the RE-AIM evaluation framework to report on key outcome and process evaluation results of theory-guided eHealth interventions and shows how RE-AIM can be used to evaluate two or more alternative interventions.

North Carolina BEAUTY and Health Project

Attempting to reach and engage individuals where they live, work, play, and receive services (such as beauty salons) is an important strategy for ensuring high participation in community-based interventions. Beauty salons are located in all communities; there are more than 219,000 beauty salons in the United States. Moreover, licensed stylists and customers share a unique and important bond that may be mobilized to promote health. Linnan and colleagues convened an advisory board to assess the feasibility of partnering with beauty salons and licensed cosmetologists to promote health using a community-based participatory research (CBPR) approach (Linnan and others, 2007). CBPR involves community members in the planning, delivery, and evaluation of services that can address community concerns, including disparities in health (Whitelaw and others, 2001; Viswanathan and others, 2004). In this example, SCT was used as a foundation, and formative research results were used to develop a multi-level and contextually appropriate theory-based intervention to promote health in beauty salons. Over a two-year period, a series of formative evaluation studies was implemented: (1) a survey of licensed stylists (Linnan and others, 2001), (2) an observational study in ten beauty salons (Solomon and others, 2005), (3) a pilot test of an intervention in two salons (Linnan and others, 2005), and (4) focus groups with salon customers. Consistent with CBPR, members of the "community" (salon owners, stylists, customers) were involved in all aspects of generating the research questions, developing measurement tools, determining intervention priorities, and deciding on appropriate intervention strategies, and are active participants in interpreting and evaluating the results of the research. The BEAUTY Advisory Board guided the project and included the president of the North Carolina State Cosmetology Association, directors of one private and two public beauty schools, salon owners, licensed stylists, and beauty product distributors.

An overview of the BEAUTY Project and baseline results are described in detail elsewhere (Linnan and others, 2005), but here we summarize SCT and important findings from a series of formative research efforts, as they informed the development of three interventions developed for the larger randomized trial: training of stylists, materials for customers, and salon-based interventions. Following a literature review to appreciate the historical, social, political, and economic realities of working in African American beauty salons (Linnan and Ferguson, 2007), a survey of licensed stylists was conducted (Linnan and others, 2001).

Survey results revealed that stylists routinely talk with their customers about everything, including health, were interested in getting specialized training to talk with their customers about health messages, and shared preferences about health topics they were most comfortable discussing and the ways they would like to receive additional training (such as local workshops and in-person consultations). Stylists reported that physical activity, healthy eating, and maintaining and achieving a healthy weight were topics they were most interested in and willing to discuss with their customers; because these behaviors are preventable causes of cardiovascular disease, cancer, diabetes, and stroke, the intervention development process focused on these behavioral risk factors. Stylist survey results revealed that although interest levels in promoting health messages were relatively high, increasing stylist self-efficacy to deliver specific health messages would be an important goal of the intervention plan; hence SCT was used to guide the development of the stylist training workshops. The curriculum for these workshops included sharing facts, dispelling myths, holding demonstrations of health talk, and asking stylists to role play exchanges between stylists and customers that weave health messages into a typical visit—all in the service of increasing self-efficacy to deliver health messages.

An observational study in ten beauty salons collected insights that helped the research team plan contextually appropriate salon-based interventions (Solomon and others, 2005). Observational study results confirmed that salon customers talk openly about many subjects, including health, and that health conversations were initiated equally by stylists and customers. Using these results and guided by SCT, in-salon educational displays were created to trigger customers to "talk with your stylist" to get additional health information. By using triggers in the salon for customers *and* training stylists to "weave" health messages into typical conversations, the intervention was consistent with the principle of "reciprocal determinism"—a hallmark of SCT. Specifically, the intervention included a "cue to action" or reinforcer in the salon environment that encouraged customers to ask the stylist for health information (displays), and the stylist training workshops encouraged stylists to deliver key messages to their customers. SCT helped guide the development of specific interventions that operated on three levels of the social ecological framework: intrapersonal, interpersonal, and organizational (McLeroy, Bibeau, Steckler, and Glanz, 1988).

The prototype intervention was tested in two salons, with five stylists, and consisted of a four-hour training workshop for stylists, an educational display for the salon, and print materials for the customers (Linnan and others, 2005). Briefly, we learned that (1) 81 percent of responding customers read information on the health education displays, (2) 86 percent of customers talked with their cosmetologist about the BEAUTY Project, and (3) all trained cosmetologists reported increased self-efficacy to deliver targeted health messages and that they would continue delivering health messages beyond the pilot intervention. At a twelve-month follow-up, 55 percent of customers reported making changes in at least one of the targeted health behaviors because of conversations they had with their cosmetologists, and those who reported more conversations with stylists also reported increased readiness to attempt health behavior changes and more actual self-reported changes in targeted health behaviors (Linnan and others, 2005). Results from a series of formative research studies and the application of SCT provided the guidance required to develop, implement, evaluate, and refine a multi-level intervention that was ready for broader testing in a larger, randomized controlled trial described in further detail elsewhere (Linnan and others, 2007).

RE-AIM Evaluation of Two Interactive Technology Programs to Enhance Diabetes Care and Self-Management

The number of theory-based health education and promotion programs being delivered in whole or in part by computer is growing rapidly (Strecher, 2007). Arguments in support of health applications such as Web-based behavior change, automated telephone calls, touchscreen computers, and other information technology programs suggest that they have the potential to reach more users, to consistently deliver tailored materials, and to do so effectively and efficiently. Unfortunately, far fewer eHealth studies have systematically and comprehensively evaluated these claims (Glasgow, 2007). This example illustrates use of the RE-AIM framework to compare two theory-based eHealth interventions for diabetes patients.

Both programs employed a SCT model, combined with a social ecological model of environmental support to enhance maintenance. Though they were evaluated in separate randomized effectiveness studies, they employed very similar measures of both process and outcomes and were targeted at similar adult primary care diabetes patients using the same recruitment methods, thereby enhancing the ability to draw comparisons (Glasgow and others, 2005; Glasgow and others, 2006b). The programs differed, however, in their intensity, their implementation, and other features. The first program, here referred to as "In-Office Self-Management," involved use of a touchscreen computer program prior to regular primary care visits, followed by a brief nurse review of the behavior change action plan generated, and follow-up phone calls. The entire intervention took about thirty-five to forty minutes (only about five minutes from the nurse) and was conducted by regular office staff in thirty diverse primary care clinics throughout Colorado.

The second program, called "Linked Health Coach Self-Management," focused on essentially the same self-management issues but involved two separate visits with a health educator, each visit approximately two hours in length. At each session, the patient first worked through a problem-solving-based, computer-administered program to produce an individually tailored action plan. This required additional visits outside of the patient's usual care, as "referrals" to diabetes educators are often conducted.

The In-Office program produced better reach (estimated at 50 percent versus 38 percent of all eligible diabetes patients invited to participate). The Linked Health Coach program produced slightly less improvement on the common measures of physical activity and healthy eating (effect size .17 versus .23) but produced substantially larger improvement in quality of life than did the In-Office program. The results of the two programs are described in detail by Glasgow and colleagues (Glasgow, Nelson, Strycker, and King, 2006; Glasgow and others, 2006a).

The largest difference between the two approaches was in adoption—with 20 percent of all physicians approached being willing to participate in the Linked Health Coach program, compared to only 6 percent of those in the In-Office program. Both approaches produced excellent implementation (97 percent and 100 percent completion of key program elements delivered), with no differences in implementation consistency across staff. Based on the RE-AIM summary index of efficiency (Glasgow, Nelson, Strycker, and King, 2006), the programs also differed in their cost. The In-Office program cost an average of $222 per participant ($57 more than its usual care comparison), whereas the Linked Health Coach, a more time-consuming program, cost an average of $547 per participant ($271 more than its randomized usual care comparison).

Maintenance data were not collected in the same way and are not comparable, but process analyses indicated that both programs were successful in improving hypothesized process measures of diabetes self-efficacy, perceived support from one's health care team, and social-environmental support relative to randomized controls. Mediation analyses, however, revealed few relationships between the hypothesized mediators and key study outcomes, suggesting that other factors may have been primarily responsible for the results observed.

In summary, the RE-AIM analysis indicated that both approaches appeared effective and practical to implement. Both appeared to produce improvements in quality of life despite the added burden of additional goals and action plans. It is likely that more health plans would decide to adopt the In-Office program due to its lower cost and great cost-effectiveness. However, the comparatively lower adoption rate of the In-Office program by physicians would need to be addressed. Additional research is needed to identify the theoretical mechanisms responsible for improvements.

CHALLENGES TO CONDUCTING AND EVALUATING THEORY-BASED HEALTH BEHAVIOR RESEARCH IN APPLIED SETTINGS

Table 21.3 summarizes several key challenges faced when delivering or evaluating health behavior interventions in applied settings. It uses the RE-AIM model to consider both common challenges and possible solutions, but these issues apply to all types of intervention and policy evaluations. The chief challenge to assessing "reach" is that, too often, evaluations include only participants who are easy to access or are especially motivated, and thus recruitment expectations for future work are unrealistically high. Another danger is of casting too narrow a net in evaluating results, focusing only on very restricted outcomes and omitting measures of potential mediating variables and other process measures that can help us understand how intervention effects (or lack of effects) occur. Table 21.3 presents a list of ways to broaden this perspective. Similarly, decision makers are most often concerned about a program's impact on participants like those in their setting. Moderator analyses, or evaluations of whether a program is differentially effective across subgroups differing on important psychosocial and demographic factors, can help to clarify subgroup effects (Glasgow and others, 2006b).

Too few health behavior research projects have been conducted in representative or low-resource real-world settings. Researchers should pay as much attention to the recruitment and representativeness of settings as they do to the representativeness of individual participants. Another frequent problem is that of "Type III error" (Basch, Sliepcevich, and Gold, 1985), or inappropriately concluding that an intervention is not effective when, in fact, the program was not delivered or implemented as intended. Collecting appropriate process and implementation measures can help to avoid this type of inferential error.

Three key implementation issues often present challenges to interpretation or research translation. The first is failure to identify the characteristics of staff who are able to intervene successfully. Staff characteristics may include expertise, education, training, age, race or ethnicity, gender, or experience as potential moderating factors. A related issue is that estimates of the program costs are often not available. Third, resolving the tension between fidelity to a program protocol—both operationally and theoretically—and adaptation to local settings, culture, and history are among the most important challenges (Linnan and Ferguson, 2007). Recommended approaches include specifying in advance key or critical components of a program that must be delivered and specifying the theoretical principles or mechanisms that are hypothesized to lead to desired outcomes. As mentioned earlier, conceptual or logic models are quite useful for depicting those relationships and in guiding intervention and measurement decisions.

TABLE 21.3. Common Challenges Encountered in Evaluating Health Behavior Interventions.

Challenge	Remedy
R: Not including a relevant, high-risk, or representative sample	Use population-based recruitment or over-recruit high-risk subgroups Report on representativeness Avoid too many exclusion criteria
E: Not thoroughly understanding outcomes or how they come about: No knowledge of mediators Conflicting or ambiguous results Inadequate control conditions to rule out alternative hypotheses	Assess broad set of outcomes, including possible negative ones. Include measures of hypothesized mediators. Conduct subgroup analyses to identify moderator effects. Design control condition to fit your question.
A: Program only studied in high-functioning optimal settings Program not ever adopted or endorsed, only used in academic settings	Involve potential adoptees using CBPR principles, beginning with initial design phase. Approach a representative or broad group of settings early on when revision is still possible and report on setting exclusions, participation, and representativeness.
I: Protocols not delivered as intended ("Type III" error) Not able to answer key questions about costs, time, or staff requirements Deciding if a program adaptation or customization is good or bad	Assess if treatment is too complicated, too intensive, or not compatible with other duties. Systematically vary staff characteristics and evaluate staff impact as well as costs. Specify a priori the critical theoretical components. Identify essential elements that cannot be changed and those that can be adapted.
M: Program or effects not maintained over time Substantial attrition of settings, delivery staff, and participants over time	Include maintenance phase in both protocol and in evaluation plan. Plan for institutionalization, sustainability, and dissemination. Take steps to minimize attrition, address attrition using appropriate methods, evaluate and report impact of attrition.

There is a dearth of information on maintenance of health behavior programs at the setting level. We need much greater understanding of the extent to which settings will move beyond program adoption to consider continuing implementation, adaptation, and long-term maintenance of an intervention once the initial program evaluation is completed. We need new theories or better use of current theories, and new measurement and analysis approaches to understand these important factors.

Finally, participant attrition is a common challenge at both the individual and organizational levels. A two-fold approach is recommended to evaluate the impact of attrition on results: (1) use theory to design procedures to maximize participant engagement, satisfaction, and retention, and (2) analyze the characteristics of those who participate (versus nonparticipants) at follow-up assessments to help clarify interpretation of results.

The key to successfully overcoming the challenges summarized in Table 21.3 is to plan for, develop, and evaluate theory-based interventions that have the potential to improve practice or policy. These issues can be addressed, using RE-AIM or other comprehensive planning frameworks, regardless of the phase of a particular research study. Program effects are often context-dependent. Evaluations should reflect the complexity of the programs and the intended audiences and settings, and reports should transparently describe program challenges, adaptations, and contextual issues so that both internal and external validity concerns are carefully considered.

SUMMARY

This chapter has summarized some of the key benefits, challenges, and realities of evaluating theory-based programs intended to address a variety of health issues, applied in a wide range of settings, and for different populations. These key issues were discussed:

- An important challenge to evaluating theory-based interventions is to determine the extent to which a program produces specified outcomes for certain types of persons, under certain conditions, and whether theory-based constructs contributed to the outcomes.
- Collection of formative evaluation and process data is important to maximize chances of programs being effective, and to understand how interventions work. Conceptual or logic models can be helpful in specifying theoretical assumptions.
- It is especially challenging to evaluate complex programs intended to be sustained, translated into practice, and widely disseminated. To enhance translation, it is recommended that evaluation efforts measure intervention reach, delivery implementation, robustness, effectiveness, and cost.
- Evaluation of setting and contextual effects is important because the types of settings and contextual factors (for example, personnel, resources, and delivery conditions) have important effects on outcomes and processes of change.

We strongly recommend that program developers and evaluators begin planning evaluations early, work closely with users and decision makers, think and measure broadly, and report clearly, accurately, and transparently to contribute to improvements in programming, policy, and theory development.

REFERENCES

Abrams, D. B., Emmons, K. M., and Linnan, L. A. "Health Behavior and Health Education: The Past, Present, and Future." In K. Glanz, F. M. Lewis, and B. K. Rimer (eds.), *Health Behavior and Health Education: Theory, Research, and Practice.* (2nd ed.) San Francisco: Jossey-Bass, 1997.

Abrams, D. B., and others. "Integrating Individual and Public Health Perspectives for Treatment of Tobacco Dependence Under Managed Health Care: A Combined Stepped Care and Matching Model." *Annals of Behavioral Medicine,* 1996, *18,* 290–304.

Basch, C. E., Sliepcevich, E. M., and Gold, R. S. "Avoiding Type III Errors in Health Education Program Evaluations." *Health Education Quarterly,* 1985, *12,* 315–331.

Des Jarlais, D. C., Lyles, C., Crepaz, N., and TREND Group. "Improving the Reporting Quality of Nonrandomized Evaluations of Behavioral and Public Health Interventions: The TREND Statement." *American Journal of Public Health,* 2004, *94,* 361–366.

Flay, B. R. "Efficacy and Effectiveness Trials (and Other Phases of Research) in the Development of Health Promotion Programs." *Preventive Medicine,* 1986, *15,* 451–474.

Glasgow, R. E. "eHealth Evaluation and Dissemination Research." *American Journal of Preventive Medicine,* 2007, *32,* S119–S126.

Glasgow, R. E., and Emmons, K. M. "How Can We Increase Translation of Research into Practice?" *Annual Review of Public Health,* 2007, *28,* 413–433.

Glasgow, R. E., Lichtenstein, E., and Marcus, A. C. "Why Don't We See More Translation of Health Promotion Research to Practice? Rethinking the Efficacy to Effectiveness Transition." *American Journal of Public Health,* 2003, *93,* 1261–1267.

Glasgow, R. E., McKay, H. G., Piette, J. D., and Reynolds, K. D. "The RE-AIM Framework for Evaluating Interventions: What Can It Tell Us About Approaches to Chronic Illness Management?" *Patient Education and Counseling,* 2001, *44,* 119–127.

Glasgow, R. E., Nelson, C. C., Strycker, L. A., and King, D. K. "Using RE-AIM Metrics to Evaluate Diabetes Self-Management Support Interventions." *American Journal of Preventive Medicine,* 2006, *30,* 67–73.

Glasgow, R. E., Vogt, T. M., and Boles, S. M. "Evaluating the Public Health Impact of Health Promotion Interventions: The RE-AIM Framework." *American Journal of Public Health,* 1999, *89,* 1322–1327.

Glasgow, R. E., and others. "The Future of Health Behavior Change Research: What is Needed to Improve Translation of Research into Health Promotion Practice?" *Annals of Behavioral Medicine,* 2004, *27,* 3–12.

Glasgow, R. E., and others. "Randomized Effectiveness Trial of a Computer-Assisted Intervention to Improve Diabetes Care." *Diabetes Care,* 2005, *28,* 33–39.

Glasgow, R. E., and others. "Evaluating the Overall Impact of Health Promotion Programs: Using the RE-AIM Framework to Form Summary Measures for Decision Making Involving Complex Issues." *Health Education Research,* 2006a, *21,* 688–694.

Glasgow, R. E., and others. "Robustness of a Computer-Assisted Diabetes Self-Management Intervention Across Patient Characteristics, Healthcare Settings, and Intervention Staff." *American Journal of Managed Care,* 2006b, *12,* 137–145.

Goodman, R. M., and Steckler, A. "A Model for the Institutionalization of Health Promotion Programs." *Family and Community Health,* 1987, *11,* 63–78.

Green, L. W., and Kreuter, M. W. *Health Promotion Planning: An Educational and Ecological Approach.* (3rd ed.) Mountain View, Calif.: Mayfield Publishing Co., 1999.

Green, L. W., and Kreuter, M. W. *Health Program Planning: An Educational and Ecological Approach.* (4th ed.) New York: McGraw-Hill, 2005.

Greenwald, P., and Cullen, J. W. "The New Emphasis in Cancer Control." *Journal of the National Cancer Institute,* 1985, *74,* 543–551.

Kleages, L. M., Estabrooks, P. A., Glasgow, R. E., and Dzewaltowski, D. "Beginning with the Application in Mind: Designing and Planning Health Behavior Change Interventions to Enhance Dissemination." *Annals of Behavioral Medicine,* 2005, *29,* 66S–75S.

Kraemer, H. C., Wilson, G. T., Fairburn, C. G., and Agras, U. S. "Mediators and Moderators of Treatment Effects in Randomized Clinical Trials." *General Psychiatry,* 2002, *59,* 877–883.

Lichtenstein, E., and Glasgow, R. E. "Smoking Cessation: What Have We Learned Over the Past Decade?" *Journal of Consulting and Clinical Psychology,* 1992, *60,* 518–527.

Linnan, L., and Ferguson, Y. O. "Beauty Salons: A Promising Health Promotion Setting for Reaching and Promoting Health Among African American Women." *Health Education and Behavior,* 2007, *34,* 530.

Linnan, L., and Steckler, A. "Process Evaluation and Public Health Interventions: An Overview." In A. Steckler and L. Linnan (eds.), *Process Evaluation in Public Health Interventions and Research* San Francisco: Jossey-Bass, 2002.

Linnan, L., and others. "Working with Licensed Cosmetologists to Promote Health: Results from the North Carolina BEAUTY and Health Pilot Study." *Preventive Medicine,* 2001, *33,* 606–612.

Linnan, L., and others. "Results of the North Carolina BEAUTY and Health Pilot Project." *Health Promotion Practice,* 2005, *6,* 164–173.

Linnan, L., and others. "The North Carolina BEAUTY and Health Project: Overview and Baseline Results." *The Community Psychologist,* 2007, *40,* 61–66.

Lomas, J. *Improving Research Dissemination and Uptake in the Health Sector: Beyond the Sound of One Hand Clapping* (Rep. No. C97–1). Montreal: McMaster University Centre for Health Economics and Policy Analysis/Policy Commentary, November, 1997.

MacKinnon, D., Fairchild, A. J., and Fritz, M. D. "Mediation Analysis." *Annual Review of Psychology,* 2007, *58,* 593–614.

McKinlay, J. B. "More Appropriate Evaluation Methods for Community-Level Health Interventions." *Evaluation Review,* 1996, *20,* 237–243.

McLeroy, K. R., Bibeau, D., Steckler, A., and Glanz, K. "An Ecological Perspective on Health Promotion Programs." *Health Education Quarterly,* 1988, *15,* 351–377.

Moher, D., Schulz, K. F., Altman, D. G., and CONSORT Group (Consolidated Standards of Reporting Trials). "The CONSORT Statement: Revised Recommendations for Improving the Quality of Reports of Parallel-Group Randomized Trials." *Journal of the American Medical Association,* 2001, *285,* 1987–1991.

Nutbeam, D. "Achieving 'Best Practice' in Health Promotion: Improving the Fit Between Research and Practice." *Health Education Research,* 1996, *11,* 317–326.

Oldenburg, B., French, M. L., and Sallis, J. F. "Health Behavior Research: The Quality of the Evidence Base." *American Journal of Health Promotion,* 2000, *14,* 253–257.

Oldenburg, B. F., Sallis, J. F., French, M. L., and Owen, N. "Health Promotion Research and the Diffusion and Institutionalization of Interventions." *Health Education Research,* 1999, *14,* 121–130.

Orleans, C. T. "Promoting the Maintenance of Health Behavior Change: Recommendations for the Next Generation of Research and Practice." *Health Psychology,* 2000, *19,* 76–83.

Patterson, R. E., and others. "Durability and Diffusion of the Nutrition Intervention in the Working Well Trial." *Preventive Medicine,* 1998, *27,* 668–673.

Paul, G. L. "Behavior Modification Research: Design and Tactics." In C. M. Franks (ed.), *Behavior Therapy: Appraisal and Status.* New York: McGraw-Hill, 1969.

Reynolds, K. D., and others. "Mediation of a Middle School Skin Cancer Prevention Program." *Health Psychology,* 2006, *25,* 616–625.

Ritzwoller, D., Toobert, D. J., Sukhanova, A., and Glasgow, R. E. "Economic Analysis of the Mediterranean Lifestyle Program for Postmenopausal Women with Diabetes." *Annals of Behavioral Medicine,* 2005, *32,* 761–769.

Rogers, E. M. *Diffusion of Innovations.* (5th ed.) New York: Free Press, 2003.

Rohrbach, L. A., Grana, R., Sussman, S., and Valente, T. W. "Type II Translation: Transporting Prevention Interventions from Research to Real-World Settings." *Evaluation and the Health Professions,* 2006, *29,* 302–333.

Shadish, W. R., Cook, T. D., and Campbell, D. T. *Experimental and Quasi-Experimental Design for Generalized Causal Inference.* Boston: Houghton Mifflin, 2002.

Shediac-Ritzkallah, M. C., and Bone, L. R. "Planning for the Sustainability of Community-Based Health Programs: Conceptual Frameworks and Future Directions for Research, Practice and Policy." *Health Education Research,* 1998, *13,* 87–108.

Solomon, F., and others. "Observational Study in Ten Beauty Salons: Using Formative Research Results to Inform Development of the North Carolina BEAUTY and Health Project." *Health Education and Behavior,* 2005, *31,* 790–805.

Steckler, A., and Linnan, L. *Process Evaluation for Public Health Interventions and Research.* San Francisco: Jossey-Bass, 2002.

Strecher, V. "Internet Methods for Delivering Behavioral and Health-Related Interventions (eHealth)." *Annual Review of Clinical Psychology,* 2007, *3,* 53–76.

Sussman, S., and others. "Translation in the Health Professions: Converting Science to Action." *Evaluation and the Health Professions,* 2006, *29,* 7–32.

Tashakkori, A., and Teddlie, C. B. *Mixed Methodology: Combining Qualitative and Quantitative Approaches.* Thousand Oaks, Calif.: Sage, 1998.

Viswanathan, M., and others. *Community-Based Participatory Research: Assessing the Evidence. Evidence Report/Technology Assessment No. 99* (Rep. No. AHRQ Pub No. 04-E022-2). Rockville, Md.: Agency for Healthcare Research and Quality, 2004.

Weiss, C. *Evaluation.* (2nd ed.) Englewood Cliffs, N.J.: Prentice Hall, 1998.

Whitelaw, S., and others. "Settings Based Health Promotion: A Review." *Health Promotion International,* 2001, *16,* 339–353.

CHAPTER

PERSPECTIVES ON USING THEORY

Past, Present, and Future

Karen Glanz

Barbara K. Rimer

KEY POINTS

This chapter will

- Look back on health behavior theory over past decades and at present and identify ways to anticipate future challenges.
- Propose key cross-cutting propositions to put the use of health behavior theory in perspective.
- Identify commonalities in how the first four chapters in Part Five describe tools, strategies, models, and issues for applying theory in health education and health behavior.
- Challenge readers to use theory effectively in developing and evaluating interventions to improve the health of individuals and populations.

In the first edition of *Health Behavior and Health Education,* Rosenstock said, "it would be the height of folly to predict the future needs of health education [and health behavior] research and practice, at least without the assistance of an outstanding

California astrologer or the Great Kreskin" (Rosenstock, 1990). Times have changed, and scientific advances and new technology have dramatically altered our lives. Every day, we live with the astonishing pace of new technologies. They have changed our understanding about the health risks we confront, the information we can obtain, day-to-day priorities and worries, relationships, and the ways we communicate.

People around the world are using this book, and it has been translated into multiple languages, including recent Japanese and Korean editions. Around the world, health professionals daily try to change the health behaviors of people to improve their lives; health education and behavior interventions transcend settings and countries. The speed of globalization has dramatically changed the landscape for health behavior, and now the audience is truly global. Theory developers and theory users must consider more than ever how culture, context, and health problems can and should affect their choices of theory and interventions. Professionals designing interventions have more options than ever before, yet our theories have improved only incrementally while our technologies have changed exponentially. This should be a wake-up call to health professionals to think more expansively and deeply about theory.

The modern field of health behavior and health education dates back only about eighty years, and progress has accelerated most rapidly in the past thirty years. As the chapters in this book have shown, many of the early ideas of social and behavioral theorists serve as solid foundations for our work today. To accelerate progress, we should stand on the shoulders of the pioneers in the field, equip ourselves to be explorers, address today's problems with new tools, and anticipate the challenges of the future.

CROSS-CUTTING PROPOSITIONS ABOUT USING THEORY

To begin, we offer some key cross-cutting propositions to readers to put the use of health behavior theory in perspective. These ideas are germane to the review and discussion of each of the chapters in this section.

1. We should not confuse *using* or *applying* theory with testing theory or developing theory. We need all of these, but they are fundamentally different activities, although complementary.

2. Testing the efficacy or effectiveness of theory-based interventions does not constitute testing a theory or theories, per se.

3. As multiple authors in this book have argued, it is likely that the strongest interventions will be built from multiple theories. We encourage researchers and practitioners alike to consider this proposition and to build interventions and their evaluations in a way that the contributions of each theory can be understood.

4. When combining theories, it is important to clearly think through the unique contribution of different theories to the combined model. If this is not done carefully or well, the "new" combined approach may be redundant, overlapping, and hard to interpret in the context of established theories.

5. Rigorous tests of theory-based interventions, including measurement and analyses of mediator and moderators, are the building blocks of the evidence base in health education and health behavior (HEHB).

6. Theory use, testing, and development will be enhanced by the use of shared instruments and reporting. The editors believe that the science of HEHB has been hampered by a lack of systematic work that is replicable and reproducible. We encourage HEHB researchers and practitioners to use open-source tools, as many biologists have adopted, and to put their instruments, interventions, and results in the public domain. Since the last edition of this book, the Internet increasingly has been used to facilitate communication across cultures and countries. The more we can build on past efforts, the more we are likely to advance the public's health. Far too often, an investigator develops an entirely new assessment tool rather than use validated questions that have been posed in many previous studies. This is only partly the fault of such investigators. It can often be a laborious process to find previously used measures and instruments. Yet, when different interventions and measures are used by different investigators using the same theory, it becomes difficult to disentangle intervention from measures. We recommend adaptations of the protocol concept used in clinical research so that it is much more transparent and accessible—in other words, so it is clear what measures were used to accompany particular theories and how theory was turned into interventions.

7. Theory, research, and practice are part of a continuum for understanding the determinants of behaviors, testing strategies for change, and disseminating effective interventions (Kerner, Rimer, and Emmons, 2005; Rimer, Glanz, and Rasband, 2001; Flay, 1986).

8. There is as much to learn from failure as there is to learn from success. Researchers and practitioners who develop and test theory-based interventions should publish their findings when they are negative, as well as when they are positive.

9. There is no substitute for knowing the audience. This applies to the conduct of fundamental research to understand determinants of health behavior as much as it applies to developing health promotion programs for specific individuals, groups, and communities. Participatory research and program design improve the odds of success.

The authors of the first four chapters in Part Five describe tools, strategies, models, and issues for applying theory in HEHB. This section of *Health Behavior and Health Education* tackles the complexity of health behavior and health promotion at its multiple levels. A basic theme is that if intervention strategies are based on a carefully researched understanding of the determinants of behavior and environments, and if systematic approaches to tailoring, targeting, implementing, and evaluating are used, the chances are good that programs will be effective. And if they are not, there should be good information about why an intervention did not work. Understanding past failure is critical to future success.

Three chapters—the PRECEDE-PROCEED Planning Model (Chapter Eighteen), Ecological Models of Health Behavior (Chapter Twenty), and Evaluation of Theory-Based Interventions (Chapter Twenty-One)—are updated versions of chapters from the preceding edition, written by the same authors. The chapter, Social Marketing (Chapter Nineteen), is a substantial revision of a chapter in the second edition; it is written by new authors.

This chapter reviews highlights from each of the other chapters in this section, discusses emerging developments and challenges, and comments on the state of the art in the use of theory in HEHB theory, research, and practice. The discussion aims to provoke thought and debate and stimulate further reading, rather than provide definitive answers or prescriptions for the field.

THE PRECEDE-PROCEED PLANNING MODEL

In Chapter Eighteen, Gielen, McDonald, Gary, and Bone present an overview of PRECEDE-PROCEED, describe each of its phases, and apply the model in case studies of child injury prevention and diabetes self-management. They explicitly illustrate the ways that behavior change theories can be applied and incorporated into a systematic planning process. They further note the challenges of using PRECEDE-PROCEED, which, when fully applied, can be a demanding and laborious process for practitioners and community groups. But when mastered, it can lead to the development of effective, appropriate health education programs.

Although health behavior theories are critical tools, professionals in health behavior and health education should not substitute theory for adequate planning and research. However, theories help us interpret problem situations and plan feasible, promising interventions. Theory also plays an important role in program evaluation. Because it identifies assumptions behind intervention strategies, theory can pinpoint intermediate steps that should be assessed in evaluation. The PRECEDE-PROCEED Model has as its raison d'être the systematic application of theory and previous research to assessment of local needs, priorities, circumstances, and resources (Green and others, 1994). It owes its robustness, in part, to the fact that it is intuitively appealing and logical but also immensely practical.

Theory is most likely to be informative during Phase 3 of the planning process suggested by PRECEDE-PROCEED: educational and ecological assessment. This phase focuses on examining factors that shape behaviors and environmental factors. Theories help guide the examination of predisposing, enabling, and reinforcing factors for particular behaviors. For example, constructs from the Health Belief Model (HBM) might help us understand why some women do not get mammograms (see Chapter Three). PRECEDE-PROCEED can also be used in conjunction with the Transtheoretical Model (TTM) of change to design stage-appropriate health education messages (see Chapter Five). This approach to using theory to guide data collection can be used to focus on specific leverage points that might best influence desired behaviors. Throughout the educational and ecological assessment, both literature reviews and information collected directly from a community or program audience are important (Alciati and Glanz, 1996). Levers are sought among predisposing factors, such as motives, reinforcing factors such as rewards, and enabling factors or barriers, such as insurance or access to care. The concepts of priority, changeability, and community preferences should be considered along with analytical and empirical findings about health behavior determinants. For example, health educators concerned with effecting the distribution of safe water must understand how people in developing countries think about water sources and what beliefs might be amenable to change. These ideas are also consistent with concepts presented in earlier chapters on community organization, diffusion of innovations, and organizational change.

Bartholomew, Parcel, Kok, and Gottlieb (2006) describe Intervention Mapping as a framework for developing theory- and evidence-based health education programs. Intervention Mapping is composed of five steps that are complementary to the planning phases of the PRECEDE-PROCEED Model. Readers may find Intervention Mapping helpful in guiding them toward an explicit specification of how to use both theory and empirical findings to develop effective health education interventions.

SOCIAL MARKETING

Social marketing is a process that promotes desired voluntary behaviors among members of a target market, by offering attractive benefits and reducing barriers associated with healthful choices. It involves the adaptation of commercial marketing technologies to promote socially desirable goals. In Chapter Nineteen, Storey, Saffitz, and Rimón take a fresh look at social marketing. They emphasize how social marketing can be applied within a strategic health communication framework and link key theories of health communication and health behavior to the effective practice of social marketing.

With social marketing, success is most likely when marketers accurately determine the perceptions, needs, and wants of target markets and satisfy them through the design, communication, pricing, and delivery of appropriate, competitive, and visible offerings. The process is consumer-driven, not just expert-driven. This orientation is consistent with principles of community organization, and its product development approach parallels the innovation development process of diffusion theory. At the same time, it shares an economic perspective with "behavioral economics"— a field of inquiry that relates individual behaviors to economic variables (Bickel and Vuchinich, 2000). Concepts from behavioral economics, including the notion of trade-offs considered when making decisions, deserve further attention along with social marketing and other theories of health behavior.

As with the PRECEDE-PROCEED Model, social marketing provides a framework to identify what drives and maintains behavior, and what factors might drive and maintain behavior change. It also requires identification of potential intermediaries, channels of distribution and communication, and actual and potential competitors. As the authors indicate, theories of health behavior can help guide the analytical process in social marketing and aid in the formulation of intervention strategies and materials. They explicitly illustrate four theories that contribute well to social marketing approaches: the Theory of Planned Behavior (TPB), the extended parallel processing model, Social Cognitive Theory (SCT), and its observational learning construct, and diffusion of innovations. Because of the focus on understanding consumers (or target audiences) from their own point of view, social marketing models are robust for use in diverse and unique populations, including disadvantaged groups and ethnic minorities, and in many countries. In fact, it is often thought that social marketing programs tend to be inherently culturally sensitive because they follow a consumer-oriented process.

The authors of Chapter Nineteen stress that social marketing draws our attention to factors beyond individual behavior change more than do some other approaches. It stresses how communication can affect the market structure itself through policy, legislative, and social normative change, thereby facilitating the adoption of beneficial health behaviors. Even so, in social marketing it is always important to identify and fulfill demand—that is, to "start where the people are."

ECOLOGICAL MODELS

In Chapter Twenty, Sallis, Owen, and Fisher update the 2002 chapter by Sallis and Owen and describe the aims and core concepts of ecological models for health education and health behavior change. As shown in Chapter One and emphasized in recent authoritative publications from the scientific community (Smedley and Syme, 2000) and public health organizations around the world, the basic tenets of ecological perspectives—of multi-level determinants of behavior and environments and transactions between individuals and their environments—are widely recognized as useful and appropriate orientations for contemporary health promotion. Although there is a shift toward lower-cost, broad-reach programs and away from intensive, costly face-to-face interventions to reduce risky health behaviors, much more work remains to be done (Orleans and others, 1999). It is likely that staged or tiered approaches that allocate intensive interventions to those who have not benefited from minimal approaches will work best.

Sallis, Owen, and Fisher outline the historical foundations of ecological models of human behavior. Ecological models also have a long tradition and a controversial place in the science of epidemiology, where critiques of the "ecological fallacy" demonstrate the often-found lack of correspondence between individual-level associations and group-level associations of the same or similar variables. MacIntyre and Ellaway (2000) provide a thoughtful articulation that argues for the revitalization of an ecological perspective, with links to epidemiology, medical geography, and sociology. New methods of statistical analysis, including multi-level modeling, make it possible to better understand people's relationships to their surroundings, to identify leverage points to improve population health, and to test multi-level interventions in cluster-randomized trials (Bingenheimer and Raudenbush, 2004).

Tobacco control is one of the applications of ecological models discussed in the chapter by Sallis and colleagues. The implementation of policies and programs to reduce tobacco use have now been consistent with ecological models for more than fifteen years, and during that time smoking in the United States has declined markedly. However, projections of global mortality indicate that worldwide, tobacco is expected to kill 50 percent more people in 2015 than HIV/AIDS and to be responsible for 10 percent of all deaths (Mathers and Loncar, 2006). Clearly, there remains much work to be done to reduce the global burden of tobacco-related diseases at multiple levels of the ecological model.

An important point that deserves attention is that, despite many calls for multi-level interventions, proposed interventions are often based solely on data regarding cross-sectional associations between environmental factors and behaviors. We need to understand the *causes* of health behavior problems before we can design success-ful interventions. The challenge to conduct better research on ecological interven-tions remains an important one for health education and health behavior. These studies are expensive and demanding, and therefore require substantial collaboration across areas of expertise. Most likely, a combination of inductive and deductive approaches, using both qualitative and quantitative techniques, will reveal the rich texture of an ecological perspective, while allowing assessment of their impact on valued outcomes.

EVALUATION OF THEORY-BASED HEALTH BEHAVIOR INTERVENTIONS

In Chapter Twenty-One, Glasgow and Linnan emphasize how evaluation results may contribute to the development of new knowledge and, in turn, help to create new the-ory, refine existing theory, and build the evidence base for intervention effectiveness. The chapter describes the RE-AIM Model as a guide for impact or outcome evalua-tion of theory-based health behavior interventions. The acronym RE-AIM stands for Reach, Efficacy/Effectiveness, Adoption, Implementation, and Maintenance (Glas-gow, Vogt, and Boles, 1999). A key idea behind the RE-AIM Model, and the message of its first two components (the "RE"), is that the public health impact of interven-tions is a function of both their efficacy and reach. Glasgow and Linnan remind us to consider this equation and to also take a traditional public health perspective that con-siders possible negative or unintended consequences on quality of life.

The second half of the RE-AIM Model emphasizes Adoption, Implementation, and Maintenance. These concepts invoke other theories such as the diffusion of in-novations and organizational change at the organizational level, as well as the TTM Model at the intrapersonal level. The RE-AIM Model as a whole also aligns well with various models of the phases of research described in Chapter Twenty-One.

Chapter Twenty-One does not attempt to provide a text on research design, meas-urement, or statistical analysis. Rather, it raises important issues for HEHB researchers and practitioners to incorporate into the "big picture" of their efforts to improve the health of specific risk groups and large populations. An important contribution of Glas-gow and Linnan's chapter is the emphasis on clear and complete reporting of partici-pation in intervention research, including both randomized and nonrandomized studies, following guidelines in the CONSORT (Moher, Schulz, and Altman, 2001) or TREND (Des Jarlais, Lyles, Crepaz, and TREND Group, 2004) statements. Use of these meth-ods will make it possible to more readily analyze completed studies in systematic ev-idence reviews (Sweet and Moynihan, 2007) and to better evaluate the relevance and applicability of research on health behavior interventions (Green and Glasgow, 2006).

MOVING FORWARD

After becoming familiar with some contemporary theories of health behavior, the challenge is to use them within a comprehensive planning process. Planning models like PRECEDE-PROCEED and processes like social marketing increase the odds of success by examining health and behavior at multiple levels. At its simplest, an ecological perspective emphasizes two main options: change people, or change the environment. The most powerful approaches will use both of these options together (Smedley and Syme, 2000). The activities most directly tied to changing *people* are derived from individual-level theories like the HBM, TTM, and the Precaution Adoption Process Model (PAPM). In contrast, activities aimed at changing the *environment* draw on community-level theories. In between are SCT, social support and social networks, and interpersonal communication models. Each of these focuses on reciprocal relations among persons or between individuals and their environments.

Theoretical frameworks are guides in the pursuit of successful efforts; they maximize flexibility and help to apply abstract concepts of theory in ways that are most useful in diverse work settings and situations. Knowledge of theory and comprehensive planning systems offers a great deal. Other key elements of effective programs are (1) a good program-to-audience match, (2) accessible and practical information, (3) active learning and involvement, and (4) skill building, practice, and reinforcement. Strong interventions will often—but not always—be built on theory, but theory alone cannot lead to effective interventions. Theory helps one ask the right questions, and effective planning enables one to zero in on these elements in relation to a specific problem. Still, theory must be turned into effective interventions, and these must be applied with fidelity and evaluated well. A lot happens between theory and behavior change. The effective use of theory for practice and research requires practice but can yield important dividends in efforts to enhance the health of individuals and populations. In the end, we should ask ourselves whether our work has made a difference. Developing better theories is a means to that end.

REFERENCES

Alciati, M. H., and Glanz, K. "Using Data to Plan Public Health Programs: Experience From State Cancer Prevention and Control Programs." *Public Health Reports,* 1996, *111,* 165–172.

Bartholomew, L. K., Parcel, G. S., Kok, G., and Gottlieb, N. H. *Planning Health Promotion Programs: An Intervention Mapping Approach.* San Francisco: Jossey-Bass, 2006.

Bickel, W. K., and Vuchinich, R. E. (eds.). *Reframing Health Behavior Change with Behavioral Economics.* Mahwah, N.J.: Erlbaum, 2000.

Bingenheimer, J. B., and Raudenbush, S. W. "Statistical and Substantive Inferences in Public Health: Issues in the Application of Multilevel Models." *Annual Review of Public Health,* 2004, *25,* 53–77.

Des Jarlais, D. C., Lyles, C., Crepaz, N., and TREND Group. "Improving the Reporting Quality of Nonrandomized Evaluations of Behavioral and Public Health Interventions: The TREND Statement." *American Journal of Public Health,* 2004, *94,* 361–366.

Flay, B. "Efficacy and Effectiveness Trials (and Other Phases of Research) in the Development of Health Promotion Programs." *Preventive Medicine,* 1986, *15,* 451–474.

Glasgow, R. E., Vogt, T. M., and Boles, S. M. "Evaluating the Public Health Impact of Health Promotion Interventions: The RE-AIM Framework." *American Journal of Public Health,* 1999, *89,* 1322–1327.

Green, L., and others. "Can We Build On, or Must We Replace, the Theories and Models in Health Education?" *Health Education Research,* 1994, *9,* 397–404.

Green, L. W., and Glasgow, R. E. "Evaluating the Relevance, Generalization, and Applicability of Research." *Evaluation and the Health Professions,* 2006, *29*(1), 126–153.

Kerner, J., Rimer, B., and Emmons, K. "Introduction to the Special Section on Dissemination: Dissemination Research and Research Dissemination: How Can We Close the Gap?" *Health Psychology,* 2005, *24*(5), 443–446.

MacIntyre, S., and Ellaway, A. "Ecological Approaches: Rediscovering the Role of the Physical and Social Environment." In L. F. Berkman and I. Kawachi (eds.), *Social Epidemiology.* New York: Oxford University Press, 2000.

Mathers, C. D., and Loncar, D. "Projections of Global Mortality and Burden of Disease from 2002 to 2030." *PLoS Medicine,* 2006, *3*(11), 2011–2030.

Moher, D., Schulz, K. F., and Altman, D. G., for the CONSORT Group. "The CONSORT Statement: Revised Recommendations for Improving the Quality of Reports." *Journal of the American Medical Association,* 2001, *285,* 1987–1991.

Orleans, C. T., and others. "Rating Our Progress in Population Health Promotion: Report Card on Six Behaviors." *American Journal of Health Promotion,* 1999, *14,* 75–82.

Rimer, B. K., Glanz, K., and Rasband, G. "Searching for Evidence About Health Education and Health Behavior Interventions." *Health Education and Behavior,* 2001, *28,* 231–248.

Rosenstock, I. M. "The Past, Present, and Future of Health Education." In K. Glanz, F. M. Lewis, and B. K. Rimer (eds.), *Health Behavior and Health Education: Theory, Research, and Practice.* San Francisco: Jossey-Bass, 1990.

Smedley, B. D., and Syme, S. L. (eds.). *Promoting Health: Intervention Strategies from Social and Behavioral Research.* Washington, D.C.: National Academy Press, 2000.

Sweet, M., and Moynihan, R. *Improving Population Health: The Uses of Systematic Reviews.* New York: Milbank Memorial Fund, 2007.

NAME INDEX

SUBJECT INDEX

Informal relationships, examples of, 238, 272
Information exchange: and the 5-As model, 261; described, 250–251; measures of, *247–248*; model of, *242*; patients' perception of, 263
Information flow, defined with application, *372*
Information management, 251
Information Preference Scale, *247*
Information processing theories, *368*, 369–370, *413*, 421
Information seeking: defined, *215*; described, 220–221; issues with, 8, 277
Information Styles Questionnaire, *247*
Information technologies. *See* Communication and information technologies
Informational needs, sensitivity to, 279
Informational support: defined, 190, *191*; described, 192; exchange of, understanding relevant to, 197, 198; intervention offering, 204; and on-line support groups, 227; provided by community health workers, 205–206
Informed by theory, defined, 33
Informed decision making, 12, 253, 272
Informed decision-making coding, *248*
Injunctive norm, *77*, 79, 80, 84
Innovation, defined, *317*
Innovation development: defined, *317*; described, 318
Innovation planning, gap between, and diffusion planning, 316
Innovations: characteristics of, that affect diffusion, 319–320; history of, 313
In-Office program, 502–503
Institute of Medicine (IOM), 28, 31, 36, 39, 69, 70, 79, 90, 94, 205, 209, 314, 332, 365, 369, 383, 385, 409, 431, 466, 467, 479, 483
Institutionalization: and Community Coalition Action Theory, 348; and community organization, 397; defined, *317*; described, 318–319; more attention paid to, need for, 356; of organizational change, *340*, *342*; in the RE-AIM evaluation framework, 497; research on, examining, 495. *See also* Maintenance
Instrumental attitude: and elicitation interviews, *83*; in the Integrated Behavioral Model, *77*, 78, 79, 80, 84; measures of, *74*
Instrumental support: defined, 190, *191*; exchange of, understanding relevant to, 197; provided by community health workers, 205–206
Integrated Behavioral Model (IBM): adopting concept from Social Cognitive Theory, 274; appeal of the, 159; application of, to diverse behaviors and populations, 80–82; constructs, definitions, and measures in the, *74–75*; described, 77–82; and the media studies framework, *368*, 369; origin and development of the, 69–70; and patient-

centered communication, *245*; for prevention of AIDS/HIV, application of, 82–92; proposed use of an, 68, 70; and social marketing, 448, *449*; summary of the, 92; value of the, 91–92
Intensity or strength: defined, 190, *191*; of intervention using community health workers, 206
Intentions. *See* Behavioral intention
Intermediate community changes, defined, 354
Intermediate outcomes, *240*, 493, *494*
Internal consistency, as a criterion for assessing theories, 35
Internal validity, 491, 492–493, 495
Internet Systems Consortium, 365, 385
Internet, the: access to, issue of, 272, 297; advantages and limitations of, 117; and diffusion of innovations, 319, 323, 330; emergence of, 365; growth in using, 8, 106; importance of, 5, 8–9, 144; influence of, increased, 396–397; and intervention planning, 417–418; as a means of facilitating communication, 511; and media message production, 366, 382; new applications of, 183; and social marketing, 442. *See also* Online communities; Online support groups
Interorganizational relations, defined, *343*
Interorganizational Relations (IOR) Theory, *343*, 346–347, 350, 352, 357, 391, 396, 397. *See also* Community Coalition Action Theory (CCAT)
Interpersonal communication: importance of, 238; and moving forward, 516; and phases in the PRECEDE-PROCEED Model, *413*. *See also* Clinician-patient communication; Social networks and social support
Interpersonal influence: on adoption decisions, 323; and information received from the media, 373; theories involving, utility of, 34; understanding, importance of, 26
Interpersonal-level models: examining the features of and issues with, 273–279; interactions in, characteristics of, 272–273; macro-level approaches complementing, 391–392; and moving forward, 516; and phases in the PRECEDE-PROCEED Model, *413*, 415; review of, 271–272; summary on, and future directions, 279–280. *See also* Clinician-patient communication; Social Cognitive Theory (SCT); Social networks and social support; Transactional Model of Stress and Coping
Intervention alignment, *410*, *413*, 416
Intervention mapping, 416, 417, 513
Intervention research: described, 25; more, need for, 36
Intervention strategies, examples of, resources for, 37
Intervention-planning model. *See* PRECEDE-PROCEED Model